ANNALS OF THE NEW YORK ACADEMY OF SCIENCES

Volume 286

BIOCHEMICAL ACTIONS OF PROGESTERONE AND PROGESTINS

Edited by Erlio Gurpide

The New York Academy of Sciences
New York, New York
1977

Library of Congress Cataloging in Publication Data

Main entry under title:

Biochemical actions of progesterone and progestins.

(Annals of the New York Academy of Sciences; v. 286)

Includes bibliographical references.

1. Progesterone-Congresses. 2. Progestational hormones—Congresses. I. Gurpide, Erlio, 1927– II. Series: New York Academy of Sciences. Annals; v. 286. [DNLM: 1. Progesterone—Physiology—Congresses. 2. Progestational hormones—Physiology—Congresses. W1 AN626YL v. 286 / WP530 B615 1976]

Q11.N5 vol. 286 [QP572.P7] 508'.1s
ISBN 0-89072-032-0 [599'.01'6] 77-3994

SP

Printed in the United States of America

ISBN 0-89072-032-0

ANNALS OF THE NEW YORK ACADEMY OF SCIENCES
VOLUME 286
March 11, 1977

BIOCHEMICAL ACTIONS OF PROGESTERONE AND PROGESTINS*

Editor and Conference Chairman
ERLIO GURPIDE

CONTENTS

*This series of papers is the result of a conference entitled Biochemical Actions of Progesterone and Progestins, held by The New York Academy of Sciences on May 5, 6, and 7, 1976.

Part IV. Actions on the Female Genital Tract

Part V. Special Topics

Financial assistance was received from:

- ALZA RESEARCH
- THE CAMILLE AND HENRY DREYFUS FOUNDATION, INC.
- HOFFMANN-LA ROCHE INC.
- THE LILLY RESEARCH LABORATORIES
- MEAD JOHNSON
- NATIONAL FOUNDATION MARCH OF DIMES
- ORTHO PHARMACEUTICAL CORPORATION
- SCHERING CORPORATION
- SEARLE LABORATORIES
- THE UPJOHN COMPANY

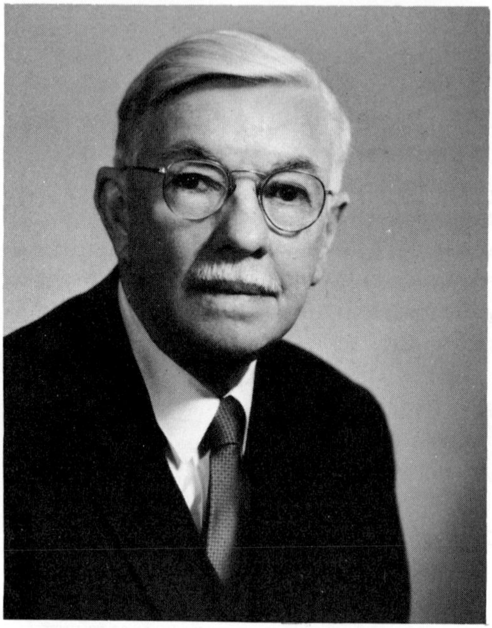

Dr. George W. Corner, Sr. (*top*) and Dr. Willard M. Allen (*bottom*), pioneers in progesterone research (see Dr. R. O. Greep's article in this volume), were guests of honor and speakers at the banquet held in occasion of the Conference on Biochemical Actions of Progesterone and Progestins, May 6, 1976.

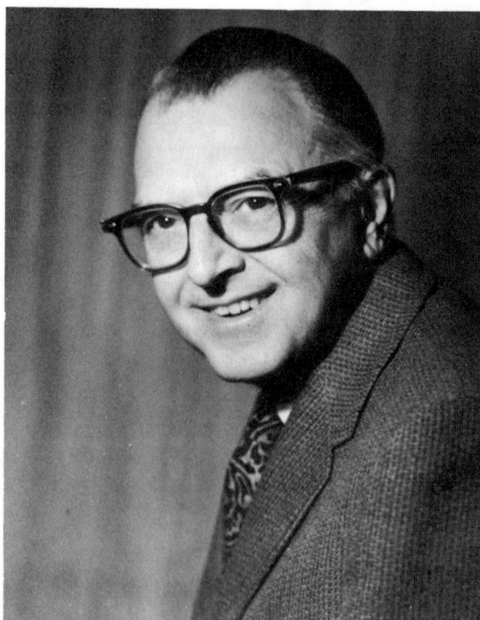

THE GENESIS OF RESEARCH ON THE PROGESTINS

Roy O. Greep

Laboratory of Human Reproduction and Reproductive Biology
Harvard Medical School
Boston, Massachusetts 02115

To this group of biochemically oriented reproductive endocrinologists, progesterone and its collective family of chemical cousins the progestins are as familiar as apple pie. Noting, too, that approximately 100 million women have at one time or another used a progestin for the prevention of conception, it might be rightfully assumed that the term "progestin" had become a household word. It is not so. Although the future welfare of humankind rests more heavily at this point in history on the progestins than it does on atomic weapons, few of the world's citizenry, even of the intelligent laity, have any knowledge as to what a progestin is or can do. Still less do they realize that without progesterone they would not have been brought into this world. Should there be among you any who disagree, I suggest that the next time your seatmate on an airplane trip inquires as to your line of work you answer *progestins* and watch the expression that comes over the face of your questioner as he or she takes your measure. The gulf that separates science and society will suddenly widen and bring the conversation to a close. What surprises me more and fills me with lamentations is that many students emerging from college and heading for a career in medicine or biology have either never heard of progesterone or have only the haziest notion as to what it really is, much less what function it serves in the biology of the mammalian world.

What the progestins *are* and what they *do* are now well understood. What occupies the attention of this body of scientists is *how* they do it. The pursuit of this line of investigation is in the hands of a new generation of progestinologists skilled in molecular biology and genetics. An old era has passed into history, and a new one has been opened. There is an old axiom to the effect that those who do not know history are doomed to repeat it. That, however, does not necessarily hold true in scientific research. Were it so, all of our new recruits to this field would initiate their research by studying the history of progestins rather than molecular biology. In science, as we know all too well, it is possible to ignore history beyond the past five years and continue to work effectively at the most advanced level of research. History is something that is left to those who have passed the menopause of their professional career and are presumed to have acquired what some are inclined to call perspective.

That brings me to the business at hand. I was asked to speak to the genesis of research on the progestins, which means that I am expected to provide some historical perspective to the substance of this conference. The dimensions of perspective vary over a very wide range, and I suspect that the answer one would get to the genesis of research on the progestins would depend on the age, experience, and interest of the respondent. The fledgling investigator would likely guess that the genesis of research on progestins occurred about five to 10 years ago with concern as to their interaction with receptors. A more advanced teacher-investigator type who had found it necessary to dig back into the ancient literature might well come across some relevant work in the early 1950s by Pincus and Chang[1] and Rock *et al.*[2] A now greying and distinguished authority having been invited to write a textbook would discover among the dust-laden and discoloring volumes dating back to the Prohibition Era works of great historical importance by such pioneering investigators as Corner and Allen,[3] Fevold and Hisaw,[4] Fels,[5] Slotta *et al.*,[6] Butenandt,[7] and Makepeace *et al.*[8] These works pertain to the extraction, purification, isolation, structure, synthesis, and function of a luteal secretion, the existence of which had already been substantiated. Let me interject here that my participation in research on the progestins around 1930 was limited to snipping thousands of corpora lutea out of sow's ovaries as raw material for the extraction studies of Hisaw *et al.*[9] What I received in return as a graduate student was the exhilarating privilege of being part of a team, plus a lot of what falls into the hopefully beneficial category of experience. Was this, then, the era in which it all began? Not at all. This was but the culminating thrust that capped a long series of important advances made during the previous 30 years by such stalwarts as Prenant, Born, Fraenkel, Marshall, Heape, Loeb, Ancel, and Bouin.

Employment of the experimental method as a means of elucidating the origin and functional significance of the luteal body stems only from the beginning of this century. Beyond that point lie 2000 years of the dialectical approach—of bewilderment, curiosity, erroneous observations, and unfounded speculation. The wheels of progress sometimes stood still for very long periods. A piece of dogma propounded in the third century B.C. by Heterophilus of Alexandria[10] held that the generative organs in women were female testes. This totally erroneous concept was still accepted as late as the sixteenth century by Andreas Vesalius,[11] the great Flemish anatomist and author of one of the early classics in anatomy, *De Humani Corporis Fabrica*. Vesalius illustrated the female testes as being connected to the uterus by a duct not unlike the male vas. Fallopius,[12] in 1561, was the first to determine that the tubes that still bear his name are not attached to the testes. Fabricius studied the hen and in 1621 reported that he could see very clearly that the structure of the generative organ of the female bore no resemblance to that of the testis and proposed the term "ovarium."[13] As is well known, it was Reinier de Graaf,[14] the Flemish physician, who in 1673 provided an authentic description of the ovarian vesicles that also still bear his name. He was a contemporary and compatriot of van Leeuwenhoek, who in 1677 observed the sperm in semen.[15] de Graaf named these large fluid-filled vesicles "ova" due to their strong resemblance to the ova seen in bird ovaries. de Graaf also took note of certain other structures on the ovarian surface, which he referred to as globules. By a stroke of what must be considered observational genius at that juncture in history, de Graaf also determined that the number of these globules corresponded with the number of fetuses in the various mammals that he dissected. These globules had also been seen somewhat earlier in human ovaries by Fallopius,[12] who described them as yellow bodies. More than 100 years later, Malpighi, in 1687, coined the term "*corpus luteum*."[16] He deduced quite incorrectly that they gave rise to the follicles and that the yellow substance, like egg yolk, served to nourish the ovum. Mind you that at this time no knowledge existed as to the true ovum or of ovulation. Nearly another 150 years were to pass before the mammalian ovum was first observed in 1827 by the Russian anatomist Karl Ernst von Baer,[17] whose observations also revealed the actual relationship of the ruptured follicle to the formation of the corpus luteum. von Baer was severely criticized by a succeeding generation of anatomists who through faulty techniques and timing failed to find the ovum in the fallopian tubes. Later, in 1857, Robin advanced the notion that the corpus luteum served only to heal the ruptured follicle and prevent the formation of scar tissue.

Following von Baer's epoch-making discoveries, a new problem arose. It concerned the presence of corpora lutea in virgins. Because the corpora lutea were known to be associated with pregnancy, it was natural to assume that their presence was related to coition. Since it was unknown that corpora lutea exist only during the second half of the cycle, their presence was reported by some observers and as vehemently denied by others.[20] As an interesting sidelight to this controversy, George Corner[21] noted an instance in which the innocence of a dead woman was once sworn away in an English court because her ovaries were found to contain a corpus luteum.

The relationship of corpora lutea to the menstrual cycle was not established until early in this century, by Meyer.[22] These bodies were first considered false or abnormal and were termed "corpus luteum spurium," as opposed to the true corpus, or luteum gravidarum or verum.

It was not until near the end of the last century that any serious attention was given to the possible physiologic significance of the corpus luteum. Keep in mind, however, that at this stage, the ovary had no known function other than the production of ova. This was an amazing circumstance, considering that an endocrine function of the male gonad had been established 50 years earlier.[23] All that was needed was a study of the effects of removing the female gonad. Similar surgical ablations had been practiced on males since ancient times. This discrepancy can no doubt be accounted for on the basis of accessibility. In fact, surgical removal of the ovaries became quite a common practice around 1895, but the results were highly controversial. In 1896–1900, Emil Knauer[24,26] reported that the involution of the genital tract seen after ovariectomy could be repaired by ovarian transplants. His results were challenged by an outpouring of reports that claimed that ovariectomy in sheep, dogs, cats, monkeys, and even women did not interrupt the cyclic appearance of heat or menstruation. Marshall[19] cites a series of clinical papers published between 1895 and 1904 that reported the occurrence of pregnancy after removal of both ovaries and in one case of the tubes as well. By hindsight, one would assume that the women were already pregnant at the time of surgery, but the recurrence of menstruation or heat is another matter. In 1905–1907, Marshall and Jolly confirmed Knauer's work and established beyond doubt that bilateral removal of the ovaries in rats and dogs led to involution of the tract and cessation of all reproductive functions.[27–29] They also proved the effectiveness of ovarian transplants and, with typical British genteelness, attributed the contrary findings of others to "inadequate surgery." Thus came the first clear evidence that the ovary exercised control over the rest of the genital system, but the mechanism was still unknown. In 1905, Walter Heape[30] postulated that a "generative ferment," probably from food or the environment, acted on the ovary, stimulating it to secrete a hypothetical material, which he termed "gonadin." His "generative ferment," of course, became the pituitary gonadotropins of today, and his postulated "gonadin" was the ethereal forerunner of our present-day estrogens.

Prenant,[31] impressed by the unfailing presence of corpora lutea during pregnancy, proposed in 1898 that these structures might be ductless glands and concurred with Beard's[32] earlier suggestion that they might also be responsible for the inhibition of ovulation during pregnancy. Much credit must go to Gustav Born, a German embryologist, who in 1900 conceived the idea that the corpus luteum might aid in the attachment of embryos to the uterus by providing a nourishing substance. Being terminally ill, Born bequeathed his idea and how to test it to his student Ludwig Fraenkel. The idea was to mate rabbits and then within the first six days remove the ovaries or destroy the corpora lutea by cautery. The experiments were performed, and the rabbits did not become pregnant. The results were published in 1903[33] and became the first firm landmark on the road to the discovery of the progestins. The choice of the rabbit for these experiments was fortuitous, because pregnancy in that species is dependent on the continuing presence of the ovaries. In several others it is not. Fraenkel came under such severe criticism by others who demonstrated that removal of the ovaries, especially from pregnant guinea pigs and monkeys, had no effect on the course of pregnancy that he was forced to repeat his work in 1910. The results were the same.[34] The key to the difficulty was species difference and the timing of the surgery during gestation. The impact of Fraenkel's work was, nevertheless, so great that it placed the corpora lutea in the position of appearing to produce the one and only ovarian hormone. Marshall[19] remained skeptical. He knew that seasonal breeders very often came into heat with no corpora lutea in their ovaries. He very cautiously proposed the possibility that the ovary might produce two kinds of secretions, one of which would induce the phenomenon of heat. The true picture was beginning to emerge, but the outline remained hazy.

What these suggestive studies at the turn of the century did was open an unsavory era of ovarian organotherapy. Saline or glycerin extracts were prepared from fresh or dried ovaries of any source and were administered to women for every conceivable reproductive dysfunction. The results were generally satisfactory, especially to the doctors. Such extracts could not have contained more than a trace of hormonal activity at best. This inglorious chapter in the history of reproductive endocrinology persisted into the 1930s, when authentic ovarian hormones became available for therapeutic use.

This bleak era was relieved by a few notable contributions. In 1907–1908, Leo Loeb demonstrated that the corpus luteum was essential for the development of deciduoma,[35,36] and in 1910, Ancel and Bouin[37] described the remarkable modification of the uterine mucosa that occurs in rabbits made pseudopregnant by mating with a vasectomized buck.

What opened the field of reproductive endocrinology to an explosion of meaningful research was the discovery by Allen and Doisy in 1923 of the estrous-inducing hormone in follicular liquor obtained from hog ovaries.[38] Asdell and Marshall[39] demonstrated that this new estrogenic hormone could not induce what Corner[40] termed "progestational proliferation." The succeeding demonstrations[3,41,42] in the late 1920s that crude extracts of corpora lutea would produce many of the normal physiologic functions attributed to that body were electrifying. They forged the final link in the chain of evidence that pointed to the existence of a luteal hormone and opened the way to its isolation. Early entrants to this second great quest of the ovarian hormones were Hisaw and Fevold, Corner and Allen, Slotta and Fels, and Parkes and Bellerby. The latter pair dropped out early but not before preparing an ether extract that inhibited estrous and ovulation in mice.[41] The extract prepared by Hisaw's group was shown to induce deciduoma formation,[42] inhibition of ovulation,[42a] and a premenstrual endometrium in monkeys.[43] Hisaw at that time was also much concerned with the effect of another luteal activity, relaxin.[44] Allen and Corner put their luteal extract to the ultimate test as a substitute for the natural hormone by showing that in rabbits castrated 18 hr after mating, it would permit implantation and sustain fetal development to term.[45,46] They also developed a suitable quantitative bioassay based on graded modification of the uterine mucosa induced in castrated adult rabbits by different dosages of the luteal extract.[3,47] This bioassay proved to be an enormous aid in their purification studies.

The hot methyl alcohol used by Corner and Allen as the initial extraction medium[3,47] was a modification of that employed much earlier with moderate but unrecognized success by Hermann.[48] Hisaw's group started out using an acid-alcohol extraction[3] medium. Although this medium gave a good yield of the relaxative hormone, the yield of progestational activity was less than optimal, whereupon they changed to a slight modification[50,51] of the extraction procedure employed by Allen and Corner.[3,47] By 1930, several laboratories were able to report progress in purifying the hormone termed "progestin" by Corner's group, "corporin" by Hisaw's group, and "luteosterone" by Slotta *et al.* The major purification efforts took place between 1930 and 1934.

Discounting the poorly characterized crystals reported by Fels[5] in 1931, credit

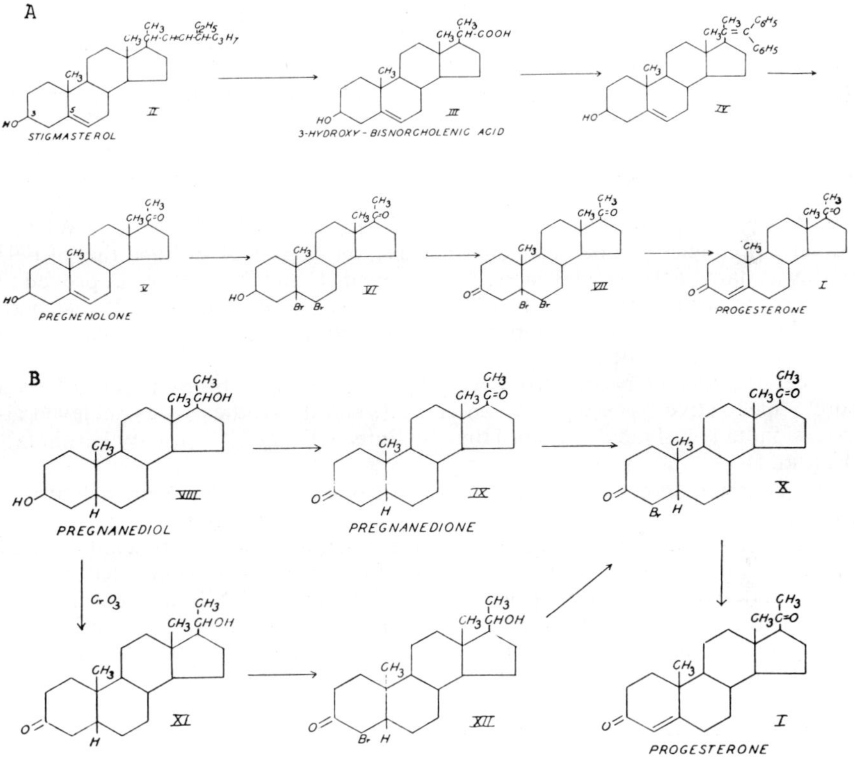

FIGURE 1. The historic synthesis of progesterone from stigmasterol and pregnanediol by the combined chemical ingenuity of Butenandt and Westphal[57] and Fernholz.[58] Stigmasterol was chosen because Fernholtz had already demonstrated a means of cleaving the side chain. Pregnanediol was an especially promising choice, because Butenandt had previously determined its chemical structure and knew that it was excreted in abundance during periods of active luteal function. A: The unsaturated diphenyl compound (IV) was produced by treatment of compound III with phenylmagnesium bromide. Oxidation yielded the 3-hydroxy-20-ketopregnene (V). The use of bromination to protect the double bond during further oxidation to progesterone was a technique conceived by Fernholz. B: The simple conversion of pregnanediol to progesterone made similar use of bromination of the diketone (IX) or the 3-keto-20-hydroxypregnene (XI) to yield the 4-bromodiketone (X). The bromine was removed with anhydrous pyridine to yield progesterone. (From Allen.[59] By permission of The Williams and Wilkins Co.)

for having achieved the first progestationally active crystalline product goes to Fevold and Hisaw,[4] as reported in 1932. The crystals proved not to be chemically pure, and further attempts at isolation of the luteal hormone by these workers were essentially discontinued. In the same year, Allen[49] also obtained a crystalline product. His crystals were of much greater potency than those of Fevold, but, again, they did not stand up to additional tests of chemical purity.

Further purification work performed by Allen left him with two crystalline products of about equal potency but with different melting points. He then turned to a collaborative effort with Wintersteiner at Columbia University. By fractional crystallization, they obtained four crystalline compounds, termed A, B, C, and D. A and D were inactive, while B and C were about equally active. B and C melted at 128° and 120–121°C, respectively. B, the luteal hormone, had the empirical formula $C_{21}H_{30}O_2$. The time was 1934, and it appeared the race had been won, but their results were not yet published. As in many dramatic situations, a glittering dark horse from the continent, Butenandt, came up from behind and sprinted to the finish line. He announced to a meeting of the Deutsche Gesellschaft für Innere Medizin on April 11th that he had obtained crystals with potent progestational activity and with a melting point of 128°C. The details of his work appeared in July[7] and gave the formula as either $C_{21}H_{30}O_2$ or $C_{20}H_{28}O_2$. A few days later, he and Westphal reported the definitive formula as $C_{21}H_{30}O_2$.[52] Allen and Wintersteiner's preliminary announcement appeared on August 24th,[53] and that of Fels *et al.* was dated only one day later.[54] Compounds C and D of Fels *et al.* proved to be identical with compounds B and C of Wintersteiner and Allen,[55] and both agreed with the findings of Butenandt.[7] The conclusion was that progesterone is a polymorphous substance.

The structure of progesterone as proposed in August by Slotta *et al.*[6] on a purely speculative basis was proven correct, and its synthesis was achieved almost simultaneously and in record time by Butenandt *et al.*[56,57] and by Fernholz[58] (FIGURE 1).

By common agreement of the Advisory Committee on the Nomenclature of Endocrine Principles of the Council on Pharmacy and Chemistry of the American Medical Association, this new jewel in the endocrine crown was officially named "progesterone."[58] Both progesterone and its related compounds that have a similar action were given the generic name "progestins."[58] There you have the genesis of research on the progestins as seen by one observer. Considering that the progestins had been in existence for hundreds of millions of years before being brought into the light of human knowledge, it is fitting and proper that we celebrate their delayed birth to science and ask now how it is that they accomplish the benefits that they have so long conferred on the mammalian world.

REFERENCES

1. PINCUS, G. & M. C. CHANG. 1953. The effects of progesterone and related compounds on ovulation and early development in the rabbit. Acta Physiol. Latinoamer. **3:** 177–183.
2. ROCK, J., C. R. GARCIA & G. PINCUS. 1957. Synthetic progestins in the normal human menstrual cycle. Rec. Progr. Hormone Res. **13:** 323–339.
3. CORNER, G. W. & W. M. ALLEN. 1929. Physiology of the corpus luteum. II. Production of a special uterine reaction (progestational proliferation) by extracts of the corpus luteum. Amer. J. Physiol. **88:** 326–339.

4. Fevold, H. L. & F. L. Hisaw. 1932. Purification of corporin. Proc. Soc. Exp. Biol. Med. **29:** 620, 621.
5. Fels, E. 1931. Zur Frage des Corpus luteum-Hormons und seines spezifischen Testes. Zentr. Gynäkol. **55:** 514–523.
6. Slotta, K. H., H. Ruschig & E. Fels. 1934. Reindarstellung der Hormone aus dem Corpus luteum. Ber. Chem. Ges. **67:** 1270–1273.
7. Butenandt, A. 1934. Neure Ergebnisse auf dem Gebiet der Sexualhormone. Wien. Klin. Wochschr. **47:** 934–936.
8. Makepeace, A. W., G. L. Weinstein & M. H. Friedman. 1937. The effect of progestin and progesterone on ovulation in the rabbit. Amer. J. Physiol. **119:** 512–516.
9. Hisaw, F. L., H. L. Fevold & R. K. Meyer. 1930. The corpus luteum hormone. II. Methods of extraction. Physiol. Zool. **3:** 135–144.
10. Heterophilus. Cited by H. B. Adelman. 1933. Heterophilus. Ann. Med. Hist. **5:** 327.
11. Vesalius, A. 1555. De Humani Corporis Fabrica Libri Septem. Baseleae, per J. Oporinum.
12. Fallopius, G. 1561. Opera ommina . . . cui nunc demun assessit tomus secundus . . . opera et studio. Petri Maphaei, Francofurti, apud. haered. A. Wecheli. Cited by A. H. F. Barbour. Edinburgh Med. J. **34:** 451–461.
13. Fabricius. Cited by J. P. Pratt. 1935. The human corpus luteum. Arch. Pathol. **19:** 380–425, 545–562.
14. de Graaf, R. 1673. On the female testes, or ovaria. R. Knox, Transl. British Record of Obstetrical Medicine and Surgery. Vol. 1, 1848. Manchester, England.
15. van Leeuwenhoek, A. 1677. Animalcula in semine masculino. Phil. Trans. Roy. Soc. London **12** (142): 1040–1043.
16. Malpighi, M. 1687. Opera omnia, seu thesaurus loupletissimus botanico-medico-anatomicus. Lugduni Batavorum. P. Vander A.
17. von Baer, K. E. 1827. De ovi mammalium et hominis genesi. Epistolam ad Academiam imperialem Scientiarum Petropolitanam, Lipsiae, L. Vossii.
18. Robin, C. 1856. Les hemorrhagies des vesicules ovariennes. Compt. Rend. Soc. Biol. **3:** 139–145.
19. Marshall, F. H. A. 1922. The Physiology of Reproduction. Longmans Green & Co. London, England.
20. Pratt, J. P. 1935. The human corpus luteum. Arch. Pathol. **19:** 380–425, 545–562.
21. Corner, G. W. 1915. The corpus luteum of pregnancy, as it is in swine. Contrib. Embryol. No. 22. Carnegie Institution. Washington, D.C.
22. Meyer, R. 1911. Über Corpus Luteum-bildung keim Menschen. Arch Gynäkol. **93:** 354–404.
23. Berthold, A. A. 1849. Transplantation der Hoden. Arch. Anat. Physiol. Wiss. Med.: 42–46.
24. Knauer, E. 1896. Einege Versuche über Ovarientransplantation bei Kaninchen. Zentr. Gynäkol. **20:** 524–528.
25. Knauer, E. 1898. Zur Ovarien transplantation. Geburt am normal Ende der Schwangerschaft nach Ovarientransplantation beim Kaninchen. Zentr. Gynäkol. **22:** 201–211.
26. Knauer, E. 1900. Die Ovarientransplantation. Arch. Gynäkol. **60:** 322–376.
27. Marshall, F. H. A. & W. A. Jolly. 1905. Contributions to the physiology of mammalian reproduction: II. The ovary as an organ of internal secretion. Proc. Roy. Soc. London Ser. B **76:** 395–398.
28. Marshall, F. H. A. & W. A. Jolly. 1906. Preliminary communication upon ovarian transplantation and its effect on the uterus. J. Physiol. **34:** XXVI.
29. Marshall, F. H. A. & W. A. Jolly. 1907. Results of removal and transplantation of ovaries. Trans. Roy. Soc. Edinburgh **45:** 589–599.
30. Heape, W. 1905. Ovulation and degeneration of ova in the rabbit. Proc. Roy. Soc. London Ser. B **76:** 260–268.
31. Prenant, A. 1898. La valeur morphologique du corps jaune. Son action physiologique et therapeutique possible. Rev. Gen. Sci. Pure Appl. Bull. Ass. Franc. Avan. Sci. **9:** 646–650.

32. BEARD, J. 1897. The span of gestation and the cause of birth. A study of the critical period and its effects in mammalia. Gustav Fischer. Jena, German Democratic Republic.
33. FRAENKEL, L. 1903. Die Function des Corpur-luteum. Arch. Gynäkol. **68:** 438–545.
34. FRAENKEL, L. 1910. Neue Experimente zur Function des Corpus luteum. Arch. Gynäkol. **91:** 705–761.
35. LOEB, L. 1907. Uber die experimentelle Erzeugung von Knoten non Decidua-gewebe in dem Üterus des Meerschweinchens nach stattgefundener Copulation. Zentr. Allgem. Pathol. Pathol. Anat. **18:** 563–565.
36. LOEB, L. 1908. The production of deciduomata, and the relation between the ovaries and the formation of the decidua. J. Amer. Med. Ass. **50:** 1897–1901.
37. ANCEL, P. & P. BOUIN. 1910. Recherches sur les fonctions du corps jaune gestatif. I. Sur le determinisme de la preparation de l'uterus a la fixation de l'oeuf. J. Physiol. Pathol. Gen. **12:** 1–16.
38. ALLEN, E. & E. A. DOISY. 1923. An ovarian hormone: preliminary report on its localization, extraction, and partial purification, and action in test animals. J. Amer. Med. Ass. **81:** 819–821.
39. ASDELL, S. A. & F. H. A. MARSHALL. 1927. On the effect of the ovarian hormone in producing pro-oestrous development in the dog and rabbit. Proc. Roy. Soc. London Ser. B **101:** 185–192.
40. CORNER, G. W. 1928. Physiology of the corpus luteum. I. The effect of very early ablation of the corpus luteum upon embryos and uterus. Amer. J. Physiol. **86:** 74–81.
41. PARKES, A. S. & C. W. BELLERBY. 1927. Studies on the internal secretions of the ovary. V. The oestrous-inhibiting function of the corpus luteum. J. Physiol. (London) **64:** 233–245.
42. WEICHERT, C. K. 1928. Production of placentomata in normal and ovariectomized guinea pigs and albino rats. Proc. Soc. Exp. Biol. Med. **25:** 490, 491.
42a. HISAW, F. L., R. K. MEYER & C. K. WEICHERT. 1928. Inhibition of ovulation and associated histological changes. Proc. Soc. Exp. Biol. Med. **25:** 754–756.
43. HISAW, F. L., R. K. MEYER & S. L. LEONARD. 1930. Production of a premenstrual endometrium in castrated monkeys by ovarian hormones. Proc. Soc. Exp. Biol. Med. **27:** 400–403.
44. HISAW, F. L. 1929. The corpus luteum hormone. Experimental relaxation of the pelvic ligaments of the guinea pig. Physiol. Zool. **2:** 59–79.
45. ALLEN, W. M. & G. W. CORNER. 1930. Physiology of the corpus luteum. VII. Maintenance of pregnancy in rabbit after very early castration, by corpus luteum extracts. Proc. Soc. Exp. Biol. Med. **27:** 403–405.
46. ALLEN, W. M. & G. W. CORNER. 1929. Physiology of the corpus luteum. III. Normal growth and implantation of embryos after very early ablation of the ovaries, under the influence of extracts of the corpus luteum. Amer. J. Physiol. **88:** 340–346.
47. ALLEN, W. M. 1930. Physiology of the corpus luteum. V. The preparation and some chemical properties of progestin, a hormone of the corpus luteum which produces progestational proliferation. Amer. J. Physiol. **92:** 174–188.
48. HERMANN, E. 1915. Über eine wirksame Substanz im Eirstocke und in der Placenta. Monatsschr. Geburtsh. Gynäkol. **41:** 1–50.
49. ALLEN, W. M. 1932. Preparation of purified progestin. J. Biol. Chem. **98:** 591–605.
50. FEVOLD, H. L., F. L. HISAW & S. L. LEONARD. 1930. Purification of hormone of the corpus luteum responsible for progestational development and other reactions. Proc. Soc. Exp. Biol. Med. **27:** 606–608.
51. FEVOLD, H. L., F. L. HISAW & S. L. LEONARD. 1932. Hormones of the corpus luteum. The separation and purification of three active substances. J. Amer. Chem. Soc. **52:** 254–263.
52. BUTENANDT, A. & U. WESTPHAL. 1934. Zur Isolierung und Charackterisserung des Corpus-luteum-Hormons. Ber. Deut. Chem. Gesellsch. **67:** 1440–1442.
53. ALLEN, W. M. & O. WINTERSTEINER. 1934. Crystalline progestin. Science **80:** 190, 191.
54. FELS, E., K. H. SLOTTA & H. RUSCHIG. 1934. Die Reindarstellung der Hormone aus dem Corpus luteum. Klin. Wochschr. **13:** 1207, 1208.

55. WINTERSTEINER, O. & W. M. ALLEN. 1934. Crystalline progestin. J. Biol. Chem. **107:** 321–326.
56. BUTENANDT, A. & J. SCHMIDT. 1934. Überfuhrung des Pregnandiols in Corpus-luteum-Hormon. Ber. Deut. Chem. Gesellsch. **67:** 1901–1903.
57. BUTENANDT, A. & U. WESTPHAL. 1934. Über die Darstellung des Corpus-luteum-Hormons aus Stigmasterin: die Konstition des Corpus-luteum-Hormons. Ber. Deut. Chem. Gesellsch. **67:** 2085–2087.
58. FERNHOLZ, E. 1934. Zur Synthese des Corpus-luteum-Hormons. Ber. Deut. Chem. Gesellsch. **67:** 1855.
59. ALLEN, W. M. 1939. Biochemistry of the corpus luteum hormone, progesterone. *In* Sex and Internal Secretions. E. Allen, C. H. Danforth & E. A. Doisy, Eds. 2nd edit.: 901–928. The Williams & Wilkins Co. Baltimore, Md.
60. ALLEN, W. M., A. BUTENANDT, G. W. CORNER & K. H. SLOTTA. 1935. Nomenclature of corpus luteum hormone. Science **82:** 153.

PROGESTERONE BINDING TO SERUM PROTEINS*

Ulrich Westphal,† Stephen D. Stroupe, and Su-Li Cheng

Department of Biochemistry
University of Louisville School of Medicine
Louisville, Kentucky 40201

Progesterone is bound in the blood serum of humans and most other mammalian species to three proteins: albumin; corticosteroid-binding globulin (CBG), or transcortin; and α_1-acid glycoprotein (AAG), or orosomucoid. Whereas human serum albumin (HSA) consists of a folded polypeptide chain free of carbohydrate, AAG and CBG are glycoproteins with relatively high sugar content (TABLE 1). The binding of the steroid hormones to the serum proteins is mediated essentially by hydrophobic forces and hydrogen bonds; noncovalent complexes are formed that are dissociable. The rate of dissociation increases with rising temperature.

An inverse relationship exists between the serum concentrations of the three proteins and their affinity for progesterone. The association constant of CBG for progesterone at 37°C is approximately 500 times higher than that of HSA, but there are about 800 HSA molecules for each molecule of CBG in normal blood serum. This is the reason why the participation of HSA in the binding of steroid hormones is substantial[1,2]; about half of the progesterone in pregnancy serum is associated with albumin (TABLE 2). A smaller percentage is albumin bound in the case of cortisol, a steroid of more hydrophilic nature than is progesterone.

The biologic significance of protein binding of the steroid hormones[3] is seen in several ways. The steroids are being transported by the serum proteins. This function does not include, however, the need for solubilization, because the maximal levels[4] of even the least soluble progesterone are within the limits of aqueous solubility.[5] An important aspect of the protein complex formation is the protection of the steroid hormones from chemical or enzymatic attack, resulting in decreased metabolic clearance. This steroid-conserving mechanism has been emphasized recently[6] for the progesterone-binding globulin (PBG) of the pregnant guinea pig, a serum glycoprotein to be discussed below. The steroids are biologically inactive as long as they are associated with protein; they can be "activated" by dissociation to the unbound hormone. In this manner, a relatively large amount of steroid can be carried in an indifferent storage form and can be made available immediately at the target tissue. For progesterone, nearly all of the hormone circulates in the body as a biologically inactive species (TABLE 2).

The most desirable objective of the study of steroid hormone interaction with proteins would be the investigation of steroid receptor proteins.[7,8] Unfortunately, none of these receptors has been available in purified form in sufficient amounts to make such study practical. Therefore, we have concentrated our efforts on the exploration of the chemical basis for the interaction of steroid hormones with serum proteins, preferably those of high affinity and specificity. Earlier results from our and other laboratories on the binding of progesterone to the three human proteins

*Supported by Grant AM-06369 from the National Institute of Arthritis, Metabolism and Digestive Diseases.

†Research Career Awardee of the United States Public Health Service.

TABLE 1

PROGESTERONE-BINDING PROTEINS IN HUMAN SERUM

Protein	Molecular Weight (daltons)	Carbohydrate (%)	Concentration (μM)	Association Constant (μM^{-1}) 4°C	37°C
HSA	69,000	—	550	0.36	0.18
AAG	41,000	42	18	1.5	0.6
CBG	52,000	26	0.7	700	90
PBG*	88,000	71	13	2200	350

*From pregnant guinea pig serum.

listed in TABLE 1 have been summarized[9]; additional results on HSA,[10] AAG,[11,12] and CBG,[13–16] have been published.

Studies on CBG, the serum protein that binds progesterone in human serum with highest affinity, are handicapped by its instability to heat and acidic milieu and by its low concentration in the blood. It was fortunate, therefore, that we discovered in the serum of the pregnant guinea pig a protein, different from CBG, that binds progesterone with high affinity and specificity and that occurs in relatively high quantity.[17] The existence of such a protein was postulated in independent studies.[18] In the present report, some recent results on this PBG will be discussed.

PURIFICATION OF PBG

PBG occurs in pooled serum of pregnant guinea pigs at the relatively high concentration of 1.2×10^{-5} mol of progesterone binding sites per liter,[19] which corresponds to more than 1 mg/ml. It has considerable heat stability. This feature is evident from FIGURE 1, which shows that more than 50% of the PBG activity survives a 2-day exposure to 60°C.[20] The heat resistance is greater than that of CBG, from which it can be separated.[21,22] Noteworthy also is the remarkable indifference toward acidic and alkaline milieus, as seen in FIGURE 2; incubation for 48 hr at pH 2 or 11 results in very little inactivation.[23]

Purification of PBG has been reported from several laboratories[19,24,25]; ion-exchange chromatography, gel filtration, ammonium sulfate precipitation, and electrophoresis were the principal methods applied in the initial studies. A useful simplification of the purification procedure was achieved[26] by taking advantage of the acid stability of PBG and its extremely low isoelectric point of 2.8[23]: chromatography at pH 4.5 of the serum over a column of sulfopropyl (SP)

TABLE 2

BINDING DISTRIBUTION OF PROGESTERONE AND CORTISOL IN HUMAN PREGNANCY SERUM[1,2]

Protein	Progesterone (%)	Cortisol (%)
CBG	43–48	60–80
HSA	50–54	13–32
AAG	~1	—
Unbound	1–2	7–8

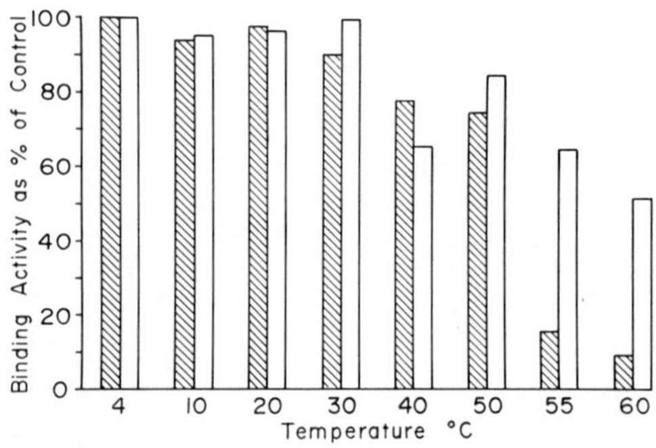

FIGURE 1. Effect of temperature on progesterone-binding activity and stability of PGB in serum diluted 1:10 with citrate-phosphate-borate buffer of pH 7.0. Specific binding was determined by charcoal adsorption at the temperatures indicated after 30 min of incubation with saturating levels of [^{3}H]progesterone at the same temperatures (hatched bars). Companion tubes were incubated for 48 hr at the temperatures indicated, and specific binding was then determined at 4°C (open bars). Binding activity is expressed as a percentage of the control value incubated for 30 min at 4°C and measured at 4°C. (From MacLaughlin & Westphal.[20] By permission of *Biochimica et Biophysica Acta*.)

Sephadex®, a strong cation exchanger, results in adsorption of most serum proteins, except PBG, which is eluted in the void volume of the column. A single run gives a PBG preparation free of albumin and of CBG, which presumably is inactivated under the acidic conditions.

The prepurified PBG preparations were subjected to affinity chromatography on columns of immobilized steroids.[27] Sepharose® 4B was activated with cyanogen bromide, coupled with diaminodipropylamine as the spacer, and the product was condensed with the 17-hemisuccinate of 19-nortestosterone, with formation of an amide bond. This steroid derivative was selected because the binding affinity of 19-nortestosterone to PBG is close to, but lower than, that of

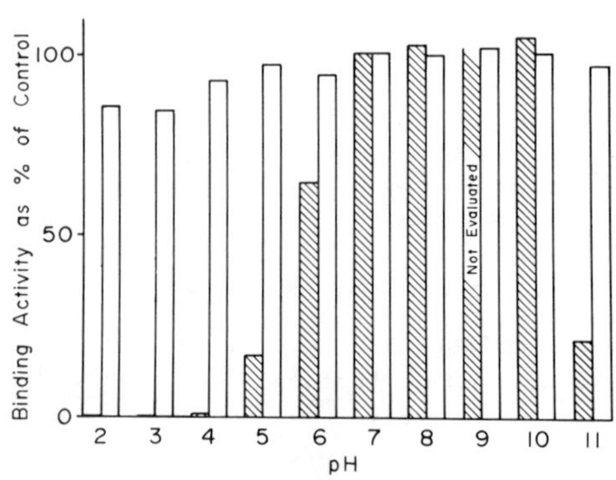

FIGURE 2. Effect of pH on progesterone-binding activity and stability of a purified PBG preparation in citrate-phosphate-borate buffer at 4°C. Binding parameters were determined by equilibrium dialysis at the pH stated (hatched bars) or at pH 7.0 after incubation for 48 hr at the pH indicated (open bars). Binding activity is expressed as a percentage of the control value determined at pH 7.0, 4°C. (From Harding *et al.*[23] By permission of *Life Sciences*.)

progesterone. Similar results were obtained with an affinity gel that was prepared by coupling the hemisuccinate of deoxycorticosterone to the diaminodipropylamino derivative of Sepharose 4B. FIGURE 3 shows that a portion of the protein applied to the column is not adsorbed and readily eluted by the starting buffer; this material (peak I) does not bind progesterone. The active PBG fraction (peak II) is obtained by elution with 10 μM progesterone or 5α-pregnane-3,20-dione, steroids that have a high affinity for PBG and are thus able to displace the protein from the steroid-Sepharose matrix. Repetition of the affinity chromatography of peak II results in one peak of pure PBG; no inactive protein can be detected.

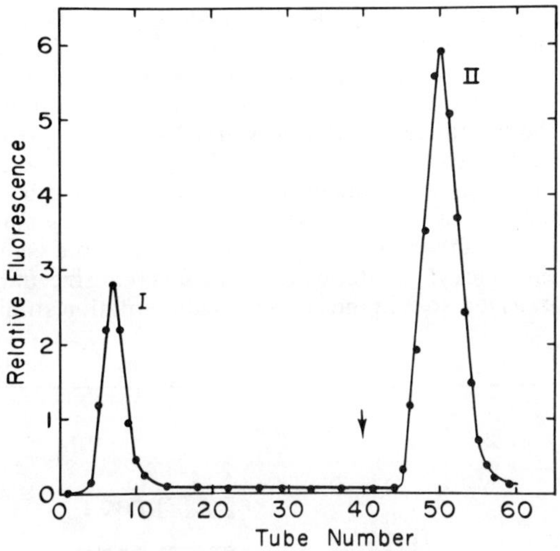

FIGURE 3. Affinity chromatography of SP-Sephadex-purified PBG on 19-nortestosterone-Sepharose gel. The arrow indicates the start of 10 μM 5α-pregnane-3,20-dione for elution. Peak I is inactive; peak II is pure PBG. (From Cheng *et al.*[27] By permission of *FEBS Letters*.)

GENERAL PROPERTIES OF PBG

Equilibrium dialysis and Scatchard analysis of the affinity-purified PBG gave an *n* value of 1.03 as an average of six determinations at different temperatures. The association constants, K_a, were 2.2×10^9 M^{-1} at 4°C and 1.1×10^9 M^{-1} at 22°C. Determination of the molecular weight by sedimentation equilibrium ultracentrifugation gave a linear Yphantis plot[28]; the apparent weight average molecular weight was 88,000. In agreement with previous results,[19] the pure PBG was found to have the unusually high carbohydrate content of about 70%, almost one fourth of which consisted of sialic acid (TABLE 3).

One of the unique properties of PBG is its polydispersity. This property can be readily demonstrated by dividing the glycoprotein peak, obtained by gel filtration, into two halves: the half fraction that elutes first has a higher molecular weight and a higher carbohydrate content than does the later portion.[19] Further subdivision by gel filtration gave active species of gradually decreasing molecular weight, forming a virtually continuous series of changing molecular sizes of PBG. This

TABLE 3

CARBOHYDRATE CONTENT OF AFFINITY-PURIFIED PBG

Carbohydrate	Percent
Sialic acid	17.0
Hexose	29.0
Hexosamine	23.5
Fucose	1.5
Total	71.0

series can be demonstrated by several independent methods: FIGURE 4 shows an electrophoretic analysis of the size distribution of two arbitrary fractions of the polydisperse active PBG species, called PBG I and PBG II, in comparison with the PBG activity of unfractionated pooled serum and of serum from an individual animal. Clearly, the full range of differently sized species is present in the pooled serum and in the serum of the individual donor; the polydispersity is, therefore, not the result of pooling. This conclusion has been verified by sucrose gradient centrifugation analysis of six individual sera from pregnant guinea pigs.[19] Polyacrylamide gel electrophoresis gives essentially the same result in the presence of sodium dodecyl sulfate, which indicates that size and not charge is the determining factor, as it also is in the gradient sedimentation studies.

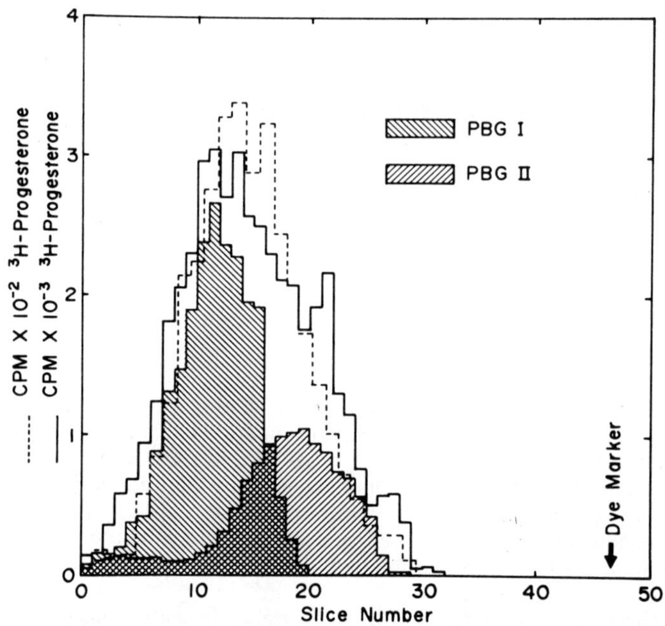

FIGURE 4. Polyacrylamide gel electrophoresis of PBG labeled with [^{3}H]progesterone. Solid line, open area, pooled pregnant guinea pig serum; broken line, serum from single animal; shaded areas, PBG I and PBG II (see text). The serum of the single animal contained about 10% of the radioactivity added to the pooled serum sample. (From Burton *et al.*[19] By permission of *Biochemistry*.)

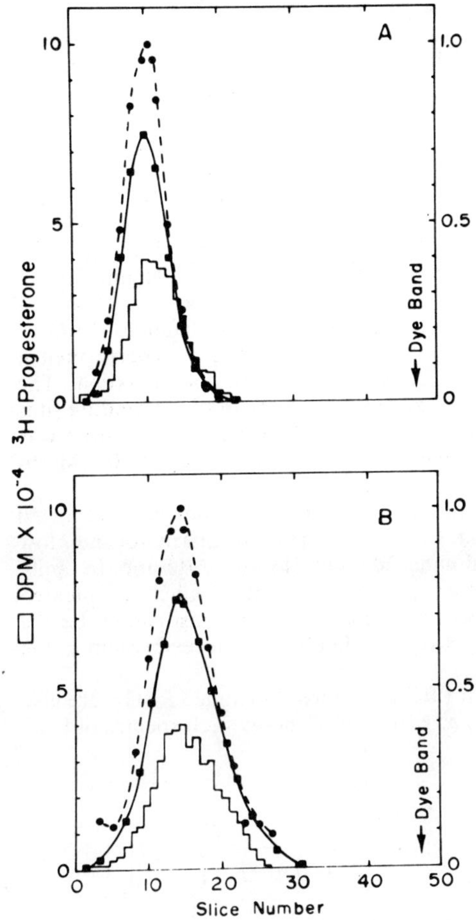

FIGURE 5. Polyacrylamide gel electrophoresis of affinity-purified PBG. Fraction A (panel A) and fraction B (panel B) were obtained by halving a symmetric gel filtration peak. One gel of triplicate runs was stained for protein with Coomassie blue and scanned at 580 nm (■); another was stained for carbohydrate with PAS and scanned at 510 nm (●); the third one was loaded with [^{3}H]progesterone-saturated PBG (—). The right ordinate shows relative absorbance. (From Cheng *et al.*[27] By permission of *FEBS Letters*.)

Purification of PBG by affinity chromatography does not affect the polydisperse nature of this glycoprotein. The polydispersity can be shown by polyacrylamide gel electrophoresis (FIGURE 5). It has been previously concluded[19] that the polydispersity of PBG results from the attachment of different amounts of carbohydrate to a polypeptide core of about 27,000 daltons molecular weight; such a polypeptide-carbohydrate relationship is known for other polydisperse glycoproteins. Assuming a peptide content of about 30% and 88,000 daltons molecular weight for the affinity-purified PBG (TABLE 3), a polypeptide core of about 27,000 daltons molecular weight can be calculated.

The unusually high carbohydrate values for pure PBG have been obtained consistently in our laboratory. It should be noted, however, that lower amounts have been found by other investigators; Milgrom *et al.*[24] reported 48.7% for their preparation, and Lea[25] determined only 42%. No definite explanation can be given for these dissimilarities, except for the possibility that different strains of guinea pigs produce variant glycoproteins. We have eliminated methodologic differences as the cause of the variations of the carbohydrate content.[19]

Conformational Changes in PBG on Steroid Binding

Only a few previous observations have been reported on the induction of conformational changes in proteins on steroid binding, involving serum albumin[29–31] and CBG.[14,32] The more readily available, and also more stable, PBG provided the opportunity to study the conformational influence of steroid binding on a high-affinity binder of high specificity.[26] Figure 6 shows the circular dichroism (CD) spectra of PBG and of the PBG-progesterone complex. Compared to free PBG, the steroid complex has a more negative ellipticity between 240 and 227 nm, where it becomes more positive. Both samples have minima at 213 and 207 nm. Zero ellipticity occurs at about 203 nm; maxima are seen at 198 nm for the progesterone complex and at 197 nm for steroid-free PBG.

To demonstrate that the CD difference between PBG and liganded PBG is, indeed, due to complex formation, a simple titration experiment was performed at 233 nm, where the percentage difference between the two curves is maximal. The CD signal changes linearly with the addition of progesterone until the binding sites are saturated (Figure 6, *inset*). The progesterone-binding site concentration was thus found to be 9.3×10^{-7} M, in agreement with the value of 8.6×10^{-7} M obtained by fluorescence quenching analysis (see below).

CD spectra of high-affinity steroid-binding proteins have not been reported previously. The spectra given in Figure 6 are noteworthy, primarily for their low ellipticity and the unusual double minima at 207 and 213 nm. Attempts to apply available methods of interpreting the PBG spectrum in terms of α helix, β-pleated sheet, and random-coil segments were unsuccessful.[26] The reason may be the contribution to the observed ellipticity of the amide chromophores present in the carbohydrate moiety of PBG.

Conformational differences between PBG and steroid-liganded PBG were also revealed by ultraviolet difference spectra.[26] Figure 7 shows such spectra of PBG

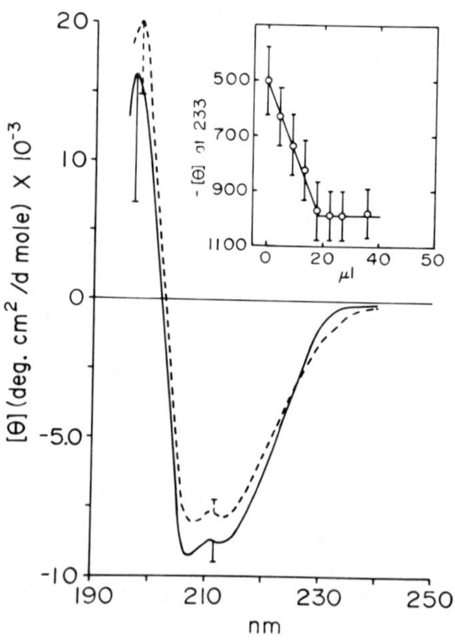

Figure 6. Circular dichroism spectra of PBG (—) and PBG-progesterone complex (- - -) at pH 7.4; progesterone-binding site concentration, 8.6×10^{-7} M. Note change of scale of ordinate. *Inset:* CD titration of PBG by progesterone. At the equivalence point, 1.08 mol of progesterone has been added per binding site. (From Stroupe & Westphal.[26] By permission of *Biochemistry*.)

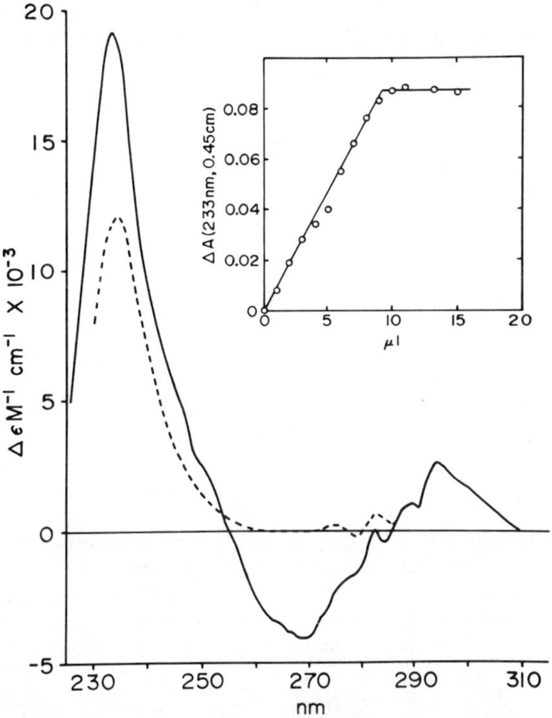

FIGURE 7. Ultraviolet difference spectra of PBG complexes with progesterone (—) and 5-pregnen-3β-ol-20-one (- - -). Between 285 and 310 nm, the difference spectra of the two complexes are identical. *Inset:* Spectral titration of PBG with progesterone at 233 nm. At the equivalence point, 1.01 mol of progesterone has been added per binding site. (From Stroupe & Westphal.[26] By permission of *Biochemistry*.)

against its progesterone and 5-pregnen-3β-ol-20-one complexes. Both steroids induce a large positive signal at 294–295 nm due to the perturbation of a tryptophan residue. Smaller peaks at 288 and 283 nm can be assigned to tyrosine and tryptophan, respectively. For the progesterone complex, the two smaller peaks and a third one at 275 nm are superimposed by a broad and intensive negative signal at 268–270 nm. This negative signal results from perturbation of the Δ^4-3-keto chromophore in progesterone; it is the basis of a previously published spectral method for measuring protein interactions with Δ^4-3-ketosteroids.[33] In accordance with this interpretation, the PBG complex with pregnenolone, a steroid that lacks the Δ^4-3-keto chromophore, does not give the 268–270 nm minimum in its difference spectrum (FIGURE 7).

The large positive peak at 233–234 nm in both difference spectra (FIGURE 7) is assumed to result primarily from perturbation of the short-wavelength transitions of aromatic amino acids.[26] However, the progesterone difference spectrum shows, in addition to this positive contribution by the protein, the signal given by the perturbed Δ^4-3-keto group. This progesterone absorption accounts almost entirely for the difference between the progesterone and pregnenolone peaks at this short wavelength; the conformational change in PBG on binding progesterone or pregnenolone is the same.

The signals at 233–234, 270, and 294–295 nm can all be used to measure the concentration of binding sites. Utilizing the short-wavelength signal, a titration of PBG with progesterone is given in FIGURE 7 (*inset*). Similar results were obtained in titrations with both progesterone and pregnenolone, following the signals at the different wavelengths. The signal changes were linear with respect to added steroid until the binding sites were saturated; no further changes were noted beyond the saturation point. This result proves that the difference spectra given by the PBG complexes of progesterone and pregnenolone result from steroid binding to a specific site on the protein and not from nonspecific solvent perturbation.

FLUORESCENCE QUENCHING OF PBG ON STEROID BINDING

The involvement of tryptophan in the steroid binding to PBG, revealed by the ultraviolet difference spectra (FIGURE 7), can also be seen in fluorometric measurements.[34] The intrinsic fluorescence spectrum of PBG shows an excitation maximum at 280 nm and an emission maximum at 340 nm, characteristic of polypeptides that contain tryptophan. Occupation of the binding site by progesterone results in strong quenching without shift of the wavelength maxima. For affinity-purified PBG, the reduction of fluorescence is more than 80%.[27] This quenching phenomenon can be utilized in a simple titration method to determine the concentration of binding sites and the association constant. Addition of small aliquots of a progesterone solution to a given PBG solution results in a gradual decrease of the relative fluorescence until the binding sites are saturated (FIGURE 8). Further addition of progesterone does not cause more quenching, except for a

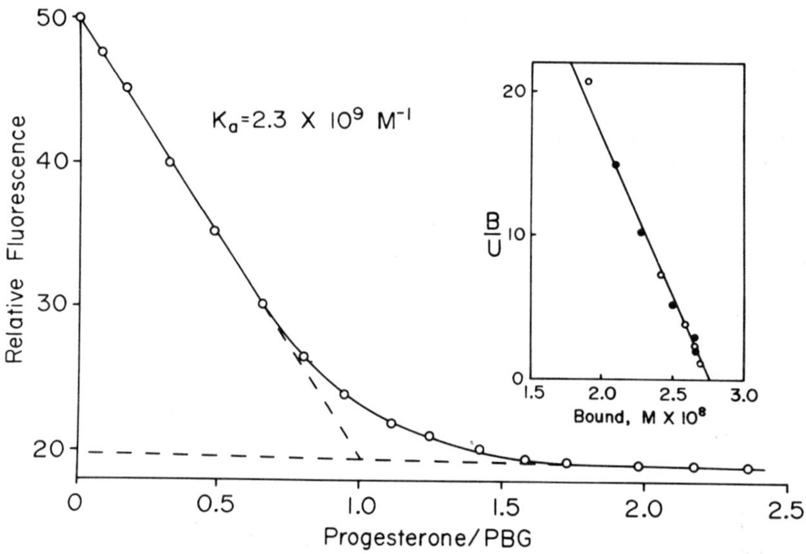

FIGURE 8. Fluorescence quenching titration of PBG with progesterone. The equivalence point gives a binding site concentration of 2.70×10^{-8} M; the solid curve yields a K_a of 2.3×10^9 M^{-1}. *Inset:* Scatchard plot of the data from the nonlinear region gives a binding site concentration of 2.77×10^{-8} M and a K_a of 2.1×10^9 M^{-1}. The solid circles correspond to the actual data points, whereas the open circles are taken from the solid curve. (From Stroupe *et al.*[34] By permission of *Archives of Biochemistry and Biophysics.*)

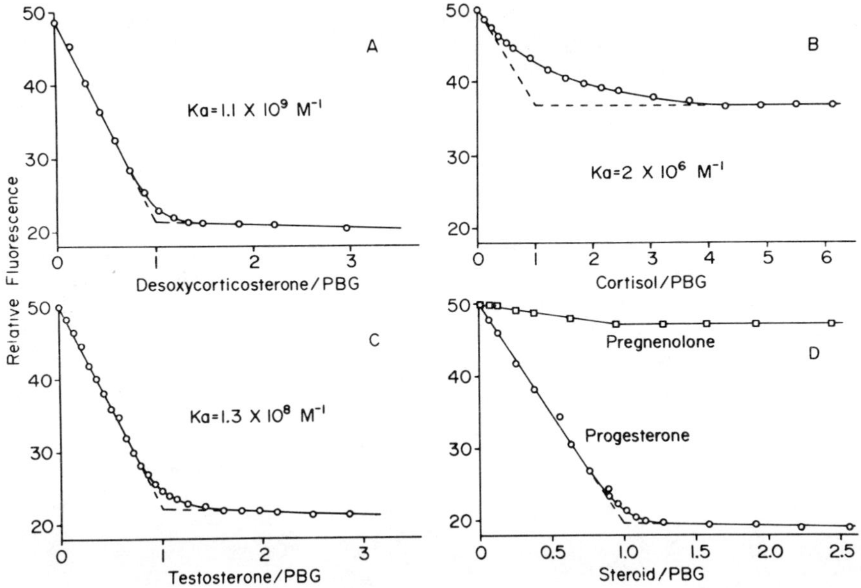

FIGURE 9. Fluorescence quenching titrations of PBG with various steroids. (From Stroupe *et al.*[34] By permission of *Archives of Biochemistry and Biophysics.*)

small contribution due to ethanol in the steroid solution and to inner filter effects. The intersect of the extended initial linear portion and the extrapolated baseline gives the equivalence point. This point determines the concentration of binding sites, because the concentration of the added progesterone solution is known.

The association constant can be determined by the expression $K_a = \alpha/(1-\alpha)^2P$, where α is the degree of association, as given by the ratio of quenching at the equivalence point over total quenching, and P is the binding site concentration at the equivalence point. Drawing a smooth curve through all data points between the two linear portions (FIGURE 8) makes it possible to base the value of α not on a single point but rather on an average. The data that represent the quenching curve between the linear portions can be presented as a Scatchard plot (FIGURE 8, *inset*). As expected, the affinity constant obtained is the same as that calculated by the simple expression given above. In a similar way, fluorescence quenching titration curves may be obtained for progesterone binding to AAG, and the concentration of binding sites and affinity constants can be determined.[34]

The main advantages of the fluorescence quenching titration method for determination of association constant and binding site concentration are the small amount of binding protein required (typically 0.1 nmol of PBG per experiment), the greater rapidity compared to equilibrium dialysis, and the possibility of using unlabeled steroids. The binding protein must be in a purified form, and the steroid must have the appropriate ultraviolet absorption. Fluorescence quenching is also a valuable method for assaying PBG activity during purification procedures without introducing radiolabeled steroids: measurement of the fluorescence of the relevant fractions in the presence and absence of a large excess of progesterone gives a value for the progesterone-induced quenching that is proportional to PBG purity.

The fluorescence quenching titration method has been applied in our laboratory for the determination of association constants of PBG complexes with a large number of steroids with Δ^4-3-keto and other absorbing groups.[34a] Examples of three Δ^4-3-ketosteroids more polar than progesterone are given in FIGURE 9 (A–C). The association constants obtained are in general agreement with those determined by a competitive equilibrium dialysis method.[35] For acceptable precision, we perform the titrations at least in quadruplicate runs. FIGURE 9,D shows the titration of two identical PBG samples with progesterone and with 5-pregnen-3β-ol-20-one. Even though pregnenolone has been reported to bind to PBG with an affinity constant more than 10 times greater than that of cortisol,[35] quenching is only minimal, and an association constant cannot be calculated. The ultraviolet difference spectra (FIGURE 7) had shown that the protein perturbation as such was virtually the same whether given by progesterone or by pregnenolone, which indicates that the same type of conformational change occurs on binding of either steroid.

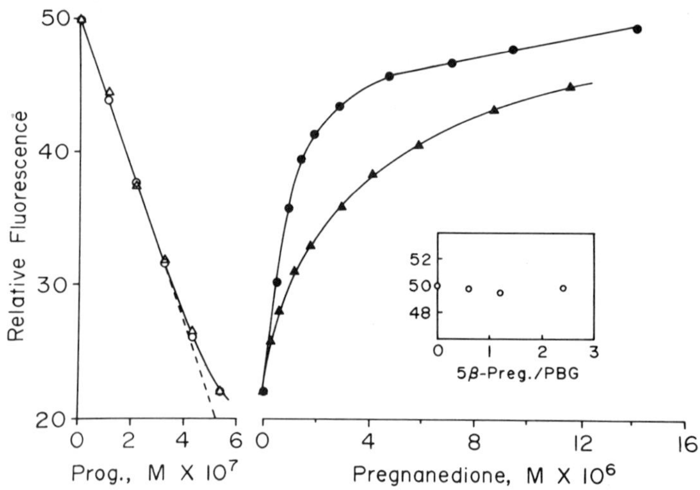

FIGURE 10. Fluorescence quenching titration of PBG with progesterone (○, Δ), followed by addition of an excess of 5α-pregnane-3,20-dione (●) or 5β-pregnane-3,20-dione (▲). Note the "unquenching" by displacement of progesterone. The inset shows that the fluorescence of PBG does not change by addition of more than 1 mol of 5β-pregnanedione per mole of PBG. (From Stroupe *et al.*[34] By permission of *Archives of Biochemistry and Biophysics*.)

If pregnenolone or any related steroid that lacks the Δ^4-3-keto group binds to the same site in PBG as does progesterone, competitive displacement of progesterone by the nonabsorbing steroid should be demonstrable. FIGURE 10 shows that this displacement, indeed, occurs: addition of 5α- or 5β-pregnane-3,20-dione to a PBG solution that is maximally quenched by a stoichiometric amount of progesterone results in restoration of fluorescence.[34] The PBG complex with the saturated pregnane derivative approaches the intrinsic fluorescence of the unbound PBG as the concentration of pregnanedione is increased. The inset of FIGURE 10 indicates that for 5β-pregnanedione, the fluorescence of PBG does not change even at a several-fold increase of the ligand over the stoichiometric amount. It is also evident from FIGURE 10 that higher amounts of the 5β steroid than of the 5α isomer are needed to displace progesterone from PBG. This phenomenon is explained by a lower binding affinity of 5β-pregnanedione. Binding studies by competitive equilibrium dialysis have shown that the association constant of the PBG complex with 5α-pregnane-3,20-dione is almost 10 times higher than that of the 5β isomer.[35] We will see below that the change of fluorescence by competitive displacement can be utilized to measure dissociation rates of PBG-steroid complexes.

A closer analysis of the fluorescence spectrum of PBG and of the spectral properties of progesterone provided insight into the protein-steroid interaction at the molecular level.[34] By utilizing the theory of radiationless energy transfer of Förster,[36,37] it was calculated that the progesterone-tryptophan distance in the complex is smaller than the corresponding distance in the complex of PBG with cortisol, which has a much lower affinity (see below; TABLE 5).

The above mechanism of fluorescence quenching by energy transfer from protein fluorophores to the $n \rightarrow \pi^*$ absorption band of a conjugated carbonyl group in the steroid requires that two conditions are met. First, the contact between steroid and protein in the complex must occur very near a fluorescent group. Second, to be a suitable acceptor, the steroid must have an absorption band that overlaps the fluorescence band of the protein. The magnitude of the quenching, then, offers information on the molecular events at the binding site.

KINETICS OF STEROID-PBG INTERACTION

Most of our present knowledge on interactions between steroids and proteins[9] has been attained under the viewpoint of systems in equilibrium. Serum proteins with high affinity for steroid hormones have been isolated and characterized, and the strength of their association with steroids has been determined under various conditions. The emphasis has been on the end products of the reversible binding reaction, that is, the steroid-protein complex and the unbound components formed by dissociation. For a meaningful interpretation of the interactions as they occur *in vivo* between hormones and proteins, and for an understanding of their biologic significance, the association complex has to be viewed as a dynamic system; detailed information is required on the rates of association and dissociation and on thermodynamic parameters. In the area of steroid-binding serum proteins, only a few quantitative kinetic studies on the interactions have been reported, as will be discussed below.

The unusual stability,[23] ready availability in pure form,[27] binding affinity for a wide variety of steroids,[24,35,38,39] and suitable fluorescence properties[34] make PBG a very useful protein to study the rates of association and dissociation for progesterone and other steroids.[40] Quenching of the strong fluorescence signal of PBG on binding a Δ^4-3-ketosteroid provides a sensitive indicator for the association; the high affinity of PBG for progesterone, androgens, and other steroids permits the use of dilute reactant solutions to slow down the rapid bimolecular association reaction while still attaining complete association. Displacement of the quenching steroid from the complex by an ultraviolet-transparent steroid, such as 5α-pregnanedione or dihydrotestosterone, results in restoration of the intrinsic PBG fluorescence, so that the dissociation rate of the PBG-Δ^4-3-ketosteroid complex can be measured. These unique features allow the use of stopped-flow fluorometry for the determination of association and dissociation rates of PBG-steroid complexes, thereby providing the first reported example in which a physical parameter of the binding protein is monitored to establish the time course of steroid binding and dissociation.

FIGURE 11 shows a representative determination of the association rate between PBG and progesterone at pH 7.4, 20°C.[40] A half-time of 22.5 msec was obtained at an equimolar concentration of 0.52 μM, which corresponds to a rate constant of 8.6×10^7 M^{-1} sec^{-1}. An average value (± standard deviation) of k_{on} = $8.7 \pm 1.9 \times 10^7$ M^{-1} sec^{-1} was calculated from 32 experiments, each of which was the mean of four runs. The association rate constant was found to be independent of concentration over a range from 33.5 nM to 1.65 μM.

To measure the dissociation rates, the PBG-Δ^4-3-ketosteroid complex was mixed at pH 7.4 with a large excess of nonquenching steroid. The inset in FIGURE 12 presents the oscilloscope trace of the photomultiplier voltage, indicating the "unquenching" of fluorescence that occurs after the displacement of progesterone by 5α-pregnanedione as a function of time. The same result was obtained with dihydrotestosterone as the competing steroid. In this trial, the dissociation rate constant, k_{off}, was 0.053 sec^{-1}, with a half-time of 13.1 sec. The

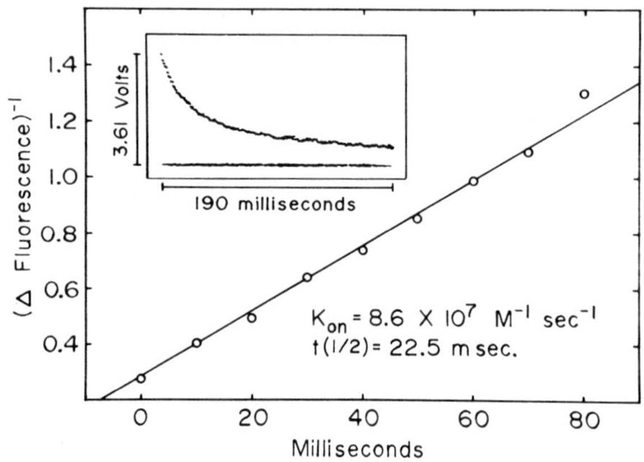

FIGURE 11. Stopped-flow fluorescence measurement of association of PBG with progesterone. The decrease in photomultiplier voltage, that is, fluorescence, was recorded as a function of time, and the data were calculated by computer. The inset is a photograph of the oscilloscope trace of the decrease in photomultiplier voltage with time. (From Stroupe & Westphal.[40] By permission of *The Journal of Biological Chemistry*.)

average value from 25 experiments of four runs each over a PBG-progesterone complex concentration of 12.5–500 nM was $k_{off} = 0.060 \pm 0.005$ sec^{-1}.

The rate of association of PBG and progesterone was measured over the temperature range from 5.9° to 41.2°C; the corresponding dissociation rate was determined from 20.0° to 41.4°C. An Arrhenius plot of the data obtained (FIGURE 3 in Reference 40) shows that the temperature dependencies of the two reactions are quite different. The association reaction has a relatively low energy of activation of 10.0 kcal/mol, being constant over the entire range measured. The temperature dependency of the dissociation reaction is greater, with an activation energy that rises from 17 kcal/mol at 20°C to 24 kcal/mol at 40°C.

With the association and dissociation rate constants available over a rather wide temperature range, the general relationship $K_a = k_{on}/k_{off}$ was compared with the association constant measured by equilibrium dialysis.[40] TABLE 4 gives the rate constants of the progesterone-PBG complex and the k_{on}/k_{off} ratios at various

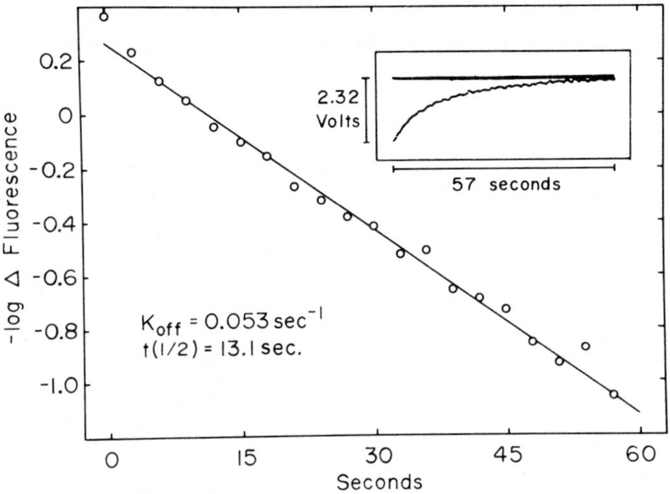

FIGURE 12. Stopped-flow fluorescence measurement of dissociation of the PBG-progesterone complex. Displacement of progesterone by a ninefold molar amount of 5α-pregnanedione produced an increase in photomultiplier voltage that was utilized to compute k_{off} and $t_{1/2}$. The inset is a photograph of the oscilloscope trace of the photomultiplier voltage as a function of time. (From Stroupe & Westphal.[40] By permission of *The Journal of Biological Chemistry*.)

temperatures. The K_a values determined by the two independent procedures agree at all temperatures. The close coincidence between the kinetic and the equilibrium association constants gives assurance that the observed fluorescence changes provide a true measure for complex formation and dissociation.

Introduction of hydroxy groups into the progesterone molecule results in a decrease of binding affinity to PBG,[35] in proportion to the number of hydroxy groups involved. This binding behavior is in accordance with the polarity rule,[9] which indicates that the PBG-steroid interaction is predominantly of a hydrophobic nature. The association and dissociation rate constants, including their ratios, are given in TABLE 5 for progesterone, deoxycorticosterone, corticosterone, and cortisol, in addition to testosterone, its acetate, and medrogestone

TABLE 4

ASSOCIATION CONSTANTS OF PBG-PROGESTERONE COMPLEX FROM KINETIC AND EQUILIBRIUM DATA[40]

Temperature (°C)	k_{on} (M^{-1} sec^{-1} × 10^{-7})	k_{off} (sec^{-1})	k_{on}/k_{off} (M^{-1} × 10^{-9})	K_a* (M^{-1} × 10^{-9})
4	2.2	0.0095†	2.4	2.2
14	4.3	0.031	1.4	1.4
23	7.4	0.083	0.89	1.0
37	16.2	0.39	0.41	0.35
45	24.6	1.05	0.23	0.22

*Equilibrium dialysis.

†A value of 0.011 sec^{-1} was determined separately by radiolabeled steroid displacement by use of gel filtration.

TABLE 5

ASSOCIATION AND DISSOCIATION RATE CONSTANTS OF PBG AND VARIOUS STEROIDS AT 20°C[40]

Steroid	k_{on} (M^{-1} sec^{-1} × 10^{-7})	k_{off} (sec^{-1})	k_{on}/k_{off} (M^{-1} × 10^{-8})	K_a (M^{-1} × 10^{-8})
Progesterone	8.8*	0.060	14.5	20†,‡
Deoxycorticosterone	8.3	0.12	6.7	10†
Corticosterone	~5§	1.4	0.4§	0.2¶
Cortisol	~5§	90‖	—‖	0.02†
Testosterone	7.8	0.43	1.8	2.9¶
Testosterone acetate	9.3	0.15	6.1	9.2¶
Medrogestone	8.5	0.024	35.3	45.5¶

*This value was determined in the experiment that compared the first four steroids.
†Reference 34.
‡$K_a = 11 \times 10^8$ M^{-1} at 20°C by extrapolation of the equilibrium dialysis data in TABLE 4.
§This value is less precise than the constants for the other steroids, because the reaction did not go to completion under the conditions used.
¶Determined by fluorescence quenching at 23°C.[34a]
‖The cortisol dissociation was biphasic, with a slower reaction (1–2 sec^{-1}) contributing about half of the fluorescence increase. None of the other dissociation reactions was biphasic.

(6,16α-dimethyl-4,6-pregnadiene-3,20-dione). For comparison, the association constants determined independently by fluorescence quenching titration are listed. The association of PBG with the various steroids occurs at a very rapid rate, which is essentially the same for all steroids, with an affinity constant greater than 10^8 M^{-1}. Complexes of lower affinity appear to associate at a somewhat slower rate. The value for binding of progesterone to PBG, $k_{on} = 8.7 \times 10^7$ M^{-1} sec^{-1} at 20°C, is similar to those of a great number of protein-ligand associations reported[41] to be in the range of 10^6–10^8 M^{-1} sec^{-1}. The association rates of the PBG-steroid complexes are not limited by diffusion.[40]

In contrast to the relatively invariant rates of association, the dissociation rate constants show considerable differences among the steroids studied, covering a relative range of 1–3750 (TABLE 5). The dissociation rate thus becomes the controlling factor in steroid binding to PBG, conferring specificity to the interaction. The slightly higher affinity constants given by fluorescence quenching for deoxycorticosterone, testosterone, testosterone acetate, and medrogestone are in accordance with our previous observation[34] that the fluorescence method somewhat overestimates the affinity constants when compared with equilibrium dialysis results. Several comparisons are of interest. Medrogestone binds to PBG with an affinity two to three times that of progesterone, yet both steroids associate at the same rate. It is the three-fold slower dissociation of medrogestone that gives it the higher affinity. Similarly, testosterone acetate binds three times more tightly than does testosterone and dissociates about three times more slowly. Again, the ratio between the affinity constants of progesterone and deoxycorticosterone is about 2:1, with a ratio of dissociation of 1:2. All of these steroids associate with PBG at the same rate. The phenomenon of the dissociation rates controlling complex stability is similar to observations with antibody-hapten systems.[42]

Because the dissociation rate of the serum protein complex determines the availability of the steroid hormone to the target cell, it is of interest to compare association and dissociation rates of various steroid complexes with serum proteins. Considering the different function of steroid binding to receptor proteins, it is worthwhile to examine in which proportions association and dissociation rates contribute to the steroid-receptor affinity constants. TABLE 6 gives the association and dissociation rates for steroid complexes with PBG, CBG, and testosterone estradiol-binding globulin (TeBG) and with several cytosol receptor proteins from chick and rat. It is evident that the k_{on} value for progesterone and PBG is about two orders of magnitude greater than any other association rate constant reported. On the other hand, the dissociation of the PBG-progesterone complex is faster than that of any other protein-steroid complex. Therefore, for PBG it is the high association rate that determines the high affinity constant, k_{on}/k_{off}. In contrast, for most other high-affinity steroid binders, especially the cytosol receptors, it is the slow rate of dissociation that yields association constants about as high as or higher than those of the PBG complex. The relatively slow association rates are thus counteracted by low dissociation rates. The low level of these association rates is noteworthy, considering that a diffusion-limited rate for steroid-protein association at 0–4°C would be three to four orders of magnitude higher.

In discussing the kinetic properties of PBG in comparison with the other data in TABLE 6, it must be remembered that purified proteins have been used only in two other studies.[15,49] Furthermore, in all other investigations, procedures have been used that disturb the equilibrium when bound and free steroids are separated. Both the use of protein mixtures in which the binder is only a minor component and the use of an interfering separation technique could result in erroneous kinetic constants, thereby weakening the validity of the comparison with the PBG system.

The characteristic kinetic differences between the steroid complexes with transport proteins and those with receptor proteins appear to be in accordance

TABLE 6

ASSOCIATION AND DISSOCIATION RATE CONSTANTS FOR VARIOUS STEROID BINDERS AT 0–4°C

Protein	Steroid*	k_{on} (M^{-1} sec^{-1} × 10^{-4})	k_{off} (sec^{-1} × 10^{5})	k_{on}/k_{off} (M^{-1} × 10^{-8})	Reference
PBG, guinea pig	P	2200	950	24	TABLE 4
CBG, human	C	20	41	4.9	43
CBG, human	C	—	45	—	44
CBG, human	C	—	230	—	15
CBG, rat	C	—	50	—	45
TeBG, human	T	—	90	—	46
TeBG, human	DHT	—	15	—	46
TeBG, rabbit	DHT	—	220	—	47
Chick progesterone					
Receptor A	P	28	1.9	150	48
Receptor B	P	63	2.4	260	48
Receptor, purified	P	—	1.6	—	49
Rat liver cytosol					
Protein A	C	—	38	—	45
Protein G	D	1.4	2.0	7.3	45
Rat uterus receptor	E	—	3.9	—	50

*P, progesterone; C, cortisol; T, testosterone; DHT, dihydrotestosterone; D, dexamethasone; E, estradiol.

with physiologic function. At late-term pregnancy concentrations of progesterone and PBG, the half-time of association at 37°C is 0.36 msec; that of dissociation of the complex is 1.8 sec.[40] The corresponding half-time values for the CBG-cortisol complex at 37°C are 44 msec and 1.1 sec. By comparison, the uptake of progesterone by the chick oviduct receptors and that of dexamethasone by the rat liver binder are rather slow. The half-time of dissociation for all three complexes is of the order of 10 hr at 0–4°C; the half-time of dissociation for the dexamethasone-binding receptor protein at 37°C is about 13 min.

The slow dissociation rate of the cytosol receptor complexes is in accord with their postulated role in mediating cellular responses to steroid hormones. It assures that the steroid remains bound to the cytosol receptor protein for a sufficiently long time, so that the subsequent reactions that lead to nuclear hormonal effects can occur. In contrast, the requirements of a hormone-transporting protein in the blood serum are different: rapid dissociation of the complex is necessary to provide immediate availability of the steroid at the target site. At the same time, the association must be fast, resulting in a high affinity, so that the major portion of the circulating hormone is present in bound form, for the protection of the organism and of the steroid hormone.

Acknowledgment

The authors appreciate the generous cooperation of Dr. Robert D. Gray in making the stopped-flow measurements possible.

References

1. Westphal, U. 1966. Z. Physiol. Chem. **346:** 243–256.
2. Rosenthal, H. E., W. R. Slaunwhite, Jr. & A. A. Sandberg. 1969. J. Clin. Endocrinol. **29:** 352–367.
3. Westphal, U. 1971. Steroid-Protein Interactions.: 434–445. Springer-Verlag New York Inc. New York, N.Y.
4. Heap, R. B., J. S. Perry & J. R. G. Challis. 1973. *In* Handbook of Physiology, Section 7, Vol. II, Female Reproductive System, Part 2. R. O. Greep, Ed.: 217–260. American Physiological Society. Washington, D.C.
5. Batra, S. 1975. J. Pharm. Pharmacol. **27:** 777–779.
6. Heap, R. B. & D. V. Illingworth. 1974. Symp. Zool. Soc. London **34:** 385–415.
7. Westphal, U. 1961. *In* Mechanism of Action of Steroid Hormones. C. A. Villee & L. L. Engel, Eds.: 33–89. Pergamon Press. New York, N.Y.
8. King, R. J. B. & W. I. P. Mainwaring. 1974. Steroid-Cell Interactions. University Park Press. Baltimore, Md.
9. Westphal, U. 1971. Steroid-Protein Interactions. Springer-Verlag New York Inc. New York, N.Y.
10. Westphal, U. & G. B. Harding. 1973. Biochim. Biophys. Acta **310:** 518–527.
11. Ryan, M. F. & U. Westphal. 1972. J. Biol. Chem. **247:** 4050–4056.
12. Kute, T. & U. Westphal. 1976. Biochim. Biophys. Acta **420:** 195–213.
13. Rosner, W. & H. L. Bradlow. 1971. J. Clin. Endocrinol. Metab. **33:** 193–198.
14. Chader, G. J., N. Rust, R. M. Burton & U. Westphal. 1972. J. Biol. Chem. **247:** 6581–6588.
15. Rosner, W., R. Darmstadt & S. J. Tauster. 1973. J. Steroid Biochem. **4:** 249–255.
16. LeGaillard, F., A. Racadot, N. Racadot-Leroy & M. Dautrevaux. 1974. Biochimie **56:** 99–108.
17. Diamond, M., N. Rust & U. Westphal. 1969. Endocrinology **84:** 1143–1151.
18. Heap, R. B. 1969. J. Reprod. Fertil. **18:** 546–548.

19. Burton, R. M., G. B. Harding, W. R. Aboul-Hosn, D. T. MacLaughlin & U. Westphal. 1974. Biochemistry **13:** 3554–3561.
20. MacLaughlin, D. T. & U. Westphal. 1974. Biochim. Biophys. Acta **365:** 373–388.
21. Milgrom, E., M. Atger & E.-E. Baulieu. 1970. Nature (London) **228:** 1205, 1206.
22. Burton, R. M., G. B. Harding, N. Rust & U. Westphal. 1971. Steroids **17:** 1–16.
23. Harding, G. B., R. M. Burton, S. D. Stroupe & U. Westphal. 1974. Life Sci. **14:** 2405–2412.
24. Milgrom, E., P. Allouch, M. Atger & E.-E. Baulieu. 1973. J. Biol. Chem. **248:** 1106–1114.
25. Lea, O. A. 1973. Biochim. Biophys. Acta **317:** 351–363.
26. Stroupe, S. D. & U. Westphal. 1975. Biochemistry **14:** 3296–3300.
27. Cheng, S. L., S. D. Stroupe & U. Westphal. 1976. FEBS Lett. **64:** 380–384.
28. Yphantis, D. A. 1964. Biochemistry **3:** 297–317.
29. Alfsen, A. 1963. Compt. Rend. Trav. Lab. Carlsberg Sér. Chim. **33:** 415–431.
30. Ryan, M. T. 1968. Arch. Biochem. Biophys. **126:** 407–417.
31. Ryan, M. T. & G. Gibbs. 1970. Arch. Biochem. Biophys. **136:** 65–72.
32. Chader, G. J. & U. Westphal. 1968. Biochemistry **7:** 4272–4282.
33. Westphal, U. 1957. Arch. Biochem. Biophys. **66:** 71–90.
34. Stroupe, S. D., S. L. Cheng & U. Westphal. 1975. Arch. Biochem. Biophys. **168:** 473–482.
34a. Blanford, A. T. & W. L. Wittman. 1975. Unpublished results.
35. Lea, O. A. 1973. Biochim. Biophys. Acta **322:** 68–74.
36. Förster, T. 1948. Ann. Phys. **2:** 55–75.
37. Förster, T. 1959. Discuss. Faraday Soc. **27:** 7–17.
38. Tan, S. Y. & B. E. P. Murphy. 1974. Endocrinology **94:** 122–127.
39. Kontula, K., O. Jänne, E. Rajakoski, E. Tanhuanpää & R. Vihko. 1974. J. Steroid Biochem. **5:** 39–44.
40. Stroupe, S. D. & U. Westphal. 1975. J. Biol. Chem. **250:** 8735–8739.
41. Eigen, M. & G. G. Hammes. 1963. Advan. Enzymol. **25:** 1–38.
42. Smith, T. W. & K. M. Skubitz. 1975. Biochemistry **14:** 1496–1502.
43. Paterson, J. Y. F. 1973. J. Endocrinol. **56:** 551–570.
44. Dixon, P. F. 1968. J. Endocrinol. **40:** 457–465.
45. Koblinsky, M., M. Beato, M. Kalimi & P. Feigelson. 1972. J. Biol. Chem. **247:** 7897–7904.
46. Heyns, W. & P. DeMoor. 1971. J. Clin. Endocrinol. Metab. **32:** 147–154.
47. Hansson, V., E. M. Ritzen, S. C. Weddington, W. S. McLean, D. J. Tindall, S. N. Nayfeh & F. S. French. 1974. Endocrinology **95:** 690–700.
48. Schrader, W. T. & B. W. O'Malley. 1972. J. Biol. Chem. **247:** 51–59.
49. Kuhn, R. W., W. T. Schrader, R. G. Smith & B. W. O'Malley. 1975. J. Biol. Chem. **250:** 4220–4228.
50. Katzenellenbogen, J. A., H. J. Johnson, Jr. & K. E. Carlson. 1973. Biochemistry **12:** 4092–4099.

Discussion

Dr. R. J. B. King: With the quenching of the tryptophan fluorescence that you're getting by interaction of the steroid $\Delta^4$3-keto group, can one infer that the tryptophan is actually near the steroid-binding site?

Dr. Westphal: Yes, we assume that it is near the site. We have unpublished results that Dr. T. Kute obtained when he was a graduate student in our laboratory, which show the involvement of tryptophan by chemical data. Reaction of the tryptophan residue in PBG with hydroxynitrobenzyl bromide results in a decrease of the binding affinity. We can partially protect the binding site from chemical modification and inactivation by first complexing with progesterone and then performing the modification reaction. One interpretation is that a tryptophan residue is in the binding site, so that the chemical modification after complex formation occurs at a decreased rate. An alternate explanation would be a conformational change on steroid binding, resulting in altered binding affinity and chemical reactivity.

DR. W. T. SCHRADER: Dr. Westphal, you mentioned the polydispersity of this material. If I recall correctly, that's due to the polydisperse nature of the carbohydrate residues in the protein. What do you know about the involvement of the carbohydrate residues in the binding of the steroid? Have you partially removed any carbohydrate and tried to look at hormone binding to that?

DR. WESTPHAL: This is a good point that I haven't mentioned. The polydisperse species have all one polypeptide core of about 27,000 molecular weight. We have picked out and characterized several molecular species of different sizes. When we analyzed the data, we always found that the molecular weight of the polypeptide core is about 27,000. Concerning the significance of carbohydrate for binding, we do not have complete data. We assume from some observations that carbohydrate is not involved in the binding of the steroid. We know that sialic acid, the last carbohydrate residue at the end of the oligosaccharide chains, is definitely not essential, because we can remove sialic acid and find no measurable effect on binding.

DR. M. R. SHERMAN: It is intriguing that you find a core polypeptide of about 27,000 daltons for all of the serum binding proteins, because we have characterized a 20,000 molecular weight steroid-binding fragment of the chick oviduct progesterone receptor (1974. J. Biol. Chem. **249:** 5351) and, more recently, steroid-binding units of similar size (about 25,000 daltons) from the rat kidney aldosterone receptor and the human breast tumor estrogen receptor.

DR. WESTPHAL: Thank you very much for that interesting comment. It would be so good if we could see the sequence of these various polypeptide cores.

DR. W. ROSNER (*The Roosevelt Hospital, New York, N.Y.*): I think that the choice of a proper experimental model is of paramount importance in trying to answer the question of the physiologic significance of the binding of steroids to albumin or CBG; most of the published experiments bear little relationship to the situation *in vivo*. With Dr. Dancis and Dr. Levitz, we have looked at the transport of cortisol across the human placenta with perfusates that contained cortisol alone, cortisol plus CBG, and cortisol plus albumin. While physiologic concentrations of CBG had no effect on the transport of cortisol, as compared to buffer, physiologic concentrations of albumin retarded cortisol transport. Although these results are somewhat contrary to the dogma in the steroid-binding field, they will not surprise those who investigate the binding of various drugs to albumin. The low association constant between albumin and cortisol is compensated for by the extremely high concentration of albumin in serum.

DR. WESTPHAL: Have you published those data?

DR. ROSNER: The manuscript is being written.

BINDING OF ATP TO PROGESTERONE RECEPTORS: PROPERTIES AND FUNCTIONAL SIGNIFICANCE OF THIS INTERACTION*

David Toft, Virinder Moudgil, Phoebe Lohmar,†
and Josephine Miller

Department of Molecular Medicine
Mayo Clinic
Rochester, Minnesota 55901

In recent years, the avian progesterone receptor has been characterized by purification and physicochemical analysis,[1-3] but the actual biochemical function of this protein remains unknown. Insight into the function of steroid receptors might be gained by studying their ability to interact with various cellular constituents. This approach has been used to demonstrate the ability of the progesterone receptor to bind to DNA and chromatin.[4,5] More recently, the interaction of the receptor with a nucleotide was demonstrated by the use of ATP-Sepharose® affinity chromatography.[6] This interaction was shown to be a reversible process with a preference for ATP among the nucleotides tested, and the results suggested that ATP may play a role in some aspect of receptor function.

Efforts have been made to identify a biologic role for this interaction with ATP. One possibility is that the progesterone-receptor complex may utilize ATP in a biochemical process during, or subsequent to, the nuclear translocation of receptor. This possibility is suggested by the present studies, which indicate a relationship between ATP binding by the receptor and the extent of *in vitro* activation and nuclear uptake of the progesterone-receptor complex.

Materials and Methods

All reagents were of analytic grade and were made up in glass-distilled water. Nucleotides were from Schwarz/Mann; Sepharose 4B and dextran T-70 from Pharmacia, Uppsala, Sweden; *o*-phenanthroline from Fischer Scientific; thioglycerol and activated charcoal from Sigma; and [1,2,^{3}H] progesterone (50 Ci/mmol) from New England Nuclear. Rifamycin AF/013 was provided by Gruppo Lepetit, Milan, Italy.

Preparation of ATP-Sepharose

ATP was covalently linked to Sepharose 4B as described previously.[6] In this process, ATP was attached to Sepharose 4B through the hydroxyl groups of its ribose via a six-carbon bridge of adipic acid dihydrazide. Our preparations contained 5–13 μmol of nucleotide per milliliter of packed Sepharose, as de-

*Supported by National Institutes of Health Contract HD-3-2769 and by the Mayo Foundation.

†Present address: Lederle Laboratories, Pearl River, N.Y. 10965.

termined by phosphate analysis.[7] Chromatography on ATP-Sepharose was performed as described previously.[6] Specific conditions for labeling or pretreating the receptor samples are described in the figure legends.

Preparation of Progesterone Receptor

Freshly excised oviducts from White Leghorn laying hens were frozen in liquid nitrogen and stored at −70°C until use, with little or no loss of hormone binding activity. The tissue was rinsed with cold 0.9% saline and homogenized with a Waring blender and then a "tissumizer" (Tekmar model SDT) in three volumes (w/v) of buffer [10 mM Tris-HCl, 12 mM thioglycerol, 1 mM EDTA, 10% glycerol, 0.01 M KCl (pH 8)]. The homogenate was first centrifuged at 12,000*g* for 10 min and then at 100,000*g* for 90 min to obtain the cytosol fraction. In some cases, the cytosol was fractionated by ammonium sulfate precipitation, as described previously,[6] and the precipitates were stored at −70°C.

White Leghorn chicks were primed with diethylstilbestrol for 2 weeks as described previously.[8] Cytosol was prepared from freshly removed oviducts as described above but with two volumes of buffer that contained either 40 mM Tris-HCl and 12 mM thioglycerol (pH 7.5) or 40 mM Tris-HCl, 12 mM thioglycerol, and 10% glycerol (pH 8) (as indicated in the figure legends).

Receptor Activation and Binding to ATP-Sepharose

In these experiments, elevated temperature (23°C) or high salt conditions were employed as a means of receptor activation. For incubations at elevated temperatures, aliquots of chick oviduct cytosol were preincubated at 4°C for 2 hr with 20 nM [^{3}H]progesterone and then incubated at room temperature for varying periods of time. The samples were then cooled on ice and tested for the binding of receptor to ATP-Sepharose (1-ml columns). For incubation in high salt, aliquots of cytosol that contained 20 nM [^{3}H]-progesterone were incubated at 4°C with 0.01–0.5 M KCl. After a 1-hr incubation, each sample was diluted 1:1 with buffer [40 mM Tris-HCl, 12 mM thioglycerol, 10 mM KCl (pH 8)] before determining the binding of receptor to ATP-Sepharose.

Preincubation and Nuclear Binding Assay

Each experiment consisted of two main parts: preincubation of the [^{3}H]progesterone-receptor sample, followed by a nuclear binding assay. In the preincubation, 0.4 ml of cytosol, labeled with 20 nM [^{3}H]progesterone, was incubated at 23° or 0°C with 0.15 ml of 42% glycerol and 0.1 ml of additive (nucleotide). For the nuclear binding assay, the preincubation solutions were all cooled to 0°C and incubated for an additional 1 hr with 0.2 ml of buffer [40 mM Tris-HCl, 12 mM thioglycerol (pH 7.5)] and 0.15 ml of purified oviduct nuclei that contained 50–100 μg of DNA. The nuclei had been prepared and stored according to method II of Spelsberg *et al.*[9] (omitting the use of Triton® X-100), and they were suspended in a buffer of 0.01 M Tris, 25% glycerol, and 0.002 M $MgCl_2$ (pH 7.5). At the end of the nuclear incubation, 3.5 ml of a wash [0.01 M Tris, 10% glycerol, 0.001 M $MgCl_2$, and 0.1% Triton X-100 buffer (pH 7.5)] were added to each tube, and the nuclei were sedimented at 1000*g* for 5 min. Supernatants were aspirated off, the nuclei resuspended in 3.5 ml of the wash, and again recovered by centrifugation. Each nuclear pellet was then suspended in 0.5 ml of H_2O and transferred to a scintillation vial. Ten milliliters of scintillation fluid, which consisted of Beckman Bio-Solv® BBS-3, Spectrofluor® PPO-POPOP, and toluene (2:1:16, v/v/v) were added. Radioactivity was determined with 40% efficiency. To measure nuclear binding, experimental points were determined from duplicate or triplicate incubations, and additional replicate incubations were performed to assess the recovery of DNA. DNA was determined by the method of Burton.[10]

Other Methods

Unless otherwise indicated, radioactivity was determined by combining aqueous samples with 5 ml of a cocktail that consisted of toluene (Baker), Triton X-100 (RPI), and Spectrofluor (Amersham-Searle), 100:521:42 (v/v/v). The counting efficiency for tritium was 33% in a Beckman LS-250 Liquid Scintillation counter. Protein concentration was determined by the method of Lowry *et al.*[11] with bovine serum albumin used as the standard.

RESULTS

Binding of Receptor to ATP-Sepharose

In our earlier report, the binding of progesterone receptor to ATP-Sepharose was demonstrated with receptor preparations that were fractionated by ammonium sulfate precipitation.[6] These receptor preparations could be readily bound to the affinity resin and then eluted either with buffer that contained ATP, as illustrated in FIGURE 1, or with a high-salt buffer (e.g., 1 M KCl). Therefore, the interaction of receptor with ATP-Sepharose is reversible and dependent on ionic conditions. Additional experiments (not shown) revealed that a relatively high salt concentration (>0.5 M KCl) is needed to release receptor from the affinity column. Therefore, in most of our studies, total elution was accomplished with 1 M KCl.

When salt-fractionated receptor was used, 80–100% of the receptor could be bound to, and subsequently recovered from, the affinity column. In contrast to the above preparation, freshly prepared cytosol had little or no affinity for ATP-Sepharose. This observation suggested that the receptor may first require an activation step similar to the activation process that is needed to bind the progesterone-receptor complex to isolated nuclei.[12] To test this hypothesis, aliquots of cytosol labeled with [^{3}H]progesterone were incubated at room temperature for varying periods of time as a means of receptor activation. The samples were then chilled and applied to columns of ATP-Sepharose. The binding of receptor to ATP-Sepharose was greatly enhanced by preincubation of receptor at room temperature, as illustrated in FIGURE 2. With this procedure (temperature activation), the extent of receptor binding to ATP-Sepharose was found to be as high as 60% of the total cytosol receptor (determined by charcoal adsorption).[8] Studies on the time course of incubation showed a close relationship between the capacities of receptor to bind both ATP-Sepharose and isolated nuclei (data not shown). Therefore, the same activation processes may be required for both binding activities.

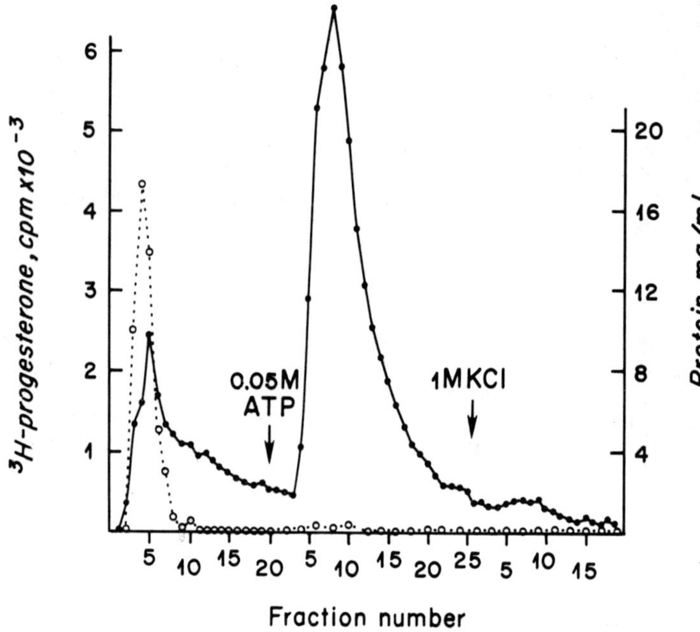

FIGURE 1. Elution of [³H]progesterone-receptor complex from an ATP-Sepharose column with ATP. Cytosol receptor from hen oviduct was precipitated with ammonium sulfate and redissolved in 1/10 the cytosol volume of buffer [10 mM Tris-HCl, 1 mM EDTA, 12 mM thioglycerol, and 20% glycerol (pH 8)] that contained 10 nM [³H]progesterone. After 2 hr at 4°C, the sample (9 ml) was applied to a 10-ml column of ATP-Sepharose with a flow rate of 0.2 ml/min. The column was washed with the same buffer that contained 0.1 M KCl, and 20 4.2-ml fractions were collected. The adsorbed receptor was eluted with buffer that contained 0.01 M KCl and 0.05 M ATP, and 25 1.8-ml fractions were collected. The column was then washed with buffer plus 1 M KCl, and 1.8-ml fractions were collected. Radioactivity (•) and protein content (○) were determined from 0.1-ml portions of each fraction.

Receptor activation can also be accomplished by a brief exposure to high-salt conditions.[13] The binding of receptor to ATP-Sepharose was also enhanced by high-salt treatment, as illustrated in FIGURE 3. Maximum binding was observed after treating the cytosol receptor with 0.5 M KCl, followed by dilution to 0.25 M KCl. Under these conditions, 80–100% of the progesterone-receptor complex acquires the ability to bind ATP-Sepharose. Because this procedure avoids temperature elevation, it can be carefully controlled and can be used to activate almost all of the receptor complex.

Effect of Nucleotides on Receptor Activation

A second approach toward understanding the relationship between nucleotides and receptor activity was to study the effects of added nucleotides on the receptor activation process. The protocol for these experiments was as follows: Oviduct cytosol labeled with 20 nM [³H]progesterone was incubated at 23°C for various periods of time to activate the hormone-receptor complex. After this incubation, the cytosol aliquots were chilled in ice, mixed with isolated oviduct nuclei, and incubated at 4°C for 60 min. The nuclei were washed and analyzed for [^{3}H]progesterone uptake to measure the extent of cytosol receptor activation. Various nucleotides were added during the 23°C incubation period to observe their effects on receptor activation. When oviduct cytosol, labeled with [^{3}H]progesterone, was incubated for various lengths of time at 23°C, maximal receptor activation occurred at approximately 2 hr (FIGURE 4). With longer incubation times, the amount of activated receptor began to decline. The decline in activated receptor during prolonged incubation can be accounted for, at least in part, by the heat lability of the receptor complex. The time course of receptor activation was markedly altered when a nucleotide was added to the cytosol. ADP at concentrations of 0.2 and 1 mM inhibited receptor activation (FIGURE 4). The finding that prolonged incubation overcame much of the inhibitory effect of 0.2 mM ADP suggests that the inhibition may primarily be a rate-altering phenomenon.

The stability of the [^{3}H]progesterone-receptor complex was not significantly

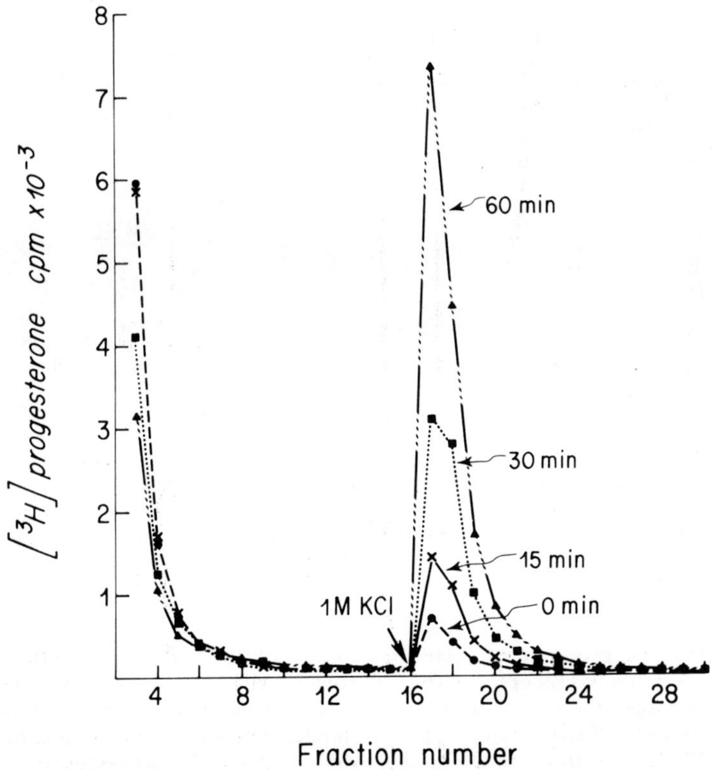

FIGURE 2. The effect of room temperature activation on the binding of progesterone receptor to ATP-Sepharose. Chick oviduct cytosol was prepared in buffer that contained 40 mM Tris-HCl, 12 mM thioglycerol, and 10% glycerol (pH 8). Aliquots (0.5 ml) of cytosol were preincubated at 4°C for 2 hr with 20 nM [^{3}H]progesterone and were then incubated at room temperature for the periods indicated. The amount of ATP binding by the 60-min sample represents 42% of the total progesterone receptor applied to the column.

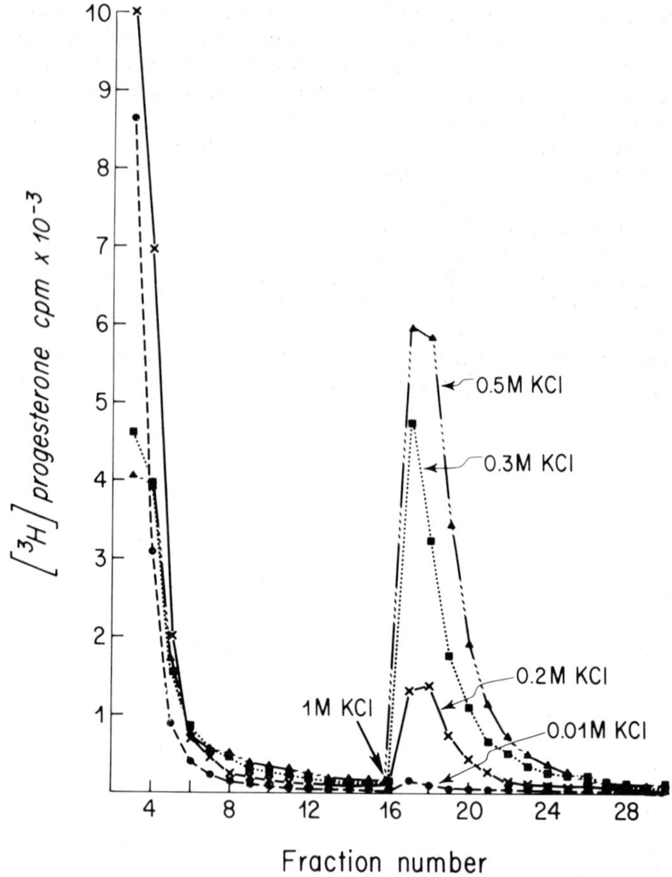

FIGURE 3. The effect of salt activation on the binding of progesterone receptor to ATP-Sepharose. Aliquots (1.5 ml) of chick cytosol were incubated at 4°C in buffer that contained 20nM [^{3}H]progesterone and the indicated concentrations of KCl. After a 1-hr incubation, each sample was diluted 1:1 with buffer before determining binding to ATP-Sepharose. The amount of ATP binding by the 0.5 M KCl sample represents about 100% of the total progesterone receptor.

affected by the presence of ADP and could not account for the difference in amounts of activated receptor in the control and ADP-containing cytosol (FIGURE 4). Furthermore, the effect of ADP could not be accounted for by interference with the binding of activated receptor to nuclei, nor did the nucleotide have any effect on "deactivating" receptor that was already in the activated form.[14] Although used for illustrative purposes here, ADP is not unique in its effect. Other nucleotides were found to produce similar results, with the triphosphates exhibiting the greatest potency of the nucleotides examined.[14]

The inhibitory effects of adenine nucleotides on receptor activation could be observed with a nucleotide concentration range of 0.01–1.0 mM. However, higher concentrations of nucleotide (>1 mM) did not inhibit activation but caused a stimulation of this process. This stimulatory effect of relatively high nucleotide concentrations, again, appeared to be an effect on the rate of receptor activation, because with sufficiently long incubation, the amount of activated receptor produced in control cytosol approached that in nucleotide-treated cytosol (FIGURE 5). When adenine nucleotides were examined at concentrations of 1.5 and 3 mM, ATP and ADP were found to stimulate activation in a concentration-dependent manner, although AMP was ineffective at the concentrations shown (FIGURE 6). Under the conditions employed, 3 mM ATP caused a stimulation of about fourfold and was clearly the most potent of the nucleotides tested. Incubation of ATP with fully activated receptor had little additional effect on the nuclear binding activity of the receptor, and when receptor was preincubated at 0° rather than 23°C, the stimulatory effect of ATP was greatly diminished.[14]

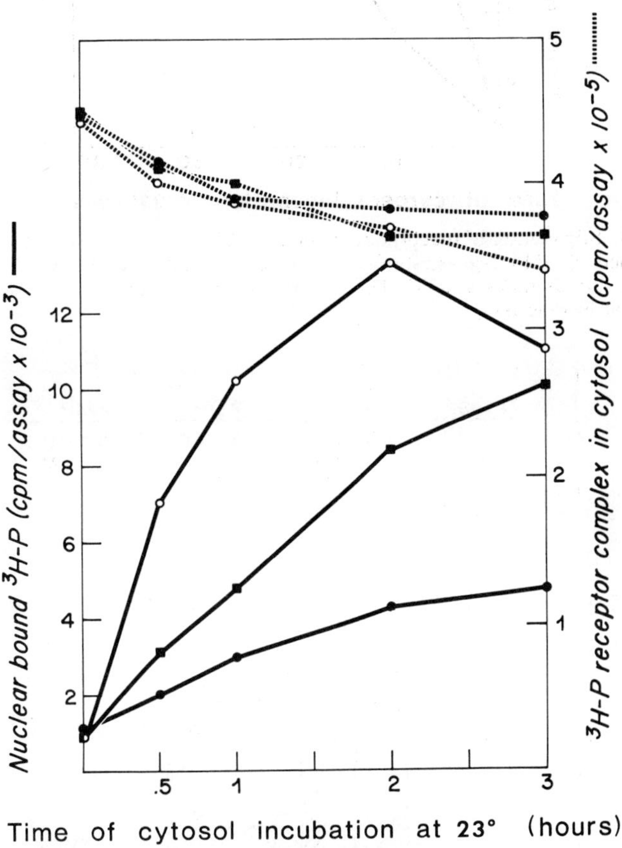

FIGURE 4. Inhibition of receptor activation by ADP. Chick oviduct cytosol was prepared in buffer that contained 40 mM Tris-HCl and 12 mM thioglycerol (pH 7.5). Cytosol aliquots that contained 20 nM [^{3}H]progesterone and ADP as indicated were incubated for various times at 23°C. The extent of receptor activation was then determined with a nuclear binding assay (see METHODS AND MATERIALS). In addition, the total [^{3}H]progesterone binding was determined in each cytosol sample by charcoal adsorption (broken lines). ○, No ADP; ●, 1 mM ADP; ■, 0.2 mM ADP.

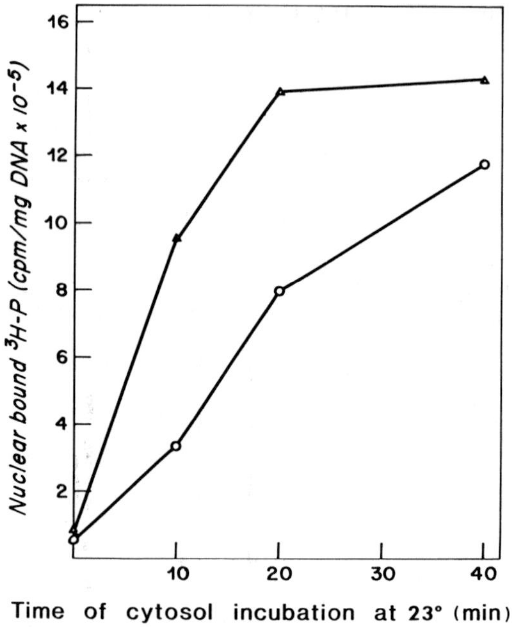

FIGURE 5. Stimulation of receptor activation by ATP. Aliquots of chick oviduct cytosol that contained 20 mM [^{3}H]progesterone and either no ATP (○) or 3 mM ATP (△) were incubated for various times at 23°C. The extent of receptor activation was then determined with a nuclear binding assay.

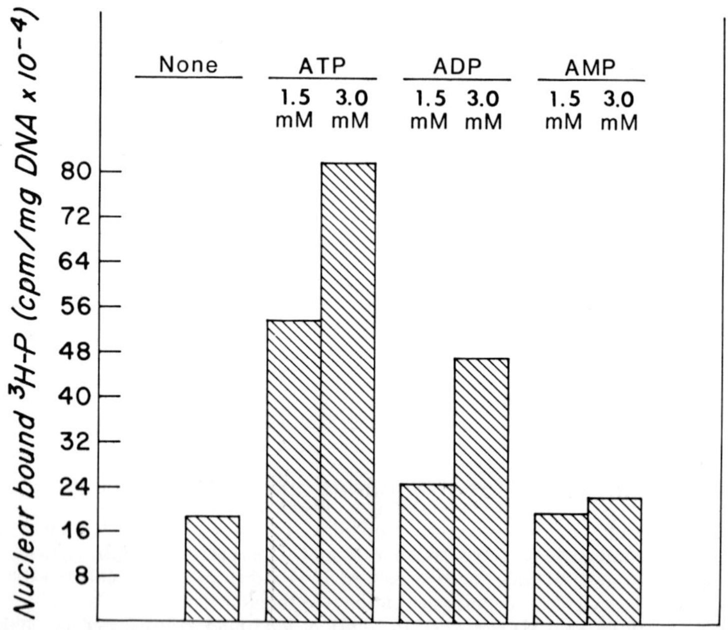

FIGURE 6. Stimulation of receptor activation by adenine nucleotides. The effects of adenine nucleotides were examined by the procedures described in FIGURES 4 and 5. The cytosol samples contained ATP, ADP, or AMP as indicated and were incubated at 23°C for 15 min to achieve receptor activation.

More recent studies from this laboratory have shown that adenine nucleotides are not unique in the effects described above. Other ribonucleotides and deoxyribonucleotides produce inhibition and stimulation at concentrations effective for ATP.[14] In all cases, nucleoside triphosphates are the most effective agents, and the purine nucleotides seemed to be somewhat more potent than the pyrimidine nucleotides.

Inhibition of the Receptor-Nucleotide Interaction

A recent report from this laboratory described the use of two inhibitors that block binding of the [^{3}H]progesterone-receptor complex to isolated nuclei.[15] One of these inhibitors, *o*-phenanthroline, is an organic metal chelator, and its effectiveness toward progesterone and estrogen receptor suggests that these receptors may be metalloproteins.[15,16] The other inhibitor, rifamycin AF/013, is an antibiotic derivative that is best known for its ability to inhibit DNA and RNA polymerases.[17,18]

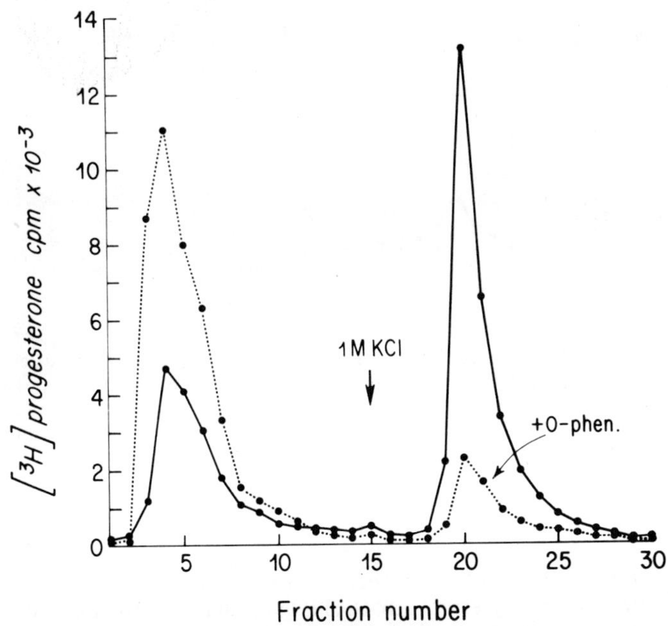

FIGURE 7. Effect of *o*-phenanthroline on the binding of progesterone receptor to ATP-Sepharose. Ammonium sulfate-precipitated receptor from hen oviduct was dissolved in buffer [10 mM Tris-HCl, 12 mM thioglycerol, and 20% glycerol (pH 8.0)], and preparations that contained 200 μl of receptor, 12 nM [^{3}H]progesterone, and 5 mM *o*-phenanthroline were incubated at room temperature for 30 min. The final concentration of glycerol in the sample was 15%, and volume was made up to 0.5 ml with the above buffer. Following this incubation, the samples were brought to 4°C for 2 hr before layering on 1-ml ATP-Sepharose columns. The columns were washed with buffer that contained 0.01 M KCl and then with 1 M KCl. Fifteen fractions (0.6 ml/fraction) were collected in each case at a flow rate of 2 ml/min. A sample without inhibitor served as the control.

Because these inhibitors block nuclear binding of the progesterone receptor, it was of interest to see if they would also interfere with binding of the receptor to ATP-Sepharose. FIGURES 7 and 8 illustrate that this is the case. Both *o*-phenanthroline and rifamycin AF/013 reduce the binding of progesterone receptor to ATP-Sepharose. In these experiments, the inhibitors were used at a concentration that would demonstrate the inhibition of ATP binding without altering the binding of steroid to receptor. At higher concentrations, these inhibitors not only block ATP binding but also reduce the binding of progesterone to receptor.

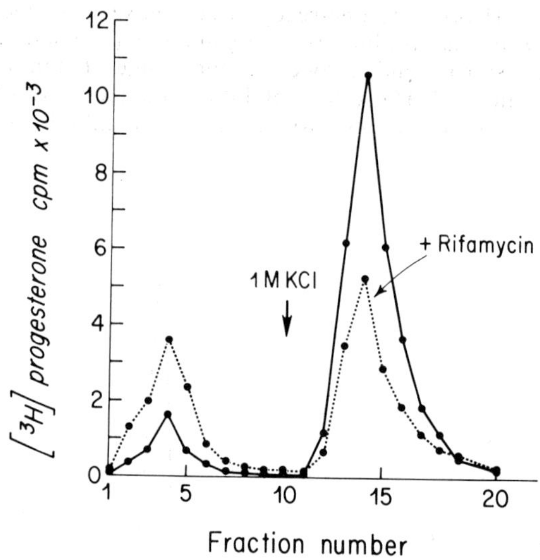

FIGURE 8. The effect of rifamycin AF/013 on the binding of progesterone-receptor complex to ATP-Sepharose. Ammonium sulfate-fractionated receptor was dissolved and labeled with [^{3}H]progesterone as described in FIGURE 7. The receptor complex was treated with rifamycin AF/013 (100 μg/ml) for 2 hr at 4°C. A sample with no inhibitor served as the control. The chromatography procedure was similar to that described in FIGURE 7.

DISCUSSION

Because the avian progesterone receptor has been shown to bind ATP, efforts were made to identify any effects that ATP might have on the functional characteristics of the receptor. The actual biochemical role of the receptor has not yet been identified; however, one can readily measure two steps that are believed to be important functions of the receptor.[1,19] These steps are activation of the receptor to a "nuclear form" and binding of the receptor to nuclear acceptor sites.

Although we could find no evidence for a direct effect of nucleotides on binding of [^{3}H]progesterone-receptor complex to isolated nuclei, nucleotides have very definite effects on the activation of the receptor complex. This process is inhibited by low concentrations of nucleotide but is stimulated when the nucleotide concentration is above 1 mM. The observation that nucleotides can both inhibit and stimulate receptor activation suggests that the relationship between the two may be quite complex, perhaps involving more than one nucleotide-binding site on the receptor. It is also possible that some of the observed effects are indirect and result from an interaction of ATP with other cytosol constituents.

While the appropriate concentration of ATP stimulates receptor activation, we also found that activated receptor has a much greater affinity for the nucleotide, when compared to nonactivated receptor, which has little or no affinity for ATP, as tested by affinity chromatography. It is possible that the binding of ATP stabilizes the receptor during the activation process in a way that enhances the extent of receptor activation. However, this hypothesis offers only a partial explanation for the results, because lower concentrations of nucleotide inhibit rather than stimulate receptor activation. Therefore, the actual mechanism by which nucleotides exert their effects remains unclear and must await further investigation.

Additional evidence for an interaction between the progesterone receptor and nucleotides is provided by studies with *o*-phenanthroline and rifamycin AF/013. These inhibitors block binding of the hormone-receptor complex to both nuclei[15] and to ATP-Sepharose. These results suggest that nucleotide-binding sites on the receptor may be closely associated with a region that participates in the nuclear binding process. However, it is also possible that two distinct sites of interaction exist that are both altered as a result of conformational changes in the receptor caused by the inhibitors. In any case, these inhibitors may prove to be useful probes for additional characterization of nucleotide-binding sites on the receptor molecule.

The present studies show that ATP and, possibly, some other nucleotides alter the rate of heat-induced receptor activation. These *in vitro* results suggest that nucleotides may be biologically important modifiers of progesterone receptor activation. On the other hand, because ATP is bound more readily by activated receptor, this interaction may be involved in a function of the receptor at sites on the nuclear chromatin. These and other possibilities will be the subject of future investigations.

Acknowledgments

The technical assistance of Nancy McMahon, Vernon Summerlin, and Bridget Stensgard is greatly appreciated.

References

1. O'Malley, B. W. & A. R. Means. 1974. Female steroid hormones and target cell nuclei. Science **183:** 610–620.
2. Schrader, W. T., R. E. Buller, R. W. Kuhn & B. W. O'Malley. 1974. Molecular mechanisms of steroid hormone action. J. Steroid Biochem. **5:** 989–996.
3. Kuhn, R. W., W. T. Schrader, R. G. Smith & B. W. O'Malley. 1975. Progesterone binding components of chick oviduct. X. Purification by affinity chromatography. J. Biol. Chem. **250:** 4220–4228.
4. Schrader, W. T., D. O. Toft & B. W. O'Malley. 1972. Progesterone binding protein of chick oviduct. VI. Interaction of purified progesterone-receptor components with nuclear constituents. J. Biol. Chem. **247:** 2401–2407.
5. Spelsberg, T. C. 1974. The role of nuclear acidic proteins in binding steroid hormones. *In* Acidic Proteins of the Nucleus. I. L. Cameron & J. R. Jeter, Eds.: 247–296. Academic Press, Inc. New York, N.Y.
6. Moudgil, V. K. & D. O. Toft. 1975. Binding of ATP to the progesterone receptor. Proc. Nat. Acad. Sci. USA **72:** 901–905.

7. King, E. G. 1932. The colorimetric determination of phosphorus. Biochem. J. **26:** 292–297.
8. Toft, D. O. & B. W. O'Malley. 1972. Target tissue receptors for progesterone: the influence of estrogen treatment. Endocrinology **90:** 1041–1045.
9. Spelsberg, T. C., J. T. Knowler & H. L. Moses. 1974. Specific methods for the isolation of nuclei from chick oviduct. Methods Enzymol. **31:** 263–279.
10. Burton, K. 1968. Determination of DNA concentration with diphenylamine. Methods Enzymol. **12**(B): 163–166.
11. Lowry, O. H., N. J. Rosebrough, A. L. Farr & R. J. Randall. 1951. Protein measurement with the folin phenol reagent. J. Biol. Chem. **193:** 265–275.
12. Buller, R. E., D. O. Toft, W. T. Schrader & B. W. O'Malley. 1975. Progesterone binding components of chick oviduct. VIII. Receptor activation and hormone-dependent binding to purified nuclei. J. Biol. Chem. **250:** 801–808.
13. Higgins, S. J., G. G. Rousseau, J. D. Baxter & G. M. Tomkins. 1973. Early events in glucocorticoid action. Activation of the steroid receptor and its subsequent specific nuclear binding studied in a cell-free system. J. Biol. Chem. **248:** 5866–5872.
14. Lohmar, P. H. & D. O. Toft. 1976. In preparation.
15. Lohmar, P. H. & D. O. Toft. 1975. Inhibition of the binding of progesterone receptor to nuclei: effects of *o*-phenanthroline and rifamycin AF/013. Biochem. Biophys. Res. Commun. **67:** 8–15.
16. Shyamala, G. 1975. Is the estrogen receptor of mammary glands a metallo-protein? Biochem. Biophys. Res. Commun. **64:** 408–415.
17. Tsai, M.-J. & G. F. Saunders. 1973. Action of rifamycin derivatives on RNA polymerase of human leukemic lymphocytes. Proc. Nat. Acad. Sci. USA **70:** 2072–2076.
18. Meilhac, J., Z. Tysper & P. Chambon. 1972. Animal DNA-dependent RNA polymerases. 4. Studies on inhibition by rifamycin derivatives. Eur. J. Biochem. **28:** 291–300.
19. Spelsberg, T. C. & D. O. Toft. 1976. The mechanism of action of progesterone. *In* Receptors and Mechanism of Action of Steroid Hormones. J. R. Pasqualini, Ed.: 261–309. Marcel Dekker Inc. New York, N.Y.

Discussion

Dr. R. W. Kuhn: Have you tried the column with an aporeceptor that hasn't been prelabeled with hormone either before or after activation procedures?

Dr. Toft: Yes, we have, after activation with preparations that have been fractionated by ammonium sulfate precipitation. In this case, the receptor is at least activated in a sense, and it will bind to the ATP-Sepharose column in the absence of hormones. The binding appears to be just as good with or without hormone. However, in the cytosol, preliminary results show that this isn't the case. The hormone is necessary to obtain the activated state and is, therefore, necessary to bind to ATP-Sepharose.

Dr. Kuhn: Have you tried other metal-chelating agents with slightly different structures, such as EDTA, to prevent the binding of receptor to ATP-Sepharose?

Dr. Toft: EDTA has no effect. In fact, EDTA is generally present in our buffered system. However, it's an ionic chelator and *o*-phenanthroline is an organic, rather nonpolar, chelator that could conceivably enter regions of the protein that are not accessible to EDTA. We have tested the analog of *o*-phenanthroline, *m*-phenanthroline, in which the structural relationship of the nitrogen groups is a bit different; *m*-phenanthroline is not a metal chelator and is not effective in these experiments.

Dr. R. J. B. King: What happens if you use something like pyrophosphate instead of the various nucleotides and nucleosides that affect receptor activation?

Dr. Toft: Pyrophosphate really isn't very effective in either inhibiting or stimulating receptor activation. Nor is just inorganic phosphate. Therefore, these effects appear to require more than just an interaction with phosphate groups.

Dr. King: As the receptor is binding to your ATP-Sepharose column, are you implying that the receptor may actually be able to carry ATP or some derivative into the nucleus with it?

Dr. Toft: It seems very conceivable that the nucleotide may have a controlling influence as to whether the receptor actually does enter the nucleus and, if so, in what state it enters the nucleus. But this is pure speculation at this point.

Dr. Kuhn: I'd like to continue asking about the specificity of the nucleotide interaction. Have you performed enough experiments to know the relative effects of the deoxynucleoside triphosphates versus the ribose; which is more effective?

Dr. Toft: In terms of the receptor activation in nuclear binding, deoxy-ATP appears to be almost equally active when compared to ATP. With ATP-Sepharose chromatography, it's a little difficult to say, and we're trying to look into this point further. In initial experiments where we were using a relatively low concentration of ATP on the column, there was a clear preference for the ribose rather than the deoxyribose. To make our columns more effective, we then changed them from about 1 mM ATP up to 10 mM, and we lost some of this specificity in the process. This may mean that there is a concentration relationship that we aren't fully appreciating, or perhaps we are observing interactions with more than one binding site.

Dr. Kuhn: How about oligonucleotides?

Dr. Toft: We've looked at a couple of synthetic oligoribonucleotides. Poly (A), for example, does not appear to interfere with the binding of receptor to ATP-Sepharose.

Dr. M. R. Sherman: Do the relative affinities of the A and B components of this receptor correlate with their relative affinities for DNA?

Dr. Toft: Although receptor component B binds to ATP-Sepharose, it does not appear to bind DNA. In addition, as far as we can tell, the A and B components don't really differ in their affinities for ATP-Sepharose. If we put a preparation that contains both A and B components on the column and elute with either a gradient of free ATP or salt, both the A and B receptors come off in a single peak.

Dr. Sherman: Have you examined the leading and trailing sides of that peak for their contents of A and B components?

Dr. Toft: We haven't examined the sides that carefully, but they cannot be separated grossly when you observe the peak that comes off the column.

Dr. W. T. Schrader: Dr. Toft, by doing ATP-Sepharose, which you called affinity chromatography, you implied that there was an ATP-binding site on the protein. Have you any direct evidence, such as showing that the material eluted from the ATP-Sepharose column will bind ATP?

Dr. Toft: We have done some experiments of that sort but not the type that I'm really satisfied with, so I have no illustrations of them. But if you take the material that comes off an ATP-Sepharose column, which is purified about 100-fold, and add [^{3}H]ATP to it, you do see bindings, as judged by Sephadex chromatography. However, you still have a large number of proteins in that preparation, and there is no way to tell whether the receptor is actually involved in the observed binding. This is something we soon hope to do with more highly purified preparations.

DR. SCHRADER: In view of your papers on this subject, we tried some of these experiments with the purified progesterone receptor. We used a doubly labeled protocol with γ-labeled [^{32}P]ATP and [^{3}H] progesterone, and we haven't been able to detect any interaction of labeled ATP with the receptor molecule. Under those circumstances, all [^{32}P]ATP can be recovered and shown to be still ATP at the end of the experiment. There is considerable question in my mind anyway that there is an ATP-binding site on the molecule. I measured the half-life of ATP in oviduct cytosol at room temperature, the conditions used for your activation studies. The half-life is less than 2 min. Have you looked at these activation experiments, monitoring the integrity of the ATP during your studies?

DR. TOFT: I agree with you regarding your last comment. The ATP would be metabolized very rapidly in our experiments. This is something we still have to look into. There is no reason to believe that it's actually ATP, rather than a metabolite of ATP, that causes the activation, except that ATP is much more effective than ADP or AMP.

In regard to the affinity chromatography, I have no doubt that the receptor does bind to ATP when it's linked to ATP-Sepharose. I think we've done enough controls for the column experiment to show this point. I think perhaps you're asking whether this is a meaningful binding: does it have high affinity, what is its true specificity, what are the reaction kinetics, and so forth? We can't test these parameters on the column very readily, so we hope we can get radioactive ATP and purified receptor together in a test tube in the near future to actually answer these questions.

DR. E. MILGROM: We have looked at the binding and activation of the glucocorticoid receptor, and there is a problem with the specificity of the acceptors, because actually you can show that the affinity of the activated receptor is raised to anything that has a negative charge. We have found that you can bind activated receptor, for instance, to carboxymethyl Sephadex or to anything like it (1973. Milgrom *et al.*, Biochemistry **12:** 5198). So in this system, we had a really difficult problem with the specificity of the acceptor. I want to make a comment on the fact that the activation rate is increased under the effect of ATP. If ATP is an acceptor in your case (I mean that once activated, the receptor binds ATP), it may be shown that this or any acceptor will speed up the rate of activation, because it will displace the equilibrium in favor of the activated form. So perhaps in your experiments, ATP plays this role. As soon as you get activated receptor, it binds to ATP, which is the acceptor in this case, and then the speed of activation is increased.

DR. TOFT: I agree that is a very possible mechanism for the stimulation. In regard to the inhibitory properties of low nucleotide concentrations, this would most likely have to be a different mechanism, but I don't know what that would be at the moment.

NUCLEAR BINDING SITES ("ACCEPTORS") FOR PROGESTERONE IN AVIAN OVIDUCT: CHARACTERIZATION OF THE HIGHEST-AFFINITY SITES*

Thomas C. Spelsberg, Robert Webster, George Pikler, Cary Thrall, and David Wells

Department of Molecular Medicine
Mayo Clinic
Rochester, Minnesota 55901

Introduction

Steroid hormones accumulate in their respective target cells due to the presence of "receptor" proteins that bind the steroid with high affinity and high specificity.[1–4] It now appears that the steroid-receptor complexes then undergo an "activation" process that is required for their transport and binding in the nucleus.[2–5] Once the nuclear binding has occurred, there is an immediate (10–15 min) alteration in RNA polymerase activity[2,6–8] and RNA processing,[9] which is followed (at 2 hr) by an alteration in the chromatin template activity and in chromatin composition.[2,6–8] The appearance of messenger RNAs and of their encoded secretory protein is also detected within 2 hr after steroid treatment.[8–14] At present, the mechanism by which steroids alter gene expression is obscure. Obviously, the events that occur between administration of the steroid and appearance of specific mRNA (2 hr posttreatment) are the ones involved in gene regulation. The exact nature of receptor activation, transport, and nuclear binding is unclear. We have been studying the earliest known event that occurs in the avian oviduct nucleus before the progesterone-receptor (P-R) complex alters gene activity, that is, the binding of the P-R complex to isolated nuclei *in vitro*. The nuclear (or chromatin) component that binds the P-R complex is being explored, because it is possible that the macromolecules that comprise this binding site may be involved in steroid-induced modifications of gene expression.

Many published studies have characterized nuclear binding for a variety of steroids.[2,3,5,15–43] These studies utilized *in vitro* assays that demonstrated many similarities to *in vivo* binding, for example, a requirement for the steroid to be complexed to its receptor and activation of the steroid-receptor complex. Practically every component in the nucleus has been suggested (with supporting evidence) as the nuclear "acceptor" that binds steroid-receptor complexes *in vitro*. Examples are the nuclear envelope,[27,28] the ribonucleoproteins,[29] basic (histone) proteins,[17,30,31] acidic (nonhistone) proteins,[2,18,23–26,32–34] and DNA.[35,39] There have also been reports of a specific binding of free steroids (not complexed with receptor) to nuclear material.[27,33,40] In short, the chemical identity of the nuclear acceptors that bind steroids *in vitro* has not yet been demonstrated. One problem is that the conditions of these *in vitro* assays have varied markedly, resulting in a saturable tissue-specific binding in some systems[18–22] but not in others.[15–17] The majority of DNA binding studies demonstrate a nonspecific, nonsaturable binding measured *in vitro*, which

*Supported by National Institutes of Health Grants HD-08441 (now HD-9140-B) and CA 14920 and by the Mayo Foundation.

probably represents nonspecific, nonsaturable binding by steroid-receptor complexes.[19,35,36,38,39] It is likely that any nonsaturable binding measured *in vitro* probably represents nonspecific adsorption, as opposed to specific binding. Before investigating the identity of the nuclear binding sites (or "acceptor"), we attempted to clarify these discrepancies between specific versus nonspecific binding *in vitro* of steroids to nuclear material.

We have found that the low ionic conditions (0.01–0.05 M KCl) in the binding assays performed by the majority of laboratories result in a pattern of nuclear binding that is neither saturable nor tissue specific. These results are obtained whether one uses the nuclear material from the oviducts of immature chicks[2,18,23] or adult hens[24–26] and either a crude or purified P-R complex. Under these low ionic conditions, the P-R complex binds to glass beads, cellulose, the surface of containers, and to all nuclear material in a nonsaturable fashion. However, when the ionic strength of the binding assays is increased to 0.15 or 0.2 M KCl, we observe a saturable tissue-specific binding that selectively measures only the highest-affinity class of binding sites.[24–26] Some of our results with respect to selection of proper conditions for assaying high-affinity specific nuclear binding will be presented in this report. We will then describe our results of purification and characterization in oviduct nuclei of high-affinity binding sites, which we term "acceptors."

Materials and Methods

The majority of materials and methods used in this report have been described previously.[24–26,41] For clarity, the more important methods will be outlined below.

Tissue Sources and Subcellular Fractions

Tissues from adult laying hens were supplied by a local produce company (Jones Produce, Rochester, Minn.). Shortly after the hens were killed, organs were removed, cleaned, sectioned, and frozen (on solid CO_2). The tissues were stored at −80°C until used. Mature erythrocytes were isolated as described by Neelin.[55] The isolation of nuclei and chromatin and the preparation of partially deproteinized chromatins were the same as previously described.[18,23,25] The final suspensions of native and treated chromatins were in 2.0 mM Tris HCl, 0.1 mM EDTA, pH 7.5 (TE buffer), at 0.2–0.8 mg of DNA per milliliter. Oviducts for preparation of the P-R complex were obtained from White Leghorn chicks that had been injected subcutaneously with 5 mg of stilbestrol for 20–25 days.

Preparation of [^3H] Progesterone-Receptor Complex

1,2-[^{3}H]Progesterone (47.8 Ci/mmol) was obtained from New England Nuclear Corporation (Boston, Mass.) and was checked for purity by thin-layer chromatography in benzene-ethyl acetate (70:30, v/v). The cytosol P-R complex from chick oviduct was labeled with [^{3}H]progesterone and partially purified by $(NH_4)_2SO_4$ precipitation, as described previously.[42] The labeled receptor preparation was stored as pellets at −80°C and dissolved in 0.01 M Tris HCl, 0.001 M EDTA, 0.012 M thioglycerol, pH 7.4 (TESH buffer) for use in the binding assays, as described elsewhere.[25]

Assays for Nuclear or Chromatin Binding of [^{3}H]Progesterone-Receptor Complex

The standard nuclear binding has been described elsewhere.[24,25] The levels of receptor and time of incubation were established to allow equilibrium with minimal breakdown of the steroid-receptor complex. In addition to the standard assay method, two new methods were used to assay for steroid-receptor binding to soluble nucleoprotein [e.g., deproteinized (soluble) chromatin and DNA]. Both techniques allow many samples of soluble deoxyribonucleoprotein or DNA to be assayed together with insoluble chromatin for steroid-receptor binding capacity in a relatively short time. The samples can be washed rapidly by use of low-speed centrifugation, as opposed to the time-consuming high-speed centrifugations used previously.[23] One method employs the antibiotic streptomycin sulfate to precipitate the DNA, together with any DNA-bound protein, including the progesterone receptor. This method has been described elsewhere.[24,26]

The other method, the cellulose method, for assaying steroid-receptor binding utilizes an insoluble matrix to which the soluble deoxyribonucleoprotein is coupled.[24,26] Chromatin was linked to cellulose in ethanol with high-intensity ultraviolet light.[24,26,43] The chromatin-cellulose preparations (2–10 mg of chromatin DNA/g of cellulose) were stored dry at room temperature (22°C) and before use were allowed to hydrate for 2 hr in the dilute Tris buffer (TE). The reactions were initiated by addition of the chromatin-cellulose (25 μg of DNA/tube) to each assay mixture. In all experiments, pure cellulose was added to separate reactions, and the resultant radioactivity used as the background (subtracted from the radioactivities of reactions that contained chromatin-cellulose). Both the streptomycin and cellulose methods yield similar results.

The chromatin material was then collected on membrane filters (0.45 μm pore size, 24 mm diameter; Millipore Corporation, Bedford, Mass.) under vacuum and washed further with dilute Tris buffer (TE) that contained streptomycin. The filters were dried and counted for radioactivity in 5.0 ml of a toluene-based scintillation solution that contained 6.0 g of 2,5-diphenyloxazole (PPO) and 0.075 g of [1,4-bis(5-phenyloxazol-2-yl) benzene] (POPOP) per liter. In all assays, complementary reaction mixtures that contained the labeled receptor, but no chromatin, were treated in the same manner to monitor background radioactivity. After radioactivity counting (30% efficiency), the filters were dried, and the DNA was hydrolyzed by incubation at 90°C for 30 min in 0.3 M $HClO_4$. The DNA in the hydrolysate was assessed by the diphenylamine reaction.[44] The radioactivity per filter was correlated with the amount of DNA on the same filter to calculate the counts per minute per milligram of DNA. In some cases, the Lowry protein assay[45] was performed on the DNA-protein complexes, and the counts per minute per milligram of protein were determined. Using the specific activity of [^{3}H]progesterone and of 2.5 pg of DNA per chick organ cell,[46] the number of molecules of [^{3}H]progesterone bound per cell nucleus was calculated.

Results

Detection of Multiple Classes of Nuclear Binding Sites in Vivo: *Identification of the Biologically Important Sites*

We have recently demonstrated the presence of more than one class of binding site in chick oviduct nuclei *in vivo* and in hen oviduct nuclei and chromatin *in vitro*.[24–26,41] By selecting a 2-hr incubation period after injection of 100 μCi (0.718

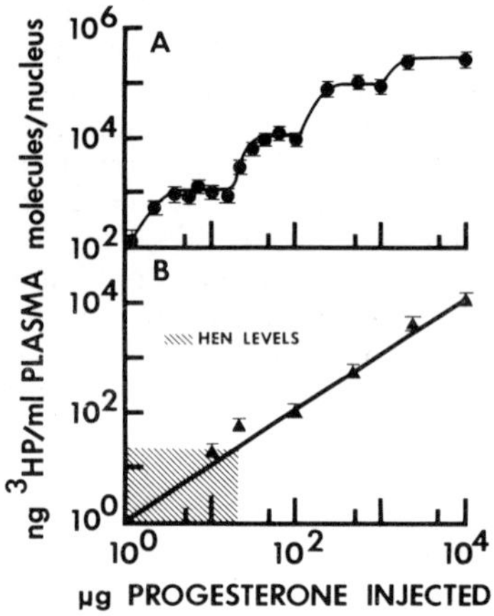

FIGURE 1. Nuclear binding versus the plasma levels of [^{3}H]progesterone *in vivo*. A: The molecules of progesterone bound to oviduct nuclei; B: serum levels of progesterone in response to the dose of the hormone given to chicks. Groups of four chicks were given subcutaneous injections of 100 μCi (or 0.718 μg) of [^{3}H]progesterone alone or in combination with specified concentrations of unlabeled hormone. Stock [^{3}H]progesterone in benzene was mixed with a specified amount of unlabeled progesterone in benzene. The solutions were frozen, freeze-dried, and resuspended in sesame oil for injection. Each chick received a 100-μl injection for doses under 100 μg and a 200-μl injection for doses over 100 μg. Two hours after injection (A), the oviducts of each group were excised and combined, and the nuclei were isolated as described elsewhere.[18,23] Their radioactivity was measured as described under MATERIALS AND METHODS. The results are plotted as molecules of [^{3}H]progesterone bound per cell nucleus, calculated as described under MATERIALS AND METHODS. The average and range of three replicates of analysis of values obtained for each group are presented. Two hours after injection of [^{3}H]progesterone (B), blood was drawn from the wing vein into heparinized capillary tubes, the tubes were centrifuged for 2 min at 200*g*, and 10–50-μl portions of the plasma were removed for measurement of radioactivity and protein analysis.[45] The amount (ng) of progesterone per milliliter of plasma was calculated from the radioactivity (dpm/ml of plasma). The average and range of two replicate analyses for each group are presented. (From Spelsberg.[41] By permission of *The Biochemical Journal*.)

μg) of labeled progesterone either alone or together with increasing concentrations of unlabeled progesterone, the number of molecules of hormone bound to oviduct nuclei was assessed. As shown in FIGURE 1 (A), use of multiple levels of unlabeled progesterone together with a fixed amount of [^{3}H]progesterone allows detection of more than one type or class of binding site in the oviduct nucleus. The saturation of the first class of binding site appears to occur when 10–15 μg of the hormone are injected and involves approximately 10^3 molecules of progesterone per cell nucleus. The saturation of the second class of binding site occurs when between 15 and 100 μg of the hormone are injected and involves about 10^4 molecules of progesterone per cell nucleus. Further increases in the dose of progesterone reveal two more classes of "weaker" binding site, which represent approximately 10^5 and 3×10^5 molecules per cell nucleus.

The physiologic concentrations of progesterone in the plasma of laying hens range between 0.88 and 17.21 ng/ml.[47,48] FIGURE 1 (B) shows the concentrations (ng/ml) of progesterone in the plasma of immature chicks 2 hr after injecting the hormone. The injection of 20 μg of progesterone into immature chicks results in concentrations of the hormone in the plasma that approximate the maximal level measured in the plasma of laying hens. This dose induces nuclear binding of progesterone that involves the two highest-affinity site classes, which represent 1000–10,000 molecules of progesterone per cell nucleus.

Comparisons between amount of nuclear binding and RNA polymerase activity by use of numerous increasing doses of progesterone were also performed. As shown in FIGURE 2, an initial enhancement of RNA polymerase-I activity over that of controls is observed, beginning at a 10-μg dose of progesterone. At doses greater than 100 μg, a decrease in RNA polymerase-I activity compared with that of controls is observed. Progesterone doses greater than 200 μg have no effect on RNA polymerase-I activity. RNA polymerase-II activity decreases, beginning at a 6-μg dose of progesterone. This decrease continues up to the 100-μg dose. Progesterone doses greater than 100 μg fail to alter further RNA polymerase-II activity. By comparing the amounts of nucleus-bound progesterone with RNA polymerase activities, it is seen that only the binding of progesterone to the two highest-affinity site classes results in some response in these enzymatic activities. Binding to the weaker classes of nuclear binding site results in no further alteration in RNA polymerase activities.

These results support the concept that the two highest-affinity classes of nuclear binding site, which bind about 10,000 molecules of progesterone per cell nucleus, represent the sites required for direct transcriptional response. The "weaker" binding sites could be involved in steroid-induced alterations in transcription but also may be artifacts obtained after tissue homogenization.

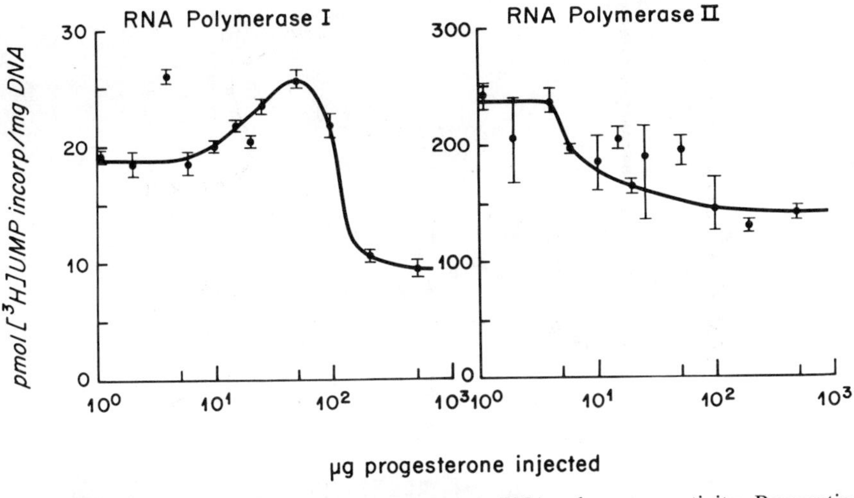

FIGURE 2. Effects of the dose of progesterone on RNA polymerase activity. Preparation of the progesterone for injections into chicks is described in the legend to FIGURE 1. Doses of 200 and 1000 μg were administered in 200 μl of sesame oil, and the lower doses were administered in 100 μl of this vehicle. These experiments were performed as described in the legend to FIGURE 1. For these polymerase experiments, groups of six to 10 chicks were each injected (subcutaneously) with a specified amount of the hormone. Two groups were injected with vehicle only and used for determining the noninjected controls. At 2 hr after injection, the oviducts from each group were excised and combined, and the nuclei were isolated as described elsewhere.[6] The activities are expressed as picomoles of [^{3}H]uridine monophosphate incorporated per milligram of DNA. The average and range of three replicates of analysis are presented for all values. (From Spelsberg.[41] By permission of *The Biochemical Journal.*)

Detection of Multiple Classes of Nuclear Binding Sites in Vitro: *Specific Binding to the Highest-Affinity Class*

A search for *in vitro* classes of binding site in oviduct nuclei similar to those found *in vivo* was then initiated. In the following experiments, isolated [^{3}H]P-R complex was incubated with various nuclear components at 4°C for 90 min, as described under MATERIALS AND METHODS and elsewhere.[24–26] The nuclear material, bound with P-R, was then separated from the free P-R, and the amount of nucleus-bound P-R was measured. The application of many different levels of P-R in the binding assays was then employed in hopes to detect the presence of more than one class of nuclear binding site. As shown in FIGURE 3, the presence of several classes of binding site with differences in binding affinities is revealed. Evidence of additional binding site classes has been obtained by use of even greater amounts of the hormone-receptor complex. The presence of these different classes of binding site may be responsible for the nonsaturability of the nuclear binding sites under the low-ionic-strength conditions.[24–26] Because increasing ionic concentrations cause a decrease in total binding of the [^{3}H]P-R complex to nuclei, it is possible that different classes of binding site are involved. The data shown in FIGURE 3 support this hypothesis, in that an increase in the

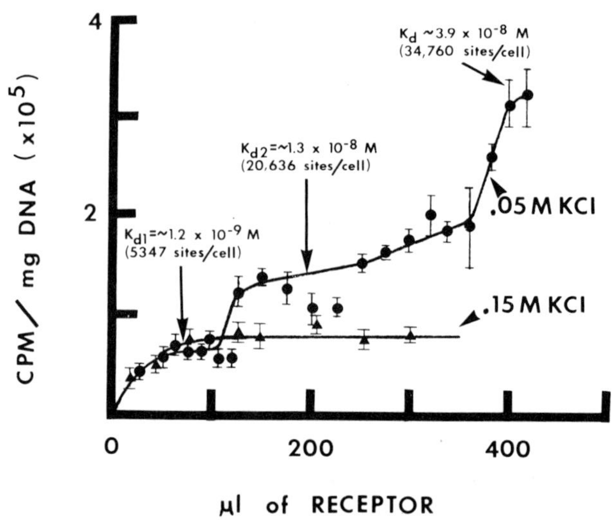

FIGURE 3. Detection of multiple classes of nuclear binding sites *in vitro* in hen oviduct: effects of ionic strength. These experiments were performed as described under MATERIALS AND METHODS and elsewhere.[24,25] The assay mixtures contained either (•) 0.05 M KCl or (▲) 0.15 M KCl (final concentration). The assays were performed with 25 μg of DNA per assay and by use of the standard assay method. The equilibrium dissociation constants and the number of binding sites per cell for the first two plateaus were calculated from Scatchard plot analysis.[25,49] The values for the third plateau were obtained from the estimated saturation (sites per cell) and half-saturation (K_d) concentrations in a plot of bound versus free [^{3}H]P-R complex. The DNA content per hen organ cell was taken as 2.5 pg per cell.[46] The range and average of three replicates of analysis for each receptor concentration are shown. (From Pikler *et al.*[25] By permission of *The Biochemical Journal.*)

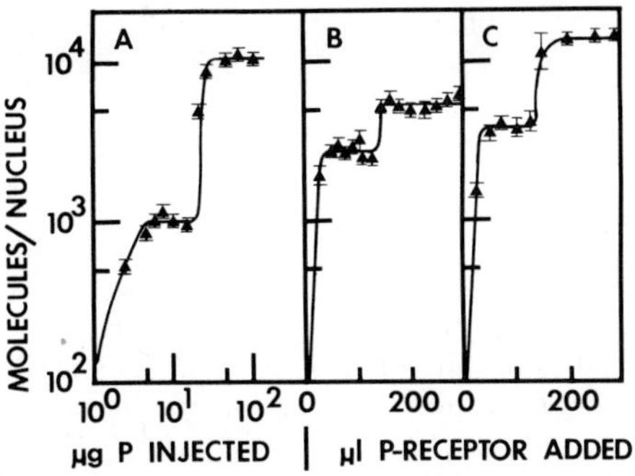

FIGURE 4. Comparison of the binding of [^{3}H]progesterone to the high-affinity sites in oviduct nuclei *in vivo* and *in vitro*. The data in A and B are taken from FIGURES 1 and 3, respectively, and represent binding to nuclei *in vivo* (A) and *in vitro* (B). Panel C represents binding to isolated chromatin, as described in the legend to FIGURE 3 for nuclei. The number of molecules per cell nucleus were calculated as described under MATERIALS AND METHODS. In A, B, and C, the range and average of three replicates of analysis for each receptor concentration are shown.

ionic strength from 0.05 to 0.15 M KCl causes the elimination of the weaker classes of binding site, leaving only a highest-affinity class. The equilibrium dissociation constants (K_d) for each class of site are also given in FIGURE 3. These constants were calculated by use of Scatchard plot analysis.[49] An equilibrium dissociation constant of 1.2×10^{-9} M, which represents approximately 5000 sites per cell nucleus, was calculated for the first (highest-affinity) class of binding site.[24,25] The second (next-highest-affinity) class of binding site has a 10-fold less affinity, with a K_d of 1.3×10^{-8} M, which represents approximately 20,000 sites per cell nucleus. Scatchard plot analysis of the third class of binding site was too variable, so estimates of the K_d ($\sim 4.0 \times 10^{-8}$ M) and the number of sites per cell (~35,000) were roughly calculated from a plot of bound versus free receptor, by use of estimated half-saturation and saturation values, respectively. In any case, more than one class of binding site is detectable both *in vitro* and *in vivo*. The interaction between P-R and oviduct nuclei in each class of site is primarily electrostatic in nature, with each class selectively dissociated at specific ionic strengths.[24] Under physiologically ionic conditions (and higher), only the highest-affinity class of binding site exists.

For better comparisons between nuclear binding *in vivo* and that which occurs *in vitro*, the data in FIGURES 1 and 3 were replotted as molecules of P bound per cell nucleus (see FIGURE 4). The levels of progesterone bound to the higher-affinity classes do not differ greatly between the *in vivo* and *in vitro* conditions (FIGURE 4, A & B). In addition, the higher-affinity classes of binding site appear to be localized with chromatin isolated from oviduct nuclei (FIGURE 4, C). In summary, studies *in vivo* and *in vitro* demonstrate more than one class of binding site, of which the highest-affinity classes bind 10,000 molecules or less of progesterone per cell nucleus. These highest-affinity sites are suspected of being the biologically important sites, because they are the only ones that bind P-R *in vitro* under physiologically ionic conditions (0.15–0.20 M KCl); they are the only ones bound *in vivo* when the steroid is at physiologic levels in the serum; and when the majority of these sites are bound *in vivo* with the P-R, the full responses of RNA polymerases I and II activities are observed.

Tissue Specificity of the High-Affinity Classes of Nuclear Binding Sites

Studies undertaken to assess the tissue specificity of the various classes of binding site revealed a marked tissue specificity with respect to the high-affinity sites. However, the lower-affinity binding sites were common to the chromatin of all tissues.[24,26,50] As shown in FIGURE 5 (A), under low-ionic-strength conditions, the higher-affinity classes of binding site are not detected in spleen chromatin, as they are in oviduct chromatin. By use of the higher ionic conditions (which selectively measure the higher-affinity classes of binding site), the differences in binding between chromatins from nontarget and target tissues are evident (FIGURE 5, B). When the ionic conditions in the binding assays reach physiologic levels (~0.18 M KCl, as shown in FIGURE 5, C), the binding of P-R is absolutely tissue specific, with binding occurring only with target tissue (oviduct) chromatin. Interestingly, while the level of binding of P-R to DNA is greater than that to oviduct chromatin under low ionic conditions (FIGURE 5, A), the situation is reversed under intermediate ionic conditions, with binding to DNA almost eliminated (FIGURE 5, B). In short, the high-affinity binding sites appear to be tissue specific. They are not found in erythrocyte, liver, spleen, or lung chromatin[26] (see FIGURE 6). DNA alone does not appear to contain the high-affinity sites. Also, the ionic conditions under which nuclear binding assays are performed appear to be very important in terms of degree of binding, class of site bound, and tissue specificity of binding.

Masking of High-Affinity Binding Sites (acceptors) in the Chromatins of Hen Tissues: Role of Acidic Proteins

From this point on, all binding assays will involve the high ionic conditions to selectively analyze the highest-affinity binding sites. This class(es) of sites was termed the "acceptor" class several years ago,[2,23,24] and this term will be used in the remaining sections of this paper.

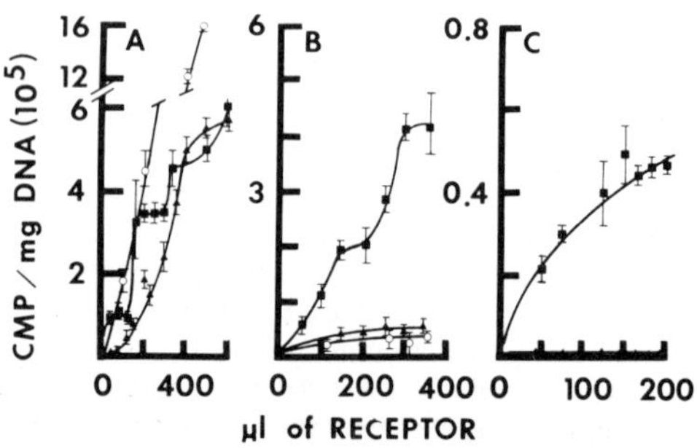

FIGURE 5. Binding of the [^{3}H]P-R complex under varying ionic conditions. Varying amounts of isolated P-R were incubated with hen oviduct chromatin (■), hen spleen chromatin (▲), and hen organ DNA (○) under 0.05 M KCl (A), 0.10 M KCl (B), or 0.18 M KCl (C) conditions. The chromatin-binding assays in A and C were performed by the standard method, while chromatin-binding assays in B and DNA-binding assays were performed by the streptomycin method.[24–26] The average and range of three replicates of analysis for each receptor concentration are given. (From Pikler *et al.*[25] and Webster *et al.*[26] By permission of *The Biochemical Journal.*)

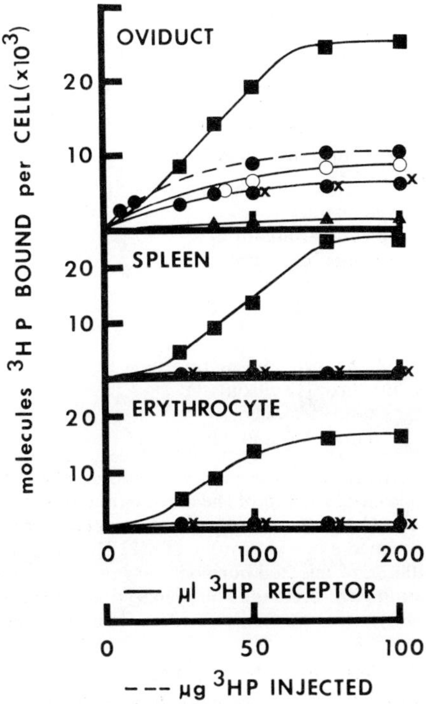

FIGURE 6. Binding of [^{3}H]progesterone to high-affinity sites in the nuclear material of oviduct, spleen, and erythrocytes of the chicken. The dashed line represents binding to nuclei of the chick oviduct performed *in vivo*, as described elsewhere.[41] The solid line represents binding under *in vitro* conditions by use of isolated nuclear components and [^{3}H]P-R complex, as described under MATERIALS AND METHODS. *In vitro* binding to the soluble DNA or DNA-protein complexes was performed by the streptomycin method or the cellulose method, as described elsewhere.[24,26] High-affinity binding *in vitro* was assayed under 0.15 M KCl conditions with 0–200 μl of labeled receptor and 50 μg of DNA (as chromatin or protein-DNA complexes). The removal of total histones and of AP_1, AP_2, or total protein has been described elsewhere.[2,18,23,26] The efficiency of removing these fractions from chromatin DNA and the integrity of the nuclear components were assayed by polyacrylamide gel electrophoresis and quantitation of the protein to DNA ratio by the Lowry[45] and diphenylamine methods.[44] The symbols represent binding to the following: isolated nuclei, ●; whole chromatin, ×; histone-deficient chromatin, ○; chromatin deficient of histone, AP_1, and AP_2, ■; and chromatin deficient of total protein (pure DNA), ▲. The number of molecules of [^{3}H]progesterone bound per cell was calculated as described under MATERIALS AND METHODS. [From Spelsberg *et al.*[50] By permission of *Nature (London)*.]

In FIGURE 6, the high-affinity binding or "acceptor" activity (i.e., binding assayed in 0.15–0.2 M KCl) of P-R to hen oviduct nuclei and chromatin *in vitro* is shown. The "acceptor" activity of chick oviduct nuclei measured *in vivo* closely approximates that measured *in vitro*. When histones are removed, the level of acceptor sites is only slightly elevated over that of whole chromatin. However, when the acidic protein (AP) fractions AP_1 and AP_2 are also removed, the number of acceptor sites in the oviduct nuclear material is enhanced four- to fivefold. A similar increase in number of acceptor sites for DNA-AP_3 complexes has previously been reported for chick oviduct chromosomal material.[18] Interestingly, the histones and AP_1 and AP_2 protein fractions can be reconstituted back to the DNA-AP_3 fraction, with reinstatement of "masking" (70–80% of the total acceptor sites) in the reconstituted chromatin, as found in the native chromatin.[2,18,50]

Also shown in FIGURE 6 is the fact that the nuclei and chromatins of nontarget tissues (hen spleen and erythrocyte) contain no acceptor sites. However, removal of histones and acidic protein fractions AP_1 and AP_2 results in a binding level that

TABLE 1

EXTENT OF MASKING OF HIGH-AFFINITY SITES*

Source	Level of Binding at Saturation (molecules/cell)	Percent of Total Sites Masked
Oviduct nuclei *in vivo*	10,600	58
Oviduct nuclei	5951	76
Oviduct chromatin	7441	71
Oviduct chromatin minus histone	9278	63
Oviduct chromatin minus histone minus AP_1 and AP_2	25,290	0
DNA	2055	—
Spleen nuclei	60	100
Spleen chromatin	48	100
Spleen chromatin minus histone minus AP_1 and AP_2	24,106	0
Erythrocyte nuclei	357	100
Erythrocyte chromatin	416	100
Erythrocyte chromatin minus histone minus AP_1 and AP_2	15,018	0

*These data were taken from the values shown in FIGURE 6. The number of binding sites measured in each of the chromatin minus histone AP_1 and AP_2 preparations was assumed to represent the total sites in the respective chromatin, and thus each of these preparations was assigned a masking value of 0%. The values of saturation for each preparation were taken at 100 μg of injected hormone for *in vivo* binding and at 200 μl of labeled receptor preparation for *in vitro* binding. The preparations of the nuclear components and of the hormone binding assays were performed as described in the legend to FIGURE 6.

approximates that of the target tissue (hen oviduct). Thus, even though the nontarget tissues appear to possess no (or a few) nuclear acceptor sites, these sites are in reality present but completely masked. TABLE 1 shows the extent of masking of these sites in the chromatins of these tissues. Assuming that all of the acceptor sites are unmasked in the chromatins devoid of histones and AP_1 and AP_2 proteins, the *in vivo* assays of oviduct nuclei show 58% masking. The *in vitro* assays of hen oviduct nuclei/chromatin exhibit about 60–80% masking, whereas those of hen spleen and erythrocyte nuclei/chromatin essentially show 100% masking.

Biologic Implications of Regulation of Nuclear Binding

The biologic need for an apparent whole animal distribution of the high-affinity binding sites and the reason for the masking of these sites remain obscure. It is possible that the extent of masking in the target tissue varies under normal biologic influences. As shown in FIGURE 7, the high-affinity binding to the chromatin of the developing oviduct of immature chicks does vary with the stage of development.[51] At 20 days of estrogen treatment, the oviduct of immature chicks is fully developed.[52] The number of acceptor sites in this fully developed oviduct of the chick closely approximates that measured in the hen oviduct. Again, chick and hen spleen display very little (or no) acceptor activity. Whether this variable level of high-affinity binding occurs during a changing endocrine state remains to be determined.

High-Affinity Binding ("acceptor" activity) in Oviduct Chromatin Associated with Acidic Proteins

As shown in FIGURE 6, removal of the remaining acidic proteins (the AP_3 fraction) results in a loss of practically all acceptor sites. Similar results are displayed in FIGURE 5 (B). These results support those reported previously for chick oviduct chromatin, wherein the "acceptor" activity (i.e., high-affinity binding) is associated with the acidic chromatin protein fraction, termed "AP_3."[23] These results strongly support a role of acidic chromatin proteins both in constituting part of the "acceptor" sites and in the masking of these sites in the oviduct (target tissue) nucleus. If the dissociated AP_3 proteins are reconstituted back to whole DNA, the high-affinity sites can be reinstated. Reconstituted whole hen oviduct chromatin displays the same relative levels of high-affinity binding as does untreated hen oviduct chromatin; that is, both the high-affinity sites and the masking are restored. This ability to restore the binding levels of reconstituted chromatins to that found in untreated chromatins was previously demonstrated for the chick oviduct system.[2,18,23] Thus, evidence is presented that suggests that one fraction of the acidic chromatin proteins (called AP_3) is involved in the high-affinity binding of P-R to hen oviduct chromatins, while another fraction (AP_1 or AP_2) is involved in masking of these binding sites. It also appears that the "acceptor" sites (high-affinity binding) also exist in the chromatins of nontarget tissues of the hen but are completely masked.

Purification and Characterization of the Nuclear "Acceptor" That Binds Progesterone-Receptor Complex

Further purification of the "acceptor" activity was desired. A chromatin-cellulose resin was prepared wherein the chromosomal proteins are eluted from the chromatographic column according to their affinity for either the DNA or other chromatin components still attached to the resin.[24] When this resin is subjected to a gradient of guanidine hydrochloride in a solvent that contains a high concentration of a reducing agent at pH 8.5, multiple peaks of protein are eluted

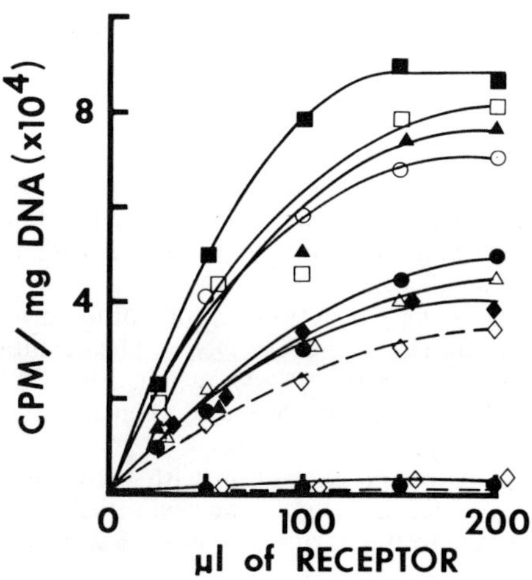

FIGURE 7. High-affinity binding of [^{3}H]P-R complex to chromatin from developing chick oviducts. The binding assay used in this experiment was the standard method,[23,25] except that crude cytosol preparation of [^{3}H]P-R complex was used, as described elsewhere.[18] The symbols represent binding to the chromatins of oviducts from chicks treated with diethylstilbestrol (DES) for 0 days (●), 4 days (○), 6 days (■), 8 days (□), 12 days (▲), 15 days (△), and 20 days (◆). At Day 0, the oviducts are undeveloped, whereas by Day 20, they are fully developed.[52] Chromatin from chick spleen (treated for 20 days with DES), ◇—◇; chromatin from hen oviduct, ◇- - -◇; chromatin from hen spleen, ○- - -○.

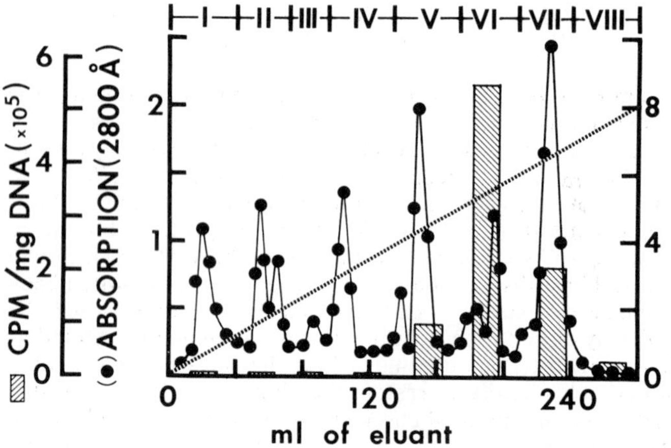

FIGURE 8. Selective dissociation of proteins and "acceptor" from chromatin-cellulose resins. Hen oviduct chromatin-cellulose resin was prepared as described in MATERIALS AND METHODS and elsewhere.[24,26] Twenty grams of this resin that contained approximately 60 mg of DNA as chromatin was resuspended in 100 ml of a cold solution that contained 0.1 M HSETOH plus 0.005 M sodium bisulfite plus 0.01 M Tris HCl (pH 8.5) and allowed to hydrate for 2–6 hr with gentle stirring at 4°C. The resin was then collected on a column, and a gradient of 0–8 M guanidine hydrochloride was passed through this column within a 4-hr period by use of constant levels of the buffered solution. The tubes were monitored by adsorption at 280 nm. The fractions were also monitored for conductivity and refractive index, and the gradient level of guanidine hydrochloride was plotted. The fractions were collected according to their elution with each unit of concentration of guanidine hydrochloride (e.g., 1 M, 2 M, and 3 M). Pooled samples were then dialyzed thoroughly against water and lyophilized. The lyophilized materials were resuspended in a small volume of water, homogenized in a Teflon® pestle glass homogenizer, assayed for protein by the Lowry method,[45] and reannealed to pure hen organ DNA. The protein to DNA ratio for these reannealings was 1:10. The reannealing consisted of a gradient dialysis from 7.0 M guanidine hydrochloride in the buffer described above to 0.0 M guanidine hydrochloride in the same buffer and finally dialysis versus 0.01 M Tris HCl (pH 7.5). The nucleoproteins were then analyzed for "acceptor" activity by the streptomycin method, subtracting the values obtained with pure DNA. This activity is presented as bar graphs. Total recoverable protein after dialysis and lyophilization was estimated to be ~50% of the total protein placed on the column as chromatin-cellulose.

from the column (FIGURE 8). As shown in FIGURE 9, the majority of the protein is eluted by ~4 M guanidine hydrochloride. The high absorption observed in FIGURE 8 under conditions of a 4–7 M guanidine hydrochloride extract, which yields only small amounts of protein, is due primarily to the elution of ribonucleoprotein and of small amounts of DNA. The protein eluted from the column was pooled according to the extraction as units of molarity of guanidine hydrochloride (see FIGURE 8) and reannealed to DNA. The resultant nucleoprotein was analyzed for high-affinity binding. As shown in FIGURE 8, only the material that elutes from the column between 5 and 7 M guanidine hydrochloride contains the high-affinity binding activity.

After the extraction with increasing unit molarity levels of guanidine hydrochloride, samples of the resin itself were removed, washed thoroughly, and subjected to the hormone-binding assay. As shown in FIGURE 9, the removal of all of the histone and most of the acidic proteins from the chromatin by 4 M guanidine hydrochloride fails to alter significantly the number of acceptor sites in the oviduct chromatin. These results support those shown previously, in which the removal of all of the histones did not unmask any more of this class of binding site. Further extraction of the chromatin-cellulose with 5 and 6 M guanidine hydrochloride does unmask many of the acceptor sites. However, the 6 M guanidine hydrochloride extraction begins to reduce the number of acceptor sites on the DNA. Therefore, as the high-affinity binding activity is lost from the resin (5–7 M guanidine hydrochloride), the majority of the "acceptor" activity is detected in the eluant. Similar studies have been performed with chromatin-hydroxyapatite resins. As shown in FIGURE 10, acceptor activity is also eluted between 5 and 7 M guanidine hydrochloride with this resin. TABLE 2 shows the estimated purification (~98,000-fold), beginning with whole tissue at this stage of purification.

Further purification has recently been achieved with molecular sieve chromatography by use of 100-cm columns that contain agarose-0.5m or agarose-1.5m, with 6.0 M guanidine hydrochloride according to the procedure of Mann

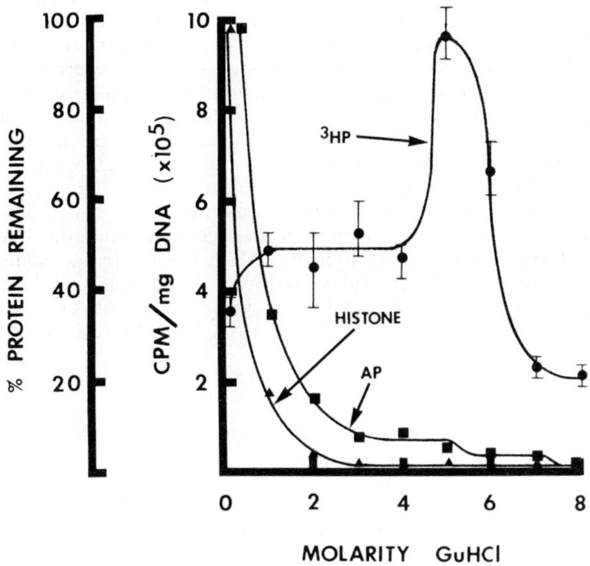

FIGURE 9. Binding of [^{3}H]P-R complex to hen oviduct chromatin-cellulose treated with guanidine hydrochloride. In this experiment, aliquots of chromatin-cellulose were washed twice in 20 vol of solution that contained 0.1 M 2-mercaptoethanol plus 0.005 M sodium bisulfate plus 0.01 M Tris HCl (pH 8.5) and a specified molarity of guanidine hydrochloride. These resins were then washed in dilute Tris-EDTA buffer several times, frozen, and lyophilized. Twenty- to 50-mg amounts of the resin were then assayed for protein content by resuspending the resin in the Tris-EDTA buffer, allowing it to hydrate several hours with gentle mixing, and assaying for histone (▲) by use of a 0.4 N H_2SO_4 extract with subsequent analysis of the acidic proteins (AP, ■) with a 0.1 N NaOH extract. These guanidine-treated resins were also tested for their acceptor activity (●) with 20–25 μg of DNA (bound to the cellulose) together with 300 μl of the hormone-receptor complex solution. The binding assay was performed essentially as described in MATERIALS AND METHODS, and the counts per milligram of DNA were calculated. The average and range of three replicates of analysis for each hormone-binding assay are shown.

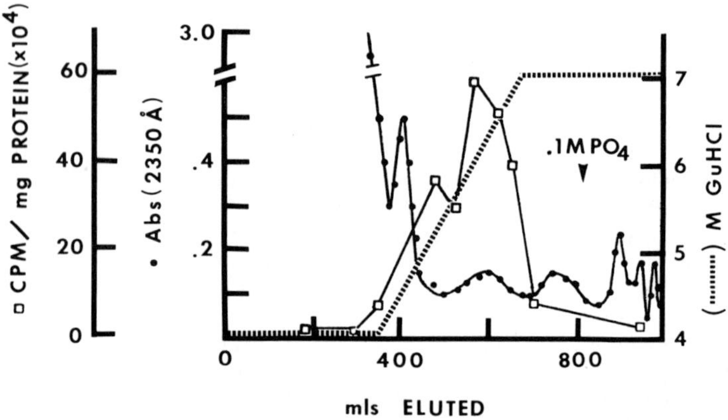

FIGURE 10. Elution of "acceptor" activity from hydroxyapatite-chromatin resins with guanidine hydrochloride. Resins of chromatin-hydroxyapatite were prepared in the presence of buffered 4.0 M guanidine hydrochloride. The resin, which contained 100 mg of chromatin DNA, was placed on the column, and the 4.0 M guanidine hydrochloride eluant was collected in 4-ml fractions. The fractions were monitored by (●) absorption at 2350 Å. When the absorption was markedly decreased, the gradient of 4–7 M guanidine hydrochloride was begun, and the eluant fractions were pooled according to the half molarity of guanidine hydrochloride between the 4 and 7 M levels. The guanidine hydrochloride determined by their refractive indices. These fractions were then reannealed to DNA at a protein to DNA ratio of 1:10 (w/w) by use of a gradient dialysis from 6 to 0.0 M guanidine in dilute Tris-EDTA buffer. The reconstituted nucleoprotein was then concentrated in dialysis bags by placing them in Aquacide® III (Calbiochem, San Diego, Calif.) and then analyzed for "acceptor" activity (○) by the streptomycin method. Values for hormone binding to pure DNA were used as background and were subtracted from the values of nucleoprotein binding. Methods for preparing the hydroxyapatite-chromatin resin and for removing the chromosomal protein and RNA without the loss of DNA from the resin have been described elsewhere.[54]

TABLE 2
SUMMARY OF PURIFICATION OF "ACCEPTOR" BINDING AT SATURATION TO HIGHEST-AFFINITY SITES

	cpm/mg of DNA	Protein/DNA	pmol/mg of Protein	Purification
Whole tissue	75,000	24.21	0.004	1
Nuclei	75,000	3.05	0.972	243
Chromatin-cellulose	362,726	2.75	5.0	1250
NAP-cellulose	877,032	0.97	36.0	8931
Chromatin-cellulose extraction with guanidine hydrochloride (M)				
1.0	496,546	0.80	24	6131
2.0	452,960	0.31	58	14,434
3.0	522,967	0.15	138	34,440
4.0	446,927	0.15	115	28,668
5.0	829,112	0.13	287	71,823
6.0	652,609	0.07	390	97,677
7.0	176,602	0.06	116	29,000

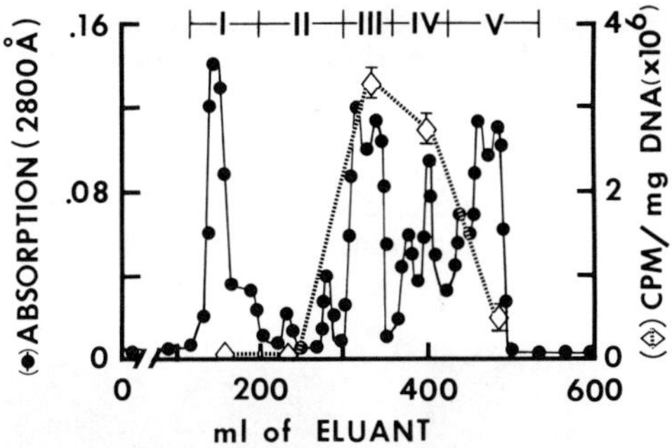

FIGURE 11. Agarose-1.5m molecular sieve chromatography of the "acceptor" protein fraction from a hydroxyapatite-chromatin column. The acceptor fraction that represented the 5–7 M guanidine hydrochloride, extract of the hydroxyapatite-chromatin resin was dialyzed against deionized water and lyophilized. The material was resuspended in 6.0 M guanidine hydrochloride solution, as described elsewhere,[53] at 2 mg of protein per milliliter. This protein solution was clarified by centrifugation at 200*g* for 10 min and then applied to a 2.6 × 94-cm column of Agarose-1.5m. The eluted fractions were pooled according to the absorbing peaks (●), as shown in the Figure. The pooled fractions were then reannealed to DNA and assayed for "acceptor" activity (◇) by the streptomycin method, as described in the legends to FIGURES 8 and 10. Values for DNA binding were subtracted from all values obtained with nucleoprotein. The average and range of three replicates of analysis are shown.

and Fish.[53] FIGURES 11 and 12 show an example of such a chromatogram (for agarose-1.5m). The eluted material was pooled according to peaks of absorbing material and was reannealed to DNA. The nucleoproteins were then analyzed for "acceptor" activity. The acceptor activity elutes with a distribution coefficient between 0.65 and 0.80, which gives a moleculear weight range of 12,000–16,000 daltons (see FIGURE 12).

After pooling fractions III and IV and performing similar chromatography on agarose-0.5m, "acceptor" activity elutes near the void volumn. Other purification approaches were tested with high success with Bio-Gel® P-100, followed by P-200

FIGURE 12. Selectivity curve for an agarose-1.5m column (2.6 × 94 cm) by use of 6.0 M guanidine hydrochloride buffered at pH 6.0 as a solvent. The standard proteins were purchased from commercial sources, and their subunit molecular weights were obtained from I.M. Klotz and D.W. Darnall, P.L. Biochemicals Chart. The hatched area represents elution of high "acceptor" activity from the column.

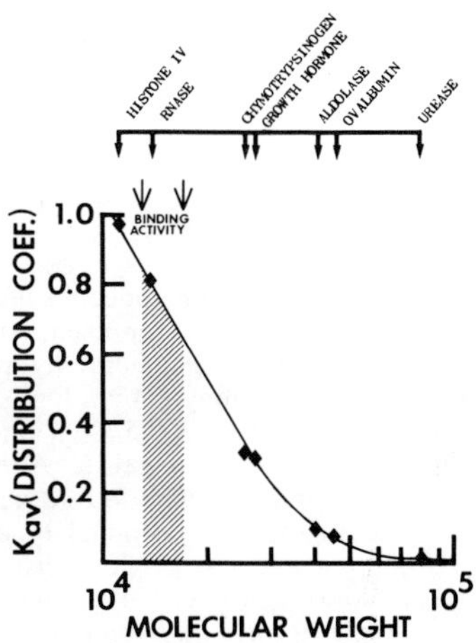

resins with 30% formic acid. In any case, successive chromatography on any two different resins results in a highly purified preparation of proteinaceous material that, when reannealed to DNA, yields a marked level of high-affinity binding. Sodium dodecyl sulfate-polyacrylamide gel electropherograms of the cleanest preparations to date are shown in FIGURES 13 and 14. Gel I represents a typical pattern of protein eluted from either chromatin-cellulose or chromatin-hydroxyapatite resins in the 5–7 M guanidine hydrochloride range. Gels II and III

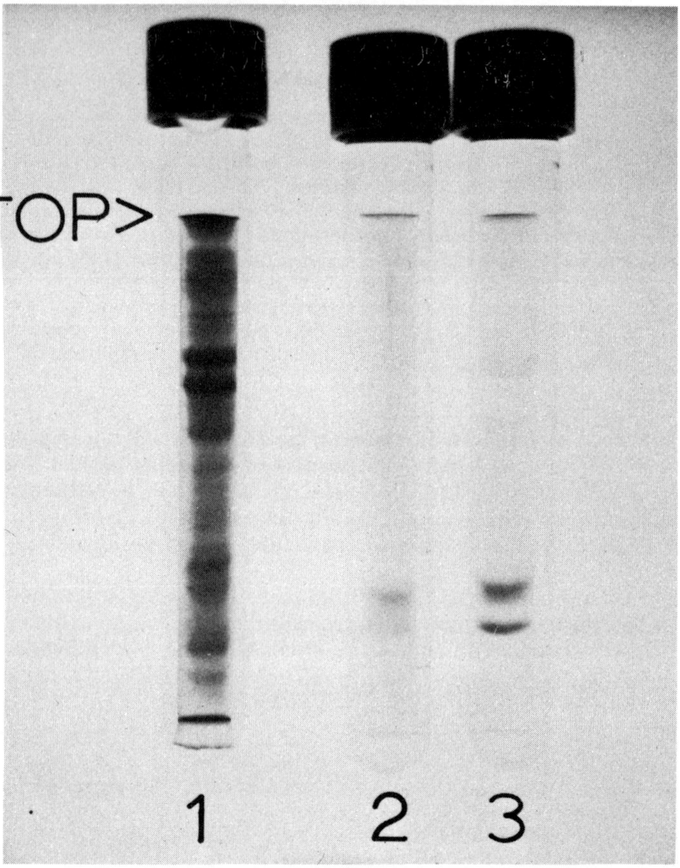

FIGURE 13. Sodium dodecyl sulfate-polyacrylamide gel electropherogram of purified "acceptor" activity. Gel 1 represents the proteins eluted from hydroxyapatite-chromatin resins between 5 and 7 M guanidine hydrochloride. This fraction was then subjected to agarose-1.5m chromatography (94 cm long), followed by rechromatography on an agarose-1.5m (30 cm long) or an agarose-0.5m (56 cm long) column. The "acceptor" proteins obtained by this approach are seen in gel 2. Alternatively, the fraction from gel 1 was subjected to chromatography in 30% formic acid on Bio-Gel P-200 (2.6 × 30 cm long), followed by rechromatography on Bio-Gel P-200 or P-100. The "acceptor" proteins obtained by this procedure are seen in gel 3. Approximately 150 μg of protein were applied to gel 1, 10 μg to gel 2, and 30 μg to gel 3. Protein was applied at the top of the gels. The gels represent 10% acrylamide (9.5 cm long) and were run until the bromphenol blue tracking dye migrated to within 0.5 cm of the bottom. The gels were stained with Coomassie blue.

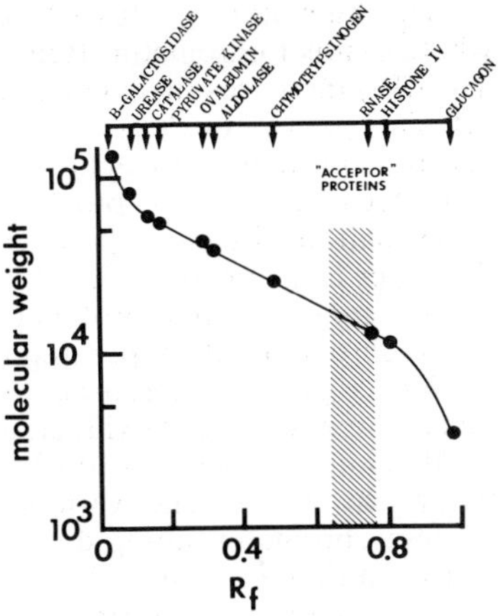

FIGURE 14. Distribution of standard-molecular-weight proteins in the sodium dodecyl sulfate-polyacrylamide gel electrophoresis described in the legend to FIGURE 13. The hatched area represents the migration of the two protein species in gels 2 and 3 of FIGURE 13.

represent the proteins eluted from the agarose and Bio-Gel P-chromatography series, respectively. In both cases, two major bands are observed with the same migration. FIGURE 14 shows that these two protein species migrate with molecular weights between 13,000 and 17,000 daltons. This molecular weight range is in close agreement with that estimated from molecular sieve chromatography (FIGURES 11 & 12).

Because the high-affinity binding activity of these preparations is destroyed by pronase, and due to the fact that reannealing to DNA is required for high-affinity binding, we conclude that the high-affinity binding of the P-R complex *in vitro*, and probably *in vivo*, is due to low-molecular-weight nonhistone proteins bound to DNA. These proteins themselves have a high affinity for DNA, information that provides a rapid effective approach to purification of the "acceptors."

DISCUSSION

The identification of the nuclear acceptors that bind steroid-receptor complexes is important, because this interaction represents the next step after steroid receptor activation and binding, and also the first step in steroid-induced changes in genetic transcription. The low-molecular-weight proteins observed in FIGURE 13 represent the only detectable protein species in the purified "acceptor" fractions. No RNA or DNA is detected in this fraction. Occasionally, minute amounts of higher-molecular-weight proteins are observed on sodium dodecyl sulfate gels. There remain the possibilities that the two isolated protein species are breakdown products of larger "native" macromolecules and that the two protein species predominant in the gels themselves are not the "acceptors" but other molecules in the preparation actually induce the "acceptor" activity. The fact that the "acceptor" activity coelutes with these proteins from a series of chromatographic resins and that the "acceptor" activity is destroyed by pronase treatment certainly supports their role as the nuclear "acceptors." Our results suggest that the "acceptor" protein must be reannealed to DNA to achieve high-affinity binding; that is, the free protein does not bind to P-R. In any case, we propose that the P-R complex migrates to the nucleus and binds to a acidic protein-DNA complex and that this step is followed by alterations in RNA polymerase activities and gene expression.[2,4,8]

The high-affinity sites ("acceptors") consist of about 6000–10,000 sites in whole oviduct chromatin. Removal of the masking acidic proteins (fractions AP_1 and AP_2) increases the number of binding sites four- to fivefold, or to 24,000–50,-000 sites per cell nucleus. Assuming one steroid-receptor complex binding to one acceptor protein, we would have 20,000–50,000 acceptor molecules per oviduct cell. Because the "acceptor" protein has an average molecular weight of about 15,000 daltons (by our experiments), and since it is known that there are 2.5 pg of DNA per hen somatic cell,[46] we have about 10^{-15} g of acceptor protein per cell, or 0.2–0.5 μg of acceptor protein per milligram of DNA. Because we obtain about 1 mg of chromatin DNA per gram of hen oviduct, it would take 5 kg of oviduct to obtain 1 mg of acceptor, assuming a 100% yield. We require about five to 10 times that amount, or 1 kg of oviduct, to obtain 20–200 μg of acceptor protein.

It is interesting that a 70–80% "masking" of acceptor sites occurs in the target tissue chromatin. The variable number of acceptor sites measured in chick oviduct chromatin during development (FIGURE 7) suggests that a regulation of steroid action on target cells may occur at the level of nuclear binding. One must wonder whether transformed cells in culture or in mammary tumors that contain steroid receptors but that do not respond to the steroids have "masked" nuclear "acceptor" sites. Thus, these cells may be nonresponsive, because the genome cannot bind the steroid-receptor complexes.

This is the first evidence of purification to possible homogeneity and characterization of an "acceptor" protein(s) that binds steroid receptors in target cell nuclei. We propose that the next step in the fate of P-R complexes after migration to the oviduct nucleus is the binding to nucleoprotein complexes that consist of DNA and low-molecular-weight proteins. Whether one or both of the protein species observed electrophoretically in our experiments are involved in the high-affinity binding of the P-R complex remains to be determined. As stated above, the possibility also exists that some other entity in the acceptor fractions is responsible for high-affinity binding in oviduct chromatin. Interesting questions arise from these studies: Are these "acceptor" proteins involved in the steroid-induced alterations of gene transcription? Are these "acceptor" proteins ubiquitous to all hen tissues? Does regulation of nuclear binding actually occur? Do specific reiterated DNA sequences bind very tightly these multiple copies of proteins? And, finally and most importantly, are these "acceptor" proteins functional *in vivo*?

Acknowledgments

The authors thank Ms. Patti Midthun, Ms. Barbara Gosse, Ms. Kay Rasmussen, Ms. Carole Laabs, and Mr. Brad Syversen for their excellent assistance in these studies.

References

1. Raspé, G. (Ed.) 1971. Advances in the Biosciences. Vol. 7. Pergamon Press. New York, N.Y.
2. Spelsberg, T. C. 1974. *In* Acidic Protein of the Nucleus. I. L. Cameron & P. R. Jeter, Eds.: 248–296. Academic Press, Inc. New York, N.Y.
3. Jensen, E. V. & E. R. DeSombre. 1972. Annu. Rev. Biochem. **41:** 203–230.
4. O'Malley, B. W. & A. R. Means. 1974. Science **183:** 610–620.

5. Pasqualini, J. R. (Ed.) 1976. *In* Receptors and Mechanisms of Action of Steroid Hormones. Marcel Dekker, Inc. New York, N.Y.
6. Glasser, S. R., F. Chytil & T. C. Spelsberg. 1972. Biochem. J. **130:** 947–957.
7. Borthwick, N. M. & R. M. S. Smellie. 1975. Biochem. J. **147:** 91–101.
8. Spelsberg, T. C. & R. F. Cox. 1976. Biochim. Biophys. Acta **435:** 376–390.
9. O'Malley, B. W., G. C. Rosenfeld, J. P. Comstock & A. R. Means. 1972. Nature [New Biol.] **240:** 45–47.
10. Chan, L., A. R. Means & B. W. O'Malley. 1973. Proc. Nat. Acad. Sci. USA **70:** 1870–1874.
11. Harris, S. E., J. M. Rosen, A. R. Means & B. W. O'Malley. 1975. Biochemistry **14:** 2072–2081.
12. Palmiter, R. D. 1973. J. Biol. Chem. **248:** 8260–8270.
13. Cox, R. F., M. E. Haines & J. S. Emtage. 1974. Eur. J. Biochem. **49:** 225–236.
14. Schimke, R. T., G. S. McKnight & D. J. Shapiro. 1975. *In* Biochemical Actions of Hormones. G. Litwack, Ed. Vol III: 245–269. Academic Press, Inc. New York, N.Y.
15. Chamness, G. C., A. W. Jennings & W. L. McGuire. 1973. Nature (London) **241:** 456–460.
16. Chamness, G. C., A. W. Jennings & W. L. McGuire. 1974. Biochemistry **13:** 327–331.
17. Puca, G. A., E. Nola, U. Hibner, G. Cicala, & V. Sica. 1975. J. Biol. Chem. **250:** 6452–6459.
18. Spelsberg, T. C., A. W. Steggles & B. W. O'Malley. 1974. J. Biol. Chem. **246:** 4188–4197.
19. King, R. J. B. & J. Gordon. 1972. Nature [New Biol.] **240:** 185–197.
20. Buller, R. E., D. O. Toft, W. T. Schrader & B. W. O'Malley. 1975. J. Biol. Chem. **250:** 801–808.
21. Buller, R. E., W. T. Schrader, & B. W. O'Malley. 1975. J. Biol. Chem. **250:** 809–818.
22. Mainwaring, W. I. P. & B. M. Peterken. 1971. Biochem. J. **125:** 285–295.
23. Spelsberg, T. C., A. W. Steggles, F. Chytil & B. W. O'Malley. 1972. J. Biol. Chem. **247:** 1369–1374.
24. Spelsberg, T. C., R. A. Webster & G. M. Pikler. 1975. *In* Chromosomal Proteins and Their Role in Gene Expression. G. Stein & L. Kleinsmith Eds.: 153–186. Academic Press, Inc. New York, N. Y.
25. Pikler, G. M., R. A. Webster & T. C. Spelsberg. 1976. Biochem. J. **156:** 399–408.
26. Webster, R. A., G. M. Pikler & T. C. Spelsberg. 1976. Biochem. J. **156:** 409–416.
27. Jackson, V. & R. Chalkley. 1974. J. Biol. Chem. **249:** 1615–1626.
28. Jackson, V. & R. Chalkley. 1974. J. Biol. Chem. **249:** 1627–1636.
29. Liao, S., T. Liang & J. L. Tymoczko. 1973. Nature [New Biol.] **241:** 211–213.
30. Sluyser, M. 1969. Biochim. Biophys. Acta **182:** 235–244.
31. Monder, C. & M. C. Walker. 1970. Biochemistry **9:** 2489–2497.
32. King, R. J. B., J. Gordon & A. W. Steggles. 1969. Biochem. J. **114:** 649–657.
33. Liang, T. & S. Liao. 1972. Biochim. Biophys. Acta **277:** 590–594.
34. Defer, N., B. Dastugue & J. Kruh. 1974. Biochimie **56:** 559–566.
35. Toft, D. 1972. J. Steroid Biochem. **3:**515–522.
36. Yamamoto, K. R. & B. Alberts. 1974. J. Biol. Chem. **249:** 7076–7086.
37. Baxter, J. D., G. G. Rousseau, M. C. Benson, R. L. Garcea, J. Ito & G. M. Tomkins. 1972. Proc. Nat. Acad. Sci. USA **69:** 1892–1896.
38. Rousseau, G. G., S. J. Higgens, J. Baxter, D. Gelfand & G. M. Tomkins. 1975. J. Biol. Chem. **250:** 6015–6021.
39. Andre, J. & H. Rochefort. 1975. FEBS Lett. **50:** 319–323.
40. Sumida, C., C. Gelly & J. R. Pasqualini. 1974. Compt. Rend. Ser. D **279:** 1793–1796.
41. Spelsberg, T. C. 1976. Biochem. J. **156:** 391–398.
42. Schrader, W. T. & B. W. O'Malley. 1972. J. Biol. Chem. **247:** 51–59.
43. Litman, R. M. 1968. J. Biol. Chem. **243:** 6222–6233.
44. Burton, K. 1956. Biochem. J. **62:** 315–323.

45. Lowry, O. H., N. J. Rosenbrough, A. L. Farr & R. J. Randall. 1951. J. Biol. Chem. **193:** 265–275.
46. Sober, H. A. 1970. Handbook of Biochemistry.: 11–111. Chemical Rubber Co. Cleveland, Ohio.
47. O'Malley, B. W., M. A. Kirschner & C. W. Bardin. 1968. Proc. Soc. Exp. Biol. Med. **127:** 521–523.
48. Gilbert, A. B. 1971. *In* Physiology and Biochemistry of the Domestic Fowl. D. J. Bell & B. M. Freeman, Eds. Vol. **3:** 1449–1468. Academic Press, Inc. New York, N.Y.
49. Scatchard, G. 1949. Ann. N.Y. Acad. Sci. **51:** 660–672.
50. Spelsberg, T. C., R. Webster & G. M. Pikler. 1976. Nature (London) **262:** 65–67.
51. Spelsberg, T. C., A. W. Steggles & B. W. O'Malley. 1971. Biochim. Biophys. Acta **254:** 129–134.
52. O'Malley, B. W., W. L. McGuire, P. O. Kohler & S. G. Korenman. 1969. Rec. Progr. Hormone Res. **25:** 105–160.
53. Mann, K. G. & W. W. Fish. 1973. Methods Enzymol. **26:** 28–42.
54. Spelsberg, T. C. 1976. In preparation.
55. Neelin, J. M. 1968. Can. J. Biochem. **46:** 241–247.

Discussion

Dr. R. J. B. King: With the design of your experiments, can you distinguish between a model in which the receptor is binding directly to the acidic protein and a situation where the acidic protein is modifying the nucleic acid and the receptor is then bound to this modified DNA?

Dr. Spelsberg: At present, we don't know, Dr. King. Our progesterone-receptor complex, based on Dr. Schrader's evidence, may consist of a combination of A and B species of receptors. We did try using B receptors, which bind protein and not DNA, and do get somewhat better results. However, the B receptor in our hands is so unstable that it gives us more headaches. We need kilograms of oviduct to get 200 μg of this material, so our time is committed just handling this problem alone. Consequently, we have not yet pursued your point.

Dr. King: I'm a little bit puzzled about the *in vivo* binding. You can destroy the binding of your receptor to the weaker classes of sites by 0.15 M KCl. How do you fit that result with the fact that you still observe receptor bound to these weaker classes of sites in nuclei after isolation with the standard sucrose solutions, which contain fairly high levels of salt?

Dr. Spelsberg: We observe the binding to several classes of sites with buffers of low ionic strength. Most buffers used for nuclear isolation do contain magnesium and potassium chloride in fairly high concentrations, adding to give ionic strengths equivalent to 0.2 M KCl or higher. Consequently, if you isolate nuclei by use of the standard buffered sucrose solutions, you do eliminate much of the weaker binding, so, to observe the weaker classes of sites, we use buffers of low ionic strength (about one-fifth of the original concentrations).

Dr. W. T. Schrader: Dr. Spelsberg, if I understand you correctly, you take the material (proteins) that you get at the end of this purification (for example, after gel filtration) and reconstitute it back to oviduct DNA to do the receptor binding assay. How much of this protein goes back on the DNA? Also, how many micrograms of this material can you put back on? One would predict that if the protein you have is really the acceptor site, only limited amounts will reanneal to the DNA at a level that you see *in vivo*.

DR. SPELSBERG: First, if we do a quick reconstitution of the protein to DNA over 10 min, as opposed to the standard 36–48 hr, the binding of the hormone-receptor complex to DNA is very low. There has to be a gradient-type dialysis over an extended period of time to reconstitute the binding. Whether we are renaturing the protein, or whether it has to find selected sites on the DNA, we don't know. Second, yes, we take this purified material and reanneal it to DNA; however, the percentage that gets reannealed depends on the protein to DNA ratio. Below a ratio of 0.02 of protein to DNA (w/w), we get between 50 and 100% recovered protein reannealed to DNA, as best we can quantitate. As we go up to higher protein to DNA ratios, we get a lower recovery of DNA-bound protein. Third, some interesting new data suggest that we need extremely low levels of protein to get maximal binding. These data indicate the possibility of preparing DNA sites specific for our acceptor preparation. We're working on that now. Another interesting point is that we estimate that there are 25,000 acceptor molecules per cell, including those that are masked. Whether there is some regulation of hormonal action with respect to masking of nuclear binding sites remains to be determined. Since we have the 25,000 or more binding sites per cell nucleus (based on the binding of one receptor to one acceptor), we may have 25,000 acceptor molecules, which makes it feasible to purify them to homogeneity, provided that they are not a heterogeneous population of species.

PURIFICATION AND PROPERTIES OF PROGESTERONE RECEPTORS FROM CHICK OVIDUCT*

William T. Schrader,† William A. Coty, Roy G. Smith, and Bert W. O'Malley

Department of Cell Biology
Baylor College of Medicine
Houston, Texas 77030

Introduction

Steroid hormone receptor proteins have been the subject of intensive study for more than 10 years. This research has clearly implicated these molecules in the process of steroid hormone-induced cell development and differentiation. These studies have also shown that receptor proteins are structurally complex, undergoing changes in aggregation, conformation, and binding activities before and during their interaction with nuclear acceptor sites.[1,2] The importance of these properties is apparent from the extensive similarities among all steroid receptor proteins studied, regardless of source or steroid-binding specificity.

Work in this laboratory has centered on the purification and characterization of progesterone receptors in chick oviduct. This research has been performed with two goals in mind. First, we have studied these proteins to gain information on the relationship between their structure and *in vivo* mechanism of action. Second, we have sought to purify these proteins to investigate their effect on gene expression *in vitro*.

Chick oviduct progesterone receptor contains two 4S components, designated A and B, which can be resolved by chromatography on a variety of ion-exchange resins.[3,4] These two components, which are present in approximately equal amounts in crude oviduct cytoplasmic extracts,[5] are not interconvertable. They have similar hormone-binding sites with respect to equilibrium and kinetic binding constants and hormonal stereospecificity.[3]

Although both receptor forms are taken up by oviduct nuclei *in vitro*,[5,6] they have distinct specificities for binding to nuclear components. The receptor A component binds only to DNA, whereas the B component binds only to chromatin.[5] Furthermore, B-component binding to chromatin is target tissue specific.[7,10]

These properties of the progesterone receptor led us to propose[5,11,12] that both chromatin- and DNA-binding forms might be necessary for receptor function *in vivo*. We have recently shown in an *in vitro* system that steroid hormones regulate gene expression in the chick oviduct at the level of messenger RNA transcription.[13] In our hypothetical model, the chromatin-binding B protein would function to specify regions in the chromatin adjacent to hormonally regulated genes. This specifier activity would then direct the A protein to its site of action, where it would bind to the DNA and thus modify transcription by RNA polymerases.

This model would suggest that aggregated forms of the receptor that contain

*Supported by National Institutes of Health Grant HD-7957 to the Baylor Center for Population Research and Studies in Reproductive Biology, NIH Grants HD-7857 and HD-8188, and Ford Foundation Grant 63-141.

†Correspondence should be addressed to this author.

both A and B subunits might be important in receptor function. The experiments described below were designed to examine the subunit structure of the progesterone receptor and the relationship this quaternary structure has to the functional activities of the A and B receptor forms. According to our model, the ultimate test of receptor activity is its effect on gene transcription. We have recently developed an *in vitro* assay for transcription of chromatin.[14] Therefore, we have also performed studies, described below, to purify the various receptor forms to test their effect in this assay.

RESULTS

Receptor Subunit Structure

A common characteristic of steroid hormone receptors is their tendency to undergo salt-dependent aggregation.[1] Chick oviduct progesterone receptor exhibits this characteristic behavior, as shown by sucrose gradient ultracentrifugation analysis.[12,15] In gradients that contain 0.3 M KCl, progesterone receptor sedi-

TABLE 1

RELATIVE STABILITY OF RECEPTOR FORMS TO DIALYSIS

Receptor Form*	Receptor in Sucrose Gradient Peak: Stored at 0°C	Dialysis (cpm)	Diluted Fivefold†
4S	1200	2100	2500
6S	1900	1400	1450
8S	1600	700	350

*Crude chick oviduct cytosol that contained [^{3}H]progesterone-receptor complex[3] was either stored at 0°C and dialyzed against 10 mM Tris (pH 7.4), 1 mM EDTA, 12 mM 1-thioglycerol (buffer A) or was diluted fivefold with buffer A prior to storage at 0°C, all for 8 hr. All three samples were then analyzed by sucrose gradient centrifugation as previously described.[3]

†Radioactivity in each peak is multiplied by five to correct for dilution.

ments as a single sharp peak at approximately 4S. In the absence of salt, however, receptor components are observed that sediment at approximately 6S and 8S. We therefore examined these aggregated receptor forms to determine their relationship to the 4S A and B components.

A major analytic tool for the study of aggregated receptor forms was provided by our discovery[12] that these proteins pass unretarded through phosphocellulose columns under conditions where 4S A and B components are quantitatively absorbed. We used this technique in combination with sucrose gradient analysis to isolate and study 6S and 8S receptor aggregates.

The results in TABLE 1 show that the 8S aggregate is unstable to dialysis and dilution. This form is apparently converted to 4S components, whereas the 6S form is relatively unaffected. This concentration dependence of receptor aggregation has been observed for other steroid hormone receptors[16] and may be due to artifactual aggregation of receptor with other cytoplasmic proteins. The relative stability of the 6S form, and the fact that its molecular weight was approximately equal to the sum of the A and B components, led us to study this aggregate further.

We isolated 6S hormone receptor complex from the unadsorbed fraction after phosphocellulose chromatography of cytosol and treated it with high salt or brief warming at room temperature. These treatments resulted in substantial conversion to receptor forms that adsorbed to phosphocellulose. Subsequent elution of this resin with a potassium chloride gradient resolved two equal peaks of radioactivity at 0.22 and 0.26 M KCl.[12] These peaks were identified as B and A components, respectively, by rechromatography on phosphocellulose and coelution with these 4S receptor forms isolated by DEAE-cellulose chromatography. These results suggest that the 6S receptor form is a dimer that contains equal amounts of A and B subunits.

The presence of progesterone had a dramatic effect on the stability of the 6S

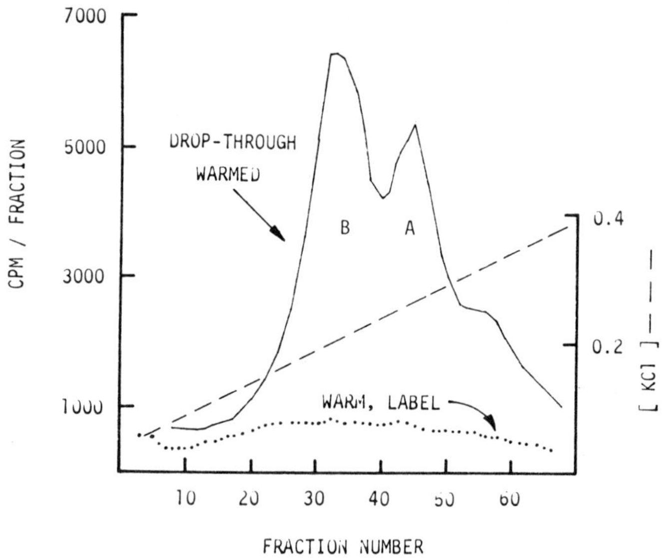

FIGURE 1. Phosphocellulose chromatography of progesterone receptor subunits. Oviduct cytosol without bound progesterone was warmed to 25°C for 30 min and then cooled and labeled before application to the column (. . . .). The drop-through fraction was then collected and rewarmed, cooled, and rechromatographed (—).

receptor dimer. Unlabeled cytosol was warmed as described above, then cooled to 0°C and labeled for 1 hr with [^{3}H]progesterone before application to a phosphocellulose column. As shown by the dotted line in FIGURE 1, the 6S receptor had not dissociated to A and B subunits and therefore did not bind to the column. The labeled column drop-through fraction was collected, rewarmed, and rechromatographed. As shown by the solid line in the Figure, the expected production of equal amounts of A and B subunits occurred.

We also tested the stability of the 6S species to dissociation by potassium chloride with sucrose gradient ultracentrifugation. Oviduct cytosol, with or without bound [^{3}H]progesterone, was run on gradients that contained various amounts of potassium chloride. As shown in FIGURE 2, apo-receptor did not dissociate at up to 0.25 M KCl. However, the labeled complex was metastable at physiologic

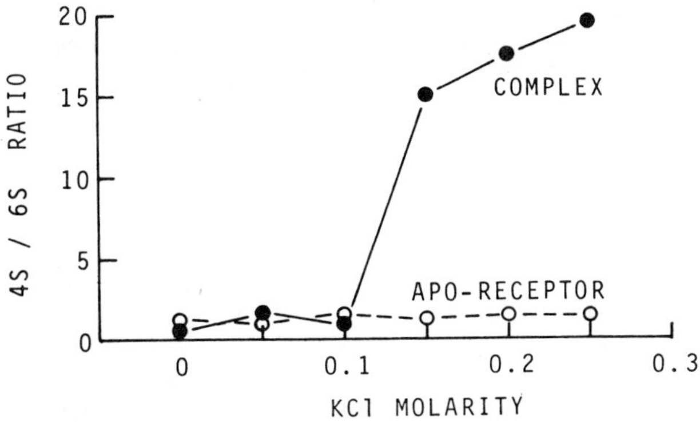

FIGURE 2. Sucrose gradient analysis of receptor dimer stability. Cytosol either unlabeled (○) or labeled (●) with [^{3}H]progesterone was run on sucrose gradients that contained the indicated amount of potassium chloride shown on the abscissa. Gradients were fractionated and assayed for receptor directly, for labeled receptor, or by the DEAE filter assay[30] after complexing with [^{3}H]progesterone for the apo-receptor. Peak heights were measured in fractions 10 (4S) and 15 (6S) after ultracentrifugation.

concentrations of potassium chloride and was completely dissociated by 0.2 M KCl. These results show that hormone binding results in destabilization of the subunit interactions in the 6S progesterone receptor dimer. Thus, hormone binding could regulate the subunit structure of both the receptor and its nuclear localization.

Because the 6S receptor contains both DNA- and chromatin-binding subunits, we examined whether these activities were expressed in the intact dimer. The results in TABLE 2 show that the 6S dimer binds to chromatin. Binding was essentially complete within 15 min at 0°C; no further binding was observed after 60 min. This finding suggests that the dimer binds directly to chromatin, because very little dissociation into subunits would be expected in this time interval.

We also examined receptor binding to DNA-cellulose, as shown in TABLE 3. Binding of the A subunit to DNA was nearly complete, whereas no significant

TABLE 2

BINDING OF INTACT 6S RECEPTOR TO OVIDUCT CHROMATIN

6S Receptor Added* (μl)	Incubation Time (min)	Receptor Bound† (cpm)	
		Control	+ Chromatin‡
100	15	3100	15,100
	60	2600	10,300
250	15	6300	24,500
	60	7400	29,500

*Labeled cytosol 6S receptors (400,000 cpm/ml) were prepared in 0.1 M KCl by phosphocellulose exclusion.

†Receptors were incubated at 0°C in a final volume of 1.0 ml, and tubes were processed according to Schrader *et al.*[29]

‡Oviduct chromatin (500 μg of DNA) was added to experimental tubes to start the binding reaction.

TABLE 3

DNA-CELLULOSE ASSAY OF RECEPTOR BINDING TO DNA

Receptor Form*	[^{3}H]Receptor Adsorbed to DNA-Cellulose (%)
A subunit	95
B subunit	5
6S intact receptor	5

*Receptor subunits were prepared and isolated as labeled complexes from cytosol by ammonium sulfate fractionation and DEAE-cellulose chromatography. Intact 6S dimers were prepared by passage through phosphocellulose.[12]

binding of the B subunit was observed, in agreement with our earlier results.[5] The 6S dimer also did not bind to DNA. Thus, the DNA binding activity of the A subunit is not expressed in the intact dimer, perhaps due to blocking or conformational alteration of the DNA-binding site through subunit-subunit interactions.

These properties of the 6S receptor dimer are consistent with our proposed model of receptor action, which suggests that both DNA- and chromatin-binding activities are required for receptor function. This property may also be a general characteristic of all steroid hormone receptors. Several researchers in our department have resolved two receptor forms by DEAE-cellulose chromatography of estrogen receptor from rat uterus and of glucocorticoid and androgen receptors from a hamster ductus deferens tumor cell line.[17] Because the latter is a cloned cell line, this finding is the first direct evidence that both receptor forms are present in the same cell.

Purification and Characterization of Receptor Forms

Our proposed model of steroid hormone action would predict that stimulation of gene transcription *in vivo* is dependent on the subunit structure of the receptor. With the development of an assay for gene transcription,[14] it became possible to examine the effect of the different receptor forms on this process *in vitro*. It is essential to use purified receptor in these studies, to avoid artifacts caused by interfering enzymatic activities[18] and to be able to relate directly any observed effect to the action of the receptor. For this reason, we have developed techniques for purification of the progesterone receptor A and B subunits and the intact 6S dimer by three independent methods.[19–21]

We have purified the receptor A subunit by a technique we have termed "differential chromatography."[21] This procedure takes advantage of the fact that the intact 6S dimer does not bind to phosphocellulose or DNA-cellulose, whereas the A subunit does. Because few proteins undergo such a dramatic alteration in binding behavior, this purification technique has proven to be an extremely powerful one.

The purification procedure for the A protein consists of the following sequence of steps: First, a crude oviduct soluble cytoplasmic extract that contains receptor aggregates is chromatographed on phosphocellulose and DNA-cellulose to remove proteins capable of binding to these resins. The receptor is then labeled by incubation with [^{3}H]progesterone and dissociated into A and B subunits by precipitation with ammonium sulfate to 30% saturation. The A and B subunits are separated by chromatography on DEAE-cellulose, and the A subunit is then subjected to the second phase of differential chromatography: rechromatography on DNA-cellulose and phosphocellulose. The A protein obtained by this procedure is purified approximately 20,000-fold to apparent homogeneity.[21]

Analysis of the purified A subunit by sodium dodecyl sulfate (SDS) gel electrophoresis shows a single protein band with an apparent molecular weight of 79,000 g/mol (FIGURE 3). This polypeptide molecular weight is in agreement with the native molecular weight of 72,000 determined by the Svedberg equation from the sedimentation coefficient and Stokes radius.[21,22] Thus, the receptor A subunit appears to be a single polypeptide chain. The purity of the A protein was verified in a second denaturing gel electrophoresis system in the presence of acid and urea.

The A protein purified by differential chromatography retained the characteristics observed in crude and partially purified preparations. Values obtained for Stokes radius, sedimentation coefficient, rate of hormone dissociation, and hormone-binding specificity were in excellent agreement with previously reported values.[21] This preparation was also active in the Millipore® filter assay for DNA

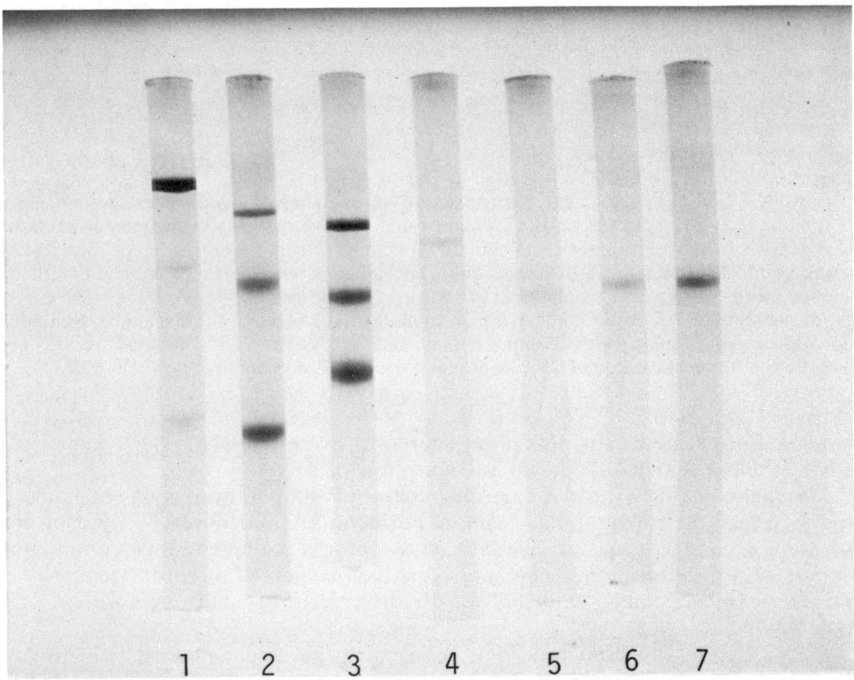

FIGURE 3. SDS polyacrylamide gel electrophoresis of purified progesterone receptor A subunit. The receptor A protein and appropriate standards were treated with 1% SDS, 1% β-mercaptoethanol at 95°C for 5 min. Electrophoresis in gels that contained 6% acrylamide was performed by the method of Weber and Osborn.[31] Gels 1–3 contain the following molecular weight standards: gel 1, *Escherichia coli* RNA polymerase subunits β, β' (160K), σ (95K), and α (39K); gel 2, β-galactosidase (130K), transferrin (90K), and ovalbumin (43K); gel 3, phosphorylase (94K), bovine serum albumin (68K), glyceraldehyde phosphate dehydrogenase (36K). Gel 4 contains a sample of hen oviduct progesterone receptor B subunit,[20] and gels 5–7 contain increasing amounts of chick oviduct progesterone receptor A subunit purified by differential chromatography.[21]

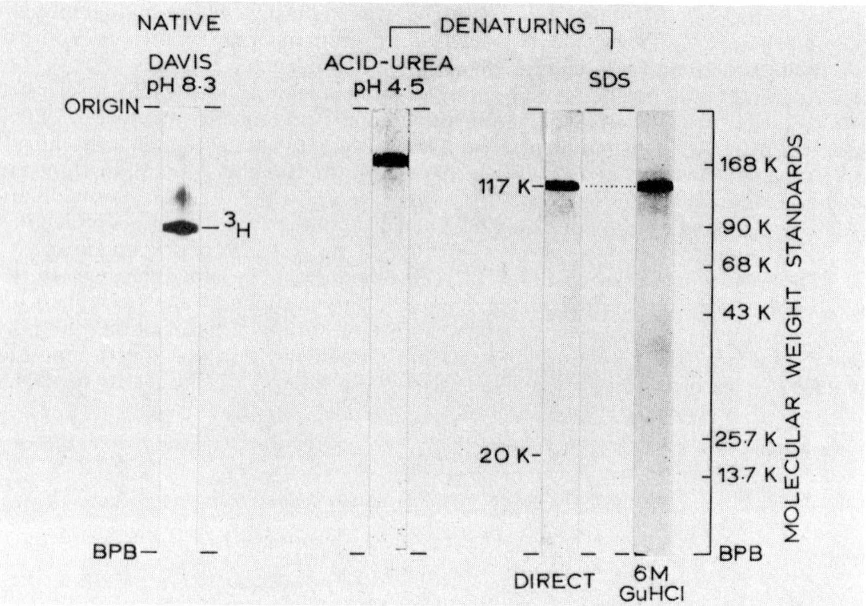

FIGURE 4. Polyacrylamide gel electrophesis of purified hen oviduct progesterone receptor B subunit.[20] *Left:* electrophoresis of receptor under nondenaturing conditions at pH 8.3.[32] One gel was heavily overloaded and stained with amido black. A companion gel was frozen, sliced, and assayed for [^{3}H]progesterone. The labeled steroid was coincident with the stained band. *Center:* electrophoresis in 10% acrylamide gels in the presence of SDS.[31] A single protein band is observed at an apparent molecular weight of 117,000 g/mol. No indication of lower-molecular-weight components is observed. *Right:* electrophoresis in SDS gels directly or after gel filtration of the receptor B protein in 6 M guanidine hydrochloride.

binding. We are now using this pure receptor A protein to study the specificity of DNA binding and its effect on transcription of DNA.

We have obtained the progesterone receptor B subunit from laying hen oviduct by a series of conventional protein purification procedures.[20] Cytosol that contains crude [^{3}H]progesterone-labeled receptor is precipitated with ammonium sulfate of 40% saturation. This material is then subjected to chromatography on DEAE-cellulose, phosphocellulose, hydroxyapatite, and agarose A-1.5m columns.

The purity of this preparation was assessed by gel electrophoresis, as shown in FIGURE 4. The B protein preparation exhibits a single stained band after electrophoresis in both a nondenaturing gel system and in the presence of SDS. In the native state, the bound [^{3}H]progesterone migrated with the same R_f as did the protein band.

The molecular weight determined by SDS gel electrophoresis is 117,000 g/mol. As for the A subunit, the B protein appears to consist of a single polypeptide chain. The receptor B protein was also denatured with guanidine hydrochloride and analyzed by gel filtration. The molecular weight by this method was in agreement with the value obtained from gel filtration and sucrose gradient ultracentrifugation.[23] After denaturation with guanidine hydrochloride and gel filtration, the B protein again migrated in SDS gels as a single polypeptide chain of molecular weight 117,000 g/mol.

The purified receptor B subunit was also tested for functional activity. The B subunit labeled with [^{3}H]progesterone bound to both nuclei and chromatin with the same affinity as that exhibited by the crude and partially purified preparations and did not bind to DNA.[23] In addition, the hormone-binding characteristics of the purified [^{3}H]progesterone-labeled B subunit were unchanged from those of the starting material.[20]

We also compared the behavior of purified A and B subunits on gel filtration chromatography to that observed with crude cytosol. The results presented in FIGURE 5 show that the two purified subunits have different Stokes radii, with the larger B subunit eluting considerably ahead of the A subunit. In crude cytosol, these two subunits chromatograph as a broad peak,[22] which can be accounted for by an equal mixture of A and B subunits.

The receptor B subunit can be prepared from laying hen oviduct in sufficient quantities for physical and chemical analysis of the protein. When we examined the B protein by electron microscopy, it appeared to have an elongated shape, with a long axis of 114Å.[23] A protein of these dimensions would have a molecular weight of 106,000 g/mol, which is in excellent agreement with values obtained by other methods. The asymmetric shape is also consistent with the hydrodynamic behavior of the B protein.

The ultraviolet spectrum of the purified receptor B subunit exhibited a feature not characteristic of most proteins. The absorbance reached a peak at 280 nm but did not significantly decline in the region between 280 and 250 nm (TABLE 2). When the protein was denatured in guanidine hydrochloride and dialyzed, the absorbance at 250 nm decreased, indicating the loss of an ultraviolet-absorbing

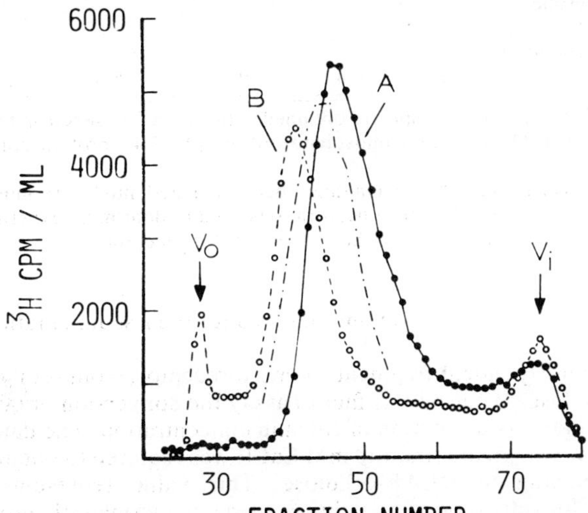

FIGURE 5. Gel filtration of the purified receptor subunits. Labeled complexes were chromatographed on a 5 × 50 cm agarose A-1.5m column in buffer A that contained 0.3 M KCl. Subunits B (○) and A (●) were run independently and compared to crude labeled cytosol mixture of A and B (— · —).

ligand, progesterone. When we added an equimolar amount of progesterone to the denatured, dialyzed receptor protein, the original ratio of absorbance at 280 and 250 nm was restored (TABLE 4). From the absorbance of receptor and progesterone, we calculated the stoichiometry of progesterone binding to be one molecule of progesterone bound per molecule of receptor B protein. If there is a similar stoichiometry of binding to the A subunit, there are two progesterone binding sites in the intact 6S dimer.

It was of interest to analyze the relationship of the A and B subunits to the smaller (mol wt 20,000 g/mol) hormone-binding component observed by Sherman *et al.*[24,25] This material is produced when oviduct cytosol is treated with high concentrations of calcium and is apparently not a subunit, as previously suggested,[24] but a proteolytic fragment. In addition to our failure to obtain a smaller subunit from the purified A or B protein by exhaustive denaturation, treatment of

TABLE 4

STOICHIOMETRY OF PROGESTERONE BINDING TO OVIDUCT RECEPTOR B SUBUNIT

Sample	Absorbance*		Concentration ($M \times 10^9$)			Steroid to Protein Molar Ratio
			Progesterone			
	250 nm	280 nm	Endogenous	Added	Protein	
Intact progesterone-receptor complex†	0.38	0.4	5.85	0	5.5	1.06:1
Receptor after Dialysis in guanidine hydrochloride‡	0.24	0.04	0	0	5.5	—
Free progesterone (1.84 μg/ml) added to denatured, receptor§	0.37	0.4	0	5.8	5.5	—

*Determined from absorption spectra obtained with a Cary 118 spectrophotometer.

†Prepared in 0.1 M potassium phosphate buffer (pH 7.4); protein concentration, 645 μg/ml.

‡Receptor dialyzed overnight in guanidine, then redialyzed into 0.1 M phosphate.

§One of a series of progesterone concentrations used to determine experimentally the extinction coefficient of progesterone in the presence of the receptor.

these purified proteins with calcium fails to alter their sedimentation or gel filtration behavior.

The calicum-dependent fragment, or mero-receptor,[22] binds extremely weakly to DEAE-cellulose. We used this fact to assay the conversion of cytosol receptor into mero-receptor as a function of calcium concentration. The data presented in FIGURE 6 show that greater than 10 mM $CaCl_2$ was required to obtain a marked reduction in binding to DEAE-cellulose. This value represents a threshold concentration for activation of a calcium-dependent cytoplasmic protease.

We also examined the effects of lower calcium concentrations on the aggregation behavior of the receptor as measured by sucrose gradient centrifugation. While concentrations of calcium below 10^{-4} had no significant effect on the receptor, treatment with 10^{-3} M Ca^{2+} resulted in a substantial shift from 6S to 8S (FIGURE 7). This shift, however, was not accompanied by the appearance of mero-

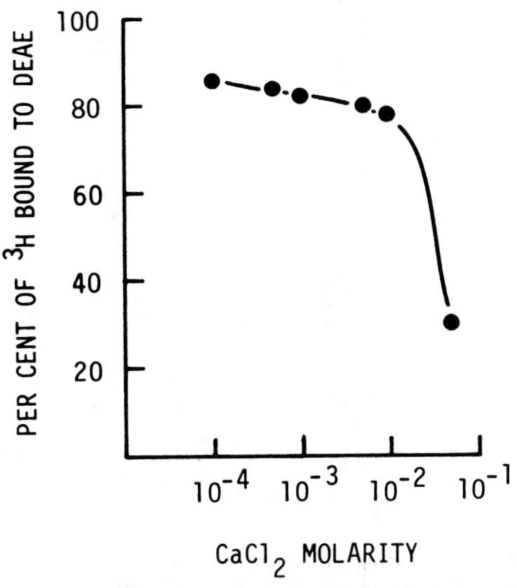

FIGURE 6. Rapid assay of progesterone receptor degradation by calcium ion-dependent protease in oviduct cytosol. Small DEAE columns (1.0 ml) were used to adsorb labeled intact progesterone receptors or their subunits. Cytosol was treated for 30 min at 0°C with the indicated calcium chloride molarities and was then diluted and adsorbed to DEAE-cellulose. The columns were washed in 0.05 M KCl in buffer A, and then receptors that remained on the columns were eluted with 0.3 M KCl and assayed for [^{3}H]progesterone.

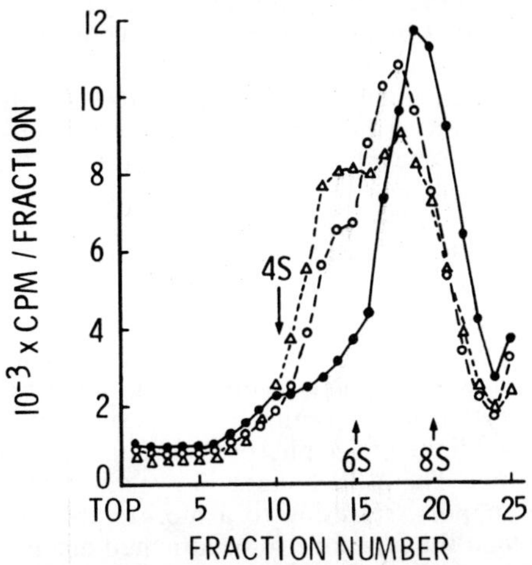

FIGURE 7. Effect of calcium on receptor aggregation state. Varying concentrations of calcium chloride were added to [^{3}H]protesterone-labeled cytosol, and samples were incubated for 1 hr at 0°C. The receptor samples were then analyzed by sucrose gradient ultracentrifugation in buffer A without potassium chloride. Profiles show results of calcium ion treatment at 10^{-5} M (△), 10^{-4} M (○), and 10^{-3} M (●). Concentrations at or below 10^{-5} M were without effect on the profile and were identical to control profile shown in FIGURE 8.

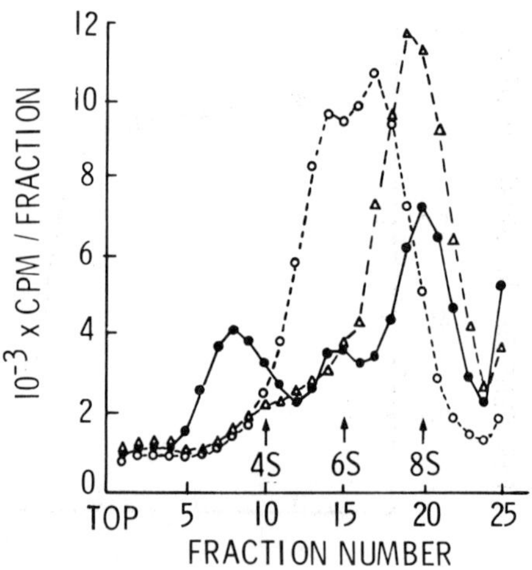

FIGURE 8. Effect of high calcium ion concentrations on proteolytic and aggregation events in chick cytosol. Experiments were performed as described in FIGURE 7. Calcium concentrations were: control (○), 1 mM (△), and 30 mM (●).

receptor sedimenting at 2.6S. When even higher concentrations of Ca^{2+} were added (FIGURE 8), production of 2.6S fragments was noted with a concomitant reduction of the 8S peak. After prolonged storage (12 hr) in 30 mM Ca^{2+}, complete conversion of all of the receptors to the 2.6S species occurred (data not shown). Thus, it appears that the calcium ion effect involves two distinct steps: a calcium ion-dependent aggregation of intact receptor 6S dimers to 8S, presumably by association of the dimer with a cytoplasmic protease, and then, at high calcium ion concentrations (or extended times), a proteolytic event that converts both A and B subunits to the 2.6S fragment.

These calcium ion-dependent events occur at calcium concentrations far greater than those observed in the cytoplasm of normal cells. However, the fact that similar behavior is observed with other steroid hormone receptors[26,27] suggests that the proteolytic cleavage of receptor may be important in receptor function *in vivo*. Preliminary evidence from this laboratory suggests that mero-receptor is no longer capable of binding to DNA or chromatin. This event may therefore relate to the mechanism of receptor release from the nucleus.

The purification procedures described above for receptor subunits are not appropriate for the intact 6S dimer, due to the high salt concentrations necessary for elution of receptor from ion-exchange columns. We therefore employed the technique of steroid affinity chromatography.[19] The resin used contains deoxycorticosterone hemisuccinate linked to Sepharose® through a denatured bovine serum albumin (BSA) backbone. This BSA linkage allows multiple attachment points for the hormone to the support, resulting to a more stable resin, and performs a spacer function, allowing the hormone to be attached distant from the Sepharose beads.

The intact 6S dimer was precipitated from oviduct cytosol with ammonium sulfate to 50% saturation.

This procedure removed enzymatic activities that cause the release to deoxycorticosterone from the affinity resin. The receptor was redissolved in buffer A and incubated with the resin overnight at 0°C. The resin was then washed to remove unbound protein and eluted with an excess of [^{3}H]progesterone (20 μM) as previously described.[19] The affinity eluate was then purified by DEAE-Sephadex® chromatography to yield receptor in homogeneous form. Two equal bands can be seen on SDS-polyacrylamide gels that comigrate with the A and B proteins prepared by the procedures described above.

One major problem encountered with this procedure has been low yield of receptor from the affinity resin. We have recently determined that this low yield is due to extremely efficient coupling of steroid to the affinity resin. The yield of receptor obtained by Kuhn *et al.*[19] from the affinity resin was approximately 70%. However, when resins that contained as much as 20-fold more bound hormone were used, the yield was reduced to about 4% (TABLE 5). One possible explanation is that the local concentration of bound steroid on the resin is so high that 20 μM [^{3}H]progesterone in the elution buffer cannot effectively compete for the hormone-binding site of the receptor attached to the affinity resin.

The yield could be improved to the original levels by dilution of the resin approximately 40-fold with unsubstituted Sepharose. However, this procedure also resulted in a substantial dilution of the receptor in the affinity eluate. Because we have not found an effective procedure for the concentration of the purified receptor, we examined a second approach for improving the efficiency of affinity resin elution. Rather than decreasing the concentration of bound steroid on the column, we increased the concentration of competing [^{3}H]progesterone in the elution mixture, from 20 to 800 μM. Progesterone is not soluble at this concentration in aqueous solution, so we added 15% dioxane to decrease the dielectric constant of the solution. Fortunately, this concentration of dioxane does not adversely affect the intact 6S receptor dimer. The resultant yield, show in TABLE 5, is comparable to previous results, and the concentration of receptor in the affinity column eluate is even greater than before, due to the higher capacity of the resin for receptor.

The purity and concentration of intact 6S receptor dimer obtained by this procedure are adequate for use in the *in vitro* assay for chromatin transcription.[14] However, because there is always dissociation of intact 6S receptor into subunits, a final purification step was employed. The affinity eluate, after removal of the

TABLE 5
EFFECT OF AFFINITY RESIN CAPACITY AND ELUTION TECHNIQUE ON RECEPTOR YIELD

Resin Capacity (nmol of receptor/ml of resin)*	Elution Technique†	Yield (%)	Receptor Concentration in Eluate (M)
0.2	20 μM [^{3}H]progesterone‡	61‡	10^{-8}
>10	20 μM [^{3}H]progesterone	4	$<10^{-9}$
>10	20 μM [^{3}H]progesterone; resin diluted 40-fold with unsubstituted agarose	70	$<10^{-9}$
>10	800 μM [^{3}H]progesterone in buffer A + 15% dioxane	70	5×10^{-8}

*Affinity resin was incubated with increasing concentrations of receptor, and the capacity was determined as the point of receptor appearance in the affinity column drop-through.

†Concentration of competing [^{3}H]progesterone added to elution buffer and other modifications.

‡Conditions and results reported by Kuhn *et al.*[19]

dioxane by Sephadex G-75 gel filtration, was passed over a small phosphocellulose column to remove the 4S subunits. The left-hand panel of FIGURE 9 shows the sucrose gradient centrifugation analysis of the afinity eluate is an approximately equal mixture of 4S and 6S receptor components, while the phosphocellulose drop-through fraction consists largely of intact 6S receptor dimer. As will be described in detail in a subsequent article in this monograph,[28] the latter fraction is extremely active in stimulating transcription of oviduct chromatin by RNA polymerase *in vitro*. The right-hand panel of FIGURE 9 shows the effect of increasing concentrations of intact 6S dimer of transcription of chromatin and DNA. Transcription of chromatin is stimulated approximately 50%, whereas DNA is not affected. The latter result is consistent with the fact that the 6S dimer does not bind to DNA.

DISCUSSION

It is evident from the results presented above that our understanding of receptor action *in vivo* is dependent on our knowledge of receptor subunit structure. Our results with the chick oviduct progesterone receptor are consistent with the model shown in FIGURE 10. The intact receptor is a protein of approximately 200,000 molecular weight, which contains two dissimilar hormone-binding subunits. Dissociation of the intact dimer into subunits can be accomplished by warming or treatment with salt and is facilitated by occupancy of the hormone-binding sites.

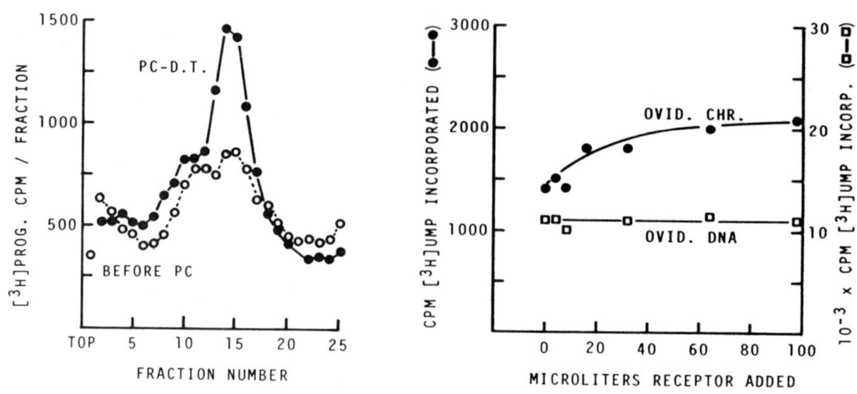

FIGURE 9. Effect of intact 6S receptor dimer on transcription of oviduct chromatin. Chick oviduct cytosol was precipitated with ammonium sulfate to 50% saturation, redissolved in buffer A, and purified by affinity chromatography.[19] *Left:* Receptor prepared by this method was analyzed by sucrose gradient ultracentrifugation in buffer A without potassium chloride. Profile after affinity chromatography (○); profile of unadsorbed fraction after subsequent chromatography on phosphocellulose (●). *E. coli* alkaline phosphatase (6.3S) was in fraction 15. *Right:* Receptors after phosphocellulose chromatography were tested for activity in regulation of chromatin transcription with the rifampicin challenge assay.[14] Receptor was added either to 5 μg of oviduct chromatin (○) from chicks stimulated with diethylstilbestrol for 14 days and then withdrawn for 14 days or to 2.5 μg of oviduct DNA (□). After incubation at room temperature, excess *E. coli* RNA polymerase was added during a second incubation. Finally, rifampicin and nucleoside triphosphates were added to start RNA synthesis, and RNA chain initiation was measured by [^{3}H] uridine monophosphate incorporation, as previously described.[14]

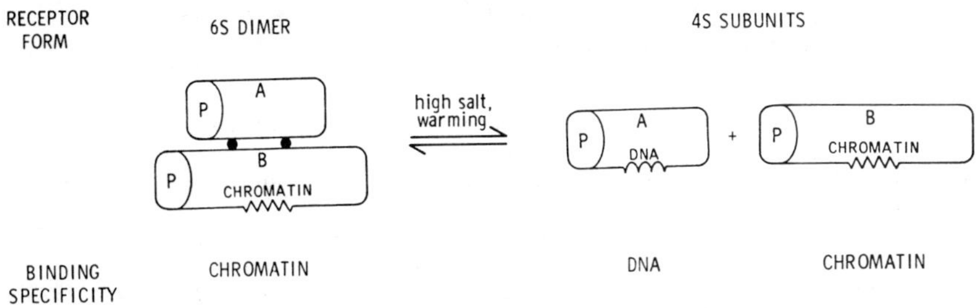

FIGURE 10. Proposed progesterone receptor subunit structure. Two 4S subunits, A and B, combine to form the intact 6S progesterone receptor dimer. Each subunit has one hormone-binding site (P). The B subunit (mol wt 115,000) has an exposed chromatin-binding site, but the DNA-binding site on the A subunit (mol wt 79,000) is not expressed. Treatment of the complex by high ionic strength or warming causes dissociation into subunits and activation of the DNA activity of the A subunit.

The two subunits have differing specificities for binding to nuclear components: the A subunit binds only to DNA, whereas B binds only to chromatin. Both activities appear to be essential for hormonal action *in vivo*. Although both subunits are present in the intact dimer, only the chromatin-binding activity of the B subunit is expressed. Dissociation of the dimer into subunits is necessary for activation of the DNA-binding site of the A subunit.

In addition to these features, the receptor subunits both contain a region that is susceptible to cleavage by a cytoplasmic calcium activated protease. We do not yet understand either the structural relationship of the hormond-binding fragment to the intact receptor subunits or the functional role of this phenomenon in receptor action.

Finally, we have succeeded in purifying both receptor subunits and the intact 6S dimer to homogeneity. These preparations can now be used to study the physical and biochemical characteristics of the receptor proteins and to investigate their effect on gene transcription in a purified *in vitro* assay system. We envision that these approaches will lead to an understanding of steroid hormone action at the molecular level.

ACKNOWLEDGMENTS

We thank S. S. Heuer and A. Johnson for their technical assistance. Thanks are also extended to Dr. R. J. Schwartz for performing the transcription assays.

REFERENCES

1. JENSEN, E. V. & E. R. DESOMBRE. 1974. Vitamins Hormones **32:** 89–127.
2. O'MALLEY, B. W. & A. R. MEANS. 1974. Science **183:** 610–620.
3. SCHRADER, W. T. & B. W. O'MALLEY. 1971. J. Biol. Chem. **247:** 51–59.
4. CLARK, J. C., E. J. PECK, W. T. SCHRADER & B. W. O'MALLEY. 1976. Methods Cancer Res. **12:** 367–417.
5. SCHRADER, W. T., D. O. TOFT & B. W. O'MALLEY. 1972. J. Biol. Chem. **241:** 2401–2407.
6. O'MALLEY, B. W., D. O. TOFT & M. R. SHERMAN. 1971. J. Biol. Chem. **246:** 1117–1122.

7. O'Malley, B. W., T. C. Spelsberg, W. T. Schrader, F. Chytil & A. W. Steggles. 1972. Nature (London) **235:** 141–144.
8. Spelsberg, T. C., A. W. Steggles & B. W. O'Malley. 1971. J. Biol. Chem. **246:** 4188–4197.
9. Spelsberg, T. C., A. W. Steggles, F. Chytil & B. W. O'Malley. 1972. J. Biol. Chem. **247:** 1368–1374.
10. Jaffe, R. C., S. H. Socher & B. W. O'Malley. 1975. Biochim. Biophys. Acta **399:** 403–419.
11. O'Malley, B. W. & W. T. Schrader. 1972. J. Steroid Biochem. **3:** 617–629.
12. Schrader, W. T., S. S. Heuer & B. W. O'Malley, 1975. Biol. Reprod. **12:** 134–142.
13. Harris, S. E., R. J. Schwartz, M.-J. Tsai, B. W. O'Malley & A. Roy. 1976. J. Biol. Chem. **251:** 524–529.
14. Tsai, M.-J., R. J. Schwartz, S. Y. Tsai & B. W. O'Malley. 1975. J. Biol. Chem. **250:** 5165–5174.
15. Sherman, M. R., P. L. Corvol & B. W. O'Malley. 1970. J. Biol. Chem. **245:** 6068–6096.
16. Stancel, G. M., K. M. T. Leung & J. Gorski. 1973. Biochemistry **12:** 2130–2136.
17. Norris, J. S. & P. O. Kohler. 1976. Science **192:** 898–900.
18. Buller, R. E., R. J. Schwartz & B. W. O'Malley. 1976. Biochem. Biophys. Res. Commun. **69:** 106–113.
19. Kuhn, R. W., W. T. Schrader, R. G. Smith & B. W. O'Malley. 1975. J. Biol. Chem. **250:** 4220–4228.
20. Schrader, W. T., R. W. Kuhn & B. W. O'Malley. 1976. J. Biol. Chem. In press.
21. Coty, W. A., W. T. Schrader & W. B. O'Malley. 1976. J. Biol. Chem. Submitted for publication.
22. Sherman, M. R., F. B. Tuazon, S. C. Diaz & L. K. Miller. 1976. Biochemistry **15:** 980–989.
23. Kuhn, R. W., W. T. Schrader, W. A. Coty, P. M. Conn & B. W. O'Malley. 1976. J. Biol. Chem. In press.
24. Sherman, M. R., S. B. P. Atienza, J. R. Shansky & L. M. Hoffman. 1974. J. Biol. Chem. **249:** 5351–5363.
25. Miller, L. K., S. C. Diaz & M. R. Sherman. 1975. Biochemistry **14:** 4433–4443.
26. Puca, G. A., E. Nola, V. Sica & F. Bresciani. 1972. Biochemistry **11:** 4157–4165.
27. Edelman, I. S. 1972. J. Steroid Biochem. **3:** 167–172.
28. Schwartz, R. J., C. Chang, W. T. Schrader & B. W. O'Malley. This monograph.
29. Schrader, W. T., R. E. Buller & S. H. Socher. 1975. Methods Enzymol. **36:** 292–313.
30. Baxter, J. D., D. V. Santi & G. G. Rousseau. 1975. Methods Enzymol. **36:** 234–239.
31. Weber, K. & M. J. Osborn. 1969. J. Biol. Chem. **244:** 4406–4412.
32. Tindall, D. J., V. Hansson, W. S. McLean, E. M. Ritzen, S. N. Nayfeh & F. S. French. 1975. Mol. Cell. Endocrinol. **3:** 83–101.

Discussion

Dr. R. J. B. King: You said that the intact 6S receptor will not bind to DNA, and yet it will promote RNA chain initiation in the chromatin assays. Is there a discrepancy here, or do you have an explanation?

Dr. Schrader: We think that there is an obligatory dissociation of the two subunits at a gene site that the receptor regulates. Dr. O'Malley will describe that model in considerable detail during his talk. We think that the initial interaction involves the intact AB dimer recognizing a chromatin acceptor site via the B subunit. Then there follows a dissociation of the A-B complex, liberating the A subunit with a functional DNA-binding activity. The DNA binder does its thing at the gene site.

DR. T. C. SPELSBERG: Dr. Schrader, I was interested in seeing that your B-binding affinity for chromatin was about the same value as we calculated by other techniques. Did you say that the affinity of the subunit for DNA was $K_d = 10^{-11}$ M?

DR. SCHRADER: Yes, I didn't show that information. The experiments are preliminary, but that's apparently what the K_d is going to turn out to be.

DR. SPELSBERG: Do you ever worry about the steroid dissociating from the receptor during those assays?

DR. SCHRADER: Fortunately, the time course for dissociation of the hormone from the receptor takes quite a while, whereas the DNA-binding reaction seems to be much more rapid. Thus, one can prepare steroid-receptor complexes with all of the hormone bound and with no free hormone present. True, that's a nonequilibrium situation, but it's going to take hours to come to equilibrium. However, the receptor binding to chromatin, to DNA, and the initiation of transcription reactions all occur much more rapidly. So it's a theoretical problem but is of no practical concern as far as I'm aware.

DR. E. MILGROM: On the slide, you showed purified receptor binding to chromatin. The pattern was very different from the one shown by Dr. Spelsberg. You showed only one class of saturable sites, whereas he showed three such classes. Is this due to the experimental conditions, to the purification of the receptor, or to other reasons?

DR. SCHRADER: I don't know how to put the two sets of information in register. At the time those experiments were done, I was not aware of Dr. Spelsberg's findings. Earlier, in a paper published by Richard Buller from our group, we looked at the kinetics of binding of receptors to nuclei and showed that the reaction was profoundly affected by the ionic strength. The number of receptors bound to nuclei changed with the conditions. Our interpretation was that the binding assay was not sufficiently precise to allow us to detect small differences in equilibrium constant for those various numbers of sites. So, I simply have not done that experiment the way Dr. Spelsberg has described it, with the purified material. However, the transcription information that Dr. O'Malley will show is consistent with the notion that the sites that we have described here are those that are functional *in vitro* during RNA chain initiation.

QUESTION: Have you been able to prepare antibodies to either A or B subunits?

DR. SCHRADER: With respect to the first question, no, I have not. I can supply to anyone who is interested a large number of rabbits injected with the purified B protein, which contains no detectable antibody!

QUESTION: In your attempts to prepare antibodies to the B protein, have you made sure that you had the protein loaded with steroid?

DR. SCHRADER: We prepared receptor that had hormone on it at the time that it was mixed with the adjuvant. This complex was then exhaustively homogenized at room temperature in a Waring blender. Such a procedure, the classic method of preparing an antigen, would be expected to cause the hormone to come off the protein. However, at the time that the protein was added into the adjuvant, there was hormone on it.

DR. KING. Are you suggesting that you need the steroid on the receptor to get a true antibody?

DR. SCHRADER: I'm not suggesting anything, Dr. King. I'm just curious as to why the attempts to prepare antibody have been unsuccessful. I think this is a rather striking situation that may have some general implications about receptors.

DR. M. LIPPMAN: With reference to Dr. Milgrom's question, if you look closely at one of your graphs, you will see inflections at almost the point that Dr. Spelsberg has them, and certainly if you look at Richard Buller's paper, you will see those same inflections, so I don't think there is any real problem there. Since progesterone receptors and corticoid receptors share affinities rather closely, is it not possible that during purification you copurify corticoid receptors that bind progesterone?

DR. SCHRADER: That's a very good point. I speculated on that some time ago, and Richard Buller did the following study. He prepared the receptors by a modification of the differential chromatography technique and did so in the absence of any hormones. He took cytosol and blindly went through the procedure. Then, at the end, he measured binding of various labeled steroids to the extract. The only one that would bind was progesterone. He has subsequently looked at hen liver glucocorticoid receptor and found that it elutes from ion-exchange columns differently than progesterone receptor does. So, although these are very similar, they do not have identical isolectric points and do not have identical behavior on a variety of systems. So, apparently, the techniques used will indeed separate the different receptors from each other.

DISCUSSION PAPER: MERO-RECEPTOR FORMATION FROM A LARGER SUBCOMPONENT OF THE OVIDUCT PROGESTERONE RECEPTOR*

Merry R. Sherman† and Soledad C. Diaz

Memorial Sloan-Kettering Cancer Center
New York, New York 10021

In the initial characterization of [^{3}H]progesterone-labeled macromolecules in chick oviduct cytosol, Sherman *et al.*[1] described two proteins, A_1 and A_2, that (1) were stimulated or diminished in parallel on administration or withdrawal of *in vivo* estrogen treatment; (2) had similar or identical affinities for progesterone, indicated by linear plots of (bound steroid)$^{-1}$ vs (free steroid)$^{-1}$ for the mixture; (3) were partially resolved and shown to have large Stokes radii by agarose gel filtration in 0.3 M KCl; (4) sedimented as a single 4S peak in KCl-containing density gradients, indicating highly asymmetric shapes in view of the large Stokes radii; and (5), in low salt media, formed large aggregates that were analyzed by gel filtration, electrophoresis, and ultracentrifugation. The next step was to analyze the complexes extracted from nuclei by KCl after oviduct slices and [^{3}H]progesterone were warmed to 37°C. Agarose filtration of the nuclear extract revealed equal quantities of the same two components, A_1 and A_2, that were found in oviduct cytosol.[2] This result implied that A_1 and A_2 were transferred to the nuclei by a concerted mechanism and that both were involved in the subsequent nuclear events. In a later study, the two [^{3}H]progesterone-labeled complexes eluted from diethylaminoethyl (DEAE) -cellulose columns by low and high KCl concentrations were identified as the A and B subunits,[3] but their relationships to forms A_1 and A_2 of Sherman *et al.*[1] were not established.

More recently, Sherman *et al.*[4] showed the correlations among the complexes detected by gel electrophoresis, chromatography on DEAE columns or filters, protamine precipitation, and gel filtration. They numbered the receptor forms in order of elution from agarose in high-salt buffer, starting with the aggregates at the void volume, I, followed by the two included peaks II and III (A_1 and A_2 of the earlier publication[1]). With the electrophoretic procedure of Miller *et al.*,[5] they demonstrated the apparent identity of form II from gel filtration with the high-salt eluate from DEAE (B)[3] and the similarity of form III from gel filtration with the low-salt eluate from DEAE (A).[3]

A further step in the analysis of this receptor was the demonstration by Sherman *et al.*[6] that all of the determinants of specific, high-affinity steroid binding resided in a portion of the receptor with a molecular weight of about 20,000. This moiety, later termed the "mero-receptor" by analogy with the fragments of myosin,[4] had the following properties: it was obtained in the presence of specific divalent cations, including Ca^{2+} but not Mg^{2+}; it had the same equilibrium dissociation constants for a wide range of steroids as does unfractionated cytosol;

*Supported in part by Grants CA-16814, CA-08748, and HL-06285 from the United States Public Health Service and by the Paul Garrett Fund.

†On leave, 1975–76, at the Cardiovascular Research Institute, University of California Medical School, San Francisco, Calif. 94143.

and it could be prepared in 77% yield from cytosol. Because forms II and III each contribute 50% of the progesterone-binding sites in cytosol,[1] these findings implied that the mero-receptor was formed from both of the larger components. The present report describes the direct conversion of a partially purified preparation of form II (B) into the mero-receptor in the presence of Ca^{2+}.

Materials and Methods

Rhode Island Red chicks were injected with diethylstilbestrol, oviducts were excised, cytosol was prepared, labeled with 4×10^{-8} M [^{3}H]progesterone, and frozen, as previously described.[1,6] All procedures were performed at 4°C. The homogenization buffer was 10 mM *N*-tris(hydroxymethyl)methyl-2-aminoethanesulfonic acid (Tes), 12 mM thioglycerol, pH 7.4 at 4°C (Tes-thioglycerol), that contained 0.25 M sucrose. The cytosol contained about 17 mg of protein per milliliter, as measured by the method of Waddell[7] with bovine serum albumin (BSA) used as the standard. L-[^{14}C]-Valine (260 mCi/mmol) was obtained from Schwarz/Mann, and [1,2,6,7-^{3}H]progesterone (105 Ci/mmol) came from New England Nuclear. [^{3}H]Progesterone of this high specific activity was stored at 4°C in benzene rather than ethanol, because polar impurities were detected in the latter solutions by thin-layer chromatography in cyclohexane:ethyl acetate (1:1). Radioactivity was measured as previously described.[6] In double-isotope experiments, the counting efficiencies in the two channels were 42 and 0% for tritium and 24 and 68% for ^{14}C. The net counts per minute contributed by [^{3}H]progesterone were calculated by the channels ratio method. Bound steroid in labeled samples was evaluated by treatment with dextran-coated charcoal.[6]

Preparative ion-exchange filtration was performed on DEAE filters (Whatman DE-81) in a Hoefer model FH-204 manifold.[4,8] Labeled cytosol (0.1 ml) was adsorbed to filters, and unbound steroid and proteins were removed by five 1-ml washes with Tes-thioglycerol. Some filters were counted to assess total adsorbed steroid; others were extracted with 0.5 ml of 0.5 M KCl or sequentially with 0.5 ml of 0.15 M KCl, twice with 1 ml of 0.15 M KCl, 0.5 ml of 0.5 M KCl, and 1 ml of 0.5 M KCl. All extracting solutions contained Tes-thioglycerol; ovalbumin (5 mg/ml) was added to reduce differences in protein concentration among the extracts, except when endogenous proteins were being measured. Potassium chloride was added to the low-salt filter extracts to give the same salt concentration in all extracts during tests of mero-receptor formation.

In preliminary experiments, aliquots of the first low-salt, first high-salt, and the 0.15–0.5 M KCl extracts were incubated at 4°C for various times with various concentrations of $CaCl_2$ or ethylene glycol bis(β-aminoethyl ether)-*N,N'*-tetraacetate (EGTA). Mero-receptor formation after various treatments of each extract (e.g., $\pm$ $CaCl_2$) was assessed by filtration on duplicate columns (24×1.27 cm) of agarose A-0.5m (BioRad®) mounted on opposite sides of an LKB UltroRac® fraction collector. The columns were eluted with 0.4 M KCl, 10% (w/v) glycerol in TES-thioglycerol, and standardized with BSA, ovalbumin, and myoglobin. The total liquid volume (V_t) was marked by [^{14}C]valine, and the void volume (V_0) was marked by the small peak of receptor aggregates or by blue dextran (Pharmacia) in experiments without receptors. The distribution coefficients (K_D) of standards or receptors were calculated from their elution volumes (V_e) as usual: $K_D = (V_e - V_0)/(V_t - V_0)$.[9]

Results and Discussion

Charcoal-dextran treatment of oviduct cytosol labeled with 4 × 10^{-8} M [^{3}H]progesterone indicated that 63% of the total steroid was bound. Aliquots of this cytosol were adsorbed to DEAE filters and eluted with various concentrations of KCl. The recoveries of [^{3}H]progesterone and endogenous proteins after various elution procedures are summarized in Table 1. When the filters were extracted twice with 0.5 M KCl (direct high-salt elution), about 85% of the bound steroid was recovered in the extracts, but little purification of the receptors was achieved. In the sequential elution procedure, 71% of the bound steroid was recovered in the combined extracts. While the receptors in the first 0.15 M KCl extract had lower specific activity (0.69 pmol of [^{3}H]progesterone/mg of protein) than in cytosol, those in the subsequent high-salt extract were purified about 2.6-fold.

Table 1

Fractionation of Receptors by Adsorption to and Elution from DEAE Filters

Preparation	Cytoplasmic Protein (mg/ml ± SEM) (*n*)*	[^{3}H]Progesterone (% of total ± SEM) (*n*)*	[^{3}H]Progesterone (pmol/mg of protein)
Cytosol-untreated,		100.	
charcoal-treated	16.9 ± 0.4 (4)	63.1 ± 0.3 (4)	1.49
Direct high-salt elution			
Combined washes		39.1 ± 1.3(12)	
0.5 M KCl Extract 1	1.81 ± 0.00 (4)	45.9 ± 3.8 (3)	2.03
Extract 2		7.9 ± 1.2 (3)	
Left on filter		3.2 ± 0.8 (3)	
Total bound†		57.0	
Total recovered		96.1	
Sequential elution			
Combined washes		39.1 ± 1.3 (12)	
0.15 M KCl Extract 1	1.29 ± 0.01 (4)	11.2 ± 0.6 (9)	0.69
Extract 2		6.1 ± 0.2 (9)	
Extract 3		3.2 ± 0.1 (2)	
0.5 M KCl Extract 1	0.43 ± 0.00 (4)	21.4 ± 0.8 (7)	3.98
Extract 2		2.8 ± 0.2 (7)	
Left on filter		4.2 ± 0.3 (7)	
Total bound†		48.9	
Total recovered		88.0	

*Number of experiments, each including two to five filters.

†Total bound was calculated from the sum of all extracts and residual steroid on the filter; the combined washes are assumed to contain the free steroid.

The receptors in the sequential low- and high-salt filter extracts have previously been resolved from each other and identified as forms III and II, respectively, by filtration on long agarose columns (110 × 1.27 cm).[4,10] On the shorter columns used in the present study (24 × 1.27 cm), forms II and III had distribution coefficients of 0.33 and 0.42, respectively, but were not clearly resolved from each other (Figure 1, a and b, open symbols). The labeled complexes in the direct

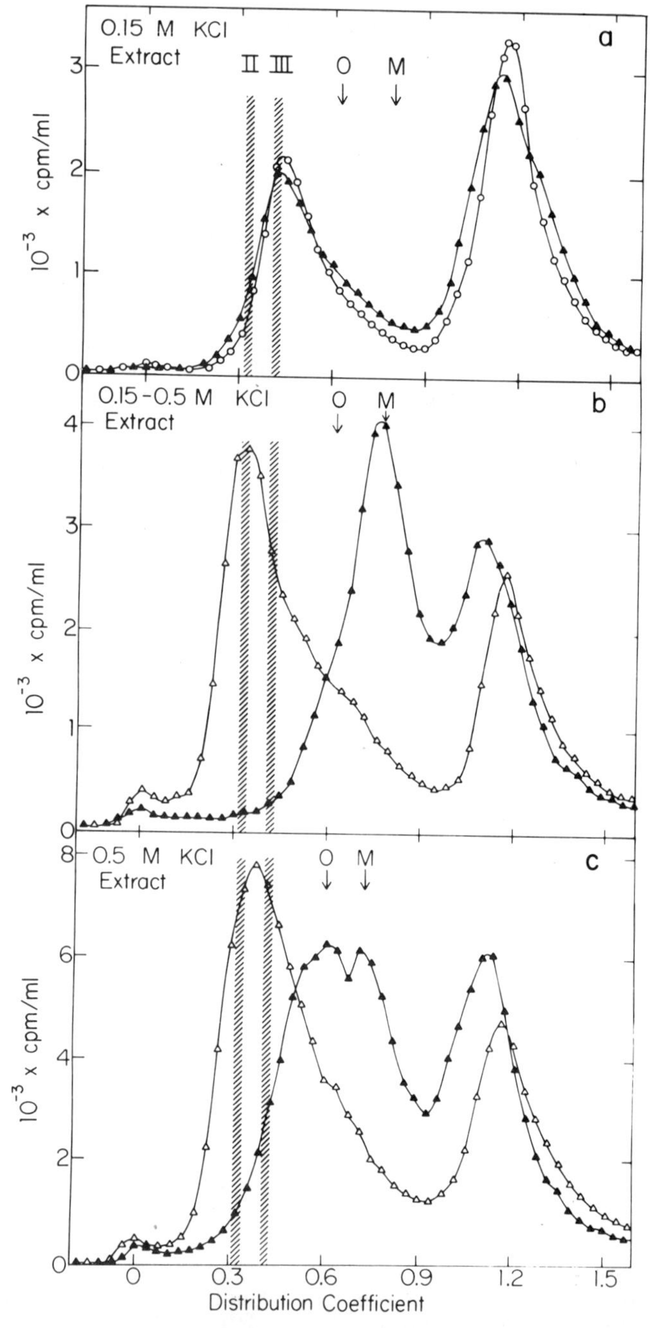

FIGURE 1. Mero-receptor formation in DEAE filter extracts of progesterone receptors analyzed by gel filtration. All procedures were performed at 4°C; all extracts contained 5 mg of ovalbumin/ml in Tes-thioglycerol. [^{3}H]Progesterone-labeled oviduct cytosol was adsorbed to DEAE filters (0.1 ml of cytosol/filter). The filters were washed with Tes-thioglycerol and extracted with 0.5 ml of either (a) 0.15 M KCl (low salt), (b) 0.5 M KCl (high salt)

high-salt filter extract, which contains both forms II and III, were eluted as a single broad peak (FIGURE 1, c, open symbols). On the other hand, these large receptor forms were clearly separated from the mero-receptor, K_D = 0.76, which cochromatographed with myoglobin (FIGURE 1, b, solid symbols).

FIGURE 1, a shows that incubation of the low-salt filter extract with 20 mM $CaCl_2$ for 2 hr did not alter the gel filtration pattern. Higher concentrations of $CaCl_2$ (up to 0.1 M) were similarly ineffective. By contrast, the labeled complexes in the 0.15–0.5 M KCl filter extract were nearly completely converted to the mero-receptor by 20 mM $CaCl_2$ (FIGURE 1, b). A 2-hr incubation without added $CaCl_2$ resulted in a broad distribution of complexes of intermediate size. The latter changes were minimized by addition of the chelating agent, EGTA. The elution profiles of both the $CaCl_2$- and the EGTA-treated samples had a shoulder of radioactivity in the region of the standard protein ovalbumin.

Several interpretations of the foregoing results were considered. (1) Receptor form II is more susceptible than III or is uniquely susceptible to the direct or protease-mediated effects of $CaCl_2$ under these conditions. (2) Both forms II and III are susceptible, but the low-salt filter extract contains some inhibitor(s) of the conversion process. (3) The 0.15–0.5 M KCl extract contains a Ca^{2+}-activated protease that is absent from the low-salt extract.

The results in FIGURE 1, c permitted a preliminary choice among these alternatives. The direct high-salt filter extract contains both receptor forms II and III and presumably all of the proteases and/or inhibitors that are present in the sequential extracts. Gel filtration of the total extract after exposure to $CaCl_2$ indicated a loss of the largest component, form II, a partial conversion to the mero-receptor, and a mixture of components of intermediate size. The observation of significant mero-receptor formation in the total extract provided evidence against alternative 2 above. If an inhibitor were present in the low-salt extract, its presence in sufficient concentration in the total extract could have blocked the formation of mero-receptor from both forms II and III.

The effect of Ca^{2+} on the direct high-salt extract resembled its effect on whole cytosol: a portion of the receptors were converted to the mero-receptor (form V) and the remainder to a complex of intermediate size (form IV).[4,6] The present study showed that the transforming activity is adsorbed to DEAE filters, is retained after the elution of receptor form III by 0.15 M KCl, but is eluted together with form II by 0.5 M KCl. Form II (B)[3] is converted to the mero-receptor in various states of purification. In contrast, form III (A)[3] is converted to the mero-receptor in the precipitated state (after protamine treatment or isoelectric focusing)[6] but to form IV in whole cytosol or in the total filter extract.

These results support the notion that the mero-receptor is formed by a cleavage process and does not exist as a separate polypeptide chain in the native

---

after three low-salt extractions, or (c) 0.5 M KCl without prior extraction. Corresponding extracts from replicate filters were pooled, and 0.4-ml aliquots were incubated for 2 hr after the following additions: (a) The KCl concentration of the low-salt extract was brought to 0.5 M, to match that of the extracts in (b) and (c). One aliquot (▲) was made 20 mM in $CaCl_2$, the other (○) was not treated further. (b) Aliquots of the 0.5 M KCl extract, after low-salt extraction, were made 20 mM in either $CaCl_2$ (▲) or EGTA (Δ). (c) Aliquots of the high-salt extract, without prior extraction, were treated as in (b). The treated extracts were analyzed simultaneously in 30-ml columns of agarose A-0.5m in 0.4 M KCl, 10% (w/v) glycerol, Tes-thioglycerol. Standard proteins ovalbumin (O) and myoglobin (M) were monitored optically, and distribution coefficients (K_D) were calculated as described in MATERIALS AND METHODS. The average K_Ds for forms II (B),[3] III (A),[3] and the mero-receptor were 0.33, 0.42, and 0.76, respectively.

receptor. Its potential importance lies in the fact that it should permit the isolation of the intact steroid-binding site in a complex of manageable molecular size. Determination of the amino acid sequence and crystallographic analyses of the three-dimensional structure of the mero-receptor, both with and without the bound steroid, would vastly increase our understanding of the strength and specificity of the steroid-protein interaction.

References

1. Sherman, M. R., P. L. Corvol & B. W. O'Malley. 1970. Progesterone-binding components of chick oviduct. I. Preliminary characterization of cytoplasmic components. J. Biol. Chem. **245:** 6085–6096.
2. O'Malley, B. W., D. O. Toft & M. R. Sherman. 1971. Progesterone-binding components of chick oviduct. II. Nuclear components. J. Biol. Chem. **246:** 1117–1122.
3. Schrader, W. T. & B. W. O'Malley. 1972. Progesterone-binding components of chick oviduct. IV. Characterization of purified subunits. J. Biol. Chem. **247:** 51–59.
4. Sherman, M. R., F. B. Tuazon, S. C. Diaz & L. K. Miller. 1976. Multiple forms of oviduct progesterone receptor analyzed by ion exchange filtration and gel electrophoresis. Biochemistry **15:** 980–989.
5. Miller, L. K., S. C. Diaz & M. R. Sherman. 1975. Steroid-receptor quantitation and characterization by electrophoresis in highly cross-linked polyacrylamide gels. Biochemistry **14:** 4433–4443.
6. Sherman, M. R., S. B. P. Atienza, J. R. Shansky & L. M. Hoffman. 1974. Progesterone receptors of chick oviduct. Steroid-binding "subunit" formed with divalent cations. J. Biol. Chem. **249:** 5351–5363.
7. Waddell, W. J. 1956. A simple ultraviolet spectrophotometric method for the determination of protein. J. Lab. Clin. Med. **48:** 311–314.
8. Santi, D. V., C. H. Sibley, E. R. Perriard, G. M. Tomkins & J. D. Baxter. 1973. A filter assay for steroid hormone receptors. Biochemistry **12:** 2412–2416.
9. Gelotte, B. J. 1960. Studies on gel filtration. Sorption properties of the bed material Sephadex. J. Chromatog. **3:** 330–342.
10. Sherman, M. R. & L. K. Miller. 1976. Fractionation of diverse steroid-binding proteins: basic and clinical applications. *In* Steroid Hormone Action and Cancer. K. M. J. Menon & J. R. Reel, Eds.: 51–67. Plenum Publishing Corporation. New York, N.Y.

RECEPTORS IN BREAST CANCER: AN INTRODUCTION

J. P. Raynaud

Centre de Recherches Roussel UCLAF
93230 Romainville, France

Human breast cancer is a field in which fundamental studies on hormone-receptor interactions seem to have a particularly close bearing on problems that impinge on our daily lives today. It is now a virtually accepted notion that, in the absence of a significant level of cytoplasmic estrogen receptor, breast cancer patients are most unlikely to respond to available hormonal therapy, whether ablative or additive. It would seem that a simple assay of receptor sites in a biopsy can spare the trauma of surgical or chemical castration to many women.

One of the aims of the pharmaceutical industry, apart from the ultimate goal of designing new drugs for the cure of disease, is to find methods, whether tests or reagents, for diagnostic purposes. The search for both new drugs and for new methods, however, is based on the development and refinement of experimental models derived from fundamental research. At present, in our laboratories as in many others, considerable attention is being given to the introduction of a simple receptor assay in human breast cancer and to the interpretation of the results obtained, because, regardless of the techniques used by different teams for receptor measurement, only 50–60% of estrogen receptor-positive patients respond to hormonal therapy. Recently, we have perfected an assay for the measurement of progestin-binding sites in animal tissues, which is now being applied, after appropriate controls, to specimens from breast cancer patients.

For a long time, a major problem in the detection of progestin-specific binding in many species was the interference of progesterone binding to specific plasma proteins, for example, transcortin. Due to this interference and also to the lability of the 7S progesterone-receptor complex, it was extremely difficult to detect, let alone measure, progestin-binding sites. It seemed to us that a simple and effective way of disregarding the interference binding was to use a synthetic radioligand, in this instance R 5020 (17,21-dimethyl-19-norpregna-4,9-diene-3,20-dione), not bound by transcortin and that, due to the slow dissociation rate of the complex formed with progestin receptor, as determined in studies on animal uterus, "stabilizes" this receptor. This approach introduced the notion of the use of synthetic molecules as receptor "tags" not bound by plasma proteins and entirely specific to the receptor corresponding to a single class of hormone. We have, in fact, shown that R 5020 is virtually totally specific for progestin receptor; it competes slightly (13%) for binding to the dexamethasone-labeled glucocorticoid receptor, a result that has been confirmed by other teams, but not for binding to the estrogen, androgen, or mineralocorticoid receptors. At present, we also have available a highly specific tag for the estrogen receptor, R 2858 (11β-methoxy-19-nor-17α-1,3,5(10)-pregnatrien-20-yn-3,17-diol), that is not bound by sex steroid-binding plasma protein and that is being used in preliminary assays for estrogen receptors in breast tumors, comparatively with estradiol, with fairly interesting results. Regarding the androgen receptor, although our radioligand R 1881 is not bound by SBP, it competes very markedly for binding to the progestin receptor. These molecules are now being used to measure total cytoplasmic binding sites by exchange assays in various tissues (e.g., rabbit uterus and rat and human prostate).

Under the assumption that measurement of cytoplasmic binding sites would be of diagnostic value to the consulting physician, it is necessary that the assay for the hospital laboratory should meet the following requirements. It should be specific, reproducible, sensitive, and, if possible, adaptable for use on a microscale. It should be preferably simple, rapid, and inexpensive. In our opinion, a method that involves measurement of binding sites by a dextran-coated adsorption exchange assay and use of the above-mentioned synthetic ligands meets the above practical requirements more satisfactorily than do sucrose density gradient ultracentrifugation and agar gel electrophoresis. At present, biochemical controls for extrapolation of the progestin receptor assay from estradiol-primed immature rabbit uterus to human breast tissue are being carried out to determine the most suitable conditions of ligand concentration, incubation time, and temperature for a valid single-point assay that ensures that total exchange of endogenous hormone occurs in a time compatible with receptor stability.

In collaboration with a medical team from Villejuif Hospital (France), we have examined tissue specimens from more than 200 patients, with a technique that employs estradiol instead of R 2858 (and therefore does not eliminate interference from binding to contaminating plasma proteins), and conditions of exchange for both estradiol and R 5020 extrapolated directly without controls from animal data. The results are, nevertheless, interesting, particularly for 15 patients for whom not only the concentration of binding sites in the tumor, but also that in a tissue sample taken from a precise region that adjoins the nipple were measured after histopathologic examination of the specimen. The receptor level in tumor tissue was generally significantly higher than in control tissue. Except for two cases of infiltration by malignant cells, the progestin receptor level in control tissue was always equal to zero or negligible. Estrogen receptor level in control tissue, however, reached approximately 200 fmol/g of tissue in five of 15 cases. To what extent interference plasma binding is involved is being studied. These results, however, emphasize the aleatory nature of quantitative assessments when the percentage of malignant cells in the specimen is not known. This immediately brings up the point of the heterogeneity of the tumor: assays on different samples from the same tumor have given different results, and the question arises as to whether all or only some malignant cells contain receptor. Furthermore, because no information is available on the possible cyclic variations in receptor content of normal mammary gland cells, the threshold value above which the tumor may be considered receptor positive and the value above which it may be, furthermore, considered clinically hormone dependent are impossible to determine, except by correlation with hormonal therapy. Prior to the establishment of any clinical correlation, however, a full-scale statistical analysis with a highly controlled technique is required to define the sensitivity of the measurement, particularly of a one-point measurement, because the quantity of tissue is often not sufficient for several determinations. Ideally, it should be possible to perform the assays on drills.

The validity of the extrapolation of techniques from animal to man is being studied, but the condition that underlies this extrapolation is that hormone mechanisms in animal tissues and in malignant human breast tissue are similar, if not the same. To check this fundamental assumption, new experimental models have to be introduced, and one of the most promising appears to be that of tissue culture, which will enable *in vitro* analysis of receptor mechanisms directly on human tissue, in particular, malignant cells. Such a model might provide answers to a few important questions. It would eliminate such problems as heterogeneity, permit comparisons in receptor mechanisms between animal and man (translocation of the complex to the nucleus, binding to a nuclear acceptor site), and would throw some light on what is probably the most vital question, namely: To what extent is the receptor mechanism implicated in malignant growth? Moreover, this model would be ideal to test all of those molecules, which, from screening data on animal studies, have been suspected to exert antihormonal activity, for instance, by virtue of the rapid dissociation rate of the cytoplasmic complex formed and the subsequently impaired response.

A ROLE FOR PROGESTERONE IN BREAST CANCER*

William L. McGuire and Kathryn B. Horwitz

Department of Medicine
University of Texas Health Science Center at San Antonio
San Antonio, Texas 78284

Clinical Effects in Breast Cancer

Because of the cyclic changes of blood estrogen and progesterone levels that occur in females and the interrelationships among these hormones in regulating target tissue development and growth, it was inevitable that progesterone would be studied for its effect on breast cancer. Although progesterone itself is not a carcinogen, it may be a potent target-specific cocarcinogen for induction of mammary tumors by viral or chemical agents.[1] As such, the hormone has been implicated both in tumor enhancement and in tumor suppression.

That progesterone plays a role in stimulating tumor growth is suggested by the pioneering studies of Huggins *et al.*[2–4] They showed that pregnancy promoted the growth of dimethylbenzanthracene (DMBA)-induced rat mammary tumors. Administration of progesterone to intact rats accelerated the appearance of tumors, increased the numbers of tumors, and augmented the growth rate of established tumors.

If DMBA-induced mammary tumor-bearing rats are ovariectomized and simultaneous lesions are placed in the median eminence to increase prolactin release, the tumor grows at an accelerated pace for only 10–12 days and then regresses, even though prolactin levels remain elevated.[5,6] The ovarian factor responsible for maintaining tumor growth under these circumstances has not been identified, but the following experiments suggest the importance of progesterone. Pregnancy stimulates the growth of DMBA-induced mammary tumors, while parturition and weaning are followed by regression of a large number of these tumors.[2,7,8] The tumor growth-promoting factor of pregnancy is probably placental lactogen,[9] while prolactin has been implicated as being responsible for the maintenance of tumor size and growth during lactation, because tumors regress if suckling is prevented.[10,11] The true situation is more complex, however, because ovariectomy blocks the stimulatory effects of endogenous or exogenous prolactin on tumor growth, and injection of progesterone removes this block.[10] One interpretation would be that prolactin stimulation of tumors under these circumstances is dependent on progesterone or, alternatively, that the high levels of circulating progesterone found in the lactating rat, which are under prolactin control,[12] are responsible for the tumor growth. This does not necessarily mean that progesterone alone is responsible for maintaining rat mammary tumor growth, because in these experiments the animals had both high prolactin levels and intact adrenal glands. On the other hand, they do suggest that progesterone plays an important physiologic role in stimulating tumor growth.

In contrast to the stimulatory effects of progesterone described above, progesterone can induce rat mammary tumor regression or prevent tumor appearance when combined with moderate to large doses of estrogen.[2,13] In humans, the percentage of breast tumor regressions to a progesterone-estrogen combina-

*Supported in part by United States Public Health Service Grants CA-11378 and CB-23862 and by American Cancer Society Grant BC-23D.

tion is generally higher than with progesterone alone.[14] The significance of these observations is somewhat obscured by the fact that moderate to large doses of estrogens alone can cause mammary tumor regression in rats[15–17] and humans,[18] so that it is necessary to ask whether addition of the progestational agent accomplishes more than does estrogen alone. The answer would seem to be "yes," for the following reasons. Patients whose tumors have failed to regress after treatment with high-dose estrogen alone have responded to a combination of estrogen-progesterone.[19–21] Postmenopausal patients with endogenous estrogen levels (presumably of adrenal origin) sufficient to cornify the vaginal mucosa have a 29% tumor remission rate with progesterone therapy, whereas patients with an atrophic vaginal smear experience only a 6% remission rate with progesterone alone.[22] These data would support a requirement for estrogen in progesterone-mediated tumor regression and may be due to estrogen's stimulation of progesterone receptor synthesis (see below). The mechanism by which progesterone promotes tumor regression is not clear. Large doses of synthetic progestins can cause significant lowering of serum luteinizing hormone and cortisol levels, which suggests that alteration of pituitary function may be involved,[23] but at least four previously hypophysectomized patients are reported to have had breast tumor regression after combinations of estrogen-progesterone.[24,25] This finding is in contrast to the lack of tumor response to estrogens alone in hypophysectomized patients.[26–28]

In summary, the specific mechanisms involved in progesterone-mediated breast tumor growth and regression are poorly understood. However, the hormone's metabolism, its binding to specific receptor proteins, and its effect on the actions of other steroid hormones have been extensively studied in several target tissues.

Subcellular Metabolism of Progesterone

Progesterone is a precursor common to estrogens, androgens, and adrenal hormones. The uptake and metabolic fates of progesterone have been extensively investigated in uteri,[29–45] mammary gland,[46,47] and other target tissues.[48–52] The results and interpretations of these studies have often been quite contradictory, for the following reasons. They have been performed in a variety of different tissues from different species under *in vivo, in vitro,* or cell-free conditions. In some cases, the progesterone concentration has been high, and in others it has been low. Certain studies deal with normal animals, others with pseudopregnant or pregnant animals. Metabolic patterns differ in estrogen treated versus castrated animals. It is perhaps understandable, then, that a simple representative metabolic scheme cannot be presented. Despite these limitations, certain observations are pertinent to the present discussion.

Although studies of progesterone metabolism and excretion in breast cancer patients reveal no major differences from control patients, the intracellular metabolism of progesterone by the breast tumor itself may be quite important. It has been shown that certain breast tumors can synthesize progesterone from pregnenolone, which means that the tumor itself can control intracellular hormone concentration.[53]

In contrast to estrogens, for which intracellular metabolism does not seem to play an important regulatory role, progesterone can be extensively metabolized in a manner analogous to that for androgens, where testosterone is converted intracellularly to an active metabolite, dihydrotestosterone, and an inactive product, androstanediol.[54,55]

Lawson and Pearlman[46] administered [^{3}H]progesterone as a continuous infusion and found that the mammary gland of the pregnant rat was able to concentrate tritium above plasma levels. In addition to progesterone, small amounts of 20α-hydroxypregn-4-ene-3-one (20α-OHPg) were found. The pattern of metabolites varied with the endocrine status of the gland: 20α-OHPg dominated the pregnant gland, whereas ring-A reduction was higher in the lactating gland.[47,56]

Because estrogen priming is required for full functional expression of progesterone activity, its effect on metabolite formation may provide a clue to its physiologic role. Saffran *et al.*[57] have shown that at physiologic progesterone concentrations, the effect of estrogen is to inhibit reductase activity. At high progesterone concentrations, the effect is reversed. Progesterone concentration does not effect 20α-hydroxysteroid dehydrogenase (20α-OHSD) activity, which is increased by estrogen at low or high progesterone levels.

Thus, the role of estrogen appears to be twofold. First, it increases progesterone receptor (PgR) and thereby reduces progesterone metabolism, because the hormone is protected by receptor binding. Second, it increases the concentration of reducing enzymes, particularly 20α-OHSD, thereby increasing metabolism. The net effect of estrogen treatment is balanced between increased binding and increased degradation, and the concentration of progesterone determines which effect predominates.

One serious problem in the earlier studies was that the presence and importance of an intracellular receptor for progesterone had not been appreciated. Although it is perhaps incorrect to assume that all progesterone effects must operate through a receptor mechanism, a good place to begin would be to see which metabolites in a given tissue can bind to the progesterone receptor and whether this binding correlates with biologic activity. This information could give insight as to whether a certain metabolic pathway is critical to the action of the hormone or whether the pathway is primarily a means of degradation and excretion.

If one or more intracellular metabolites mediate progestational effects, a receptor for the metabolite should be present, the metabolite should accumulate and bind, and its binding affinity should reflect its biologic activity. In mammalian tissues, [^{3}H]-5α-dihydroprogesterone (5α-DHPg) does not bind to a receptor, the unlabeled hormone does not compete for progesterone binding to PgR, and neither 5α-DHPg nor 3α-hydroxy-5α-pregnan-20-one possesses progestational activity.[58,59] Therefore, it appears that these metabolites serve little biologic function.

Strott[52] has studied the chick oviduct to show which metabolites can bind to PgR and whether this binding correlates with biologic activity. In unstimulated oviducts, essentially no bound progesterone can be found. In marked contrast to this finding, after estrogen stimulation, 70% of protein-bound hormone is unreacted progesterone. Therefore, as in mammals, in estrogen-primed chicks, progesterone is the major bound hormone, although some 5α-DHPg is also bound. In the chick, unlike the mammal, the biologic activity of 5α-DHPg may reside in its ability to compete for progesterone binding to PgR.[60]

In the absence of evidence for a functional role of progesterone metabolites in mammals, their significance remains to be determined, and their formation may simply serve to terminate the action of progesterone. One must conclude that the capacity to elicit a progestational effect resides in the progesterone molecule itself and that it acts without metabolic transformation, as supported by the demonstration of specific progesterone-binding proteins in a variety of target tissues and cells.

Progesterone Receptors

We now turn to studies of PgR and its dependence on estrogen priming. Extensive investigations in guinea pig uterus unequivocally demonstrated PgR in a mammal.[61–74] The receptor migrates at 6S to 8S in sucrose gradients and does not bind glucocorticoids. Uterine levels of PgR are maximum at proestrus and fall progressively during estrus and postestrus to a 16-fold lower level in diestrus. Injection of estrogen causes an eightfold rise in PgR within 24 hr, which can be prevented by inhibition of protein or RNA synthesis. The normal half-life of PgR is approximately 3–5 days, but an injection of progesterone will deplete the uterine cytoplasm of PgR within 3 hr. Evidence for nuclear translocation of PgR is available from direct biochemical and autoradiographic studies. Similar conclusions have been reached about PgR in the hamster,[58,75] rabbit,[76–81] mouse,[82,83] rat,[76–78,82–91] and man.[92–99] In the latter two species, PgR has been difficult to demonstrate reproducibly, because the majority of radioactive progesterone binds in the 4S region of the sucrose gradient, making it difficult to distinguish PgR from the corticosteroid-binding globulin. With incorporation of glycerol into buffers or gradients, the receptor complex is stabilized,[99] and a specific high-affinity (K_d 3–8 $\times$ 10^{-9} M) 7S binding component is seen occasionally in myometria from women treated with estrogen,[94] in endometrium obtained from proliferative (estrogen dominated) tissues,[99,100] in hyperplastic endometrium,[101] and in endometrial carcinoma.[100]

The receptor is precipitated by ammonium sulfate,[102] and this property has been used to purify it.[103] The pure receptor (which migrates as a single band of molecular weight 110,000 on sodium dodecyl sulfate polyacrylamide gels) sediments at 3.7S on sucrose gradients (after elution with hypertonic salt), has a K_d of about 10^{-9} M, and does not bind hydrocortisone. The purified receptor-hormone complex will bind to nuclei; the nuclear bound form also sediments at 3.7S.

The most exhaustive studies of PgR have been performed in estrogen-primed chick oviduct. In this tissue, administration of a single dose of progesterone *in vivo* stimulates chromatin template capacity, DNA-dependent RNA polymerase activity, and synthesis of a specific messenger RNA, culminating with induction of the specific protein, avidin.[104–108] Unlabeled progesterone, its active metabolites, and testosterone (a good inducer of avidin) block [^{3}H]progesterone binding to the receptor.[109] Progesterone receptor concentration is increased 20-fold by estradiol.[110] The receptor has been purified to homogeneity and found to consist of two similar subunits that have distinctly different affinities for DNA and chromatin.[111]

Although the breast is also a target of progesterone action, virtually no information about receptor binding of the hormone exists. After injection, an apparent selective accumulation of progesterone by the normal human breast has been described.[112] This property is lost in neoplastic tissue.[113] Terenius[114] used charcoal-resistant radioactivity of cytosols that contained [^{3}H]progesterone and excess hydrocortisone to show a progesterone binder in human and rat mammary carcinomas. Attempts to demonstrate receptors in normal mammary tissue with progesterone have been unsuccessful, despite the fact that glucocorticoid receptors (which are often difficult to distinguish from PgR) are present.[115,116]

This survey of PgR in various tissues fails to explain progesterone-induced regression and stimulation of experimental and human breast cancers, but it may provide important clues about the estrogen requirement for progesterone's effects. Most important is the stimulation of PgR after estrogen priming. Estrogen modulation of PgR levels is probably a direct effect on the target cell and not mediated by the pituitary, because in ovariectomized, adrenalectomized, and hypophysectomized rats, uterine PgR levels are restored by estradiol but not by prolactin injections.[117] In addition to controlling PgR levels, the estrogen requirement for progesterone action may be due to estrogen's role in regulating progesterone metabolism.

Progesterone Interrelationships with Other Steroid Hormones

Progesterone may control breast tumor growth or regression in several ways. The simplest mechanism involves a direct effect of the hormone on the tumor. However, progesterone can also modify the actions of the other steroid hormones that influence the mammary gland, and this modifying effect may form the basis for interhormonal control mechanisms.

Estrogens

The ability of progesterone is antagonize and/or modify the action of estrogen is well documented.[118,119] Tamoxifen® and Nafoxidine®, two widely used antiestrogens, exhibit progesterone-like effects.[120–122] Hsueh *et al.*[122] have shown that after depletion of cytoplasmic estrogen receptor (ER) by high-dose estrogen treatment, progesterone blocks the overshoot of ER seen during replenishment. They propose that this reduction of ER is correlated to reduced sensitivity of the uterus to estrogen. There is no evidence, however, that progesterone affects replenishment of ER after physiologic estrogen treatments or that it alters basal ER levels. In summary, estrogen and progesterone may exert feedback control on each other at the target tissue. Estradiol pretreatment enhances tissue sensitivity to progesterone correlated with increased PgR levels. Progesterone, in turn, may modify cytoplasmic ER and redirect the cells' ability to respond to estradiol.

Androgens

The androgenic properties of progestins are well known, and fetal virilization can result from their use in man.[123] Progestins can masculinize the reproductive tract of rat fetuses[124] and can mimic androgens' effects in several organs.[125–128] Recently, Bullock *et al.*[127] and Mowszowicz *et al.*[125] have demonstrated that progestins can be either synandrogenic (by potentiating androgen effects) or antiandrogenic (by inhibiting these effects), depending on the steroid structure, dose, and tissue. If androgens have similar modifying effects on progesterone's actions, it may be one reason why they are effective in treatment of hormone-dependent breast cancer. Although the mechanism of androgen-induced regression of breast tumors is not known, androgens cause regression of fetal mammary buds[129] and may have similar effects on dedifferentiated malignant cells. It is possible that progestin-induced tumor regression is a reflection of the progestins' androgenic properties.

Glucocorticoids

By far the most familiar model for the interaction of two differing steroids is that proposed by Rousseau *et al.*[130] to explain the inhibitory effects of progestins and the stimulatory effects of glucocorticoids on tyrosine aminotransferase production in rat hepatoma tissue culture (HTC) cells. Competition by progestins for glucocorticoid binding has also been demonstrated in mammary carcinomas[131,132] and lactating mammary glands.[115,116] Because glucocorticoids are involved in mammary gland maturation, it is possible that progestins may affect mammary tumors by modifying glucocorticoid action.

We have recently shown that MCF-7, a stable cell line derived from a human mammary carcinoma, contains receptors for progestins, androgens, glucocorticoids, and estrogens. These cells may prove useful for studying interrelationships among the binding and biologic actions or these four steroids and their role in tumor endocrine response.[133]

Progesterone Receptors in Human Breast Cancer

Although metastatic breast cancers have long been treated by endocrine therapies, responsive tumors constitute only 20–40% of cases. The success rate can be improved to 55–60% by selecting for endocrine therapy only patients whose tumors contain ER. Our concern now is to identify the 40% of ER-positive but endocrine-resistant tumors, whose growth cannot be inhibited by either ablative or additive endocrine manipulation.

Normal target tissues for any hormone contain specific receptors for that hormone, and when malignant transformation occurs, the cell may retain all or part of its normal complement of receptors. The assumption has been implicit that when ER is present in malignant mammary cells, tumor growth is regulated by the hormonal environment and that a change in this environment will cause tumor regression. However, because binding to receptors is only an early step in hormonal action, it is possible that in ER-positive tumors where endocrine manipulations fail, the lesion is at a later step. An ideal marker of an endocrine-responsive tumor would, therefore, be a measurable product of hormonal action rather than the initial binding step.

Because in estrogen target tissues the synthesis of PgR depends on the action of estrogen,[73] we investigated the possibility that PgR might be such a marker. If so, it would be expected that PgR would be rare in tumors that lack ER. The presence of PgR in tumors that contain ER would indicate that the tumor is capable of synthesizing at least one end product under estrogen regulation and that the tumor remains endocrine responsive. As a corollary, the prospect of a successful response to therapy would be low in tumors with ER but no PgR.

We have used 8S binding of a synthetic progestin [^{3}H]R 5020[83] to identify PgR in human breast cancer tissue.[134,135] We have now determined PgR and ER in 236 human mammary tumors. Of 64 ER-negative tumors, only five (8%) had PgR, whereas 107 of 172 (62%) ER-positive tumors had PgR. These percentages approximate the response rate to endocrine therapy based on ER, so that this result is consistent with the hypothesis that PgR is a marker of endocrine-responsive tumors. Confirmation of this hypothesis requires direct correlation of the presence of PgR with objectively defined clinical remission. Our preliminary data on 27 patients are encouraging. We find that in cases where ER is positive and PgR is negative, the successful response rate is very low, analogous to the response rates seen with ER-negative tumors. In contrast, if both receptors are present, remissions are seen in a larger percentage of patients than would be predicted on the basis of ER alone. However, it should be emphasized that these data are very preliminary; they represent only the simplest cases in which receptor measurements were performed on a single biopsy and in which response to a single trial of endocrine therapy is involved.

Most questions remain unresolved. How does one interpret contradictory responses to two or more therapeutic trials? What is the effect of previous therapy on receptor levels in multiple biopsies or metastases? How does menopausal status or menstrual cycle affect PgR levels in biopsies? Are measurements of only cytoplasmic receptors an adequate representation of the total receptor content of the cell? And, in considering cytoplasmic receptors, what constitutes a positive assay for PgR? How are we to interpret the tumors that have no 8S but considerable suppressible 4S binding? Finally, we have shown that human breast tumor cells can contain receptors for four steroid hormones. How are we to incorporate androgen and glucocorticoid receptor data in estimating the response potential of a tumor? Hopefully, the current efforts by many laboratories, including ours, will resolve these questions.

Acknowledgment

We thank Dr. J.-P. Raynaud of Roussel UCLAF for generously providing the R 5020.

References

1. Poel, W. E. 1968. Brit. J. Cancer **22:** 867–873.
2. Huggins, C., R. C. Moon & M. Sotokichi. 1962. Proc. Nat. Acad. Sci. USA **48:** 379–386.
3. Huggins, C. & N. C. Yang. 1962. Science **137:** 257–262.
4. Huggins, C. 1965. Cancer Res. **25:** 1163–1175.
5. Clemens, J. A., C. W. Welsch & J. Meites. 1968. Proc. Soc. Exp. Biol. Med. **127:** 969–972.
6. Sinha, D., D. Cooper & T. L. Dao. 1973. Cancer Res. **33:** 411–414.
7. Dao, T. L. & H. Sunderland. 1959. J. Nat. Cancer Inst. **23:** 567–586.
8. McCormick, G. M. & R. C. Moon. 1965. Brit. J. Cancer **19:** 160–166.
9. Nagasawa, H. & R. Yanai. 1973. Int. J. Cancer **11:** 131–137.
10. McCormick, G. M. & R. C. Moon. 1967. Cancer Res. **27:** 626–631.
11. McCormick, G. M. 1972. Cancer Res. **32:** 1574–1576.
12. Tomogane, H., K. Ôta & A. Yokoyama. 1975. J. Endocrinol. **65:** 155–161.
13. McCormick, G. M. & R. C. Moon. 1973. Eur. J. Cancer **9:** 483–486.
14. Muggia, F. M., P. A. Cassileth, M. Ochoa, F. A. Flatow, A. Gellhorn & G. A. Hyman. 1968. Ann. Intern. Med. **68:** 328–337.
15. Pearson, O. H. & H. Nasr. 1970. Excerpta Med. Int. Congr. Ser. **219:** 602–606.
16. Nagasawa, H. & R. Yanai. 1971. Int. J. Cancer **8:** 463–467.
17. Meites, J., E. Cassell & J. Clark. 1971. Proc. Soc. Exp. Biol. Med. **137:** 1225–1227.
18. Council on Drugs. 1960. J. Amer. Med. Ass. **172:** 1271–1283.
19. Growley, L. G. & I. MacDonald. 1965. Cancer **18:** 436–446.
20. Stoll, B. A. 1967. Brit. Med. J. **3:** 338–341.
21. Stoll, B. A. 1967. Brit. Med. J. **1:** 150–153.
22. Stoll, B. A. 1967. Cancer **20:** 1807–1813.
23. Sadoff, L. & W. Lusk. 1974. Obstet. Gynecol. **43:** 262–266.
24. Landau, R. L., E. N. Ehrlich & C. Huggins. 1962. J. Amer. Med. Ass. **182:** 632–636.
25. Kennedy, B. J. 1965. Cancer **18:** 1551–1557.
26. Pearson, O. H. & B. S. Ray. 1959. Cancer **12:** 85–92.
27. Lipsett, M. B. & D. M. Bergenstal. 1969. Cancer Res. **20:** 1172–1178.

28. KENNEDY, B. J. & L. FRENCH. 1965. Amer. J. Surg. **110:** 411–414.
29. WICHMANN, K. 1967. Acta Endocrinol. **55**(Suppl. 116): 1–98.
30. BRYSON, M. J. & M. L. SWEAT. 1967. Endocrinology **81:** 729–734.
31. BRYSON, M. J. & M. L. SWEAT. 1969. Endocrinology **84:** 1071–1075.
32. ARMSTRONG, D. T. & E. R. KING. 1971. Endocrinology **89:** 191–197.
33. MILGROM, E. & E.-E. BAULIEU. 1970. Endocrinology **87:** 276–287.
34. HASHIMOTO, I., D. M. HENDRICKS, L. I. ANDERSON & R. M. MELAMPY. 1968. Endocrinology **82:** 333–341.
35. HOWARD, P. D. & W. G. WIEST. 1972. Steroids **19:** 35–46.
36. LAUMAS, K. R. & A. FAROOG. 1966. J. Endocrinol. **36:** 95–96.
37. LAUMAS, K. R. & A. FAROOG. 1967. Indian J. Exp. Biol. **5:** 12,13.
38. FALK, R. J. & C. W. BARDIN. 1970. Endocrinology **86:** 1059–1063.
39. SAFFRAN, J., B. K. LOESER, B. M. HAAS & H. E. STAVELY. 1974. Steroids **24:** 839–848.
40. EGERT, D. & H. MAASS. 1974. Acta Endocrinol. **77:** 135–149.
41. EGERT, D., W. JONAT & H. MAASS. 1974. Acta Endocrinol. **77:** 150–159.
42. EGERT, D. & H. MAASS. 1974. Acta Endocrinol. **77:** 160–170.
43. WIEST, W. G. 1971. *In* The Sex Steroids. K. W. McKerns, Ed. Chap. 10: 295–313. Appleton-Century-Crofts. New York, N.Y.
44. COLLINS, J. A. & D. M. JEWKES. 1974. Amer. J. Obstet. Gynecol. **118:** 179–185.
45. WIEST, W. G. 1963. Endocrinology **73:** 310–316.
46. LAWSON, D. E. M. & W. H. PEARLMAN. 1964. J. Biol. Chem. **239:** 3226–3232.
47. CHATTERTON, R. T. 1971. *In* The Sex Steroids. K. W. McKerns, Ed. Chap. 12: 345–382. Appleton-Century-Crofts. New York, N.Y.
48. PODRATZ, K. C., T. W. MUNNS & P. A. KATZMAN. 1974. Steroids **24:** 775–792.
49. TABEI, T., H. HAGA, W. L. HEINRICHS & W. L. HERRMANN. 1974. Steroids **23:** 651–666.
50. O'MALLEY, B. W., W. L. MCGUIRE, P. O. KOHLER & S. G. KORENMAN. 1969. Rec. Progr. Hormone Res. **25:** 105–160.
51. MORGAN, M. D. & J. D. WILSON. 1970. J. Biol. Chem. **245:** 3781–3789.
52. STROTT, C. A. 1974. Endocrinology **95:** 826–837.
53. DESHPANDE, N. 1975. J. Steroid Biochem. **6:** 735–741.
54. BRUCHOVSKY, N. & J. D. WILSON. 1968. J. Biol. Chem. **243:** 2012–2021.
55. WILSON, J. D. 1972. N. Engl. J. Med. **287:** 1284–1291.
56. CHATTERTON, R. T., A. J. CHATTERTON & L. HELLMAN. 1969. Endocrinology **85:** 16–24.
57. SAFFRAN, J., B. K. LOESER, B. M. HAAS & H. E. STAVELY. 1974. Steroids **23:** 117–131.
58. LEAVITT, W. W. & C. J. GROSSMAN. 1974. Proc. Nat. Acad. Sci. USA **71:** 4341–4345.
59. COFFEY, J. C. 1973. Steroids **22:** 561–566.
60. O'MALLEY, B. W. & W. T. SCHRADER. 1972. J. Steroid Biochem. **3:** 617–629.
61. MILGROM, E., M. ATGER & E.-E. BAULIEU. 1970. Steroids **16:** 741–754.
62. FALK, R. J. & C. W. BARDIN. 1970. Endocrinology **86:** 1059–1063.
63. MILGROM, E., M. ATGER, M. PERROT & E.-E. BAULIEU. 1972. Endocrinology **90:** 1071–1078.
64. MILGROM, E., M. PERROT, M. ATGER & E.-E. BAULIEU. 1972. Endocrinology **90:** 1064–1070.
65. CORVOL, P., R. FALK, M. FREIFELD & C. W. BARDIN. 1972. Endocrinology **90:** 1464–1469.
66. FABER, L. E., M. L. SANDMANN & H. E. STAVELY. 1972. J. Biol. Chem. **247:** 8000–8004.
67. MILGROM, E., L. THI, M. ATGER & E.-E. BAULIEU. 1973. J. Biol. Chem. **248:** 6366–6374.
68. ATGER, M., E.-E. BAULIEU & E. MILGROM. 1974. Endocrinology **94:** 161–167.
69. WAREMBOURG, M. 1974. Endocrinology **94:** 665–670.
70. SAR, M. & W. E. STUMPF. 1974. Endocrinology **94:** 1116–1125.
71. MACLAUGHLIN, D. T. & U. WESTPHAL. 1974. Biochim. Biophys. Acta **365:** 372–388.

72. Kontula, K., O. Janne, E. Rajakoski, E. Tanhuapaa & R. Vihko. 1974. J. Steroid Biochem. **5:** 39–44.
73. Freifeld, M. L., P. D. Feil & C. W. Bardin. 1974. Steroids **23:** 93–103.
74. Philibert, D. & J.-P. Raynaud. 1974. Endocrinology **94:** 627–632.
75. Leavitt, W. W., D. O. Toft, C. A. Strott & B. W. O'Malley. 1974. Endocrinology **94:** 1041–1053.
76. Reel, J. R., S. K. VanDeward, Y. Shih & M. R. Callantine. 1971. Steroids **18:** 441–461.
77. McGuire, J. L. & C. D. Bariso. 1972. Endocrinology **90:** 496–506.
78. Faber, L. E., M. L. Sandmann & H. E. Stavely. 1972. J. Biol. Chem. **247:** 5648,-5649.
79. Faber, L. E., M. L. Sandmann & H. E. Stavely. 1973. Endocrinology **93:** 74–80.
80. Rao, B. R., W. G. Wiest & W. M. Allen. 1973. Endocrinology **92:** 1229–1240.
81. Davies, J., J. R. G. Challis & K. J. Ryan. 1974. Endocrinology **95:** 164–173.
82. Feil, P. D., S. R. Glasser, D. O. Toft & B. W. O'Malley. 1972. Endocrinology **91:** 738–746.
83. Philibert, D. & J.-P. Raynaud. 1973. Steroids **22:** 89–99.
84. McGuire, J. L. & C. DeDella. 1971. Endocrinology **88:** 1099–1103.
85. Milgrom, E. & E.-E. Baulieu. 1970. Endocrinology **87:** 276–287.
86. Davies, J. & K. J. Ryan. 1972. Endocrinology **90:** 507–515.
87. Davies, I. J. & K. J. Ryan. 1973. Endocrinology **92:** 394–401.
88. Saffran, J., B. K. Loeser, B. Haas & H. E. Stavely. 1973. Biochem. Biophys. Res. Commun. **53:** 202–209.
89. Hsueh, A. J. W., E. J. Peck & J. H. Clark. 1974. Steroids **24:** 599–611.
90. John, P. N. & A. W. Rogers. 1972. J. Endocrinol. **53:** 375–386.
91. Stumpf, W. E. & M. Sar. 1973. J. Steroid Biochem. **4:** 477–481.
92. Verma, V. & K. R. Laumas. 1973. Biochim. Biophys. Acta **317:** 403–419.
93. Batra, S. 1973. J. Endocrinol. **57:** 561,562.
94. Kontula, K., O. Janne, T. Luukkainen & R. Vihko. 1973. Biochim. Biophys. Acta **328:** 145–153.
95. Haukkamaa, J. 1974. J. Steroid Biochem. **5:** 73–79.
96. Smith, H. E., R. G. Smith, D. O. Toft, J. R. Neergaard, E. Burrows & B. W. O'Malley. 1974. J. Biol. Chem. **249:** 5924–5932.
97. Guerigvian, J. L., M. E. Sawyer & W. H. Pearlman. 1974. J. Endocrinol. **61:** 331–345.
98. Rao, B. R., W. G. Wiest & W. M. Allen. 1974. Endocrinology **95:** 1275–1281.
99. Young, P. C. M. & R. E. Cleary. 1974. J. Clin. Endocrinol. Metab. **39:** 425–439.
100. Pollow, K., H. Lubbert, E. Boquoi, G. Kruezer & B. Pollow. 1974. Endocrinology **96:** 319–328.
101. Haukkamaa, M. & T. Luukkainen. 1974. J. Steroid Biochem. **5:** 447–452.
102. Kontula, K., O. Janne, T. Luukkainen & R. Vihko. 1974. J. Clin. Endocrinol. Metab. **38:** 500–503.
103. Smith, R. G., C. A. Iramain, V. C. Buttram & B. W. O'Malley. 1975. Nature (London) **253:** 271,272.
104. McGuire, W. L. & B. W. O'Malley. 1968. Biochim. Biophys. Acta **157:** 187–194.
105. O'Malley, B. W. & W. L. McGuire. 1968. J. Clin. Invest. **47:** 654–664.
106. Tuohimaa, P., S. J. Segal & S. S. Koide. 1972. Proc. Nat. Acad. Sci. USA **69:** 2814–2817.
107. Korenman, S. G. & B. W. O'Malley. 1968. Endocrinology **83:** 11–17.
108. O'Malley, B. W., G. C. Rosenfeld, J. P. Comstock & A. R. Means. 1972. Nature (London) **240:** 45–48.
109. Sherman, M. R., P. L. Corvol & B. W. O'Malley. 1970. J. Biol. Chem. **245:** 6085–6096.
110. Toft, D. O. & B. W. O'Malley. 1972. Endocrinology **90:** 1041–1045.
111. Schrader, W. T., D. O. Toft & B. W. O'Malley. 1972. J. Biol. Chem. **247:** 2401–2407.
112. Deshpande, N., R. D. Bulbrook & F. O. Belzer. 1966. Excerpta Med. Int. Congr. Ser. **132:** 750–753.

113. Ellis, F. G., T. V. Berne, N. Deshpande, F. O. Belzer & R. D. Bulbrook. 1969. Surg. Gynecol. Obstet. **128:** 975–984.
114. Terenius, L. 1973. Eur. J. Cancer **9:** 291–294.
115. Shyamala, G. 1973. Biochemistry **12:** 3085–3090.
116. Gardner, D. G. & J. L. Wittliff. 1973. Biochim. Biophys. Acta **320:** 617–627.
117. Horwitz, K. B. 1975. Progesterone Receptors and Hormone Dependent Breast Cancer. Doctoral Dissertation: 80–85. University of Texas Southwestern Medical School at Dallas. Dallas, Texas.
118. Hsueh, A. J. W., E. J. Peck & J. H. Clark. 1975. Nature (London) **254:** 337,338.
119. Bullock, D. W. & G. F. Wellen. 1974. Proc. Soc. Exp. Biol. Med. **146:** 294–298.
120. Armstrong, E. M. & I. A. R. More. 1974. Cytobios **11:** 13–16.
121. Heuson, J.-C., C. Waelbroeck, N. Legros, G. Gallez, C. Robyn & M. L'Hermite. 1971–1972. Gynecol. Invest. **2:** 130–137.
122. Hsueh, A. J. W., E. J. Peck & J. H. Clark. 1976. Endocrinology **98:** 438–444.
123. Voorhess, M. L. 1967. J. Pediat. **71:** 128–131.
124. Suchowsky, G. K. & K. Junkmann. 1961. Endocrinology **68:** 341–349.
125. Mowszowicz, I., D. E. Bieber, K. W. Chung, L. P. Bullock & C. W. Bardin. 1974. Endocrinology **94:** 1589–1599.
126. Fabim, M. S. & D. G. Hall. 1970. Amer. J. Obstet. Gynecol. **106:** 183–186.
127. Bullock, L. P., P. L. Barthe, I. Mowszowicz, D. N. Orth & C. W. Bardin. 1975. Endocrinology **97:** 189–195.
128. Naqvi, E., M. X. Zarrow & V. H. Dennberg. 1969. Endocrinology **84:** 669,670.
129. Kratochwil, K. 1971. J. Embryol. Exp. Morphol. **25:** 141–153.
130. Rousseau, G. G., T. D. Baxter & G. M. Tomkins. 1972. J. Mol. Biol. **67:** 99–115.
131. Gardner, D. G. & J. L. Wittliff. 1973. Brit. J. Cancer **27:** 441–444.
132. Shyamala, G. 1974. J. Biol. Chem. **249:** 2160–2163.
133. Horwitz, K. B., M. E. Costlow & W. L. McGuire. 1975. Steroids **26:** 785–795.
134. Horwitz, K. B. & W. L. McGuire. 1975. Steroids **25:** 497–505.
135. Horwitz, K. B., W. L. McGuire, O. H. Pearson & A. Segaloff. 1975. Science **189:** 726,727.

Discussion

Dr. R. J. B. King: Do I understand it that the assays that you presented for the breast tumors were measuring basal progesterone receptor levels?

Dr. McGuire: You mean did we use a provocative test? The answer is "no." These were basal unstimulated levels of progesterone receptor.

Dr. King: In that case, isn't it going to be more important to know whether a receptor actually can be translocated when you give a steroid?

Dr. McGuire: Yes, I think it would be fairly straightforward. First, you have to convince the ethical review committee at your institution. I can foresee a provocative test for the translocation of receptor performed prior to a biopsy. One could use a single injection of estradiol, then biopsy the tumor at a specific time interval, and you would have all of the receptor in the nucleus. You would not only have a receptor measurement but you would also know that it was functional, at least with regard to translocation. For this measurement, you have to have a good assay for nuclear receptor. That's been the thrust of our recent work, and the application of a provocative test I think is in the future.

Dr. King: The other question concerns the ER-negative PgR-positive patients that you demonstrated. Our experience is very similar to your own with smaller numbers. We've found that these patients tend to have very high progesterone levels and tend to be in the postmenopausal group, which suggests that whatever the reason, it is not due to estrogenic stimulation.

DR. P. K. SIITERI: There is less estrogen being produced by menopausal females than by ovulatory females, yet you have just as many PgR-positive patients older than 50 years on your slide as you have younger than 50 years, and that doesn't make sense to me.

DR. MCGUIRE: I think we need some information about the minimal level of estrogen in the environment needed to support a PgR level in a given target tissue.

DR. SIITERI: Your estrogen receptor studies have suggested that you need a lot, because most of it was in the cytoplasm and not in the nucleus.

DR. MCGUIRE: I don't think anybody has any data that would bear directly on that point. All we can do is revert back to an animal model in which the synthesis of PgR seems to be linked directly to the presence of estrogen.

DR. E. GURPIDE: The levels of PgR in human endometrium peak at the time of ovulation. It seems, therefore, that they might be responsive to changes in estradiol concentration that occur during the follicular phase of the cycle. Are the estradiol receptor levels measured in cytosol greatly affected by the concentrations of hormones in the plasma?

DR. MCGUIRE: Yes, the values obtained from a premenopausal patient will depend on the circulating estradiol concentration. Dr. Saez, from Lyon, examined several dozen patients and had simultaneous blood estrogen measurements and then, by an exchange procedure, determined the contribution of the endogenous estrogen in her receptor measurement. It turned out that the absolute value corresponded to the amount of estrogen in the environment, but in no case was the value changed from a positive to a negative. Now, theoretically, that should occur at sometime, and I think as we refine our methods and do routine exchange assays, we may pick up the occasional patient whom we would have misclassified based on just measuring unoccupied sites.

DR. SIITERI: It is perhaps a little dangerous to consider the amount of unextractable nuclear radioactivity as being reflective of some important biologic phenomenon. We've shown that in the guinea pig, you can manipulate the amount of extractable receptor from the nuclei after *in vivo* injection simply by the medium in which you homogenized the tissue. Specifically, if you homogenize it in sucrose media, you can extract virtually no radioactivity by the usual 0.4 M KCl procedure. You get about 5 or 10%.

DR. E. MILGROM: In animal models in the absence of estrogen, you still have a measurable level of progesterone receptors that increases when you inject estrogen.

I have a question about how to interpret results on PgR-positive or -negative tumors. As we have more and more sensitive assays, we find more and more tumors that contain receptors, the decision over what's positive and what's negative becomes difficult. How do you decide what level of receptor is positive or negative?

DR. MCGUIRE: Our initial data for PgR analyses were the finding of greater than 2 fmol/mg of protein in the 8S region of a sucrose gradient by use of R 5020. However, we find that if we take the total suppressible R 5020 binding throughout the whole gradient, we have a cut off of about 8 fmol. It gives essentially the same result. In other words, there is some 4S suppressible material on most of these gradients. This is very different from what other people have tried to do: take the response data on responders and nonresponders and then draw an arbitrary line. I think it depends on whether you want an assay that predicts for responsiveness or whether you want an assay that tells you the amount of receptor irrespective of responsiveness. We prefer to draw the line at the lower limits of confidence in the sensitivity of the assay.

PROGESTERONE AND GLUCOCORTICOID INTERACTIONS WITH RECEPTOR IN BREAST CANCER CELLS IN LONG-TERM TISSUE CULTURE

Marc Lippman, Karen Huff, and Gail Bolan

Medicine Branch
National Cancer Institute
Bethesda, Maryland 20014

It has long been appreciated that the clinical course of breast cancer can be altered by a variety of hormonal manipulations.[1] Despite an awareness that a variety of ablative and additive hormonal therapies may be accompanied by objective tumor regressions in some cases, the exact mechanism whereby these therapeutic interventions cause tumor regression is unclear. While clinical studies of breast cancer and investigation of hormone-dependent breast cancer in animals have contributed much to our understanding, the inherent complexities of studying hormonal regulation of tumor growth *in vivo* led us to attempt to investigate this process in long-term tissue culture lines of human breast cancer. By using defined media in which single hormones could be added to well-characterized uniform populations of cells, we hoped to avoid some of the difficulties intrinsic in more complexly organized systems. Thus, effects of hormone mediated by alterations in levels or activity of other trophic hormones, or effects of hormone on supporting stromal elements or the immune system, could be eliminated from consideration.

In addition, some recent work has suggested that determination of progesterone receptor activity may be helpful in predicting which patients with breast cancer might benefit from hormonal therapy,[2] much as the knowledge of estrogen receptor levels has also been shown to be of value.[3] We have previously reported that some lines of human breast cancer in long-term tissue culture contain glucocorticoid and progesterone receptors,[4,5] and this finding has been confirmed by others.[6] Because of the biologic interactions of glucocorticoids and progesterone, the availability of new compounds, such as R 5020, for receptor quantification (see below), and the need to establish assays that would unambiguously measure each of these receptors independently, we undertook a series of experiments aimed at studying progesterone-glucocorticoid interactions with human breast cancer in long-term culture.

To substantiate the likelihood that observations made on such tissue culture systems bear any relevance to breast cancer *in vivo,* it is important to review the criteria that suggest that these cells resemble those found in the tumor *in vivo*. Four lines of evidence suggest that these cells,* which were initially derived from breast cancer specimens, continue to manifest properties characteristic of the primary tumor. First, morphologically, all of the cell lines employed have epithelial characteristics. In some cell lines, such as the MCF-7,[7] the tendency of

*The ZR-75-1 cell line was initially established by Young *et al.* at the National Cancer Institute.[7a] The MCF-7 cell[7] line was provided by Dr. Marvin Rich of the Michigan Cancer Foundation. The Evsa T-cell line was established in our laboratory, as previously described.[10] MDA-231, HT-39, BT-20, G-11, and 496 were provided by Dr. Ronald Herberman of the National Cancer Institute. All of these cell lines have been shown repeatedly to be free of mycoplasma contamination.

these cells to arrange themselves in glandular arrays is striking. An example of the MCF-7 cells grown on artificial capillary culture units in collaboration with Dr. Richard Knazek is shown in FIGURE 1. Electron microscopic examination reveals desmosomes, microvilli, and secretory granules. Second, these cell lines have been shown to have a human chromosomal karyotype, and for the ZR-75-1 and the Evsa T-cell line,[8] the chromosomal pattern after more than 6 months in culture is similar to that of fresh malignant material from which the lines were derived. Third, these cells synthesize a variety of proteins associated with breast cancer, including α-lactalbumin[8,9] and carcinoembryonic antigen.[10] Finally, we have previously demonstrated the hormone-responsive nature of some of these cell

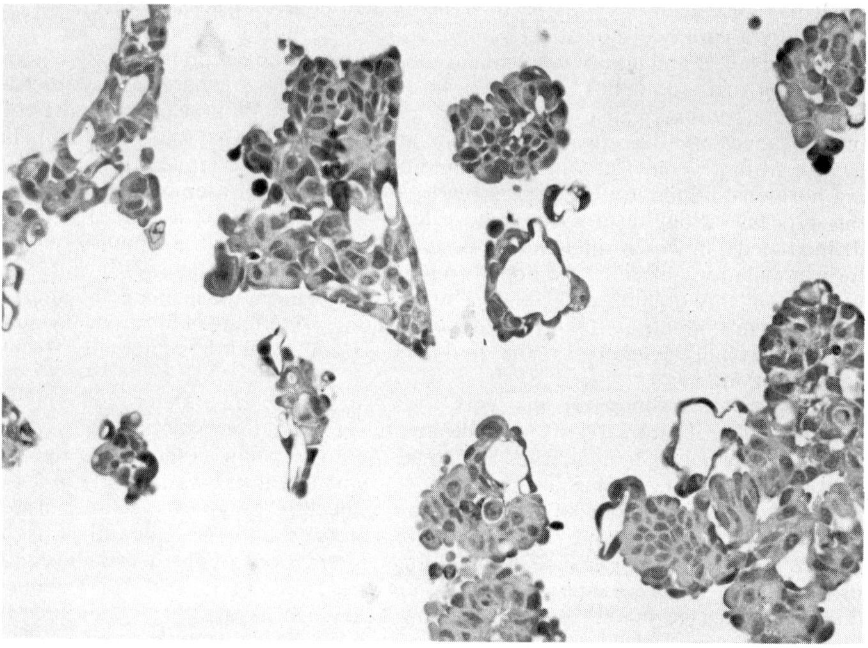

FIGURE 1. MCF-7 human breast cancer grown on an artificial capillary culture unit. These studies were performed in collaboration with Dr. Richard Knazek.[20,20a] The tendency of these cells to arrange themselves in glandlike structures is readily apparent. Hematoxylin and eosin stain; ×150.

lines.[5,8,10,11] Both the ZR-75-1 and the MCF-7 cell lines are strongly estrogen[8] and insulin[12] responsive, and MCF-7 is also androgen responsive.[11] Thus, morphologic, chromosomal, and biochemical data support the contention that these cells are human and breast in origin.

Because of the known requirement of glucocorticoids for mammary gland morphogenesis,[13] the occurrence of specific glucocorticoid receptors in some rodent mammary carcinomata,[14] the induction by glucocorticoids of enhanced mammary tumor virus in tissue culture,[15] and the palliative effects of glucocorticoids in a small proportion of patients with breast cancer,[16] we initially examined the effects

TABLE 1

EFFECTS OF DEXAMETHASONE ON THYMIDINE AND LEUCINE INCORPORATION IN MCF-7 HUMAN BREAST CANCER*

Dexamethasone Concentration (M)	Thymidine Incorporation (dpm × 10^{-2}/μg of protein/hr ± 1 SD)	Leucine Incorporation (dpm × 10^{-2}/mg of protein/hr ± 1 SD)
0	52.3 ± 5.1	39.6 ± 0.68
10^{-9}	49.7 ± 3.2	39.1 ± 2.3
10^{-8}	40.4 ± 3.6	46.6 ± 6.8
10^{-7}	30.8 ± 2.4	37.3 ± 2.9
10^{-6}	32.1 ± 3.1	37.3 ± 2.9

*Cells growing in log phase in Eagle's minimal essential medium (MEM) supplemented with 5% fetal calf serum, 0.6 g/liter of glutamine, and antibiotics (complete MEM) were harvested with trypsin-EDTA solution and replicately plated into multiwell Linbro dishes. After 24 hr, the medium was changed to serum-free MEM. Twenty-four hours later, hormones as noted above were added, and after 36 hr, radiolabeled precursors were added. Two hours later, cells were harvested with trypsin-EDTA after washing the dish with iced phosphate-buffered saline (PBS), pH 7.4. Cell pellets were collected by centrifugation, suspended in water, sonicated briefly, and aliquots were taken for acid precipitation and protein determination by the Lowry technique.[19] Acid-insoluble counts were collected and washed on 0.45-μm Millipore® filters, dried, and counted in Aquasol® in a liquid scintillation counter with an efficiency of about 35% for tritium and 62% for ^{14}C.

of glucocorticoids on incorporation of precursors into macromolecules in these cell lines. Dexamethasone inhibits thymidine incorporation in the MCF-7 cell line by approximately 50% at a concentration of 10^{-6} M, as shown in TABLE 1. Lower concentrations are less inhibitory. Under similar conditions, inhibition of labeled leucine incorporation into acid-insoluble material is not significant. The inhibition of thymidine incorporation is reflected by a markedly decreased rate of cell division. The data supplied in TABLE 2 show that 10^{-6} M dexamethasone slows cell division to less than one-third of control rates. Despite this slowing of cell division,

TABLE 2

EFFECT OF 10^{-7} M DEXAMETHASONE ON CELL DIVISION IN MCF-7 HUMAN BREAST CANCER*

	Cell Number per Dish (× 10^{-4} ± 1 SD)	
Time (days)	Control	Dexamethasone
0	8.1 ± 1.1	8.0 ± 0.8
1	11.4 ± 2.2	9.1 ± 0.9
2	17.2 ± 2.4	10.4 ± 0.4
3	22.6 ± 2.9	11.5 ± 0.5
4	28.5 ± 2.1	13.1 ± 0.6
5	32.8 ± 3.2	14.9 ± 1.0

*Forty-eight hours prior to the start of the experiment, MCF-7 cells growing in log phase in complete MEM were harvested with trypsin-EDTA solution and replicately plated into 60-mm petri dishes. Twenty-four hours later, the medium was replenished with fresh complete MEM. Twenty-four hours later, 10^{-7} M dexamethasone as a 1000-fold concentrate in ethanol was added to half of the dishes; a similar amount of vehicle was added to the other half. Thereafter, three dishes from each group were harvested daily with trypsin-EDTA solution, and cells were counted in a hemocytometer.

TABLE 3
EFFECTS OF DEXAMETHASONE ON THYMIDINE INCORPORATION IN SEVERAL HUMAN BREAST CANCER CELL LINES

Cell Line	Percentage of Inhibition of Thymidine Incorporation* in the Presence of 10^{-7} M Dexamethasone (± 1 SD)	Glucocorticoid Receptor Activity‡ (fmol of dexamethasone bound/mg of cytoplasmic protein)
MCF-7	46 ± 7†	199
MDA-231	23 ± 6	77
G-11	76 ± 4	146
ZR-75-1	43 ± 2	102
EVSA T	0 ± 6	0
496	4 ± 8	5.3

*Thymidine incorporation was measured in the presence or absence of 10^{-7} M dexamethasone, as described in TABLE 1.

†Results are expressed as the percentage of nonhormone-treated incorporation.

‡Glucocorticoid receptor activity was determined with a dextran-coated charcoal competitive binding assay, as previously described.[8]

10^{-6} M dexamethasone is not lethal to the cells, and they continue to grow slowly to confluency.

Other cell lines show one of two responses to glucocorticoids: either inhibition or no effect. Stimulation is not seen at any concentration of glucocorticoid tested. As shown in TABLE 3, inhibition of thymidine incorporation correlates well with the presence or absence of glucocorticoid receptor proteins. The ZR-75-1 cell line also contains glucocorticoid receptor and is inhibited by glucocorticoids.

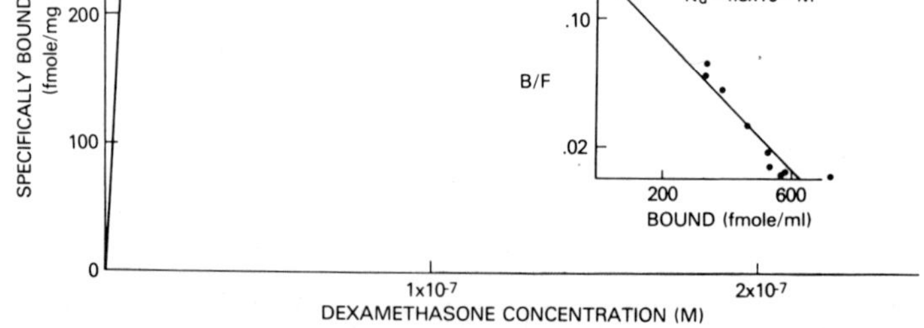

FIGURE 2. Binding of [^{3}H]dexamethasone to glucocorticoid receptor in MCF-7 human breast cancer. Cells growing in complete MEM were switched to serum-free MEM 24 hr prior to harvesting. Cells were harvested with trypsin-EDTA solution and washed in PBS at 0°C. Cells were homogenized, and cytoplasmic extracts were prepared as previously described.[8] Binding data are replotted according to Scatchard analyses in the inset.

Having observed the inhibition of some of these cell lines by glucocorticoids, it appeared worthwhile to examine the steroid receptor proteins of these cell lines in detail. By use of a dextran-coated charcoal competitive binding assay, a glucocorticoid receptor protein was demonstrable in cytoplasmic extracts obtained from the MCF-7 cell line; the data are shown in FIGURE 2. Scatchard analysis of the binding data is shown in the inset. The straight line obtained is consistent with a single class of receptor sites of uniform affinity being detected in the assay. This receptor also appears to have binding specificities characteristic of glucocorticoid

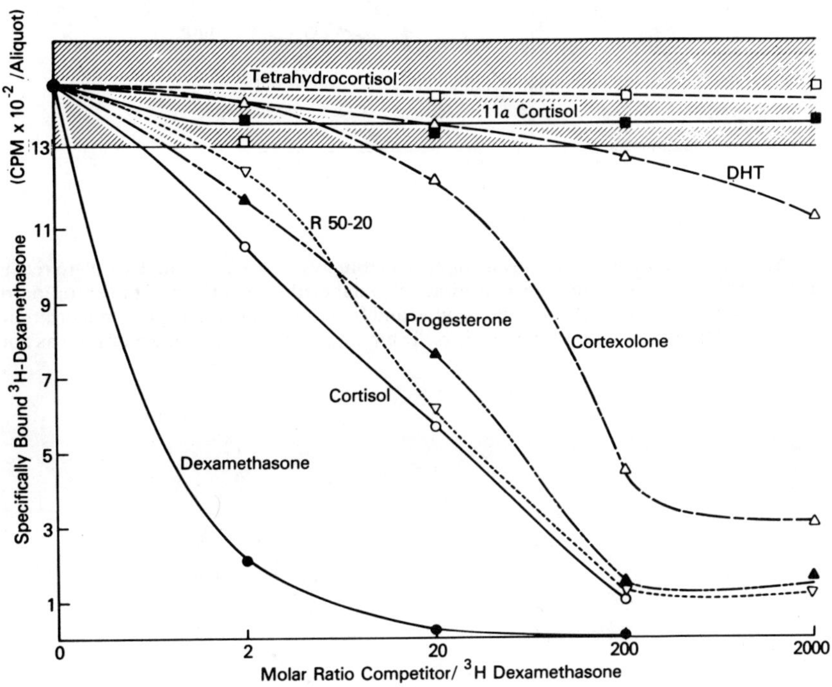

FIGURE 3. Specificity of the glucocorticoid receptor in MCF-7 human breast cancer. Cytoplasmic extracts were incubated with 10^{-8} M [^{3}H]dexamethasone in the presence of various concentrations of unlabeled steroid. After an overnight incubation at 0°C, specific binding was determined by use of dextran-coated charcoal to separate unbound [^{3}H]dexamethasone from protein-bound radioactivity. Points represent means of triplicate determinations.

receptor. In the experiments shown in FIGURE 3, the ability of various unlabeled steroids added simultaneously to block [^{3}H]dexamethasone binding to receptor is portrayed. As expected, unlabeled glucocorticoids, such as dexamethasone and cortisol, prevent [^{3}H]dexamethasone binding, whereas biologically inactive reduced metabolites or stereoisomers, such as tetrahydrocortisol or 11α-hydroxycortisol, show little ability to compete with dexamethasone. Of considerable interest are the results obtained with two progestational agents, progesterone and 17,21-dimethyl-19-norpregn-4,9,dien-3,20-dione (R 5020). The

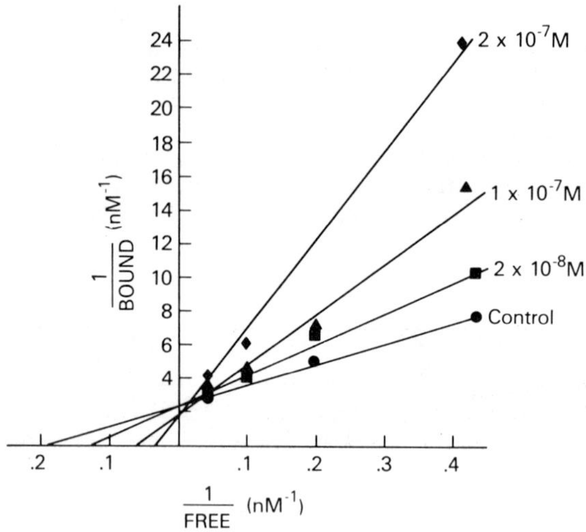

FIGURE 4. Double-reciprocal analysis of specific binding of [^{3}H]dexamethasone to receptor in the presence of various concentrations of unlabeled cortisol. The concentration of cortisol is given to the right of each line. Bound and free [^{3}H]dexamethasone concentrations are in units of femtomoles per milliliter. Specific binding was measured and analyzed as outlined in FIGURE 2.

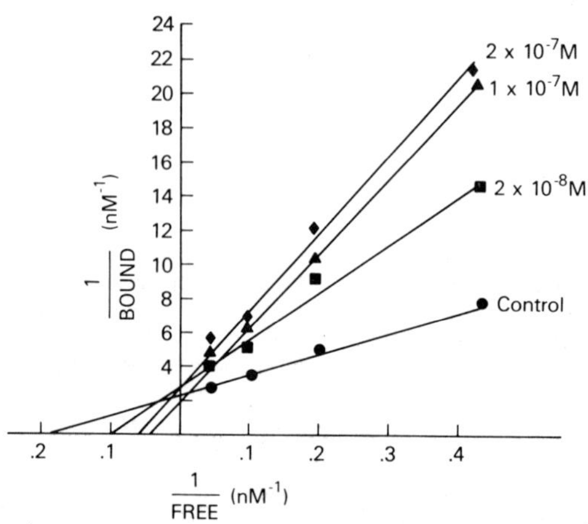

FIGURE 5. Double-reciprocal analysis of specific binding of [^{3}H]dexamethasone to receptor in the presence of various concentrations of unlabeled progesterone. The concentration of progesterone is given to the right of each line. Bound and free [^{3}H]dexamethasone concentrations are in units of femtomoles per milliliter. Specific binding was measured and analyzed as outlined in FIGURE 2.

latter compound is a synthetic progestational agent, prepared (and kindly provided) by the Roussel Corporation, that shows high affinity for progesterone receptor but essentially none for corticosteroid-binding globulin or transcortin.[17] Note that both of these compounds readily block [^{3}H]dexamethasone binding to receptor. The fact that an unlabeled steroid reduces binding of [^{3}H]dexamethasone does not necessarily indicate that the unlabeled steroid is competing for an identical binding site. For example, if a nonhomologous unlabeled steroid simply increased the nonspecific binding of the labeled ligand, a decrease in specific binding would be observed. A similar effect could be induced by any compound that inactivated the receptor.

The exact nature of the interaction of either unlabeled cortisol, progesterone, or R 5020 with the binding of [^{3}H]dexamethasone to its receptor sites is shown by the binding studies summarized in FIGURES 4–6. In FIGURE 4, double-reciprocal

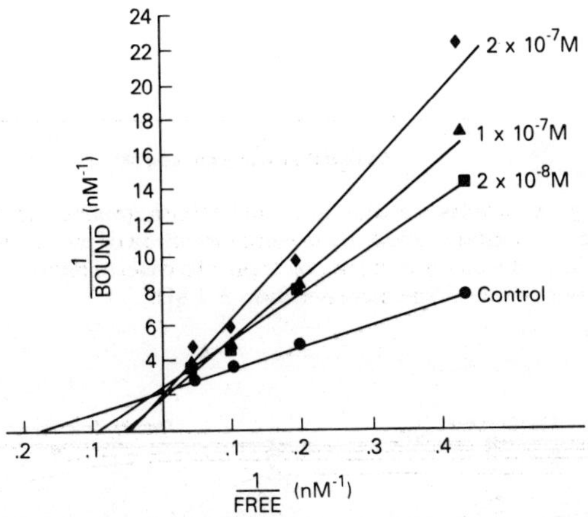

FIGURE 6. Double-reciprocal analysis of specific binding of [^{3}H]dexamethasone to receptor in the presence of various concentrations of unlabeled R 5020. The concentration of R 5020 is given to the right of each line. Bound and free [^{3}H]dexamethasone concentrations are in units of femtomoles per milliliter. Specific binding was measured and analyzed as outlined in FIGURE 2.

plots of [^{3}H]dexamethasone binding in the presence of various concentrations of unlabeled cortisol are shown. The expected competitive inhibition is obtained, as shown by the extrapolation of the lines to a constant number of binding sites at infinite [^{3}H]dexamethasone concentration. In FIGURE 5, the same experiment is repeated, except that various concentrations of unlabeled progesterone are employed instead of cortisol. Competitive inhibition is, again, seen. Finally, in FIGURE 6, [^{3}H]dexamethasone binding is measured in the presence of various concentrations of unlabeled R 5020, and, once again, competitive inhibition is seen. Thus, clearly both progestational agents behave similarly to cortisol, in that both can compete for a site to which [^{3}H]dexamethasone can bind. Thus, progestational agents appear to bind to glucocorticoid receptors in human breast cancer.

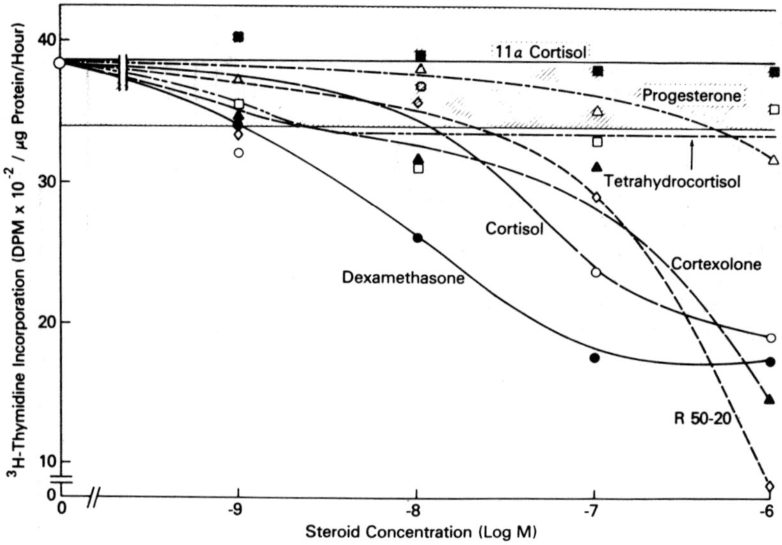

FIGURE 7. Ability of various steroids to inhibit [^{3}H]thymidine incorporation in MCF-7 human breast cancer. Conditions used to measure inhibition of nucleoside incorporation are as outlined in TABLE 1. Results are means of triplicate determinations. The shaded area at the top represents control thymidine incorporation ± 1 SD.

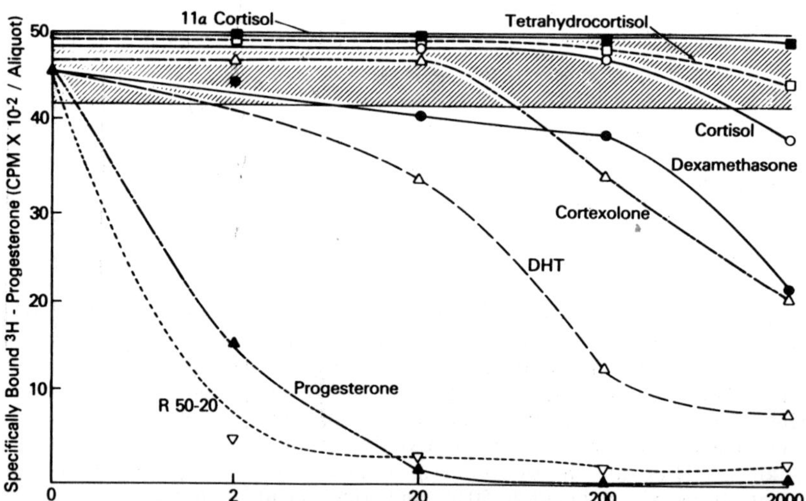

FIGURE 8. Competition of various steroids with [^{3}H]progesterone for binding sites. Cytoplasmic extracts prepared as previously described were incubated with [^{3}H]progesterone (10^{-8}M) with various concentrations of unlabeled steroids as noted in the Figure. At the end of an overnight incubation at 0°C, specific binding was assessed as described in FIGURE 3.

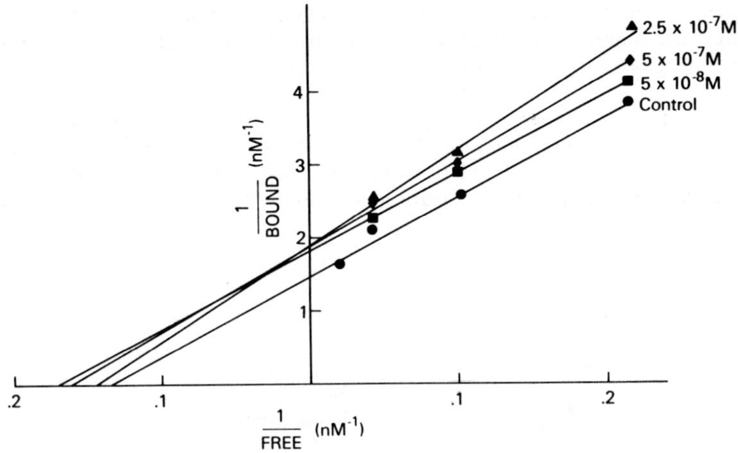

FIGURE 9. Double-reciprocal analysis of [^{3}H]progesterone to receptor in the presence of various concentrations of unlabeled cortisol. Concentrations of unlabeled cortisol employed are given to the right of each line. Bound and free [^{3}H]progesterone concentrations are given in units of femtomoles per milliliter.

If the biologic activities of various steroids are compared, results very different from those seen for binding are obtained. As shown in FIGURE 7, when thymidine incorporation is measured in the presence of increasing steroid concentrations, glucocorticoids, such as cortisol and dexamethasone, give the inhibitory responses previously described in TABLES 1–3. Note that tetrahydrocortisol and

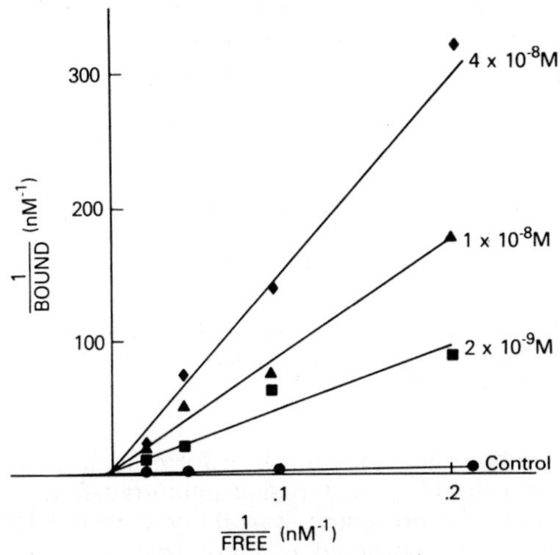

FIGURE 10. Double-reciprocal analysis of [^{3}H]progesterone to receptor in the presence of various concentrations of unlabeled R 5020. Concentrations of unlabeled R 5020 employed are given to the right of each line. Bound and free [^{3}H]progesterone concentrations are given in units of femtomoles per milliliter.

11α-cortisol, which failed to compete with [^{3}H]dexamethasone for glucocorticoid receptor, are inactive. R 5020 appears to be about as inhibitory as cortisol, whereas progesterone is essentially noninhibitory, except at extremely high concentrations. Thus, R 5020 appears to both compete with [^{3}H]dexamethasone for binding and to be biologically active as a glucocorticoid, whereas progesterone can also compete with [^{3}H]dexamethasone for binding activity but has essentially no glucocorticoid activity. The latter result is exactly the same as that previously reported in hepatoma tissue culture cells, in which it has been shown that

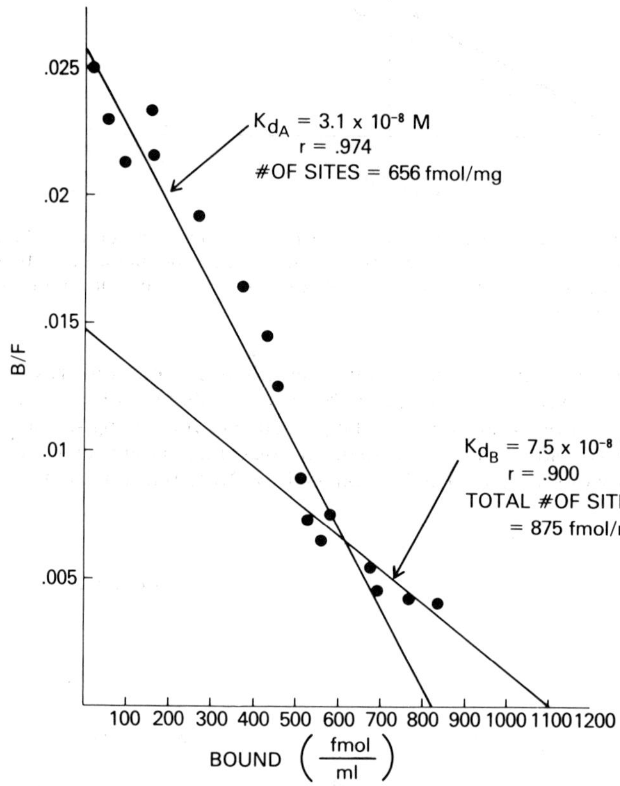

FIGURE 11. Scatchard analysis of the binding of [^{3}H]progesterone to receptor sites in cytoplasmic extracts of MCF-7 human breast cancer. Specific binding was measured and analyzed as described in FIGURE 2.

progesterone can bind to, but does not transform, glucocorticoid receptor and therefore is not an inducer of hepatic tyrosine aminotransferase.[18]

From the results thus far presented, it might be concluded that the MCF-7 cell line contains a single glucocorticoid receptor that also has some affinity for progestational agents. Two lines of evidence suggest that this might not be the case. First, if quantities of "receptor" are estimated and compared for labeled glucocorticoid and progesterone by using relatively high concentrations of labeled steroid (10^{-7} M), there is invariably an excess number of sites obtained in at least

TABLE 4
BINDING OF [^{3}H]PROGESTERONE TO RECEPTOR SITES IN MCF-7 HUMAN BREAST CANCER

	Component A*			Component B*		
Experiment	Dissociation Constant ($K_d \times 10^9$)	Correlation Coefficient (r)	Number of Sites (fmol/mg of protein)	Dissociation Constant ($K_d \times 10^9$)	Correlation Coefficient (r)	Number of Sites (fmol/mg of protein)
I	21	0.895	256	90	0.863	705
II	27	0.993	811	90	0.927	445
III	31	0.974	656	75	0.900	219

*Quantity and affinity of binding were determined as noted in the legend to FIGURE 2.

eight experiments with [^{3}H]progesterone as compared with dexamethasone. Second, if cytoplasmic extracts are incubated with [^{3}H]progesterone at a relatively low concentration (10^{-8} M) and various unlabeled steroids are added, as shown in FIGURE 8, a curious result is obtained. As expected, unlabeled progesterone and R 5020 both compete with labeled progesterone for binding sites. But glucocorticoids compete very poorly. Thus, it appears difficult to understand if progesterone is binding to glucocorticoid receptor, why glucocorticoids would fail to compete with [^{3}H]progesterone for binding. This lack of competition by glucocorticoids with progesterone is emphasized by the detailed studies shown in FIGURES 9 and 10. In FIGURE 9, unlabeled cortisol, even at a concentration of 5×10^{-6} M, essentially shows noncompetitive binding kinetics with [^{3}H]proges-

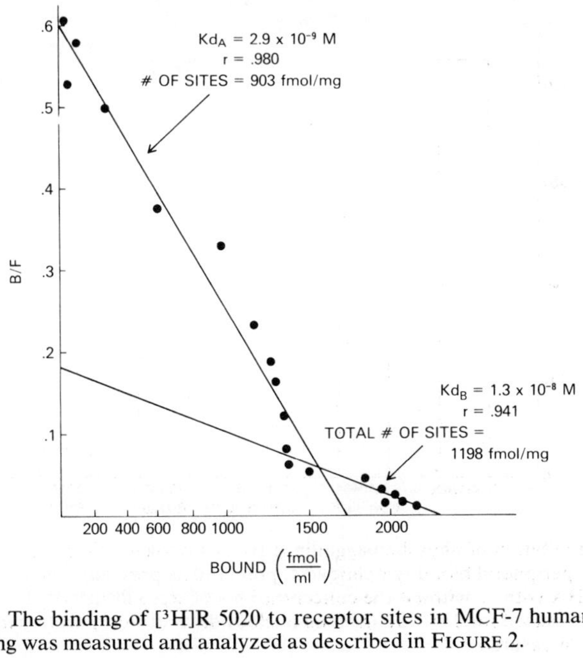

FIGURE 12. The binding of [^{3}H]R 5020 to receptor sites in MCF-7 human breast cancer. Specific binding was measured and analyzed as described in FIGURE 2.

TABLE 5
BINDING OF [^{3}H]R 5020 TO RECEPTOR SITES IN MCF-7 HUMAN BREAST CANCER

	Component A*			Component B*		
Experiment	Dissociation Constant ($K_d \times 10^9$)	Correlation Coefficient (r)	Number of Sites (fmol/mg of protein)	Dissociation Constant ($K_d \times 10^9$)	Correlation Coefficient (r)	Number of Sites (fmol/mg of protein)
I	2.9	0.980	903	13	0.941	295
II	1.0	0.963	963	17	0.903	625
III	4.2	0.938	1149	33	0.497	451

*Quantity and affinity of binding were determined as noted in the legend to FIGURE 2.

terone. In contrast, in FIGURE 10, R 5020 clearly shows competitive inhibition with labeled progesterone for binding sites. These results seem to suggest strongly that progesterone at lower concentrations might be binding to a unique site for which glucocorticoids have little affinity, while progesterone could bind at higher concentrations to glucocorticoid receptor. This model predicts that it should be possible to demonstrate two classes of progesterone-binding sites by careful Scatchard analysis if performed at a sufficiently wide range of concentrations. This result is exactly what is obtained, as shown in FIGURE 11. As indicated, two classes of binding sites are seen for [^{3}H]progesterone binding. The low bound/free ratio at which the second site becomes apparent speaks to the ease with which such lower-affinity but saturable binding sites may be missed in some studies.

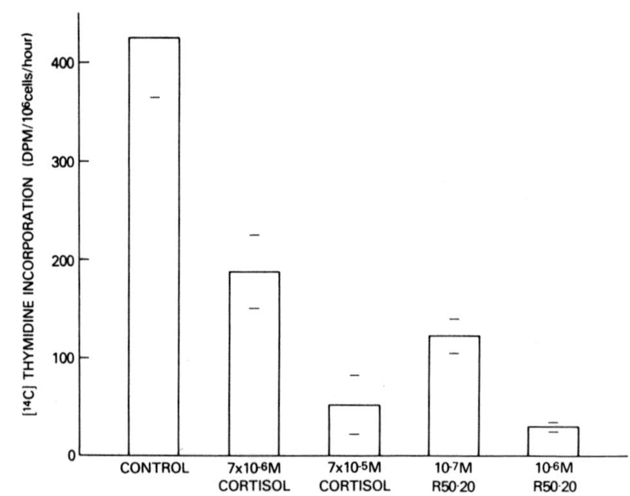

FIGURE 13. Inhibition of phytohemagglutin (PHA) -provoked mitogenesis by cortisol and R 5020. Human peripheral blood lymphocytes, prepared as previously described,[22] were incubated with PHA with or without the concentrations of steroids as noted. At the end of 24 hr the cells were pulsed for 2 hr with tritiated nucleoside, and incorporation into acid-insoluble material was measured.

TABLE 4 gives the results of two additional similar progesterone-binding experiments and emphasizes the reproducibility of this finding.

Based on the above considerations, one would presume that R 5020 would also give a two-component Scatchard plot; the results are shown in FIGURE 12. Once again, the two-component plot obtained is consistent with the idea that R 5020 binds to both progesterone and glucocorticoid receptors. TABLE 5 summarizes two additional experiments in which R 5020 was used to measure binding sites at a wide range of concentrations with essentially similar results. Note that [^{3}H]R 5020 binds to component A, the presumed progesterone receptor, about 10 times more tightly than does [^{3}H]progesterone but that it also binds about five times more tightly to component B, the putative glucocorticoid receptor. Thus, R 5020 would appear to be roughly twice as "selective" for progesterone receptor in the presence of glucocorticoid receptor as is progesterone.

We conclude from these data that the MCF-7 cell line has two receptors, one for glucocorticoid and one for progesterone (in addition to the previously described sex steroid receptors[11]). The glucocorticoid receptor has a range of binding specificities that includes progestational agents. The progesterone receptor, on the other hand, has essentially no affinity for glucocorticoids.

Our results also would seem to suggest that R 5020, aside from its progestational activity, can both bind to glucocorticoid receptor and has considerable glucocorticoid activity. The latter contention was confirmed in an experiment in collaboration with Dr. James P. Neifeld in which the abilities of cortisol and R 5020 to inhibit phytohemagglutinin (PHA) stimulation of human peripheral blood lymphocytes were compared; the results are shown in FIGURE 13. As shown, cortisol and R 5020 are about equipotent at blocking the PHA response under serum-free conditions, which obviate the effects of binding to transport proteins. Thus, in this independent assay system with human lymphocyte cells, R 5020 has glucocorticoid activity.

We conclude that measurement of progesterone receptor in the presence of glucocorticoid-binding sites, such as corticosteroid-binding globulin or glucocorticoid receptor, can be readily accomplished with either R 5020 or progesterone, provided that unlabeled glucocorticoids are added to the assay tubes to saturate the sites for which glucocorticoids and progesterone both compete.

REFERENCES

1. ATKINS, H. 1974. *In* The Treatment of Breast Cancer. H. Atkins, Ed.: 87–111. University Park Press. Baltimore, Md.
2. HORWITZ, K. B. & W. L. MCGUIRE. 1975. Steroids **25:** 497–505.
3. MCGUIRE, W. L., P. P. CARBONE, M. E. SEARS & G. C. ESCHER. 1975. *In* Estrogen Receptors in Human Breast Cancer. W. L. McGuire, P. P. Carbone & E. Vollmer, Eds.: 1–8. The Raven Press. New York, N.Y.
4. BOLAN, G., K. HUFF & M. E. LIPPMAN. 1975. Glucocorticoids inhibit human breast cancer in long term tissue culture. Proceedings of the 15th Annual Meeting of the American Society of Cell Biology. Puerto Rico.
5. LIPPMAN, M. E., G. BOLAN & K. HUFF. 1976. *In* Breast Cancer, Trends in Research and Treatment. J. C. Heuson, W. H. Mattheiem & M. Rozenzweig, Eds.: 111–139. The Raven Press. New York, N.Y.
6. HORWITZ, K. B., M. E. COSTLOW & W. L. MCGUIRE. 1975. Steroids **26:** 785–795.
7. SOULE, H. D., J. VAZQUEZ, A. LONG, A. ALBERT & M. BRENNAN. 1973. J. Nat. Cancer Inst. **51:** 1408–1413.

7a. YOUNG, N., L. L. ENGEL et al. 1976. In preparation.
8. LIPPMAN, M. E. & G. BOLAN. 1975. Nature (London) **256:** 592–593.
9. ROSE, H. N. & C. M. MCGRATH. 1975. Science **190:** 673–675.
10. LIPPMAN, M. E., G. BOLAN & K. HUFF. 1976. Cancer Res. **36:** 4595–4601.
11. LIPPMAN, M. E., G. BOLAN & K. HUFF. 1975. Nature (London) **258:** 339–341.
12. OSBORNE, C. K., G. BOLAN, M. E. MONACO & M. E. LIPPMAN. 1976. Proc. Nat. Acad. Sci. USA. In press.
13. VONDERHAAR, B. K. & Y. J. TOPPER. 1973. Enzyme **15:** 340–350.
14. GORAL, J. E. & J. WITTLIFF. 1975. Biochemistry **14:** 2944–2952.
15. PARKS, W., E. SCOLNICK & E. KUZIHOWSKI. 1974. Science **184:** 158–160.
16. STOLL, B. A. 1972. *In* Endocrine Therapy of Malignant Disease. B. A. Stoll, Ed.: 176–182. W. B. Saunders Company. Philadelphia, Pa.
17. PHILIBERT, D. & J. P. RAYNAUD. 1974. Endocrinology **94:** 627–634.
18. ROUSSEAU, G. G., J. D. BAXTER & G. M. TOMKINS. 1972. J. Mol. Biol. **67:** 99–116.
19. LOWRY, O. H., N. J. ROSEBROUGH, A. L. FARR & R. J. RANDALL. 1951. J. Biol. Chem. **193:** 265–275.
20. KNAZEK, R. A., P. M. GULLINO, P. O. KOHLER & R. L. DEDRICK. 1972. Science **178:** 65–67.
20a. KNAZEK, R. A., M. E. LIPPMAN & H. CHOPRA. 1976. J. Nat. Cancer Inst. In press.
21. SCATCHARD, G. 1949. Ann. N.Y. Acad. Sci. **51:** 660–672.
22. RABINOWITZ, Y. 1965. Blood **26:** 100–103.

DISCUSSION

DR. P. K. SIITERI: I was intrigued by the fact that the dexamethasone seemed to inhibit thymidine incorporation by about 50%, and though the R 5020 didn't bind quite as well, it seemed capable of a nearly total shutdown of thymidine incorporation.

DR. LIPPMAN: There are any number of possibilities. The first one, of course, is that R 5020 may be inhibiting the cells by some nonspecific pathways as well. The evidence against that possibility is that R 5020 does not affect breast cell lines that lack glucocorticoid receptor. The fact that a hormone has a lower affinity for receptor simply means it is less potent, but it does not mean that it cannot induce the full effect at a higher concentration.

DR. M. R. SHERMAN: The elegant demonstration of two distinct classes of binding sites does not resolve the apparent discrepancy between the competition by progesterone for the dexamethasone-binding sites and the failure of progesterone to inhibit thymidine uptake. This apparent discrepancy may be explained in terms of my model for combined steric and allosteric interactions between steroids and steroid analogs [1976. Nature (London) **260:** 288]. In this model, the receptor is assumed to equilibrate between two states, one of which is active and the other inactive, in mediating the observed response. A single class of steroid-binding sites is assumed to be present, but the relative affinities of these sites for various steroids depend on the state of the receptor. Accordingly, in your system, dexamethasone and progesterone would compete for the same class of binding sites. Dexamethasone would bind to (and thus stabilize) the active state of the receptor, and progesterone would bind to the inactive state. Since the binding of the two steroids would shift the equilibrium between receptor states in opposite directions, they would have different physiologic effects.

DR. LIPPMAN: Yes, I quite agree. I meant to imply that I think that the major interaction of progesterone with glucocorticoid receptor is via a nontransforming effect similar to that seen in studies that Guy Rousseau did in Gordon Tomkins' lab, showing that progesterone would not transform the glucocorticoid receptor of hepatoma cells.

DR. R. J. B. KING: Two different groups at our institute have obtained a different cell line from the MCF-7 from Marvin Rich. Our experience with these cells is relatively different from yours, and I would just like to offer a word of caution to anybody who is hoping to see these cells: the cell line that we have certainly doesn't seem to respond to steroids in the same way that yours do. But one feature that they do show is a very marked tendency of coming off the bottom of the dish in the absence of serum. Both of the groups at our institute have found this tendency.

Can you distinguish in your assay between a steroid inhibition, what you call proliferation, and just an increase in the rate at which the cell has come off the bottom of the dish, so they are in effect being lost to your assay[3]

DR. LIPPMAN: In our hands, by use of a mycoplasma-free MCF-7 cell line that may be different from the one you obtained, less than 4–5% of the cells are off the surface of the dish at the end of the experiment, usually considerably less. Even under totally serum-free conditions, we don't observe the effect that you describe. I would like to reemphasize that while I have shown a considerable number of experiments involving MCF-7, we have confirmed these results in at least three of the other human breast cancer cell lines, so I feel a high degree of confidence in those observations.

EFFECTS OF ESTROGEN AND PROGESTERONE ON OVALBUMIN SYNTHESIS IN THE WITHDRAWN OVIDUCT*

Robert T. Schimke, Pierre Pennequin, Diane Robins, and G. Stanley McKnight

Department of Pharmacology
Stanford University
Stanford, California 94305

The chick oviduct is an excellent system for study of the mechanism(s) of action of steroid hormone regulation of specific protein synthesis (see References 1–3 for reviews). Two distinct biologic phenomena are involved: stimulation of proliferation and cytodifferentiation, and a modulatory effect to regulate specific protein synthesis in differentiated cells. Estrogen administration to immature chicks stimulates proliferation and differentiation of tubular gland cells, which synthesize egg-white proteins. Progesterone given simultaneously inhibits estrogen-induced proliferation and cytodifferentiation. However, once tubular gland cells exist, progesterone, and estrogen, can stimulate egg-white protein synthesis. Because the synthesis of ovalbumin constitutes as much as 50% of total protein synthesis in the hormonally stimulated oviduct, the regulation of its synthesis has been studied extensively, employing the most advanced techniques available to eukaryote molecular biologists. Studies from several laboratories have concluded that the rate of ovalbumin synthesis is controlled largely by the content of ovalbumin mRNA, assayed either by its ability to drive ovalbumin synthesis in cell-free, heterologous protein-synthesizing systems[2,4] or by its ability to undergo hybridization with its complementary DNA (cDNA).[5–7] The data obtained thus far are consistent with the general model of steroid hormone action, which proposes that these hormones act directly on certain DNA sequences, presumably adjacent to the coding sequences, and regulate the rate of specific mRNA synthesis, that is, transcription.[8] In this paper, we report the effects of estrogen and progesterone on ovalbumin synthesis that do not necessarily fit such a simplistic model and suggest that the mechanism(s) may be more complex.

ARE THERE OVALBUMIN mRNA SEQUENCES IN THE WITHDRAWN OVIDUCT?

The simple model of steroid hormone action would predict that in the absence of administered hormone to chicks in which tubular gland cells exist, no ovalbumin mRNA sequences should exist. We have asked this question in chicks that have received 10 days of estrogen treatment, after which treatment no hormones have been administered for 2–6 weeks. At such time, the tissue is involuted, and although tubular gland cells comprise approximately 15% of the cells, ovalbumin synthesis in fragments is undetectable.[5] As shown in FIGURE 1, although we would predict finding no ovalbumin mRNA sequences, ovalbumin mRNA can be detected readily. We calculate that there are approximately 60

*Supported by Research Grant GM 14931 from the National Institutes of Health and Grant NP 148 from the American Cancer Society.

mRNA molecules per tubular gland cell, compared to about 50,000 per cell in the laying hen. This number of sequences is similar, regardless of whether the tissues are obtained from chicks at various intervals from 2 to 6 weeks after cessation of hormone administration.

We have characterized the properties of these sequences, employing mRNA-cDNA hybridization for identification, in an attempt to determine if they differ from those in the laying hen in cellular location or physical properties in a fashion that would indicate that hormone administration might affect some aspect of their properties. We find the following features:

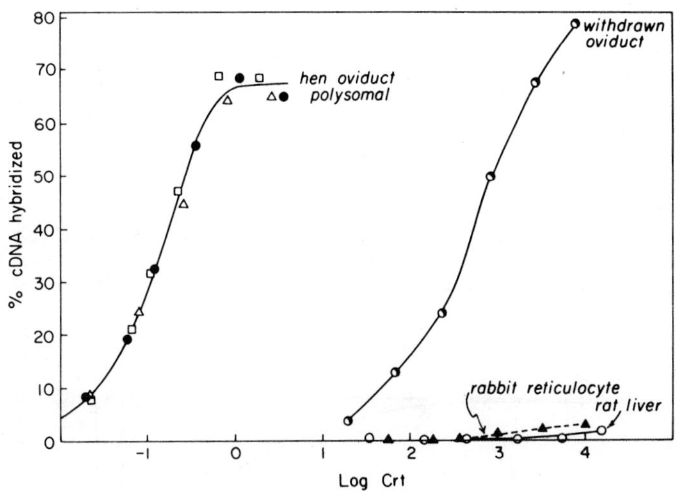

FIGURE 1. Hybridization of ovalbumin cDNA with RNA from various tissues. Withdrawn oviduct RNA (◑, 100.2 $A_{260\ nm}$/ml), rabbit reticulocyte RNA (▲, 102 $A_{260\ nm}$/ml), and rat liver RNA (○) were hybridized to 20 pg of cDNA. Three separate experiments are plotted for hen polysomal RNA. The RNA preparations were washed extensively with 3 M sodium acetate to remove DNA. The hen liver RNA was also treated with DNase. All hybridizations were performed in a total volume of 10 μl, except those for hen liver RNA, which were done in 20 μl. Unincubated controls that contained the RNA and all reaction components were treated with S_1 nuclease, and the percentage of cDNA resistance in the absence of added RNA (2–4%) was subtracted from all values. Details are given in Reference 5. (From McKnight *et al.*[5] By permission of *The Journal of Biological Chemistry*.)

1. Essentially all of the sequences are cytoplasmic, rather than nuclear.[5]
2. All of the sequences are the same size as ovalbumin mRNA isolated from laying hen polysomes, that is, 16S on denaturing sucrose gradients.[5]
3. All of the sequences are associated with the "membrane" fraction.[9] In the laying hen, 95% of total RNA and 99% of ovalbumin mRNA sequences are present in a membrane fraction, consistent with the concept that proteins destined for export are synthesized on membrane-bound polysomes. In the withdrawn oviduct, only 8% of the total RNA is membrane bound, whereas virtually all of the ovalbumin mRNA sequences are present in the membrane fraction (date not shown[9]).

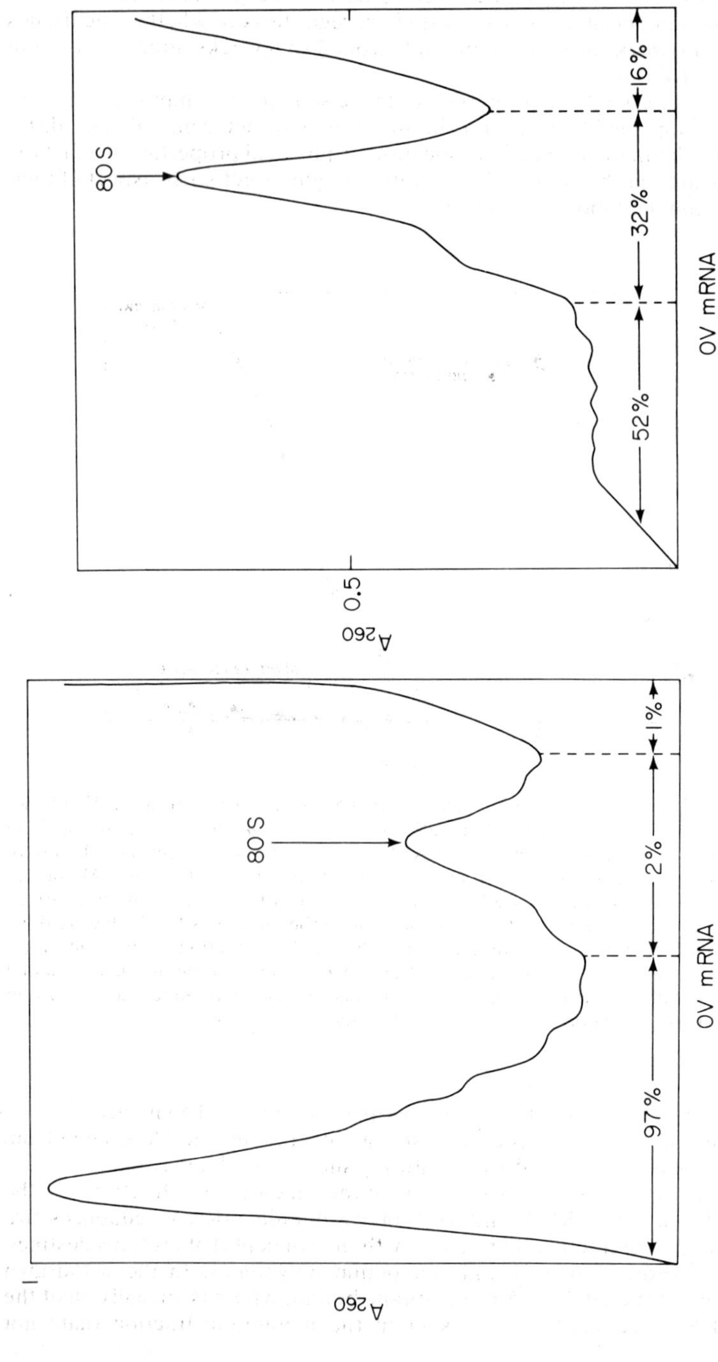

FIGURE 2. Distribution of ribosomes and ovalbumin mRNA in laying hen and withdrawn chick oviduct. Oviduct homogenates were centrifuged on concave exponential gradients. Fractions were collected as indicated on the OD profile. RNA was extracted from the fractions, washed with sodium acetate, and aliquots were hybridized with ovalbumin cDNA. The percentage figures indicate the distribution of ovalbumin mRNA sequences in the fractions. *Left*, laying hen; *right*, withdrawn chicks.

4. Ovalbumin mRNA is associated with small-sized polysomes. FIGURE 2 shows sucrose gradients of deoxycholate-solubilized homogenates of postnuclear pellets of oviduct from laying hen and withdrawn oviduct. In the laying hen, the vast majority of the RNA is present as large-sized polysomes, and 99% of the ovalbumin mRNA is associated with the polysomal fraction. In the withdrawn oviduct, monosomes predominate, and the average size of polysomes is smaller. In addition, only 52% of ovalbumin sequences is present in the polysomal fraction. One possibility in the withdrawn oviduct is that the ovalbumin mRNA is present, not on polysomes, but as mRNP particles. Using as a criterion of mRNP

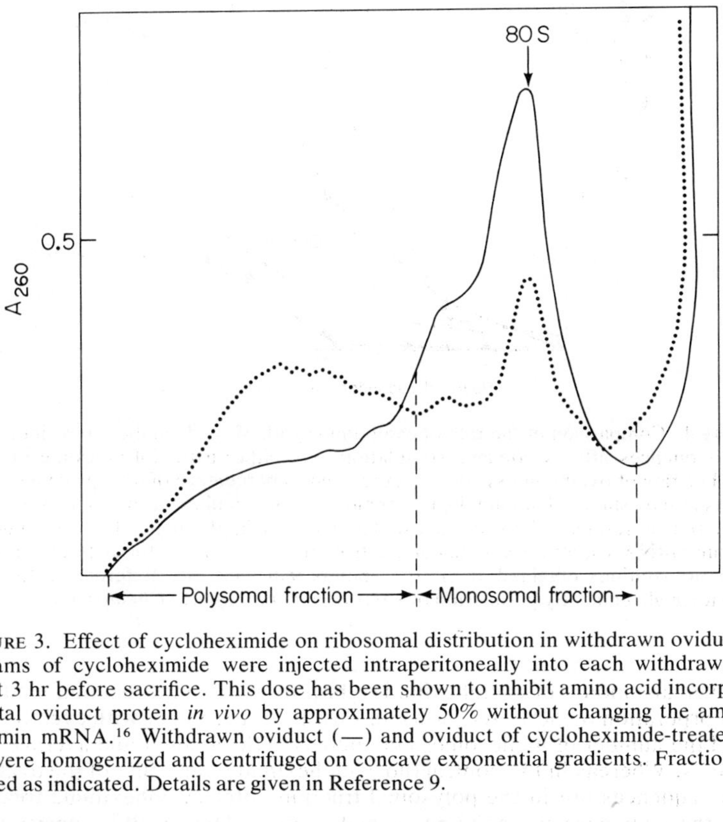

FIGURE 3. Effect of cycloheximide on ribosomal distribution in withdrawn oviduct. Five milligrams of cycloheximide were injected intraperitoneally into each withdrawn chick oviduct 3 hr before sacrifice. This dose has been shown to inhibit amino acid incorporation into total oviduct protein *in vivo* by approximately 50% without changing the amount of ovalbumin mRNA.[16] Withdrawn oviduct (—) and oviduct of cycloheximide-treated chick (. . .) were homogenized and centrifuged on concave exponential gradients. Fractions were collected as indicated. Details are given in Reference 9.

particles the fact that their sedimentation characteristics are not altered when treated with EDTA,[10] we find that they are not present as mRNP particles, because in both laying hen and withdrawn oviduct, treatment of the polysomal fraction with EDTA results in shifting of ovalbumin mRNA to a position in sucrose gradients typical of a 22S particle (data not shown; see Reference 9).

The finding of ovalbumin mRNA sequences with characteristics of those of the laying hen, except that they are present, on the average, on smaller-sized polysomes, suggests that the mRNA is poorly initiated, that is, few ribosomes per mRNA strand. This suggestion is further supported by studies in which chicks

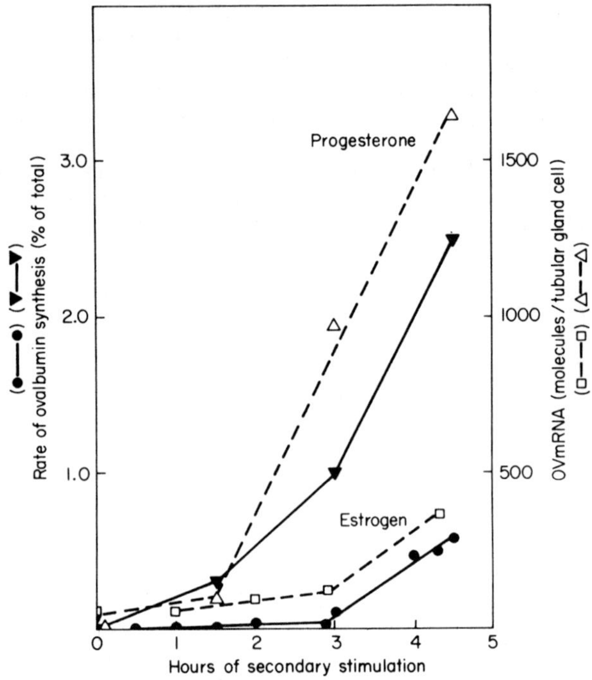

FIGURE 4. Comparison of the rate of ovalbumin synthesis and number of ovalbumin (OV) mRNA sequences after secondary stimulation with either estradiol benzoate or progesterone. The rate of ovalbumin synthesis (expressed as percentage of total protein synthesis) was measured by standard immunologic techniques. Three milligrams of each hormone were administered in sesame oil by intramuscular injection in the upper leg. The amount of ovalbumin mRNA sequences was calculated from the Crt $_{1/2}$ values for cDNA hybridization to RNA preparations obtained at the time points indicated. See Reference 5 for details. (From McKnight *et al.*[5] By permission of *The Journal of Biological Chemistry*.)

were given an amount of cycloheximide 3 hr prior to sacrifice that inhibited amino acid incorporation by 50%. As shown in FIGURE 3, treatment with cycloheximide reduced the number of monosomes and increased the amount and average size of polysomes. Whereas in the control (no cycloheximide) only 50% of the ovalbumin mRNA sequences are in the polysomal fraction, after cycloheximide treatment, 90% of the sequences are in the polysomal fraction. This result is consistent with the concept that ovalbumin sequences are present on polysomes with chain initiation rate limiting. Because cycloheximide inhibits peptide chain elongation[11] after drug treatment, initiation is no longer rate limiting, and therefore more ribosomes can be associated with each ovalbumin mRNA strand.

We conclude that the ovalbumin mRNA sequences present in the withdrawn oviduct are present in polysomes, and we cannot detect ovalbumin synthesis per se because of the low efficiency of utilization of the existing mRNA. The obvious conclusion from such studies is that the steroid hormones have effects on the efficiency of utilization of mRNAs, a conclusion reached from other considerations by Palmiter.[12]

What Is the Time Course of Initiation of Ovalbumin Synthesis and Ovalbumin mRNA Accumulation After Estrogen or Progesterone Administration?

The model of steroid hormone action in its most simple form predicts that specific mRNA should begin to accumulate as soon as the hormone becomes associated with its chromatin receptor. We have therefore examined the effects of estrogen and progesterone in the withdrawn chick on both ovalbumin synthesis and on the accumulation of ovalbumin mRNA, the results of which are summarized in Figure 4.[5] After estrogen administration, there is a 4-hr lag before ovalbumin synthesis can be detected in oviduct fragments. Inasmuch as estrogen binding to chromatin is maximal within 30 min after its administration,[13] we cannot ascribe this lag to a time-dependent binding process. One possibility for the lag is that mRNA does, in fact, begin to accumulate immediately but that it must undergo secondary processes before it can be translated. However, we also find that there is a 4-hr lag before ovalbumin mRNA sequences begin to accumulate. After progesterone treatment, the lag before ovalbumin synthesis and mRNA accumulation can be demonstrated is much shorter, that is, 90 min. With both hormones, the lag periods are not affected by the dose or route of administration. In addition, the initial rate of accumulation of ovalbumin mRNA is greater with progesterone than with estrogen.

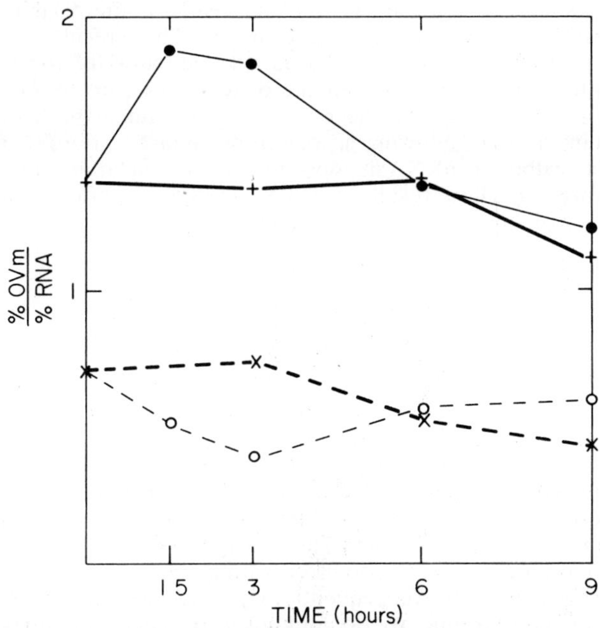

Figure 5. Relative concentration of ovalbumin mRNA in monosomal and polysomal fractions after secondary stimulation. RNA was extracted from monosomal and polysomal fractions of oviduct secondarily stimulated with 2.0 mg of estrogen or progesterone for different times, hybridized with ovalbumin cDNA, and results were expressed as the ratio of the percentage of ovalbumin mRNA to the percentage of total RNA in that fraction. Details are given in Reference 9.

After steroid hormone administration, in addition to the accumulation of specific mRNA (see FIGURE 4), there is an increase in the rate of peptide chain elongation[12] and a shift from monosomes to polysomes.[13] Therefore, we have also compared the effect of estrogen and progesterone in inducing the shift of ribosomes from inactive monosomes to active polysomes and in producing the shift of ovalbumin mRNA from the monosomal fraction to the polysomal fraction (see FIGURE 1). We have asked the question of whether either or both hormones preferentially affect the initiation of ovalbumin mRNA. We reason that a preferential shift of ovalbumin mRNA from the monosomal to the polysomal fraction relative to the shift of total RNA (ribosomal RNA) would indicate a preferential effect on utilization of these mRNAs. We administered estrogen or progesterone to withdrawn chicks and, at various times thereafter, made total polysomal preparations from which RNA was extracted from monosomal and polysomal fractions (see FIGURE 2), and the number of ovalbumin mRNA molecules and total RNA were determined. The results are summarized as follows. There is no detectable change in polysomal profiles with either hormone within the first 4 hr, after which time there is a progressive diminution in monosomes and an increase in the number and average size of polysomes. After estrogen administration, ovalbumin mRNA shifts progressively from the monosomal to the polysomal fraction, starting after 4 hr, and the proportional shift of ovalbumin mRNA and total RNA from monosomes to polysomes is similar. In contrast, after progesterone treatment, there is a more rapid shift of ovalbumin mRNA to polysomes, which can be detected as early as after 90 min, a time when ovalbumin mRNA is just beginning to accumulate. These results are summarized in FIGURE 5, which presents the data as derived ratios of the percentage of ovalbumin mRNA relative to percentage of total RNA in the monosomal and polysomal fractions.[9] Whereas the ratios are constant in both fractions after estrogen administration, following progesterone administration, there is an early enrichment in ovalbumin mRNA in polysomes and a comparable diminution in the monosomal fraction. These results indicate a preferential effect of progesterone, but not of estrogen, on the initiation of ovalbumin mRNA.

DISCUSSION

Our results raise questions concerning a simplistic model of steroid hormone action wherein specific protein synthesis is regulated solely by hormonal effects on transcription (synthesis) of specific mRNAs. First, we find a certain number of ovalbumin mRNA sequences in the withdrawn oviduct. Palmiter *et al.*[14] have recently reported that there are a considerable number of conalbumin mRNA sequences in the withdrawn oviduct. Thus, it appears that in the absence of the amounts of hormone normally associated with active synthesis of the egg-white proteins, mRNA is present. Consequently, we conclude that mRNA is being synthesized. At the present time, we do not know if the accumulation of mRNA that occurs after hormone administration results solely from an acceleration in its rate of synthesis or whether a significant factor in controlling accumulation is related to the turnover rate of the mRNA. It is interesting that Palmiter and Carey[15] have previously shown a significant hormonal effect on the half-life of ovalbumin mRNA, and, consequently, an effect of the hormones on rates of mRNA turnover is likely.

Second, there is no simple explanation for the differences in lag periods that occur after estrogen and progesterone administration and the accumulation of ovalbumin mRNA sequences. This fact becomes all the more puzzling in the light of recent studies by Palmiter *et al.*,[13] who showed that after estrogen administration, conalbumin mRNA, detected by a translational assay, accumulates immediately, whereas its accumulation after progesterone administration begins only after 4 hr. One cannot, therefore, invoke time-dependent metabolic interconversions of the hormones. Thus, we must interpose additional steps between initial hormone binding to presumed chromatin receptor sites and an effect in controlling mRNA accumulation. Presuming a transcriptional model (as opposed to one that controls only mRNA degradation), one can envisage the time dependence to involve migration of receptors to specific sites different for different DNA sequences or processes that involve more extensive alterations in chromosomal structure.

We have also demonstrated that the steroid hormones have effects on the utilization of mRNA. Thus, the ovalbumin mRNA present in the withdrawn oviduct is present as poorly initiated polysomes. It is interesting that progesterone, but not estrogen, would appear to have an effect on the initiation of this mRNA. The nature of this effect and the extent to which other egg-white protein mRNAs are differentially controlled by estrogen and progesterone are currently under active study. Clearly, the conclusions one makes concerning the mechanisms of action of steroid hormones in the oviduct are prejudiced by the steroid hormone and the specific protein (and mRNA) studied, and the multiple and different effects obtained with different combinations of the above suggest that hormonal regulation in this system is more complex than we currently envisage.

References

1. O'Malley, B. W., W. L. McGuire, P. O. Kohler, & S. G. Korenman. 1969. Studies on the mechanism of steroid hormone regulation of synthesis of specific proteins. Rec. Progr. Hormone Res. **25:** 105–160.
2. Schimke, R. T., G. S. McKnight, D. J. Shapiro, D. Sullivan & R. Palacios. 1975. Hormonal regulation of ovalbumin synthesis in the chick oviduct. Rec. Progr. Hormone Res. **31:** 175–209.
3. Palmiter, R. D. 1975. Quantitative parameters that determine the role of ovalbumin synthesis. Cell **4:** 189–197.
4. Means, A. R., J. P. Comstock, G. C. Rosenfeld & B. W. O'Malley. 1972. Ovalbumin messenger RNA of chick oviduct: partial characterization, estrogen dependence, and translation *in vitro*. Proc. Nat. Acad. Sci. USA **69**(5): 1146–1150.
5. McKnight, G. S., P. Pennequin & R. T. Schimke. 1975. Induction of ovalbumin mRNA sequences by estrogen and progesterone in chick oviduct as measured by hybridization to complementary DNA. J. Biol. Chem. **250**(20): 8105–8110.
6. Harris, S. E., J. M. Rosen, A. R. Means & B. W. O'Malley. 1975. Use of a specific probe for ovalbumin messenger RNA to quantitate estrogen-induced gene transcripts. Biochemistry **14**(10): 2072–2081.
7. Cox, R. F., M. E. Haines & J. S. Emtage. 1974. Quantitation of ovalbumin mRNA in hen and chick oviduct by hybridization to complementary DNA. Accumulation of specific mRNA in response to estradiol. Eur. J. Biochem. **49:** 225–236.
8. Jensen, E. V. & E. R. DeSombre. 1973. Estrogen-receptor interaction. Estrogenic hormones effect transformation of specific receptor proteins to a biochemically functional form. Science **182:** 126–134.
9. Pennequin, P., D. Robins & R. T. Schimke. 1976. Regulation of ovalbumin messenger RNA translating estrogens and progesterone in oviduct of withdrawn chicks. In press.

10. Morel, C., B. Kayibanda & K. Scherrer. 1971. Proteins associated with globin messenger RNA in avian erythroblasts: isolation and comparison with the proteins bound to nuclear messenger-like RNA. FEBS Lett. **18**(1): 84–88.
11. Warner, J. R., A. Rich & C. E. Hall. 1962. Electron microscope studies of ribosomal clusters synthesizing hemoglobin. Science **138:** 1399–1403.
12. Palmiter, R. D. 1972. Regulation of protein synthesis in chick oviduct. II. Modulation of polypeptide elongation and initiation rates by estrogen and progesterone. J. Biol. Chem. **247**(21): 6770–6780.
13. Palmiter, R. D., A. K. Christensen & R. T. Schimke. 1970. Organization of polysomes from pre-existing ribosomes in chick oviduct by a secondary administration of either estradiol or progesterone. J. Biol. Chem. **245**(4): 833–845.
14. Palmiter, R. D. 1976. Cell. In press.
15. Palmiter, R. D. & N. H. Carey. 1974. Rapid inactivation of ovalbumin messenger ribonucleic acid after acute withdrawal of estrogen. Proc. Nat. Acad. Sci. USA **71**(6): 2357–2361.
16. 19xx. Unpublished results.

PROGESTERONE-DEPENDENT MESSENGER RNA: IDENTIFICATION OF THE PRODUCTS OF HETEROSPECIFIC ACTIVITY *IN VIVO**

Sheldon J. Segal, Mario Burgos,† and C. Richard Lyttle‡

The Population Council
The Rockefeller University
New York, New York 10021

Introduction

The oviduct of an estrogen-primed chick will synthesize avidin in response to a single injection of progesterone.[1] The synthesis of avidin is preceded by an increase in the rate of nuclear RNA synthesis.[1] It has also been demonstrated that if poly(A)-containing RNA is isolated from estrogen-primed progesterone-treated chick oviducts and subsequently injected into the lumen of the oviduct of estrogen-primed chicks, avidin synthesis will result.[2] Treatment of the isolated RNA with ribonuclease results in the loss of activity which suggests that induction is not due to progesterone contamination.[3] Other examples of this phenomenon have been reported; RNA extracted from antigen-stimulated macrophages is capable of initiating an IgM response in both lymphoid organ and cell cultures.[4] RNA isolated from uteri of estradiol-treated rats, when injected into the lumen of ovariectomized rats, resulted in an increase in glucose 6-phosphate dehydrogenase activity.[5] These findings are examples of homologous transfer of information by isolated RNA. By use of similar techniques, we have also demonstrated heterospecific transfer.[6] If poly(A) RNA is extracted from estrogen-primed progesterone-treated chick oviducts and given via an intraoviductal injection to estrogen-primed pigeons, avidin is induced. RNA extracted from hormonally treated pigeons and given to estrogen-primed chicks also results in avidin synthesis.[3] In this paper, we will demonstrate that the avidin produced is characteristic of the species from which the poly(A) RNA has been isolated.

Materials and Methods

The techniques for isolation of poly(A) RNA, instillation of RNA in chick oviducts and the biotin-binding assay for avidin, have been published previously.[1–3,6] An immunologic assay for avidin is based on a rabbit antiserum developed with the use of chick avidin purified by affinity chromatography. This assay is described here in detail. In the prototype experience, 1-day-old chicks are treated with 0.5 mg of diethylstilbestrol for at least 5 days and are given one subcutaneous injection of 5 mg of progesterone. Eighteen hours later, the oviducts are removed and assayed for avidin. The tissue is homogenized (10% w/v) in 0.02 M phosphate buffer (pH 7.1) that contains 70 mM KC1, 70 mM NaC1, and 4 mM

*Supported by United States Public Health Service Grant HD05671.

†Present address: University of Cuyo, Mendoza, Argentina.

‡Present address: Ben May Cancer Research Laboratory, The University of Chicago, Chicago, Ill.

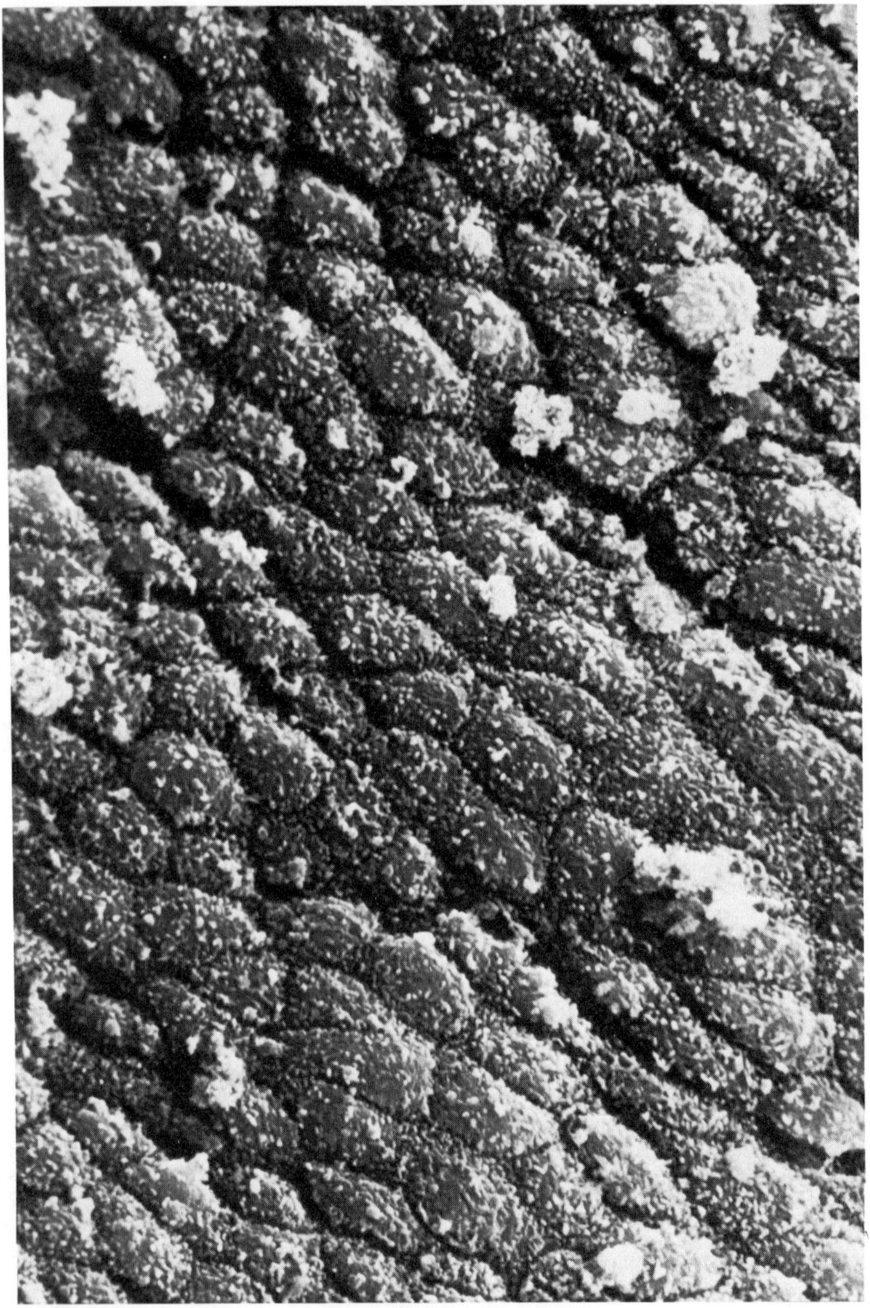

FIGURE 1. Scanning electron micrograph of a 7-day chick oviduct without hormone stimulation. ×4500.

$MgCl_2$. The homogenate is centrifuged at 105,000*g* for 30 min, and the supernatant is used for each assay. In the antibody assay, 4.0 ml of the supernatant are supplemented with 0.2 ml of D-[*carbonyl*-^{14}C]biotin (0.01 μCi; 45 mCi/mmol) and are then mixed and left to stand for 15 min; 25 μl of the antibody are then added. Two hours later, the solution is filtered on Millipore HAWP (0.45 μm) filters, which are washed 10 times with 5 ml of 0.2 M ammonium carbonate, then the radioactivity on each filter is determined by use of Aquasol® as a scintillation fluid. The bentonite assay was identical, except that instead of adding antibody after radioactive biotin, 20 mg of bentonite in 1.0 ml of the homogenizing buffer are added, mixed, and left to stand for 30 min. The precipitate is then filtered on glass fiber filters (Whatman GF/C), and the filters are washed and counted as in the antibody assay.

TABLE 1

BIOLOGIC ACTIVITY OF TOTAL RNA AND POLY(A) RNA FROM PROGESTERONE-STIMULATED CHICK OVIDUCT

Treatment on Final Day*	Dose (μg)	Avidin† (μg/g)
Chick oviduct total RNA	2500	1.78 ± 0.63
	500	0.79 ± 0.45
	50	0
washed	500	0.48 ± 0.34
RNase treated	500	0
Chick oviduct poly(A) RNA	10	0.83 ± 0.42
RNase treated	10	0

*One-day-old chicks primed for 5 days with 0.5 mg of diethylstilbestrol daily.
†± Standard deviation: $S = \sqrt{[\Sigma(x - \bar{x})^2]/n - 1}$.

RESULTS AND DISCUSSION

Total RNA or poly (A) RNA, when administered to estrogen-primed chicks, can within a 24-hr period cause avidin synthesis, as does progesterone treatment (TABLE 1). The nitrocellulose trapping procedure purifies a total RNA extract to a very high degree. When total RNA is used for stimulation, approximately 500 μg are required to induce avidin synthesis. Fifty micrograms fails to induce avidin synthesis. However, as little as 10 μg of poly(A) RNA can induce significant avidin synthesis. Thus, the nitrocellulose trapping effects a 50-fold purification. RNase treatment of either the total RNA extract or the nitrocellulose-trapped RNA causes a loss of biologic activity.

The biologic effect of poly(A) RNA can be seen also in terms of the morphologic response of the chick oviduct. FIGURE 1 is a scanning electron micrograph of a nonstimulated oviduct of a 7-day chick. It is a rather bleak surface covered with punctate microvilli and occasional single cilia or clusters of cilia. In general, however, the surface gives the impression of inactivity.

Estrogen stimulation for 5 days results in the initiation of a marked degree of ciliogenesis (FIGURE 2). The growth of cilia is clear and pronounced, but large areas of the surface are not covered with cilia and remain in the nonstimulated condition. The addition of progesterone for a final 18-hr period of treatment results in a dramatic increase in ciliogenesis. Essentially, the entire surface is

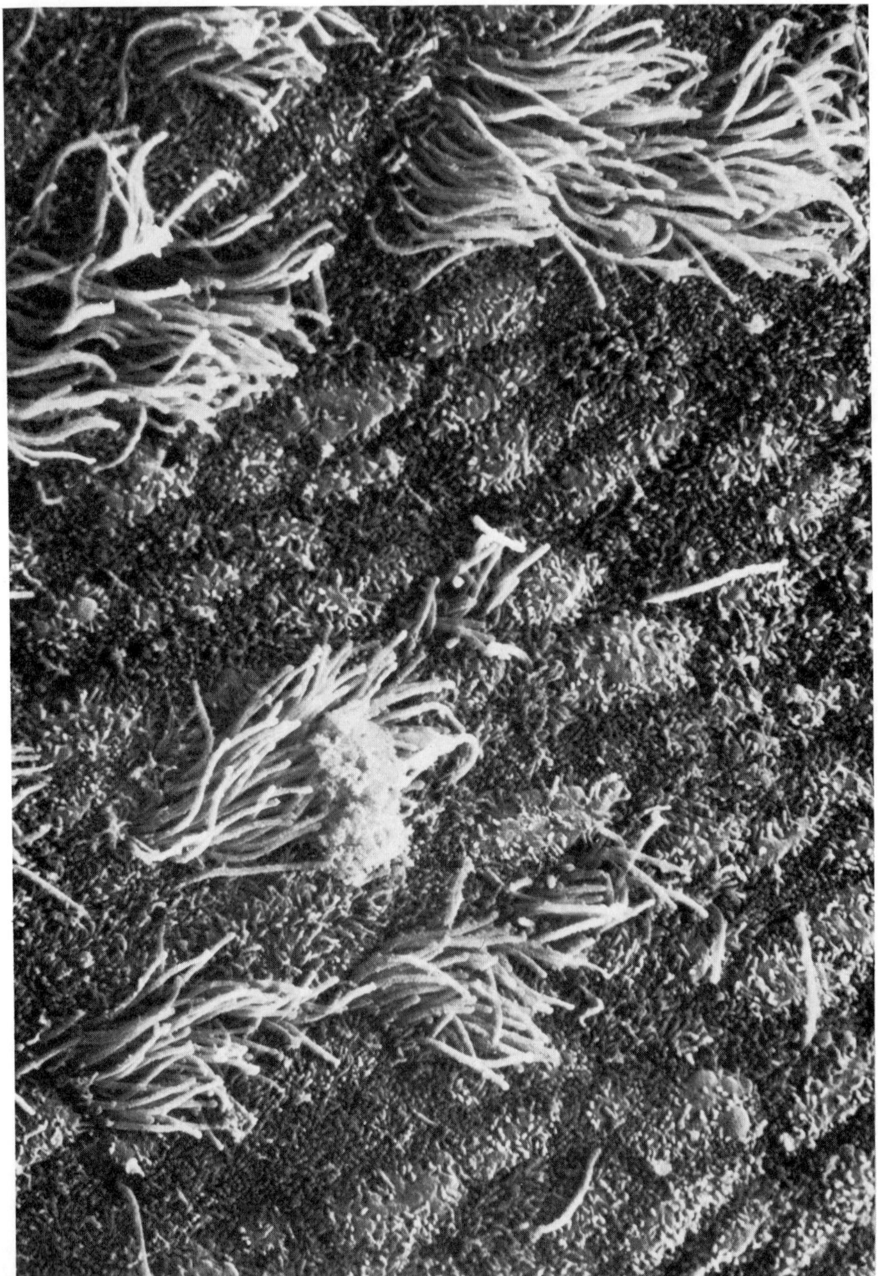

FIGURE 2. Scanning electron micrograph of a 7-day chick oviduct, treated with 0.5 mg of diethylstilbestrol daily by subcutaneous injection for 5 days (Days 2–6 posthatching). On Day 7, the chick was treated with 100 μl of saline intraoviductally and was sacrificed 12 hr later. ×4500.

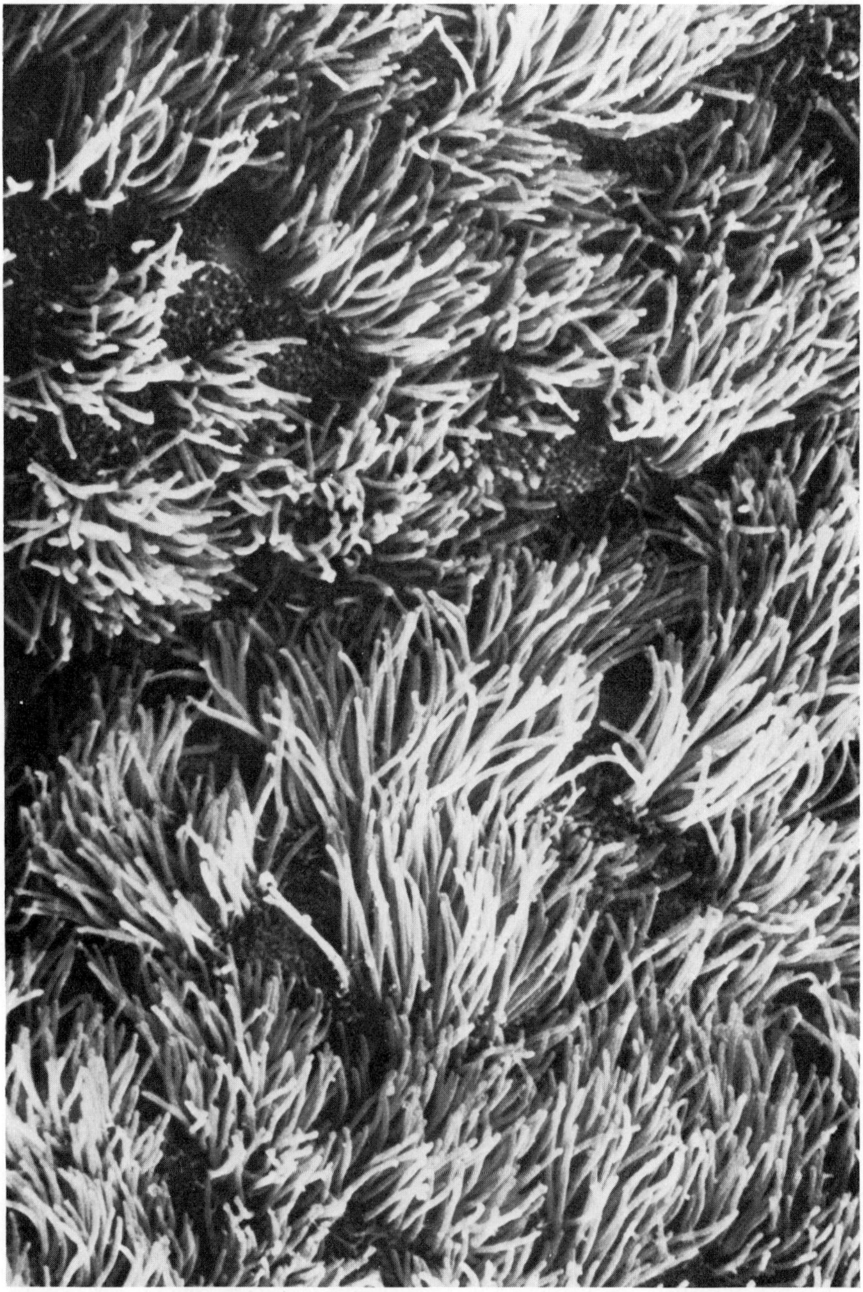

FIGURE 3. Scanning electron micrograph of a 7-day chick oviduct, treated with 0.5 mg of diethylstilbestrol daily by subcutaneous injection for 5 days (Days 2–6 posthatching). On Day 7, the chick was treated intraoviductally with 50 μg/100 liters of poly(A) RNA from progesterone-stimulated chick oviducts. ×4500.

covered with an abundance of ciliary processes. This effect of progesterone can be replicated by adding during the final 18-hr period, not progesterone, but poly(A) RNA recovered from the oviduct of progesterone-stimulated chicks, as shown in FIGURE 3. Here, a morphologic pattern develops identical to that seen when progesterone is the final treatment agent. We have demonstrated previously that progesterone or steroid contamination could not account for the activity of the mRNA fraction.[2] The activity is prevented by pretreatment with RNase.

Thus, we have demonstrated that biologically active poly(A) RNA can be extracted from progesterone-treated chicks. This RNA, when administered intraluminally into the oviducts of estrogen-primed chicks, stimulates both avidin synthesis and morphologic changes characteristic of the action of progesterone itself.

The pigeon oviduct also responds to progesterone treatment by synthesizing avidin. The time sequence of maximum avidin synthesis after progesterone treatment is essentially the same as that seen in the chick. By approximately 24 hr, avidin synthesis reaches its maximum and then begins to decline.[6] Having demonstrated the progesterone dependence for avidin synthesis in the pigeon, it has been possible to demonstrate avidin synthesis by the pigeon oviduct in response to RNA extracted from either pigeons or chicks treated with progesterone.[6] Similarly, the chick oviduct can respond to either homologous or heterologous progesterone-coded RNA by synthesizing avidin.[6] The heterospecific activity of the nitrocellulose-trapped RNA can be demonstrated not only among avian species but also among animals of different vertebrate classes. Avidin synthesis occurs in response to the administration of chick RNA into the oviduct of the adult *Xenopus* female.[6] It is of interest that neither progesterone nor 20α-hydroxyprogesterone administered into the oviduct or into the dorsal lymph sac is capable of stimulating avidin synthesis in the *Xenopus* oviduct. Subsequently, we have found that in *Xenopus*, avidin is normally synthesized within the ovary itself and not by the oviduct. Thus, it is particularly interesting to note that under these experimental conditions, the administration of heterologous

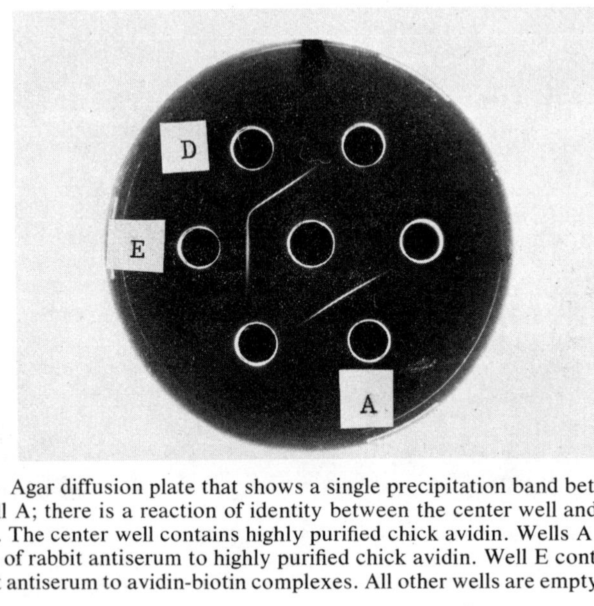

FIGURE 4. Agar diffusion plate that shows a single precipitation band between the center well and well A; there is a reaction of identity between the center well and wells D and E, respectively. The center well contains highly purified chick avidin. Wells A and D contain a 1:64 dilution of rabbit antiserum to highly purified chick avidin. Well E contains a 1:64 dilution of rabbit antiserum to avidin-biotin complexes. All other wells are empty.

TABLE 2

AVIDIN ASSAYS: ANTISERUM AND BENTONITE

Avidin Source	Treatment on Final Day	Avidin (μg/g)		Ratio AS/B	p Value
		AS*	B		
Chick oviduct	5 mg of progesterone	6.95 ± 2.70	6.24 ± 2.70	1:1	ns
Pigeon oviduct	5 mg of progesterone	0.15 ± 0.08	2.37 ± 1.60	1:15	<0.001
Xenopus ovary	5 mg of progesterone	1.70 ± 1.10	14.20 ± 5.90	1:8	<0.001
Chick oviduct	100 μg of RNA†	0.18 ± 0.05	1.75 ± 0.40	1:10	<0.001
Chick oviduct	100 μg of RNA‡	0.87 ± 0.23	0.73 ± 0.17	1:1	ns
Pigeon oviduct	100 μg of RNA‡	0.69 ± 0.28	0.91 ± 0.25	1:1	ns

*Antiserum to purified chick avidin.
†Poly(A) RNA from pigeon oviduct.
‡Poly(A) RNA from chick oviduct.

RNA that is coded for avidin results in synthesis of the protein *in vivo* by an organ not ordinarily involved in the synthesis.

An important issue raised by these observations is how the exogenous RNA, once it enters the cell, brings about the synthesis of avidin. One possibility is that there is a direct translation of the exogenously administered RNA, a phenomenon described in other systems *in vitro* and, occasionally, *in vivo*. The translation of a foreign message by *Xenopus* oocytes[7] and the ability of cell-free preparations of rabbit reticulocyte lysates[8] to translate RNA are examples. Another possibility is that the exogenous messenger RNA entering the cell initiates a process that affects the nucleus and ultimately results in *de novo* transcription of the host cell's message for avidin synthesis.

To explore this issue, concerning the stimulus for avidin synthesis once the exogenous RNA enters the cell, an immunologic approach has been used. The objective has been to determine whether the exogenous RNA is translated directly or whether it acts in some manner at the nuclear level to influence transcription of avidin-coded RNA. We have sought to determine whether there is an absolute antigenic identity among the avidin molecules produced by the different species we have used. Highly purified chicken avidin was used to immunize rabbits. A standard immunization procedure that uses Freund's complete adjuvant was employed. The purity of the antibody produced is revealed by the single band developed in the Ouchterlony agar diffusion plate (FIGURE 4). The center well contains the purified avidin used in the immunization procedure, and well A contains a 1:64 dilution of the antibody produced against purified avidin. The Figure also shows that binding with biotin does not alter the antigenic specificity of the avidin molecule. In wells D and E, equal dilutions of two different antisera are placed side by side. In well D is the antiserum to purified avidin. Well E contains antiserum from a rabbit immunized with avidin bound to biotin. There is no difference in the immunoprecipitation characteristics. The two antibodies give a reaction of identity.

With the antibody to highly purified chick avidin, it has been possible to develop an antibody assay for avidin, for comparison with the conventional [^{14}C]biotin binding method, which involves precipitation with bentonite. TABLE 2 shows a comparison of the antibody assay and the bentonite assay with an extract of oviduct from estrogen-primed chicks treated with progesterone. As can be seen, the two assays give a 1:1 ratio, which indicates that under optimal conditions, there is a quantitative recovery of all of the avidin in the sample. The amount of bentonite or of antibody added has been established by serial dilutions to assure that it is not a limiting factor in either assay.

When the same two assays are used for determining avidin in either pigeon oviduct or *Xenopus* ovary, the ratio obtained is less than 1:1. This finding indicates that the chick antibody binds only inefficiently, if at all, to the avidin present in the tissues of these foreign species. For pigeon avidin, the ratio between the two assays is 1:15. For *Xenopus* ovaries, the ratio between the two assays is 1:8. In each case, the difference is statistically significant ($p < 0.001$). From these results, it can be concluded that an immunologic difference exists among the avidin molecules produced by the three species. For chick avidin, precipitation after ^{14}C binding with either bentonite or antibody to chick avidin, which is a specific precipitating agent, results in total recovery of the avidin-biotin complex. When pigeon or *Xenopus* avidin is used, [^{14}C]biotin binding and nonspecific precipitation with bentonite proceed similarly. However, there is inefficient precipitation of the complex that involves antichick avidin antibody.

By use of the comparative assay results, it is possible to characterize the avidin synthesized in response to heterospecific RNA. In one experiment, RNA is extracted from the oviduct of pigeons treated with progesterone. The RNA is purified by nitrocellulose trapping and is administered into the chick oviduct lumen. Comparison of the two assays reveals a 1:10 ratio, indicative of the fact that the avidin in the preparation is immunologically different from native chick avidin, even though it has been produced by the chick oviduct. Thus, it appears that the heterospecific RNA is undergoing cytoplasmic translation rather than acting at the nuclear level to influence transcription of avidin-coded RNA. A similar conclusion can be drawn from experiments in which poly(A) RNA from chicks is administered intraoviductally to pigeons. The type of avidin synthesized is characteristic of the donor species (the exogenous RNA) and not the host species (the avidin-producing tissue).

Conclusions

From the immunologic analysis of these heterospecific crosses, we conclude that the experiments reported here, and previous experiments from our laboratory, are explained on the basis of *in vivo* translation of exogenously administered message.

These observations provide direct evidence for the concept, now widely accepted, that hormones act through a process of gene activation, creating a specific pattern of RNA synthesis that characterizes the conversion of the nonstimulated target cell to the stimulated state. Specific hormonal effects on both secretory function and the synthesis of structural components involved in morphologic transformation of cells can be simulated by exposure of target cells to hormone-induced RNA, thus confirming that after its role in gene activation, the hormone molecule is no longer involved in transformation of the target cell to the stimulation phase of activity.

References

1. O'Malley, B. W., W. L. McGuire, P. O. Kohler & S. G. Korenman. 1969. Rec. Progr. Hormone Res. **25:** 105–160.

2. Tuohimaa, P., S. J. Segal & S. S. Koide. 1972. Proc. Nat. Acad. Sci. USA **69**(10): 2814–2817.
3. Segal, S. J., R. O. Ige, P. Tuohimaa & M. H. Burgos. 1973. Science **181:** 569, 570.
4. Fishman, M. 1973. *In* The Role of RNA in Reproduction and Development. M. C. Niu & S. J. Segal, Eds.: 127–137. North-Holland Publishing Co. Amsterdam, The Netherlands.
5. Villee, C. A. 1973. *In* The Role of RNA in Reproduction and Development. M. C. Niu & S. J. Segal, Eds.: 167–182. North-Holland Publishing Co. Amsterdam, The Netherlands.
6. Segal, S. J., R. Ige, M. Burgos, P. Tuohimaa & S. S. Koide. 1973. *In* The Role of RNA in Reproduction and Development. M. C. Niu & S. J. Segal, Eds.: 270–283. North-Holland Publishing Co. Amsterdam, The Netherlands.
7. Knowland, J. S., J. B. Gurdon & R. A. Laskey. 1973. *In* The Role of RNA in Reproduction and Development. M. C. Niu & S. J. Segal, Eds.: 110–120. North-Holland Publishing Co. Amsterdam, The Netherlands.
8. Schimke, R. T., R. E. Rhoads, R. Palacios & D. Sullivan. 1973. *In* The Role of RNA in Reproduction and Development. M. C. Niu & S. J. Segal, Eds.: 26–42. North-Holland Publishing Co. Amsterdam, The Netherlands.

Discussion

Dr. R. T. Schimke: Do you think you have demonstrated that RNA can get into a cell and be translated? Do you think that there is any biologic relevance to this finding? Is this a way in which one cell type interacts with another?

Dr. Segal: I don't know the answer to the question, but I think it is a possibility. One of the things that strikes biologists looking at the question of mechanism of hormone action is that one really has to be able to account for a wave of activity. The vascular supply may not necessarily bring the circulating hormone to every cell in the 5- or 6-cm long oviduct. So, I believe there must be some form of cell-to-cell communication to indicate the presence of the hormone.

Dr. C. A. Villee: I would like to comment on two aspects of your talk, which I think are of general interest. Your scanning micrographs remind us that the response of a tissue to a hormone goes far beyond the synthesis of a single protein. We have to keep in mind that finding that estrogen turns on ovalbumin, or that progesterone turns on avidin, synthesis is just the first step in understanding the response of the oviduct. The other thing I would like to comment on is your beautiful experiments showing the specificity of the RNA that gets instilled and gets read out. We have performed the same kind of experiments with a different method by use of poly(U) columns or poly(dT) columns, but we get essentially the same sort of evidence that you have. We can prepare RNA from the stimulated oviduct, put it back in the lumen, and get ovalbumin if we obtained the RNA from an estrogen-treated oviduct, or get avidin if we obtained it from an estrogen-progesterone-treated oviduct. One disappointment in our experiment was that when we put the chick oviduct RNA into the rat uterus, we didn't get any ovalbumin.

Dr. Segal: Neither did we. We tried it with the mouse and the rat, with negative results.

DR. SCHIMKE: Various heterologous protein-synthesizing systems show differences in the efficiency with which they use oviduct messengers. So, it may well be that you can't see ovalbumin because the messenger is not utilized, even though it gets in.

DR. SEGAL: That may be one of the explanations. We also consider that in mammalian oviduct fluid, there may be a higher RNase activity that destroys the messenger before it can get into the cell.

STRUCTURE OF THE OVALBUMIN GENE IN CHROMATIN*

Richard Axel and Annie Garel†

Department of Pathology
and Institute of Cancer Research
College of Physicians & Surgeons
Columbia University
New York, New York 10032

The tubular gland cells of the oviduct of the laying hen produce 3×10^{19} molecules of ovalbumin per day. More than half of the protein-synthetic capacity of the oviduct cell is involved in ovalbumin synthesis, and each cell contains about 100,000 ovalbumin messenger RNA molecules associated with polyribosomes (for review, see References 1–3). The magnitude and specificity of this response to a complex hormonal stimulus are likely to result from adaptive changes that regulate transcriptional and posttranscriptional events.

In our laboratory, we have been concerned with the organization of proteins along the DNA molecule and the possible role of this nucleoprotein complex in regulating gene expression. Over the past few years, it has become increasingly clear that the proteins of chromatin specifically restrict the transcription of DNA and that this restriction is, at least in part, responsible for the differentiation of specific cell types engaged in highly specialized cell functions. It is possible that structural changes accompany transcriptional activation and that such changes may be responsible for the induction of specific genes.

We have therefore used a variety of biologic and chemical agents to probe the structure of specific genes in chromatin.[4] The ovalbumin gene is particularly amenable to this type of analysis. This gene is represented uniquely in the haploid genome of the chicken.[5,6] Furthermore, the availability of highly purified ovalbumin mRNA permits the synthesis of radioactive complementary DNA (cDNA) probes capable of detecting ovalbumin sequences in molecular hybridization reactions. In addition, expression of the ovalbumin gene is modulated by estrogen and progesterone, so that its structure may be compared in both active and inactive states. In this report, we demonstrate that although histones reside on the transcriptionally active ovalbumin genes, the organization of proteins around this gene renders it highly sensitive to DNase I. This sensitivity is not observed in tissues not actively synthesizing ovalbumin, which suggests that this parameter of chromatin structure may be related to transcriptional activity.

The Nucleosomal Subunit

Over the past year, an experimentally consistent model of chromatin structure has emerged that postulates the presence of regularly repeating nucleoprotein subunits joined by short segments of DNA. Biochemical evidence for a periodic

*Supported by Grants CA-16346 and CA-02332 from the National Cancer Institute.

†Permanent address: Institute of Molecular and Cellular Biology, National Center of Scientific Research (CNRS), Strasbourg, France.

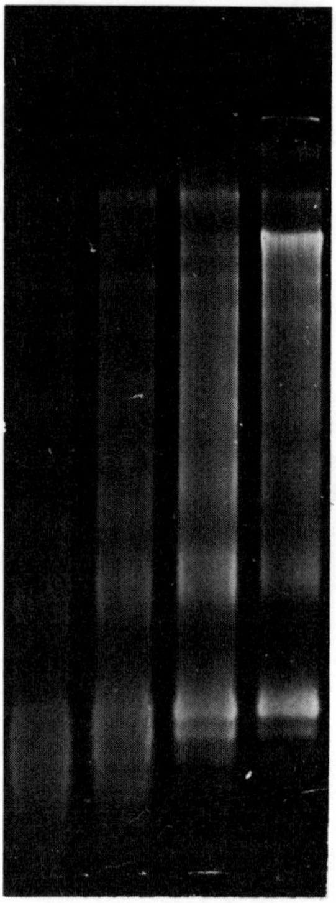

FIGURE 1. Polyacrylamide gel electrophoresis of DNA liberated by staphylococcal nuclease digestion of intact nuclei. Purified oviduct nuclei were incubated for increasing times with staphylococcal nuclease.[10] DNA was purified from the resultant nucleoprotein fragments and analyzed on composite 3% acrylamide, 0.5% agarose slab gels, as previously described.[10] Gels were stained with ethidium bromide and photographed under short-wave ultraviolet illumination. Samples from right to left represent 2.5, 10, 16, and 25% acid solubilization.

protein-DNA complex was initially introduced by Hewish and Burgoyne[7] and was subsequently confirmed in several laboratories.[8–13] These data demonstrate that mild nuclease digestion of nuclei results in the liberation of a series of nucleoprotein particles, nucleosomes, or ν-bodies that contain DNA fragments whose molecular weights are all multiples of a unit fragment 150–200 base pairs in length. Subsequent studies have revealed that the nucleosome represents a transient intermediate in the digestion process and that cleavage of DNA within the nucleosome results in the generation of a true-limit digest that reflects the internal structure of the monomeric subunit.[14]

Electron microscope observations[15,16] are in accord with the biochemical data and reveal the existence of spherical nucleoprotein particles that are joined by a short filament of DNA. These particles can be observed closely opposed to one another in gently disrupted nuclei, providing evidence that these nucleoprotein particles reflect a level of structure characteristic of the chromatin fiber *in vivo*.

It should be noted that this basic repeating structure has been observed in all eukaryotic nuclei examined and is present both in yeast and in man.[17] Furthermore, this subunit structure is not restricted to a specific stage in the cell cycle. While most studies have been performed on interphase nuclei, nucleosomes have also been observed in metaphase chromosomes.[18,19] Approximately 20 million nucleosomal subunits exist per mammalian nucleus, which suggests that we are dealing with a basic aspect of structure responsible for at least one level of chromosomal organization.

Attempts to analyze the distribution of proteins around the ovalbumin genes initially required that we examine the gross organization of proteins along the total genomic DNA of oviduct cells. To this end, nuclei were obtained from the magnum portion of oviducts from laying hens. The nuclei were incubated with staphylococcal nuclease, and the resultant DNA fragments were analyzed at various times during the digestion process (FIGURE 1). As previously described, at early times in the digestion process, DNA fragments are generated whose molecular weights are integral multiples of a single monomeric unit, 185 base pairs in length. At 2.5% solubilization, DNA bands are observed at 185, 370, 550, 735, and 910 base pairs. As the digestion proceeds, the relative proportion of the monomeric fragment increases at the expense of the multimeric components. These data would suggest that the proteins of chromatin arrange the DNA in a regular conformation that repeats itself every 185 base pairs. The repeating subunit is punctuated by regularly spaced nuclease cleavage sites, presumably due to a region relatively free of protein and sensitive to nuclease attack.

These studies merely demonstrate that a nuclease cleavage site exists at regular intervals along the DNA backbone. Evidence that such a repeating unit results from a regular arrangement of nucleoprotein subunits, however, requires that we demonstrate the liberation of such particles that contain both protein and DNA, 185 base pairs in length. To this end, oviduct nuclei were partially digested with nuclease, and the resultant nucleoprotein fragments were sedimented in sucrose gradients (FIGURE 2). The absorbance profiles reflect the particles generated on 5, 8, and 15% solubilizations of nuclear DNA. In FIGURE 2 we observe a series

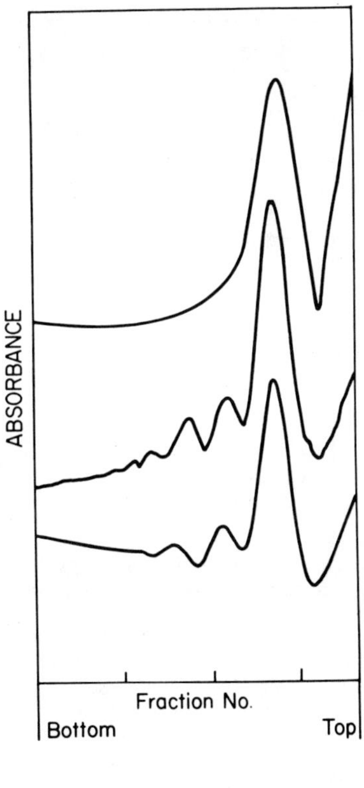

FIGURE 2. Sucrose gradient fractionation of nucleosomal subunits. Purified oviduct nuclei were digested with staphylococcal nuclease to generate 5, 8, and 15% solubilization of nuclear DNA. The resultant nucleoprotein fragments were layered directly on a 5–20% sucrose gradient in 5 mM EDTA (pH 7.0). Gradients were centrifuged at 25,000 rpm for 17 hr in an SW41 rotor. The absorbance at 260 nm was monitored in a flow-through cuvette.

of five absorbance peaks. The DNA from each of these components represents a multimeric form of a 185 base pair monomeric fragment.

Previous analyses of the proteins within each nucleoprotein peak derived from rat liver reveal the presence of H2A, H2B, H3, and H4 in proportions identical to those observed in unfractionated chromatin. Histone H1 is present in equal proportions in the dimeric through pentameric fractions but appears to be reduced in the monomeric subunit. The degree of loss of histone H1 in the monomeric form appears to be related to the extent of digestion, which suggests that excision of the interbead DNA results in a concomitant loss of histone H1.

Structure of the Ovalbumin Gene in Chromatin

From the nuclease digestion data, we observe that more than 85% of the genomic DNA of the chicken oviduct is organized within nucleosomal structures. In accord with this observation, the kinetic complexity of the nucleosomal DNA of nuclei is indistinguishable from the complexity observed in total nuclear DNA.[14] These observations, however, do not exclude the possibility that a small, but biologically significant, subset of sequences is excluded from monomeric DNA. Interesting candidates for such a population of DNA are the sequences actively expressed within the genome. It is possible that there is a unique distribution of chromatin proteins around transcriptionally active segments of the genome and

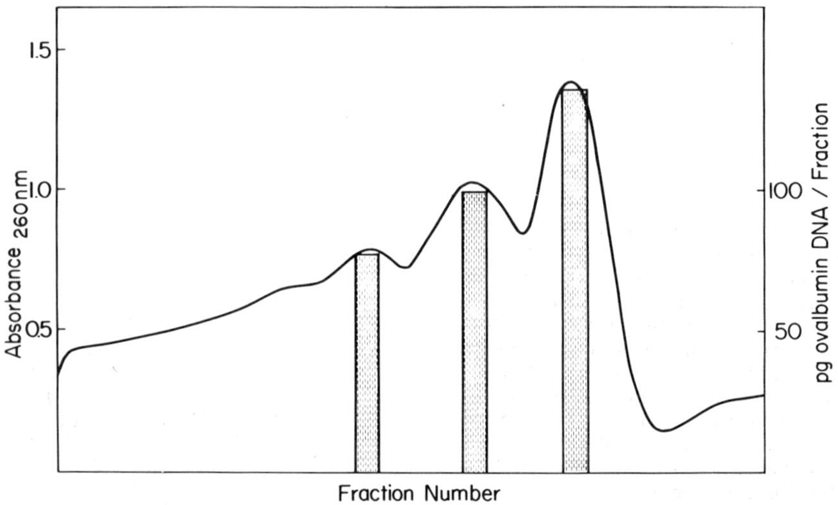

FIGURE 3. Quantitation of the ovalbumin genes in nucleosomal subunits. Oviduct nuclei were digested with staphylococcal nuclease to 8% solubilization of DNA. The resultant nucleosomal subunits were fractionated on sucrose gradients. DNA was purified from the monomeric, dimeric, and trimeric nucleosomal fractions and annealed with ovalbumin cDNA under conditions described in the legend to FIGURE 4. The solid curve represents the absorbance profile of fractionated nucleosomes. The bars represent the quantity of ovalbumin sequences in the three nucleoprotein fractions. These values are obtained from the kinetic data shown in FIGURE 4.

TABLE 1

$C_0t_{1/2}$ OF ANNEALING OF OVALBUMIN AND AMV cDNA WITH CHROMATIN DNA PREPARATIONS

	Oviduct Nucleosomal DNA	DNase I-Treated	
		Oviduct DNA	Liver DNA
Ovalbumin cDNA	650*	2000 (5%)† 2000 (15%) 2000 (21%)	600 (15%)
AMV cDNA	—	600 (15%)	600 (15%)

*All values represent $C_0t_{1/2}$ of annealing reactions shown.
†Values in parentheses represent extent of digestion prior to isolation of resistant DNA.

that this organization of proteins differs from that observed on unexpressed DNA sequences.

To investigate this possibility, we initially asked whether proteins reside on the ovalbumin genes in a tissue that actively expresses this gene as mRNA. To this end, oviduct nuclei were digested to a limit with staphylococcal nuclease, and the resistant DNA was analyzed for the presence of ovalbumin sequences by molecular hybridization. Nuclease digestions of chromatin or nuclei reach a well-defined limit, with about half of the DNA resistant to nuclease action.[20] The resistant DNA presumably results from the association of histone with DNA, rendering the resultant nucleoprotein insensitive to nuclease attack. If proteins are bound to the ovalbumin genes in chromatin, we would predict that these genes should be present in the nuclease-resistant fraction of chromatin DNA. Annealing of ovalbumin cDNA to this DNA fraction reveals the presence of ovalbumin sequences at concentrations identical to those of total sonicated nuclear DNA. These data indicate that histones are present on the ovalbumin gene and that the mere presence of proteins along a given sequence is not sufficient to restrict its transcription.

We now asked whether the ovalbumin genes are organized in a nucleosomal array in a manner analogous to that observed for total DNA, in a tissue in which they are actively transcribed. Oviduct nuclei were therefore subjected to mild staphylococcal nuclease digestion, solubilizing only 8% of the nuclear DNA. The resultant nucleoprotein fragments were then fractionated on sucrose velocity gradients. The absorbance profile shown in FIGURE 3 reveals discrete peaks of nucleoprotein that correspond to the monomeric and multimeric forms of the 11S nucleosomal subunit. DNA was extracted from monomeric, dimeric, and trimeric peaks, and the ovalbumin gene content was determined by annealing this DNA to ovalbumin cDNA. In these annealing reactions, the nucleosomal DNA is in vast excess (10^7:1) such that the rate of annealing is solely dependent on the concentration of ovalbumin genes in nucleosomal DNA. The kinetics of annealing of monomeric, dimeric, and trimeric DNA all fit a single second-order curve, with a $C_0t_{1/2}$ of 650. This value is quite close to that observed with total undigested chicken DNA. These data indicate that the ovalbumin genes are organized in a repeating subunit structure in a manner analogous to that observed for total nuclear DNA.

An alternative annealing experiment was performed in which the ovalbumin genes were titrated in monomeric and total DNA with an excess of ovalbumin cDNA. In these experiments, increasing quantities of either total nuclear or

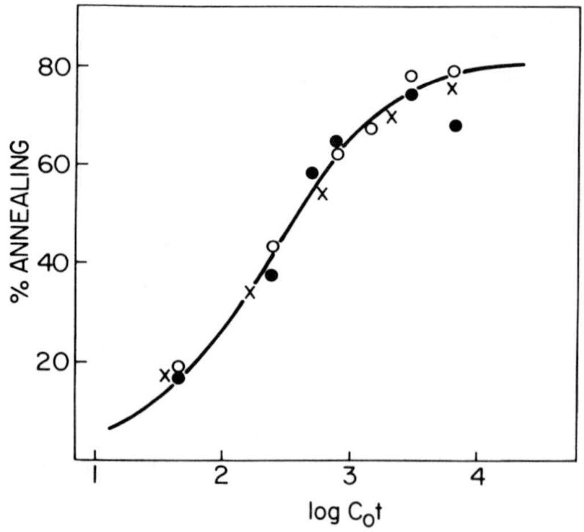

FIGURE 4. Kinetics of annealing of ovalbumin cDNA with DNA obtained from isolated nucleosomal subunits. DNA was purified from monomeric (○), dimeric (●) or trimeric (×) nucleosomes, as described in FIGURE 3. DNA fractions (1.6 mg each) were then annealed with 0.18 ng (9000 cpm) of [^{3}H]ovalbumin cDNA. Annealing reactions were performed at a DNA concentration of 20 mg/ml in 1 mM Tris-HCl (pH 7.9), 0.1 mM EDTA, and 0.4 M NaCl at 69°C. Duplex formation was assayed with the single strand-specific nuclease, S_1. $C_0t_{1/2}$ = moles of nucleotide × seconds/liter.

monomeric DNA from oviducts are added to a fixed excess quantity of ovalbumin cDNA under conditions that allow completion of the annealing reaction. From the initial slope of this curve, the concentration of ovalbumin genes can be determined directly. We find that the ovalbumin genes are present as a single copy in both monomeric and total DNA (data not shown).

These findings are in accord with similar observations for the globin gene in avian erythroblasts[14] and indicate that the template-active regions of the genome appear to participate in the basic repeat structure characteristic of chromatin. Transcription through protein-covered regions of the genome must therefore occur, and the presence of histone on a specific gene does not appear to be sufficient to block polymerase action.

A note of caution should be added here. It is possible that cleavage by nuclease results in distortion of the native structure over transcriptionally active genes. If these regions of the chromatin are physically restrained in an extended conformation, nuclease action may relieve this restraint, thereby allowing nucleosomes to reform over the liberated fragments. Such a model still requires the presence of histone over active genes. It implies, however, that these genes are not organized in a compact subunit but only assume the more stable nucleosomal conformation after nuclease cleavage.

DNase I Digestion of the Ovalbumin Genes

It is apparent from the previous studies that the arrangement of nucleosomes along the DNA may not be related in a straightforward way to the specific transcription observed with chromatin. It is possible that more subtle alterations characterize the template-active regions of chromatin and that these structural aspects are not recognizable in a simple analysis of the nucleosomal DNA. In support of this contention, Weintraub and Groudine[21] have demonstrated that the globin genes in avian erythroblasts are selectively sensitive to digestion with pancreatic DNase I. This study revealed that levels of digestion capable of solubilizing only 10% of the nuclear DNA resulted in complete and specific digestion of the globin genes. This exceedingly important observation now provides a structural parameter that distinguishes active from inactive segments of the genome.

We have therefore examined the sensitivity of the ovalbumin genes in chromatin to DNase I digestion in the liver and oviduct of the laying hen. In initial studies, intact nuclei from liver and oviduct were digested with DNase I, solubilizing 15% of the nuclear DNA. The ovalbumin gene content of the resistant DNA samples was then determined in annealing reactions with ovalbumin cDNA. FIGURE 5 presents the kinetics of annealing of cDNA to a large excess of liver and oviduct DNA after DNase I treatment. The $C_0 t_{1/2}$ value observed with digested liver DNA is 600, a value consistent with no specific sensitivity of the ovalbumin genes in this tissue. The $C_0 t_{1/2}$ value observed with digested oviduct DNA, however, is 2000, which is 3.3 times higher than the value observed with either digested liver DNA or total DNA. These data indicate that the ovalbumin genes are sensitive to DNase I digestion only in tissues that are actively engaged in ovalbumin synthesis.

These values were obtained with samples of DNA after 15% DNase digestion. It was of interest to determine at what point in the digestion process the

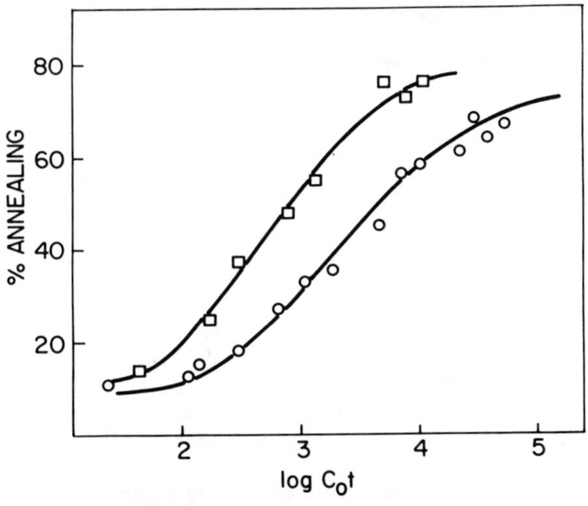

FIGURE 5. Kinetics of annealing of ovalbumin cDNA with DNase I-treated nuclear DNA. Oviduct (○) and liver (□) nuclei were digested with DNase I, liberating 15% of the DNA as acid-soluble oligomers. The resistant DNA was purified free of protein and annealed with ovalbumin cDNA, as described in the legend to FIGURE 4. Annealing reactions contained 4 mg of oviduct or liver DNA and 0.18 ng of ovalbumin cDNA. Duplex formation was monitored with S_1 nuclease.

ovalbumin genes are solubilized. To this end, aliquots of oviduct nuclei were digested to various levels with DNase. The concentration of ovalbumin sequences was measured by annealing these DNA fragments to ovalbumin cDNA (TABLE 1). We observe that even at the earliest time of digestion assayed, with only 5% of the DNA solubilized, 75% of the ovalbumin sequences are liberated as acid-soluble oligomers. These data provide further evidence for the specificity of DNase action on the transcriptionally active ovalbumin gene.

It is evident from TABLE 1 that even at high levels of digestion, it is not possible to digest specifically all of the ovalbumin sequences. About 25% of these sequences do not appear to be sensitive to DNase I action. This resistant DNA does not represent a specific region of the ovalbumin genes, because annealing to this DNA saturates the cDNA probe at a value identical to that observed with total DNA, albeit at a higher $C_0 t_{1/2}$ value. It appears, then, that subsets of ovalbumin

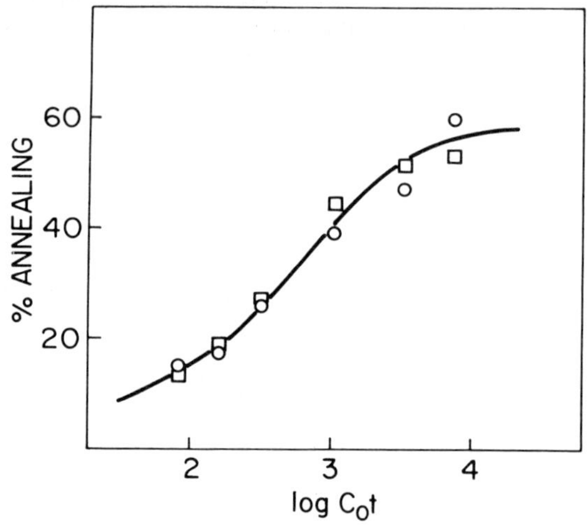

FIGURE 6. Kinetics of annealing of AMV cDNA with DNase I-treated nuclear DNA. Oviduct and liver nuclei were digested with DNase I, and the resistant DNA was purified free of protein. The resistant DNA (2.5 mg) from oviduct (○) and liver (□) nuclei was annealed to 0.5 ng of AMV cDNA under the conditions described in FIGURE 4.

genes within the oviduct are not sensitive to DNase attack and behave in these experiments as if they were transcriptionally inactive. These observations are in accord with histologic findings that demonstrate that only 75–80% of the oviduct cells are tubular gland cells actively expressing ovalbumin.[24]

These studies confirm the observations of Weintraub and Groudine[21] for the globin genes and reveal that the template-active segments are organized in chromatin in such a way as to render them exceedingly sensitive to DNase I attack. We would predict, then, that genes inactive in both liver and oviduct should be present in DNase-treated preparations at concentrations identical to that of undigested total DNA. One such genome amenable to this analysis is the sequence of the avian myeloblastosis virus (AMV). Sixty percent of the AMV genome is integrated in uninfected chick cells, but these sequences are not normally expressed in adult liver or oviduct. We therefore annealed AMV cDNA to DNase-treated liver and oviduct DNAs, used in FIGURE 5. We find that there is no selective digestion of these sequences in nuclei derived from either tissue (FIGURE 6). The $C_0 t_{1/2}$ value of 600 is twice that observed with total sonicated DNA, a finding consistent with the differences in the lengths of the DNA populations. These data support our observations with the ovalbumin genes and indicate that selective sensitivity of the specific sequences to DNase I may reflect a structural parameter directly related to transcriptional activity.

CONCLUSIONS

The elucidation of a regular array of nucleosomal subunits in chromatin immediately poses the question as to the possible role of this structure in the process of transcription. Analysis of the organization of this subunit structure with respect to DNA sequence reveals that no long special sequence of nucleotides is necessary for nucleosome formation. Virtually all genomic sequences are involved in the repeat structure, with the particles randomly distributed along the genomic DNA. Similar studies that probed the distribution of proteins around specific genes in chromatin have revealed that histones are present along actively transcribing regions of the genome.[14,22] The mere presence of protein along a given sequence is therefore not sufficient to restrict transcription.

We would predict, however, that the organization of proteins around template-active genes should be distinct from that observed on unexpressed segments and that this organization may in part be responsible for transcriptional activation. The ovalbumin genes of the laying hen provide a system to examine this problem. In initial studies, we found that ovalbumin sequences are present in DNA derived from nucleosomes obtained after staphylococcal nuclease digestion of oviduct nuclei. Assuming that the nuclease does not grossly distort the native structure around these genes, it would appear that the template-active regions of the genome are organized in a nucleosomal structure similar to that observed for total nuclear DNA.

It is possible that more subtle alterations characterize the template-active regions of chromatin and that these structural aspects are not apparent in a simple analysis of the nucleosomal array. Convincing support for this idea is provided by the recent experiments of Weintraub and Groudine,[21] which demonstrate the selective digestion of the globin genes with pancreatic DNase I erythroid tissues. We have performed similar experiments that demonstrated the specific sensitivity of the ovalbumin genes to DNase I in tissues actively engaged in ovalbumin mRNA synthesis. Regions of DNA not actively transcribed, such as the endogenous viral genes of the chicken, are not selectively degraded by this enzyme.

The apparent paradox between the susceptibility of the ovalbumin genes to the two different nucleases warrants further comment. It is clear that DNase I is capable of recognizing an aspect of structure of the ovalbumin genes that is not recognized by staphylococcal nuclease. This structural property renders transcriptionally active genes sensitive to DNase I at exceedingly low levels of digestion. No such selectivity is observed with staphylococcal nuclease. A possible explanation resides in the fact that the modes of action of the two enzymes are quite different. Staphylococcal nuclease initially cleaves at sites that bridge adjacent nucleosomes and digests within the nucleosome only late in the digestion process. DNase I shows no preference for inter- or intranucleosomal DNA and results in nicking at 10-base intervals along the DNA.[23] Furthermore, the two enzymatic reactions are performed under different ionic conditions, which may alter the structure of the ovalbumin genes. These results are compatible with a model in which nucleosomes reside over template-active regions of chromatin, but the internal organization within the nucleosome itself differs over active and inactive regions.

Alternatively, specific protein complexes may reside over active segments of DNA in an extended conformation such that this structure would be highly sensitive to DNase I action. Cleavage with staphylococcal nuclease would then release segments of nucleoprotein that are no longer restrained in an extended structure. These fragments can now freely reform the more stable, condensed structure of the nucleosome, generating the pattern observed in FIGURE 3.

These observations clearly demonstrate that differences exist between the conformation of the ovalbumin gene in its active state in the oviduct and in its inactive state in the liver. It is now of obvious interest to determine what factors are responsible for the initiation and maintenance of the "active configuration" of specific genes. The regulatory effects of estrogen and progesterone on ovalbumin RNA synthesis in the oviduct provide an ideal system for the elucidation of structure-function relationships about a specific gene in chromatin.

ACKNOWLEDGMENTS

We thank Dr. H. Weintraub and Dr. M. Groudine for making their data available to us prior to publication. In addition, we thank Dr. Raymond Sweet for providing us with AMV cDNA.

REFERENCES

1. PALMITER, R. D. 1975. Cell **4:** 189–197.
2. SCHIMKE, R. T., P. PENNEQUIN, D. ROBINS & G. S. MCKNIGHT. This monograph.
3. SCHWARTZ, R. J., C. CHANG, W. T. SCHRADER & B. W. O'MALLEY. This monograph.
4. AXEL, R., H. CEDAR & G. FELSENFELD. 1975. Biochemistry **14:** 2489–2495.
5. SULLIVAN, D., R. PALACIOS, J. STAVNEZER, J. M. TAYLOR, A. J. MARAS, M. L. KIELY, N. M. SUMMERS, J. M. BISHOP & R. T. SCHIMKE. 1973. J. Biol. Chem. **248:** 7530–7539.
6. HARRIS, S. E., A. R. MEANS, W. M. MITCHELL & B. W. O'MALLEY. 1973. Proc. Nat. Acad. Sci. USA **70:** 3776–3780.
7. HEWISH, D. R. & L. A. BURGOYNE 1973. Biochem. Biophys. Res. Commun. **52:** 504–510.
8. NOLL, M. 1974. Nature (London) **251:** 249–251.
9. SAHASRABUDDHE, C. G. & K. E. VAN HOLDE. 1974. J. Biol. Chem. **249:** 152–156.
10. AXEL, R. 1975. Biochemistry **14:** 2921–2925.
11. SOLLNER-WEBB, B. & G. FELSENFELD. 1975. Biochemistry **14:** 2916–2920.
12. KORNBERG, R. & J. O. THOMAS. 1974. Science **184:** 865–868.
13. SHAW, B. R., T. M. HERMAN, R. T. KOVACIC, G. S. BEAUDREAU & K. E. VAN HOLDE. 1976. Proc. Nat. Acad. Sci. USA **73:** 505–509.
14. LACY, E. & R. AXEL. 1975. Proc. Nat. Acad. Sci. USA **72:** 3978–3982.
15. OLINS, A. L., R. D. CARLSON & D. E. OLINS. 1975. J. Cell Biol. **64:** 528–537.
16. OUDET, P., M. CROSS-BELLARD & P. CHAMBON. 1975. Cell **4:** 281–300.
17. LOHR, D. & K. E. VAN HOLDE. 1975. Science **188:** 165,166.
18. WIGLER, M. H. & R. AXEL. 1976. Nucl. Acid Res. **3:** 1463–1471.
19. RATTNER, J. B., A. BRANCH & B. A. HAMKALO. 1975. Chromosoma **52:** 329–338.
20. CLARK, R. J. & G. FELSENFELD. 1971. Nature [New Biol.] **229:** 101–106.

21. WEINTRAUB, H. & M. GROUDINE. 1976. Science **193:** 848–856.
22. GOTTESFELD, J. M., R. F. MURPHY & J. BONNER. 1975. Proc. Nat. Acad. Sci. USA **72:** 4404–4408.
23. NOLL, M. 1974. Nucl. Acid Res. **1:** 1573–1578.
24. SCHIMKE, R. T. 1976. Personal communication.

DISCUSSION

DR. R. T. SCHIMKE: Dr. Axel, do you feel that the histones are coming on or off the gene as polymerase is reading down it, or do you feel that they are being pushed along in the railroad style?

DR. AXEL: I don't think they are being pushed along. I can envisage a mechanism in which extension of the nucleosome occurs to permit polymerase action without dissociation of the histone complex from DNA.

DR. E. MILGROM: Did you compare the active oviduct with the nonactive oviduct?

DR. AXEL: That's a very important experiment, but I think it's logistically difficult. Dr. Schimke has pointed out that the withdrawn oviduct is no longer 80% tubular cells, but perhaps 20% tubular cells. So, at best, you would expect to remove only 20% of the genes, and your annealing kinetics would be shifted only 20%. I'm not willing, considering the accuracy of annealing reactions, to interpret a 20% shift as significant. In the case of untreated oviducts, again, you're dealing with different cell types. Furthermore, preparing the amounts of DNA that are required to do these kinds of experiments, I think, would prohibit doing these experiments.

DR. MILGROM: I realize that it is difficult, but I think that it is a very important experiment, because you have two possibilities: the gene is more accessible to the DNase either due to differentiation of the tissue or to the level at which the gene is transcribed at the moment.

DR. AXEL: There is some evidence bearing on that point from Hal Weintraub's lab. He examined the globin genes in the immature erythroblast, and in the adult erythrocyte he found that the gene is DNase accessible in both tissues. Therefore, the sensitivity does not seem to be due to the presence of polymerase molecules on the given gene.

DR. W. T. SCHRADER: There is one way you can do what Dr. Milgrom recommended. If you just don't withdraw the hormone for quite such a long time, the number of tubular gland cells will remain reasonably high. My question is about the staphylococcal nuclease experiments. You showed that the nucleosomes contained ovalbumin structural gene sequences. Do you have any estimate in comparison, for example, with work done by Brian McCarthy's lab? Perhaps these nucleosomes can, in fact, move around in the gene. The other side of the coin is to ask how many ovalbumin sequences were destroyed in the staphylococcal nuclease digestion.

DR. AXEL: There is no specific destruction of the ovalbumin genes with staphylococcal nuclease, so that the relative concentration of ovalbumin genes in resistant DNA is identical to that of untreated total DNA. The second question on movement is really difficult to answer. To my mind, the best *in vitro* experiments on movement would suggest that it is not occurring under the conditions of transcription reactions. These experiments, from Howard Cedar's lab, involve methylation of DNA in protein-free regions and then examination of protection of methylated groups.

DR. SCHIMKE: Do you think that the nucleosomes attach rather specifically to certain sites in the DNA, or is attachment relatively arbitrary?

DR. AXEL: That's a very hard question to answer. I would predict random attachment, on the basis of the following evidence. First, you can form nucleosomes on virtually any DNA. We have prepared nucleosomes with histones of duck reticulocyte and λ DNA and *E. coli* DNA. If there are sequence-specific attachment sites, those sites are likely to be present, then, on λ DNA as well. On the other hand, you could readily argue that, indeed, nucleosomes form anywhere but that there are high-affinity sites that phase nucleosome formation.

EFFECT OF PROGESTERONE RECEPTORS ON TRANSCRIPTION*

Robert J. Schwartz, Christina Chang, William T. Schrader, and Bert W. O'Malley

Department of Cell Biology
Baylor College of Medicine
Houston, Texas 77030

The chick oviduct provides an excellent model system for the hormonal control of cellular differentiation and gene expression. Chronic administration of estrogen over a period of 10–14 days results in growth and differentiation of the chick oviduct. Previous studies from this laboratory have shown that estrogen-mediated growth and differentiation of the chick oviduct involve significant alterations in gene transcription. Competition hybridization experiments have demonstrated qualitative changes in the repetitive sequences of nuclear RNA synthesized during estrogen-mediated differentiation.[1] More recent studies have also demonstrated increased transcription of unique sequence DNA during oviduct growth.[2] Concomitant with steroid-mediated oviduct differentiation, increased levels of nuclear RNA,[3] RNA polymerase activity,[4,5] chromatin template capacity, and changes in chromatin nonhistone proteins[6,7] were also found in the oviduct. Preceding the well-documented specific changes in protein synthesis,[8,9] previous studies have demonstrated an unequivocal net accumulation of specific, biologically active messenger RNA, coding for ovalbumin.[10–12]

When estrogen treatment of the chicks is discontinued, a reduction in the overall level of RNA and protein synthesis occurs, and the cells' ability to synthesize specific proteins, such as ovalbumin, decreases.[11,13] After 12 days of hormone withdrawal, the rate of ovalbumin biosynthesis is less than 1% of that observed in hormonally stimulated chicks.[10] If either estrogen or progesterone is readministered (secondary stimulation), there is a rapid increase in the production of ovalbumin mRNA, and the induction of other egg-white proteins begins again.[13] Therefore, the chick oviduct provides a system in which to study a specific endocrine response where overall gene expression can be dramatically altered while a specific marker for measuring changes in the transcriptional rate of a single gene is also available.

It thus appears that the pattern of steroid hormone action may include the following events in a time-dependent manner: First, steroids are taken up by the target cells and bind to a specific cytoplasmic receptor protein; second, the steroid-receptor complex is translocated into the nuclear compartment; third, receptor-hormone complex binds to acceptor sites on nuclear chromatin; and, finally, activation of the transcriptional process occurs, followed by the appearance of specific new RNA species.

To elucidate further the mechanism of steroid hormone action, it is necessary to examine the process by which biochemical information held by the steroid-receptor complex is transferred to the transcriptional apparatus. Of the many

*Supported by National Institutes of Health Grants HD-8118, HD-7857, and HD-7495-02 and by a Ford Foundation Grant to the Cell Biology Department, Baylor College of Medicine.

possible approaches to this problem, our recent efforts have centered on direct examination of the effects of steroid receptors on chromatin transcription in cell-free systems. Since the initial identification and characterization of the oviduct progesterone receptor by Sherman *et al.*,[14] we have sought to obtain this important regulatory molecule in pure form. Our recent success in this venture[15] now allows us to directly assess the effect of a pure steroid hormone-receptor complex on gene expression under cell-free conditions. Initial efforts in our laboratory were directed at characterizing the interaction of purified RNA polymerase with intact chromatin. The process of initiation of RNA synthesis has received special attention, because this step appears to be regulated by steroids.[16] In this article, we will discuss our recent evidence on progesterone-dependent transcription of chromatin in the chick oviduct.

Formation of Initiation Complexes on Chick DNA and Chromatin

The capacity of oviduct chromatin to serve as a template for *Escherichia coli* RNA polymerase has previously been shown to increase after estrogen administration to the immature chick.[7,17] While chromatin template activity measurements may generally reflect the amount of DNA sequences made available to RNA polymerase, the components of such a reaction are so complex that these experiments shed little light on the biochemical mechanisms of hormone-induced alterations in gene transcription. To determine the effect of steroids on gene transcription in the chick oviduct, it appeared necessary to monitor and control all of the parameters involved in RNA synthesis.

Procedures for measuring the initiation of RNA chains *in vitro* were adopted from studies initially performed in bacterial and bacteriophage systems.[18,19] The initiation of RNA synthesis can be divided into two basic processes. First, RNA polymerase binds randomly and reversibly to DNA to form a series of nonspecific complexes. However, after sufficient time and at a proper temperature, RNA polymerase binds proximal to an initiation region and forms a stable binary complex with DNA.[20,21] This complex has undergone a transition that involves the local destabilization of the DNA duplex structure[21] and is now capable of rapidly initiating an RNA chain.[22] The second process is the actual initiation step, in which RNA polymerase catalyzes the formation of the first phosphodiester bond between two nucleoside triphosphates.

The existence of stable RNA polymerase-DNA initiation complexes was elucidated through the use of the drug rifampicin.[24,25] Rifampicin is a competitive inhibitor of RNA synthesis that acts prior to the formation of the first phosphodiester bond but that has no effect on RNA chain elongation. RNA chain initiation by RNA polymerase bound to DNA in a stable initiation complex is so rapid that it can occur in the presence of the drug.[23] The fraction of RNA polymerase in stable complexes can be determined after the simultaneous addition of a mixture of rifampicin and the four ribonucleoside triphosphates.[26] RNA polymerase molecules that are free in solution or randomly bound to DNA will be inhibited by rifampicin. Under these conditions, reinitiation of RNA transcription will be completely inhibited, and thus each RNA polymerase at a stable initiation site can synthesize one and only one RNA chain. By measuring the number of RNA chains made, the rifampicin challenge assay provides a method for quantitating the number of RNA polymerase initiation sites for a given template.

To test for the formation of stable RNA polymerase-DNA initiation complexes, increasing amounts of *E. coli* RNA polymerase were preincubated with a fixed amount of chick DNA at 37°C for 15 min. The binary complexes were challenged by the addition of rifampicin (40 μg/ml) together with ribonucleoside triphosphates and were allowed to synthesize RNA in the presence of heparin for an additional 15 min at 37°C.[5,27] The number of RNA chains synthesized was determined from the amount and length of the RNA chains produced. The number of chains is equivalent to the number of initiation sites at which RNA polymerase was bound. By adding increasing amounts of RNA polymerase to a fixed amount of template, the total number of available initiation sites can be determined from the saturation level of RNA synthesis.[16,27,29]

Acute Progesterone Stimulation of Initiation of RNA Synthesis

Although incapable of inducing egg-white protein synthesis in the oviduct during primary stimulation, progesterone not only reestablishes ovalbumin protein synthesis but appears generally to also mimic estrogen as a secondary stimulant to

Table 1

Effect of Progesterone Administration *in Vivo* on RNA Polymerase Transcription of Withdrawn Oviduct Chromatin *in Vitro*

Hours After Progesterone Administration*	Size of RNA Product (nucleotides)	Initial Elongation Rate (nucleotides/sec)†	Picomoles of RNA Chains Initiated per 5 μg of Chromatin‡	Number of Initiation Sites per Picogram of DNA
0	820	7.2	0.072	8600
0.5	730	7.0	0.132	15,900
1.0	750	7.8	0.191	23,000
2.0	750	6.7	0.134	16,100
6.0	800	8.0	0.123	14,800
24.0	750	8.0	0.112	13,500

*Chicks were stimulated for 12 days with DES, withdrawn from hormone treatment for 10 days, and then injected with 2 mg of progesterone.

†Initial elongation rate was determined for 1 min of chain propagation, as previously described.[16]

‡The amount of initiated chains was calculated from the total nucleotides incorporated at the transition point of RNA polymerase titration curves, assuming that RNA contained 25% UMP, divided by the number average chain size of 770 nucleotides, as previously described.[16]

hormonally withdrawn chicks.[13,28] Furthermore, the similarity in the extent of egg-white protein synthesis induced by progesterone suggests that the time course of induction of RNA synthesis during secondary stimulation is similar to that induced by estrogen and is not influenced by the cytodifferentiation of new tubular gland cells.[13] Therefore, it was of interest to understand the manner by which progesterone can substitute for estrogen in hormone-withdrawn chicks.

Estrogen-treated chicks were withdrawn from hormone treatment for 12 days and then restimulated with a single injection of progesterone (2.0 mg). Oviduct chromatin was isolated after secondary stimulation and assayed by the rifampicin challenge technique. The number of initiated RNA chains was calculated as described above. As shown in Table 1, withdrawn chromatin had the capacity to support the initiation of 8600 RNA chains/pg of DNA. After a single injection of progesterone, a rapid increase in the number of initiation sites was found. Within 30 min of hormone treatment, the number of initiation sites had nearly doubled to 15,900 sites. After 1 hr of progesterone stimulation, a maximum of 23,000 initiation sites was detected. Thereafter, the number of initiation sites declined, so that by 24 hr after progesterone administration, 13,500 sites were observed. During this time of intense transcriptional activity, the parameters of the RNA chain propagation rate (~7.5 nucleotides/sec) and the number average chain length of the RNA product (~770 nucleotides) did not vary significantly from those of withdrawn oviduct chromatin (TABLE 1). Therefore, the progesterone-induced increase in chromatin transcription in the oviduct was mainly due to a modulation in the number of available RNA polymerase initiation sites.

To investigate further the mechanism by which progesterone augments increased chromatin transcription in withdrawn chicks, we tested the possibility that nuclear progesterone receptors acted at sites on chromatin that were identical to those affected by estrogen. Withdrawn chicks were given single injections that contained increasing doses of progesterone. Chromatin was then isolated from oviduct tissue 1 hr after restimulation and was assayed for the number of RNA polymerase initiation sites (TABLE 2). The number of initiation sites increased in a dose-dependent fashion from a control value of about 9100 (sites/pg of DNA) to a maximum value of ~22,500 sites at a dose of 1.25 mg of progesterone. We have previously reported a dose-dependent estrogen stimulation of RNA polymerase initiation sites.[27] In the present experiments, a maximal response occurred 1 hr after the *in vivo* injection of 1.25 mg of diethylstilbestrol (DES) and resulted in the formation of ~23,000 initiation sites (TABLE 2). Thus, the same dose of either steroid was effective in stimulating the same number of initiation sites.

We then tested the possibility that these steroids induced the initiation of transcription at the same sites. Both DES (1.25 mg) and progesterone (1.25 mg) were administered together to withdrawn chicks. If estrogen and progesterone acted at different chromatin RNA initiation sites, the stimulation of RNA synthesis by the two hormones would be additive. The results in TABLE 2 show that the number of RNA chain initiations was not additive when both hormones were simultaneously administered. These data suggest that in the withdrawn chick

TABLE 2

EFFECT OF THE COMBINED ADMINISTRATION OF PROGESTERONE AND DIETHYLSTILBESTROL ON INITIATION SITES FOR RNA SYNTHESIS IN OVIDUCT CHROMATIN

Hormone Dose* (mg)	RNA Chains Initiated (pmol/5 μg of DNA)	Initiation Sites per Picogram of DNA†
Control	0.076	9100
Progesterone, 0.25	0.135	16,200
Progesterone, 1.25	0.187	22,500
Progesterone, 2.0	0.196	23,600
DES, 1.25	0.191	23,000
Progesterone, 1.25 + DES, 1.25	0.180	21,600

*Chicks were stimulated for 12 days with DES, withdrawn from hormone treatment for 10 days, and then injected with various doses of hormones.

†The amount of initiated chain was calculated as described in the legend to TABLE 1.

TABLE 3

EFFECT OF PROGESTERONE ADMINISTRATION ON LEVELS OF OVALBUMIN MRNA IN OVIDUCTS OF WITHDRAWN CHICKS

Hours After Progesterone Administration	Number of Molecules of $mRNA_{ov}$ per Tubular Gland Cell
0	5–10
4	1200
10	2400
24	5400

oviduct, estrogen and progesterone may act at similar chromatin RNA initiation sites to enhance transcription.

A qualitative measure of the intracellular levels of ovalbumin mRNA was obtained by hybridizing [^{3}H]DNA complementary to ovalbumin mRNA ($cDNA_{ov}$) with RNA extracted from chick oviducts. The tritiated $cDNA_{ov}$ hybridization to $mRNA_{ov}$ sequences in the RNA samples constituted a specific probe to estimate the concentration of these sequences. This method is essentially the same as that described by Young *et al.*[30] Briefly, a fixed concentration of [^{3}H]$cDNA_{ov}$ is allowed to hybridize with an excess of either pure $mRNA_{ov}$ standards or with isolated RNA. From the kinetics of the $cDNA_{ov}$-$mRNA_{ov}$ reassociation reaction at various RNA concentrations, the $mRNA_{ov}$ concentration in the extract can be determined.[31,41] In withdrawn chicks, there is no detectable synthesis of ovalbumin protein, and less than 10 ovalbumin mRNA molecules were present per tubular gland cell (TABLE 3). Within 4 hr after a single injection of progesterone (2 mg) to withdrawn chicks, we observed an accumulation of 1200 additional ovalbumin mRNA molecules per gland cell in the oviduct. The number of mRNA molecules continued to increase, reaching a level of 5400 molecules by 24 hr, as shown in TABLE 3. Thus, like estrogen, progesterone induces accumulation of ovalbumin mRNA in oviduct cells of withdrawn chicks. This increase in the level of ovalbumin mRNA follows temporarily the steroid-induced increase in chromatin initiation sites for RNA synthesis. These experiments demonstrate that during secondary hormonal stimulation of withdrawn chicks, progesterone is an adequate substitute for estrogen with respect to its effect on gene expression.

PURIFIED PROGESTERONE RECEPTOR STIMULATES INITIATION OF TRANSCRIPTION OF OVIDUCT CHROMATIN *in Vitro*

During the course of investigating the mechanism of action of steroid hormones, we have identified the progesterone receptor proteins in the chick oviduct.[12,32,33] We have recently purified the cytoplasmic progesterone receptor to homogeneity.[15] The receptor appears to function by complexing with progesterone in the cytoplasm, followed by translocation of the steroid-receptor complex to the nuclear compartment.[32,34,35] The steroid-receptor complex binds, then, to a limited number of nuclear acceptor sites, which are present in greater numbers in oviduct nuclei than in nontarget cell nuclei.[36] Although the subsequent events are not yet completely defined, stimulation of nuclear RNA synthesis occurs and leads to mRNA synthesis and ultimately to the induction of synthesis of cell-specific proteins. Because an increase in RNA chain initiation sites was detected within 30 min of progesterone administration to withdrawn chicks

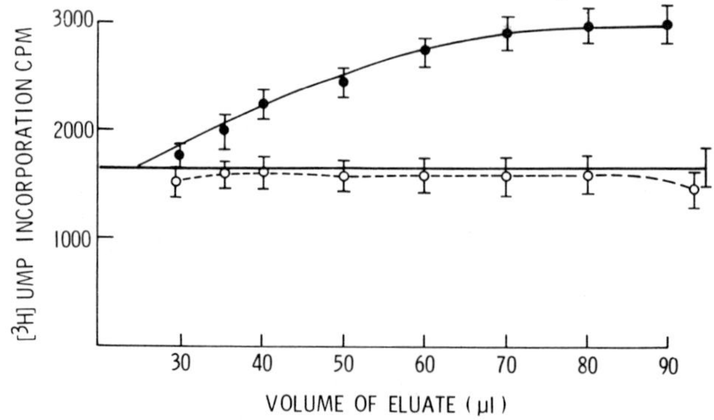

FIGURE 1. Effect of purified progesterone-receptor complexes on oviduct chromatin RNA synthesis *in vitro*. Chick oviduct ammonium sulfate cytosol[15] was divided into two parts. Progesterone was added to one-half (○), while the other half remained untreated (●). Both fractions were separately incubated with a deoxycorticosterone hemisuccinate bovine serum albumin-Sepharose® affinity resin and eluted as previously described.[16] The eluted fraction pretreated with progesterone did not contain any progesterone receptors, whereas the untreated fraction contained progesterone receptor (1.5×10^{-8} M). Various amounts of the eluted fractions in 10 mM Tris-HCl (pH 7.4), 1 mM Na_2EDTA, 12 mM 1-thioglycerol, and 50 mM KCl were added in a maximum volume of 100 μl to 25 μl of a withdrawn oviduct chromatin suspension (5 μg of DNA) and incubated for 30 min at 22°C. A saturating amount of *E. coli* RNA polymerase (15 μg) was then added, together with 20 μmol of Tris-HCl (pH 7.9), 1.0 μmol of $MnCl_2$, 0.5 μmol of β-mercaptoethanol, and 100 μg of bovine serum albumin, and incubated for an additional 30 min at 22°C. At the end of the preincubation period, RNA synthesis was initiated by the addition of 37.5 nmol of ATP, GTP, CTP, and UTP and 10 μCi of [^{3}H]UTP, 10 μg of rifampicin, 0.1 μmol of potassium phosphate (pH 7.0), and 200 μg of heparin in a final volume of 250 μl for 15 min at 37°C. Synthesized RNA was precipitated with 5% trichloroacetic acid, collected on glass fiber filters, and counted in scintillation fluid at an efficiency of 19.5%. The straight line represents the level of constitutive RNA synthesis in the absence of added receptor.

(TABLE 1), these results appeared to be consistent with our hypothesis that steroid-receptor complexes enter target cell nuclei and modulate gene transcription. Nevertheless, there has previously been no proof that the steroid-receptor complex could act directly on nuclear chromatin to stimulate transcription. Toward this end, we tested the effect of purified progesterone-receptor complexes on all parameters of transcription with a reconstituted cell-free system that contained the following purified components: progesterone-receptor complex, *E. coli* RNA polymerase, ribonucleotides, cofactors, rifampicin, heparin, and chromatin from withdrawn chicks.[37]

A fixed concentration of withdrawn oviduct chromatin (5 μg) was preincubated with increasing quantities of purified progesterone-receptor complex (up to 1.1×10^{-8} M) for 30 min at 22°C. The cytoplasmic progesterone-receptor complex contains mainly 6S dimers, which are composed of A (mol wt 80,000) and B (mol wt 117,000) subunits. The intact 6S dimer was purified by the affinity chromatography procedure of Kuhn *et al.*[15] The chromatin-receptor complexes were next incubated for an additional 30 min with a saturating concentration of RNA polymerase (15 μg) to allow for the formation of stable initiation complexes. Finally, rifampicin, heparin, and nucleotides were added as before for a 15-min period of RNA synthesis. RNA synthesis in the presence of rifampicin increased in a receptor dose-dependent manner, in which half-maximal stimulation occurred at a progesterone receptor concentration of 0.5×10^{-8} M (FIGURE 1). In this experiment, RNA synthesis was stimulated to a maximum of ~75% over control values at 1.1×10^{-8} M purified progesterone-receptor complex. Shown also in FIGURE 1 are the results of an experiment in which the progesterone receptor was presaturated with nonradioactive progesterone prior to application to the affinity column used to purify the molecule. Under these conditions, all available steroid receptor-binding sites were saturated with progesterone and thus prevented progesterone receptor from subsequently interacting with the steroid covalently linked to the affinity resin. The eluted material from the affinity preparation, which was pretreated with an excess of progesterone, did not contain any detectable [^{3}H]progesterone-receptor complex and was also incapable of causing any increase in RNA chain initiation over values obtained by control chromatins. This experiment strongly indicated that the stimulation in chromatin transcription was due to the progesterone receptor and not to a contaminant that was nonspecifically bound to the affinity column.

We have previously reported that crude ammonium sulfate precipitates of cytosol fractions of eukaryotic cells can often spuriously stimulate RNA synthesis by a template-independent process that is unrelated to hormone receptor.[38] To rule out such an effect in the present study, we investigated the sensitivity of rifampicin-resistant incorporation of [^{3}H]uridine monophosphate into RNA under various conditions. TABLE 4 shows that RNA synthesized in the presence of receptor and chromatin was completely dependent on template and inhibited by actinomycin D. Furthermore, none of the components alone contained significant synthetic activity, and therefore neither the chromatin, polymerase, or receptor was contaminated with other enzymes that were capable of incorporating [^{3}H]uridine triphosphate into acid-insoluble material. In these experiments, the progesterone receptor preincubated with chromatin in the presence of *E. coli*

TABLE 4

EFFECT OF PROGESTERONE-RECEPTOR COMPLEXES ON RNA SYNTHESIS FROM OVIDUCT CHROMATIN *in Vitro*

Components Added to Assay	[^{3}H]UMP Incorporated into RNA/5 μg of Chromatin DNA* (cpm)	Activity (%)
Background		
RNA polymerase only	230	8
Progesterone-receptor complex plus RNA polymerase	400	14
Chromatin alone	200	7
Control		
Chromatin plus RNA polymerase	2730	100
Chromatin plus boiled progesterone-receptor complex	2860	105
Chromatin plus 10^{-8} M progesterone alone	2430	89
Experimental		
Chromatin plus RNA polymerase plus 10^{-8} M progesterone-receptor complex	4100	150
plus α-amanitine (10 μg)	3740	137
plus actinomycin D (10 μg)	320	12

*RNA synthesis was assayed in the presence of nucleotides and rifampicin, as described in FIGURE 1.

RNA polymerase increased RNA synthesis 50% over control values. With the addition of α-aminitine, a potent inhibitor of eukaryotic RNA polymerase II, there was little effect on the progesterone receptor-directed stimulation of RNA transcription. These data showed that the stimulation of RNA synthesis was not due to the activation of endogenous RNA polymerase, which could have been a contaminant in chromatin preparations, but, rather, was due to transcription by the added *E. coli* enzyme. Nevertheless, it should be noted that receptor-mediated stimulation of RNA synthesis also occurred in the presence of exogenously added oviduct RNA polymerase II.[39] Moreover, TABLE 4 also shows that the increased RNA synthesis was dependent on the native structure of the hormone-receptor complex, because neither free progesterone nor boiled receptor was effective in stimulating RNA synthesis. Importantly, the purified progesterone receptor does not contain any detectable proteolytic or nuclease activity that would spuriously affect the chromatin template.[37] Thus, the stimulation of [^{3}H]UMP incorporation is derived through a chromatin template-dependent process that is directly mediated by an intact progesterone-receptor complex.

TABLE 5

EFFECT OF PROGESTERONE RECEPTOR ON THE AMOUNT AND RATE OF RNA CHAIN SYNTHESIS BY OVIDUCT CHROMATIN

Concentration Progesterone Receptor (M)	Total Incorporation of Nucleotide* (pmol)	Initial Elongation Rate† (nucleotides/sec)	Number Average Chain Size‡ (nucleotides)	Picomoles of RNA Chains Initiated per 5 μg of Chromatin DNA	Number of Initiation Sites per Picogram of DNA
No receptor	62	7.9	739	0.083	10,000
10^{-8}	91	7.8	720	0.126	15,200

*RNA was synthesized in the presence of rifampicin and nucleotides, as shown in FIGURE 1, and was corrected for base composition of RNA, assuming 25% UMP.

†Measured in first minute of synthesis.

‡Measured by sucrose gradient analysis of RNA synthesized in 15 min.

Quantitation of RNA initiation sites induced by receptor-steroid complexes was determined by measuring the total incorporation of nucleotides in the presence of rifampicin and by dividing this value by the number average chain length of the RNA product. From the data in TABLE 5, it was calculated that withdrawn chromatin, in this experiment, had the capacity to code for 10,000 RNA chains per picogram of DNA. After an *in vitro* incubation with progesterone-receptor complexes, the capacity to initiate RNA synthesis was increased to 15,200 sites at 10^{-8} M receptor concentration. There were no significant differences in either the size of the RNA product or in the initial rate of elongation. Thus, the purified receptor preparation had stimulated the RNA initiation events, rather than the steps required for RNA chain elongation.

The stimulatory effect of the progesterone receptor on RNA chain initiation by chromatin was next verified by a totally independent assay. Quantitation of the number of 5′-termini present in the population of nascent RNA chains was measured by the incorporation of γ-[^{32}P]guanosine triphosphate into RNA.[48] We have previously shown that 57% of the initial 5′-tetraphosphate nucleosides (A + G) from the RNA synthesized from oviduct chromatin is guanosine.[16] As shown in TABLE 6, the number of 5′-tetraphosphate nucleosides incorporated into nascent

TABLE 6

EFFECT OF PROGESTERONE ON INCORPORATION OF γ-[^{32}P]GTP AT THE 5′-END OF RIFAMPICIN-RESISTANT RNA CHAINS

Treatment	[^{32}P]GTP (pmol)*	5′-Termini (pmol)†	Number of RNA Chains per Picogram of DNA
Control	0.048 ± 0.002	0.086	10,300
10^{-8} M Progesterone receptor	0.037 ± 0.003	0.131	15,700

*Withdrawn chick oviduct chromatin (5 μg) and 10^{-8} M progesterone-receptor complex were preincubated for 30 min at 22°C. RNA polymerase (15 μg) and the assay component described previously in FIGURE 1 were added for an additional 30 min. RNA synthesis was then initiated by the addition of 85.2 μCi of γ-[^{32}P]GTP (5000 cpm/pmol), together with nucleotides, rifampicin, and heparin. After 10 sec at 37°C, the transcription reaction was terminated by pipetting a 125-μl sample on DEAE filter paper, and the filters were washed according to the procedure of Roeder.[47] The incorporated γ-[^{32}P]GTP was identified as guanosine tetraphosphate after degradation of the RNA product with alkali.[37,48]

†Total number of initiated chains was estimated by the value of guanosine 5′-tetraphosphate nucleosides multiplied by 1.8, a factor for total chain starts.

RNA chains also increased by 50% in the presence of progesterone receptor. The incorporation of γ-[^{32}P]GTP into the 5′-termini of RNA substantiates our observations that the progesterone receptor stimulates initiation of transcription in the cell-free assay by increasing the number of chromatin initiation sites for RNA synthesis available to RNA polymerase.

The kinetics for the stimulation of chromatin transcription *in vitro* revealed a $t_{1/2}$ of 15 min.[37] This value is close to the optimal time required for receptor binding to chromatin at 22°C and is similar to the kinetics of receptor appearance in nu-

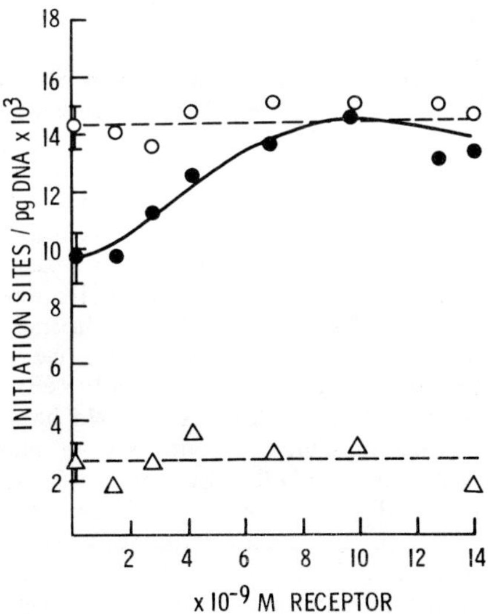

FIGURE 2. Tissue specificity for the progesterone receptor's effect on initiation sites. Chromatin from oviduct (●), erythrocyte (Δ), or liver (○), were incubated with increasing doses of the purified progesterone receptor. Conditions for RNA synthesis were identical to those described in FIGURE 1. Data are expressed as initiation sites per picogram of chromatin DNA.

clei *in vivo* and *in vitro* after progesterone administration.[32,35] A maximal increase in transcription was found to occur within 30 min after the addition of receptor. Previous studies have demonstrated a quantitative tissue specificity for binding of oviduct progesterone-receptor complexes to nuclei and to chromatin.[35,40] It was therefore of interest to investigate the ability of the receptor to modify the transcriptional response of various chromatins (FIGURE 2).

At receptor concentrations that produced maximal stimulation, there was an increase of 4700 initiation sites per picogram of DNA in oviduct chromatin but only 750 and 300 additional receptor-induced sites in liver and erythrocyte chromatin, respectively (FIGURE 2). It thus appears that the progesterone receptor-mediated effect is at least partly dependent on the presence of tissue-specific proteins in the oviduct chromatin. These proteins may be related to the nonhistone chromosomal proteins that convey quantitative tissue specificity for receptor binding and that comprise a vital part of the chromatin "acceptor sites" for steroid hormone-receptor binding.[6,36]

TABLE 7

In Vitro SYNTHESIS OF OVALBUMIN mRNA FROM CHICK OVIDUCT CHROMATIN IN THE ABSENCE OR PRESENCE OF PURIFIED PROGESTERONE-RECEPTOR COMPLEXES*

Chromatin Source	Progesterone Receptor Concentration (10^{-8} M)	Chromatin in Reaction (μg of DNA)	RNA Synthesized (μg)	$mRNA_{ov}$ in RNA (%)	mRNA Synthesized (pg × 10^{-3})	Picograms of $mRNA_{ov}$ per Microgram of DNA
Withdrawn oviduct	−	400	125	0.0015	1.9	0–4.8
Withdrawn oviduct	+	400	135	0.015	20.0	50.0

*Chromatin was preincubated with progesterone receptor for 30 min at 22°C. Bulk RNA synthesis was performed at 22°C, as described by Chang *et al.*[31] The purified RNA was hybridized with $cDNA_{ov}$ (1.5 μg) as described previously.[41]

PROGESTERONE RECEPTOR STIMULATES SYNTHESIS OF OVALBUMIN mRNA SEQUENCES FROM CHROMATIN *in Vitro*

The data presented above strongly support our proposal that direct transcriptional control is the primary locus of steroid hormone action. Because progesterone can induce ovalbumin synthesis in withdrawn chicks, it was conceivable that the purified progesterone receptors could induce the ovalbumin gene in isolated oviduct chromatin. Such a demonstration would strongly reaffirm the notion that the *in vitro* receptor-chromatin interaction mimics the events that occur *in vivo*. To test this assumption, we transcribed oviduct chromatin *in vitro* in the presence of bacterial RNA polymerase. The RNA synthesized was isolated and reacted with $[^3H]cDNA_{ov}$.[41] We have previously reported that chromatin from withdrawn chick oviduct was a poor template for the *in vitro* synthesis of ovalbumin mRNA.[41] However, within 2 hr after a single injection of progesterone to withdrawn chicks, oviduct chromatin was capable of supporting the synthesis of ovalbumin mRNA sequences.[29] Ovalbumin mRNA synthesis required addition of RNA polymerase and was only detected in the chromatin prepared from progesterone-stimulated oviducts. These results implied that the ovalbumin gene in chromatin is inaccessible to RNA polymerase or "repressed" after hormone withdrawal and prior to hormonal stimulation. In contrast, stimulation by steroid hormones alters the chromatin template of the oviduct target cells in such a manner that the ovalbumin gene is open or available to be transcribed by RNA polymerase.

To extend these studies further, we then asked whether the purified progesterone-receptor complex could directly stimulate the transcription of the ovalbumin gene in a cell-free system. The results of this experiment are shown in TABLE 7. Bulk amounts of RNA were synthesized from both withdrawn chromatin and from withdrawn chromatin incubated in the presence of progesterone receptor (10^{-8} M). Both RNA preparations were assayed for complementary sequences to [^{3}H]cDNA$_{ov}$. The RNA synthesized in the presence of receptor-hormone complex contained at least a 10-fold enrichment of mRNA sequence, as compared to that found in untreated, withdrawn chromatin controls.[29] It thus appears that a steroid-receptor complex may act directly on chromatin to enhance the number of initiation sites for RNA synthesis, leading to the synthesis of specific mRNAs for induced proteins.

DISCUSSION

The mechanism of steroid hormone action may be related to the distinctive properties of the progesterone receptor.[42,43] Our current working hypothesis for progesterone action in chick oviduct is summarized in FIGURE 3. The progesterone receptor is a dimer composed of A and B subunits that have different and unique properties. The intact dimer (6S) is located in the cytoplasm of the target cell in the absence of hormone stimulation and translocates to the nuclear compartment on administration of progesterone. Both the A and B subunits bind a molecule of hormone. The B subunit binds to the nonhistone protein-DNA complexes of oviduct chromatin but not to pure DNA, whereas the A subunit binds to pure DNA but poorly to chromatin.[33,42] Accordingly, these observations have led to the suggestion that the A subunit could be the actual gene regulatory protein and the B subunit could specify where the A protein is to localize.[33,42] In the absence of the B component of the dimers, the A subunit alone should encounter difficulty in locating the specific initiation sites (genes) it is to regulate, whereas the B subunit alone should be totally inactive as a transcriptional stimulant. Consistent with these predictions, we have found that purified A subunit protein[44] was capable of stimulating transcription on withdrawn chromatin but only at much higher concentrations (~10–50-fold) than that required for the intact dimer.[45] The isolated B subunit[46] was ineffective in stimulating transcription from oviduct chromatin at any concentration tested.[45] These observations are consistent with a model in which one part of the progesterone receptor dimer (B subunit) acts as a binding site specifier to localize the dimer in certain regions of chromatin, whereas the other subunit (A) is effective in destablizing a portion of the chromatin DNA, so that new sites are available to RNA polymerase for initiation of RNA synthesis (FIGURE 3).

In summary, the results presented in this paper are inconsistent with models of steroid hormone action that postulate a requirement for RNA or protein intermediates to be induced that then exert secondary effects on transcription. Rather, the data presented here support our proposal that direct positive regulation of nuclear gene transcription is a viable mechanism for steroid hormone action in eukaryotic cells.

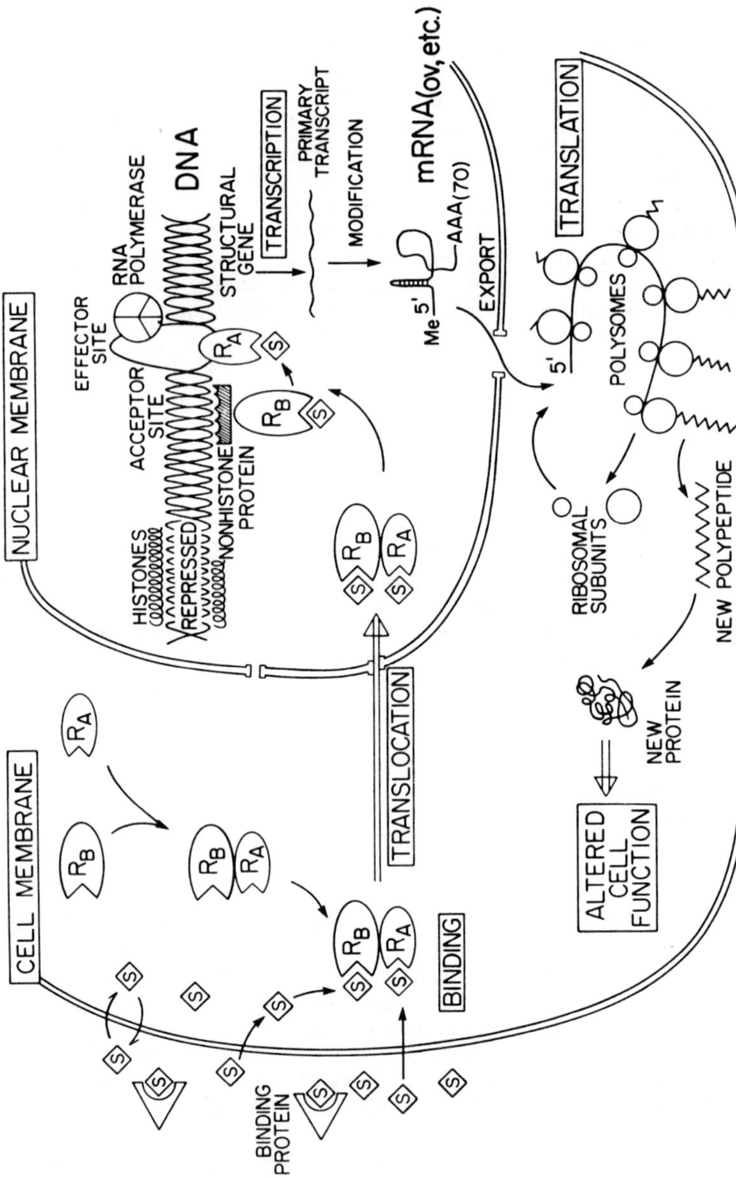

FIGURE 3. Mechanisms of steroid hormone action in the chick oviduct.

References

1. O'Malley, B. W. & W. L. McGuire. 1968. Proc. Nat. Acad. Sci. USA **60:** 1527–1534.
2. Liarakos, C. D., J. M. Rosen & B. W. O'Malley. 1973. Biochemistry **12:** 2809–2816.
3. O'Malley, B. W. & W. L. McGuire. 1968. J. Clin. Invest. **47:** 654–664.
4. O'Malley, B. W., W. L. McGuire, P. O. Kohler & S. G. Korenman. 1969. Rec. Progr. Hormone Res. **25:** 105–160.
5. Cox, R. F. 1973. J. Biochem. **39:** 49–61.
6. Spelsberg, T. C., A. W. Steggles, F. Chytil & B. W. O'Malley. 1972. J. Biol. Chem. **247:** 1368–1374.
7. Spelsberg, T. C., W. M. Mitchell, F. Chytil, E. M. Wilson & B. W. O'Malley. 1973. Biochim. Biophys. Acta **312:** 765–768.
8. Means, A. R., J. P. Comstock, G. C. Rosenfeld & B. W. O'Malley. 1972. Proc. Nat. Acad. Sci. USA **69:** 1146–1150.
9. Comstock, J. P., G. C. Rosenfeld, B. W. O'Malley & A. R. Means. 1972. Proc. Nat. Acad. Sci. USA **69:** 2377–2380.
10. Harris, S. E., J. M. Rosen, A. R. Means & B. W. O'Malley. 1975. Biochemistry **14:** 2072–2081.
11. Chan, L., A. R. Means & B. W. O'Malley. 1973. Proc. Nat. Acad. Sci. USA **70:** 1870–1874.
12. Palmiter, R. D. & L. Smith. 1973. Mol. Biol. Rep. **1:** 129–134.
13. Palmiter, R. D. 1973. J. Biol. Chem. **248:** 8260–8270.
14. Sherman, M. R., P. O. Corvol & B. W. O'Malley. 1970. J. Biol. Chem. **245:** 6085–6096.
15. Kuhn, R. W., W. T. Schrader, R. G. Smith & B. W. O'Malley. 1975. J. Biol. Chem. **250:** 4220–4228.
16. Schwartz, R. J., M. J. Tsai, S. Y. Tsai & B. W. O'Malley. 1975. J. Biol. Chem. **250:** 5175–5182.
17. Cox, R., M. Haines & N. Carey. 1973. Eur. J. Biochem. **32:** 513–524.
18. Lill, H., U. Lill, A. Sippel & G. Hartmann. 1970. *In* Lepetit Colloquium on RNA Polymerase and Transcription. L. G. Silvestri, Ed.: 55. North-Holland Publishing Co. Amsterdam, The Netherlands.
19. Bautz, E. K. F. & F. A. Bautz. 1970. Nature (London) **226:** 1219–1222.
20. Sippel, A. E. & G. R. Hartmann. 1970. Eur. J. Biochem. **16:** 152–157.
21. Zillig, W., D. Zechel, D. Rabussay, U. S. Schachner, X. Setha, P. Palm, A. Heil & W. Seifert. 1970. Cold Spring Harbor Symp. Quant. Biol. **35:** 47–58.
22. Travers, A., D. L. Baillie & S. Pedersen. 1973. Nature [New Biol.] **243:** 161–163.
23. Hinkle, D. S. & M. J. Chamberlin. 1972. J. Mol. Biol. **70:** 157–185.
24. Umezawa, H., S. Mizuno, H. Uamasaki & K. Hitta. 1968. J. Antibiotics (Tokyo) **21:** 234, 235.
25. Hartmann, H., K. O. Nonikel, F. Knusel & J. Nuesh. 1967. Biochim. Biophys. Acta **145:** 843, 844.
26. Chamberlin, M. J. & J. Ring. 1972. J. Mol. Biol. **70:** 221–237.
27. Tsai, M. J., R. J. Schwartz, S. Y. Tsai & B. W. O'Malley. 1975. J. Biol. Chem. **250:** 5165–5174.
28. McKnight, S. G., P. Pennequin & R. T. Schimke. 1975. J. Biol. Chem. **250:** 8108–8110.
29. Tsai, S. Y., M. J. Tsai, R. J. Schwartz, M. Kalimi, J. H. Clark & B. W. O'Malley. 1975. Proc. Nat. Acad. Sci. USA **72:** 4228–4232.
30. Young, B. D., P. R. Harrison, R. S. Gilmour, G. D. Birnie, A. Hell, S. Humphries & J. Paul. 1974. J. Mol. Biol. **84:** 555–568.
31. Chang, C., R. Schwartz & B. W. O'Malley. 1977. In preparation.
32. O'Malley, B. W., D. O. Toft & M. R. Sherman. 1971. J. Biol. Chem. **246:** 1117–1122.
33. Schrader, W. T. & B. W. O'Malley. 1972. J. Biol. Chem. **247:** 51–59.

34. Buller, R. E., D. O. Toft, W. T. Schrader & B. W. O'Malley. 1975. J. Biol. Chem. **250:** 801–808.
35. Buller, R. E., W. T. Schrader & B. W. O'Malley. 1975. J. Biol. Chem. **250:** 809–818.
36. Spelsberg, T. C., A. W. Steggles & B. W. O'Malley. 1971. J. Biol. Chem. **246:** 4188–4197.
37. Schwartz, R. J., R. Kuhn, R. E. Buller, W. T. Schrader & B. W. O'Malley. 1976. J. Biol. Chem. **251:** 5166–5177.
38. Buller, R. E., R. J. Schwartz & B. W. O'Malley. 1976. Biochem. Biophys. Res. Commun. **69:** 106–113.
39. Schwartz, R. J., M. J. Tsai, W. T. Schrader & B. W. O'Malley. 1977. In preparation.
40. Jaffe, R. C., S. H. Socher & B. W. O'Malley. 1975. Biochim. Biophys. Acta **339:** 403–419.
41. Harris, S. E., R. J. Schwartz, M. J. Tsai, A. Roy & B. W. O'Malley. 1976. J. Biol. Chem. **251:** 524–529.
42. O'Malley, B. W., T. C. Spelsberg, W. T. Schrader, F. Chytil & A. W. Steggles. 1972. Nature (London) **235:** 141–144.
43. Schrader, W. T., S. S. Heurer & B. W. O'Malley. 1975. Biol. Reprod. **12:** 134–142.
44. Coty, W., W. T. Schrader & B. W. O'Malley. 1977. J. Biol. Chem. Submitted for publication.
45. Buller, R. E., R. J. Schwartz, W. T. Schrader & B. W. O'Malley. 1976. J. Biol. Chem. **251:** 5178–5186.
46. Schrader, W. T., R. W. Kuhn & B. W. O'Malley. 1977. J. Biol. Chem. In press.
47. Roeder, R. G. 1974. J. Biol. Chem. **249:** 241–248.
48. Maitra, U. & J. Hurwitz. 1965. Proc. Nat. Acad. Sci. USA **54:** 815–822.

REGULATION OF ESTROGEN RECEPTOR REPLENISHMENT BY PROGESTERONE*

James H. Clark, A. J. W. Hsueh,† and Ernest J. Peck, Jr.

Department of Cell Biology
Baylor College of Medicine
Houston, Texas 77030

Introduction

The cyclic changes in female reproductive tissues have been studied extensively by reproductive biologists. The periodic variations in blood levels of estrogen and progesterone are believed to be responsible for the changes observed in uterine tissue throughout the estrous and menstrual cycles. With the discovery of steroid hormone receptors, it became apparent that variations in tissue levels of hormone receptors might also act as a regulatory step in the control of reproductive cyclicity. It has been suggested that progesterone might antagonize the action of estrogen by reducing the amount of cytoplasmic estrogen receptor, R_c.[1-3]

Recent work from our laboratory indicates that this is one of the mechanisms by which progesterone and nonsteroidal antiestrogens exert their antagonistic effects.[4-6] Another possibility is that progesterone might interfere with the nuclear binding of the receptor-estrogen complex and thus reduce or modify its effects on nucleus-mediated events. In this paper, we have examined the influence of progesterone on estrogen receptor replenishment and nuclear binding in immature and adult rats.

Materials and Methods

Preparation of Animals and Materials

Immmature (22 days old) female Sprague-Dawley rats were purchased from Texas Inbred Mice Co. and housed in a controlled environment with 13 hr of artificial light between 7 AM and 8 PM. All rats received two daily subcutaneous injections of 17β-estradiol (2.5 μg in 0.5 ml of 0.9% saline solution that contained 1% ethanol). Pretreatment with estradiol was performed to increase the sensitivity of the uterus to progesterone, presumably via estrogen's effect of increasing the synthesis of the progesterone receptor.[7,8] On the third day, rats were randomly divided into three groups. Animals in one group were injected with 2.5 μg of estradiol (E) and 0.2 ml of sesame oil. Animals in a second group were injected with 2.5 μg of estradiol plus 2.5 mg of progesterone (E + P) dissolved in 0.2 ml of sesame oil. Animals in a third group were injected with 2.5 μg of estradiol plus 1 mg of testosterone propionate (E + T) dissolved in 0.2 ml of sesame oil. In all groups,

*Supported by National Institutes of Health Grants HD-04985 and HD-08389 and by American Cancer Society Grant BC-92.

†Present address: National Institute of Child Health and Human Development, Bethesda, Md. 20014.

the sesame oil or steroids dissolved in oil were injected at a subcutaneous site separate from that of estradiol injection. Animals were killed at various intervals after injection to assess the effect of progesterone and testosterone propionate on the level of uterine estrogen receptors.

In experiments designed to test the uterine responsiveness of the various groups to subsequent estrogen treatment, animals were further injected with 2.5 μg of estradiol in 0.5 ml of saline on Day 4 and killed 24 hr later.

All animals were killed by cervical dislocation; the uteri were stripped of adhering fat and mesentery and weighed (wet weight). Some uteri were used for the determination of nuclear and cytoplasmic receptor concentrations by [^{3}H]estradiol exchange.[9,10] Some uteri were saved for protein[11] and DNA determinations[12] or dried overnight in an 80°C oven for dry weight determination.

Ovariectomized adult (body weight 200–250 g) female Holtzman-strain rats were purchased from Hormone Assay Co. (Chicago, Ill.) and used 3–5 weeks after the operation. All rats received one subcutaneous injection of 10 μg of 17β-estradiol in 1 ml of saline solution that contained 1% ethanol. On the second day, rats were randomly divided into three groups. Animals in group A were injected with 10 μg of estradiol in 1 ml of saline plus 0.5 ml of sesame oil (E). Animals in group B were injected with 10 μg of estradiol in 1 ml of saline plus 6.5 mg of progesterone dissolved in 0.5 ml of sesame oil (E + P). Animals in group C were injected with 10 μg of estradiol plus 5 mg of hydrocortisone 21-acetate dissolved in 0.5 ml of sesame oil (E + HA). In all groups, the sesame oil or steroids in oil were injected at separate subcutaneous sites. Twenty-four hours later (Day 3), the animals were sacrificed; the uteri were stripped of adhering fat and mesentery and weighed with luminal fluid (whole uterine weight). The uteri were then slit to release luminal fluid, pressed against filter paper, and reweighed (empty uterine weight) to enable the amount of fluid to be calculated by difference (luminal fluid weight). The uteri were then analyzed for cytoplasmic and nuclear receptor levels by the [^{3}H]estradiol exchange assay, as described above. To determine the uterine sensitivity to further estradiol treatment, some animals were injected with 1 ml of saline or 10 μg of estradiol in 1 ml of saline in Day 3 and analyzed for whole or empty uterine weight, dry weight, and DNA content 24 hr later.

In experiments designed to study the cytoplasmic receptor concentration in rats during the estrous cycle, Purdue Wistar virgin female rats (4–6 months old) were used. Vaginal smears were taken daily, and only adult rats that had completed at least two 4-day cycles were used. All animals were killed between 9:30 and 10:30 AM by decapitation. Their uteri were removed, and cytoplasmic receptor concentration was determined by the [^{3}H]estradiol exchange assay.[9,10]

Separation of Myometrial and Endometrial Components

To measure receptor concentration in different components of the uterine tissue, gentle scraping was used to separate myometrium from the rest of the uterine tissue. Uterine tissues stimulated with hormones were taken from castrate rats on Day 3 of hormone treatment and dissected carefully under a dissecting microscope. Endometrial tissues were gently scraped from the remaining myometrial tissues by a pair of fine forceps, and these two fractions were used for the [^{3}H]estradiol exchange assay. Histologic examination revealed that the myometrial fraction was completely devoid of endometrial components, whereas the endometrial fraction was composed of epithelial and stromal elements, in addition to small fragments of myometrium. Therefore, the latter fraction was called the enriched endometrial fraction.

Determination of Cytoplasmic Binding Sites by the [^{3}H] Estradiol Exchange Assay

The uterine tissues were homogenized in all-glass Kontes homogenizers under ice and then centrifuged at 800*g* for 10 min. The pellet fractions were used for the determination of nuclear binding sites by the [^{3}H]estradiol exchange assay.[9] The supernatant fraction was treated with an equal volume of activated charcoal

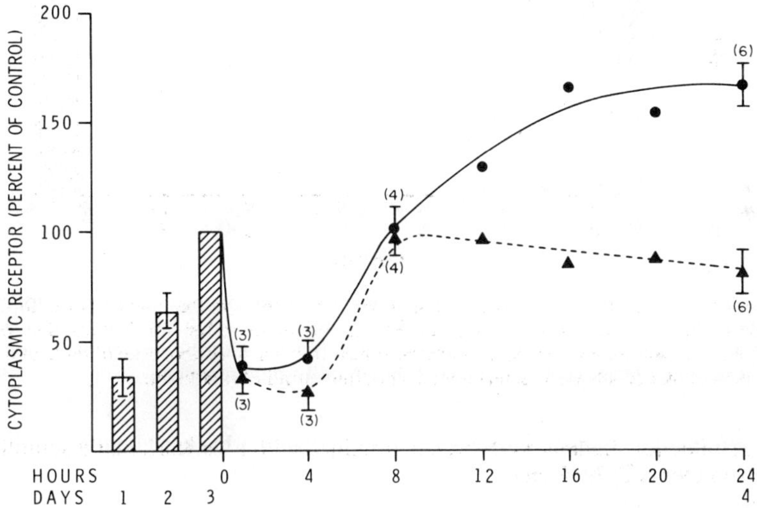

FIGURE 1. Effect of progesterone on the estrogen-induced depletion and replenishment of the cytoplasmic estrogen receptor. Immature rats received 2.5 μg of estradiol for 2 days and on the third day were injected with either estradiol (●) or estradiol plus progesterone (▲). The quantity of cytoplasmic estrogen receptor was determined on Days 0–2 and at various times after estrogen or estrogen plus progesterone treatment on Day 3. All values are expressed as the percentage of control based on the receptor concentration on Day 3. Numbers in parentheses represent the numbers of experiments with four animals per experiment.

suspension (0.5% charcoal and 0.05% dextran) at 4°C for 15 min to remove free steroids. The tubes were then centrifuged for 15 min at 800*g*. The supernatant fractions were dispensed into two series of tubes that contained either 13 nM [^{3}H]estradiol for determination of total binding or 13 nM [^{3}H]estradiol plus a 100-fold excess of diethylstilbestrol (DES) for determination of nonspecific binding. The tubes were incubated at 23°C for 18–20 hr. At the end of incubation, the tubes were cooled to 4°C for 10 min, and the charcoal suspension was added. Incubation was continued for 15 min at 4°C, and the tubes were centrifuged at 800*g* for 15 min. Aliquots of the supernatants were added to 3 ml of ethanol and 10 ml of scintillation fluid (5.5 g of Permablend® I, Packard Instruments Co., Chicago, Ill., in 1

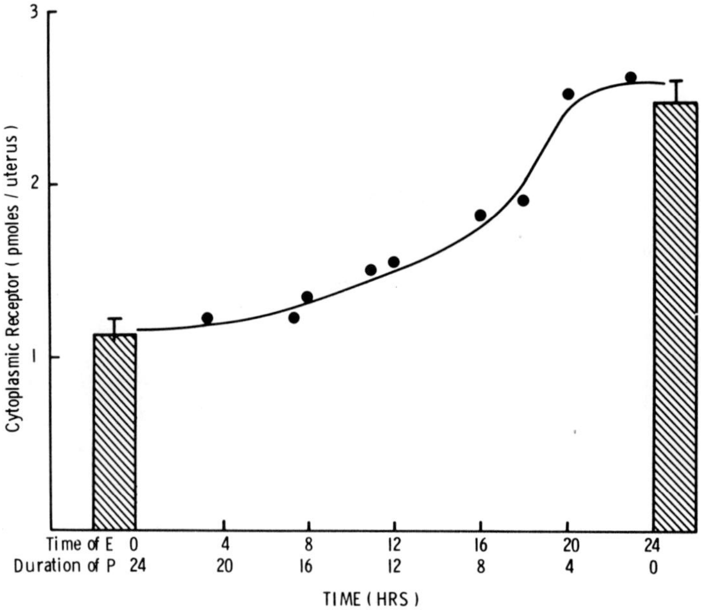

FIGURE 2. The effect of delayed progesterone treatment on the quantity of cytoplasmic estrogen receptor. Immature rats received 2.5 μg of estradiol for 2 days. On Day 3, progesterone was administered at various times after an injection of estradiol, and cytoplasmic receptor levels were determined 24 hr after estradiol treatment.

liter of toluene). Radioactivity was determined with a Packard liquid scintillation spectrometer at 25% efficiency.

RESULTS

Effects of Progesterone on Cytoplasmic Levels of Estrogen Receptor

We have previously demonstrated that progesterone treatment causes a significant reduction in the amount of cytoplasmic estrogen receptor, R_c, 24 hr after injection in estrogen-primed immature rats.[6,17] The reduced R_c also correlated with a reduced sensitivity to estrogen injection on Day 4. To gain further information on the mechanism of action of progesterone on the reduction of estrogen receptor concentration, the quantities of R_c and R_nE were determined by [^{3}H]estradiol exchange at various stages of hormonal treatment. As shown in FIGURE 1, pretreatment with estradiol on Days 1 and 2 increases the concentration of R_c in uterine tissue. On Day 3, animals were divided into two groups, and estradiol (E) or estradiol plus progesterone (E + P) were injected. The quantity of R_c fell to low levels within 1 hr of injection and began to increase gradually at 4–8 hr. During the time of R_c depletion, there was a concomitant increase in the amount of R_nE in the nucleus in both treatment groups (see FIGURE 5). However, between 8 and 24 hr after injection, the R_c level continued to increase in the E treatment group but remained constant in the E + P treatment group. This observation suggested that two separate processes were involved in the replenishment of R_c and that progesterone might inhibit the replenishment process between 8 and 24 hr after estradiol injection. No significant effect of progesterone on uterine DNA or protein content was observed on Day 4.[6]

To further study the time sequence of progestational inhibition of R_c replenishment, progesterone was injected at various intervals after estradiol treatment on Day 3, and the level of R_c was measured 24 hr after estradiol injection. As can be seen in FIGURE 2, progesterone injection at 4–8 hr after estrogen injection decreased the quantity of R_c to the level observed when progesterone was injected simultaneously with estradiol. However, when progesterone was injected between 8 and 24 hr after estrogen, the level of R_c 24 hr after E treatment increased gradually, thus suggesting an escape from the antagonistic effect of progesterone. These data suggest the existence of two separate processes for receptor replenishment.

The ability of progesterone to cause a reduction in R_c appears to be specific for estrogen antagonists. Testosterone propionate (1 mg Day 3) caused a 25% reduction in R_c and a slight decrease in estrogen-stimulated uterine weight (data not shown). Other steroids, such as hydrocortisone 21-acetate, have no effect on R_c replenishment (to appear elsewhere). Progesterone has no effect on R_c in the nonestrogen-primed uterus. Presumably, this finding reflects an insensitivity of the uterus to progesterone that results from low quantities of progesterone receptor.[7,8]

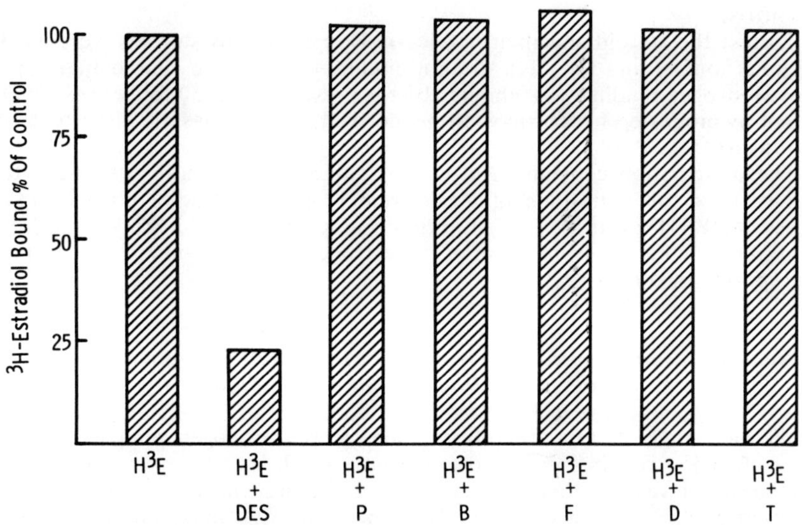

FIGURE 3. Stereospecificity of the cytoplasmic estrogen receptor after estrogen plus progesterone treatment. The ability of various compounds to compete for estradiol-binding sites was measured by competitive binding analysis of uterine cytosol obtained on Day 4 from estrogen plus progesterone-treated rats. Compounds were added to receptor assays at 100 times the concentration of [^{3}H]estradiol. Abbreviations: diethylstilbestrol, DES; progesterone, P; corticosterone, B; cortisol, F; dexamethasone, D; and testosterone, T.

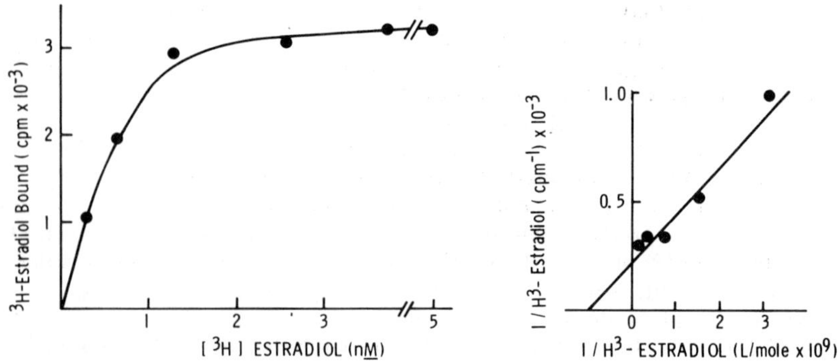

FIGURE 4. Binding parameters of the cytoplasmic estrogen receptor after estrogen plus progesterone treatment. Uterine cytosol was incubated with various concentrations of [^{3}H]estradiol, and the quantity of bound receptor was determined as described in the text. The data are plotted as a saturation curve (*left*) and a double reciprocal plot (*right*).

Properties of Cytoplasmic Estrogen Receptor After Progesterone Treatment

Progesterone could alter steroid binding parameters of R_c rather than cytoplasmic levels of R_c and thereby affect the ability of the uterus to respond to estrogen. To examine some of these properties, cytosol was prepared from estradiol plus progesterone-treated animals, as described under MATERIALS AND METHODS.

To test the steroid specificity of R_c on Day 4, various steroids were used as potential competitors for [^{3}H]estradiol binding by R_c in the charcoal adsorption assay. Estrogen binding was inhibited by the presence of a 250-fold excess of DES but not by progesterone, corticosterone, cortisol, dexamethasone, or testosterone (FIGURE 3).

The dissociation constant, K_d, was examined by incubating uterine cytosol with various concentrations of [^{3}H]estradiol or [^{3}H]estradiol plus a 100-fold excess of DES (FIGURE 4). The saturation characteristics and K_d (6×10^{-10} M) did not differ significantly from those of the estrogen receptor found in control uteri and reported by others.[4,8,9]

Nuclear Accumulation and Retention of Estrogen Receptor in Estrogen- or Estrogen plus Progesterone-Treated Animals

We have suggested that retention of the receptor-estrogen complex for longer than 4–6 hr is a requirement for true uterine growth.[13–15] Therefore, any interaction that interferes with this process is likely to be antagonistic. Accumulation and retention of R_nE were measured at 1, 6, and 24 hr after injection of estradiol on Days 3 and 4 in immature animals (FIGURES 5 & 6). On Day 3, the quantity of R_nE did not differ between either group: however, the total quantity of R_nE that was retained at the 4- and 24-hr points in the E + P-treated group was less than that in the E-treated group (FIGURE 5). On Day 4, the quantity of R_nE was significantly reduced in E + P-treated animals 1 hr after injection, as compared to estrogen-treated animals. By 6 hr, the quantity of R_nE in E + P-treated animals had declined to levels that were not significantly different from those of controls, whereas the level of R_nE in estradiol-treated rats was maintained above control levels (FIGURE 6). Because R_c in the E + P-treated group was lower on Day 4, the decrease in R_nE that was observed in this group may be caused by a reduction in the quantity of R_c that is available for translocation.

Effect of Progesterone on Quantity of Estrogen Receptor and Uterine Responsiveness in Adult Castrate Rats

As shown in FIGURE 7, progesterone treatment caused a significant decrease in cytoplasmic estrogen receptor, R_c, content. A reduction is also observed in levels of nucleus-bound estrogen receptor, although these quantities in all groups were small and therefore have little influence on the total amount of receptor. The decrease in quantity of R_c does not result from a general depressive action of progesterone on uterine protein synthesis, because the decrease is significant, even when the data are expressed as sites per milligram of protein (25.9 ± 1.9 pmol/100 mg of protein for the E pretreatment; 11.1 ± 1.7 pmol/100 mg of protein for the E + P pretreatment group, $p < 0.01$).

We have previously shown that testosterone has a weak effect on R_c replenishment and that this effect correlates with its weak antiestrogenicity.[6] To further examine the specificity of the depressive effect of progesterone on uterine R_c content, estrogen-treated adult castrate rats were injected with hydrocortisone 21-acetate, as explained under MATERIALS AND METHODS. This treatment caused no

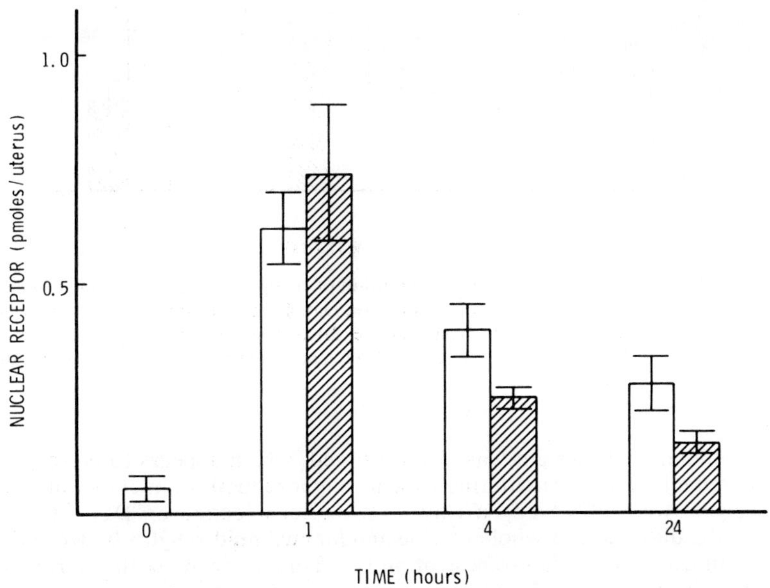

FIGURE 5. The effect of progesterone on the nuclear retention of estrogen receptor on Day 3. Immature rats received 2.5 μg of estradiol for 2 days and on the third day were injected with either estradiol (□) or estradiol plus progesterone (▨). The quantity of R_nE was determined 1, 4, and 24 hr after injection.

significant decrease in either cytoplasmic or nuclear estrogen receptor concentration (FIGURE 7). These data suggest that the depressive effect of progesterone on estrogen receptor level is hormone specific.

To demonstrate that the reduced level of estrogen receptor does reflect a decrease in uterine responsiveness in progesterone-treated animals, animals in E and E + P pretreatment groups were injected with E or saline on Day 3, and the uterine weights were measured 24 hr later. The uterine weights (whole, empty, and dry) and luminal fluid weights at various stages of treatment were measured, and the results are shown in FIGURE 8. Progesterone depressed the whole uterine weight dramatically within 24 hr after treatment (Day 3). A significant decrease in

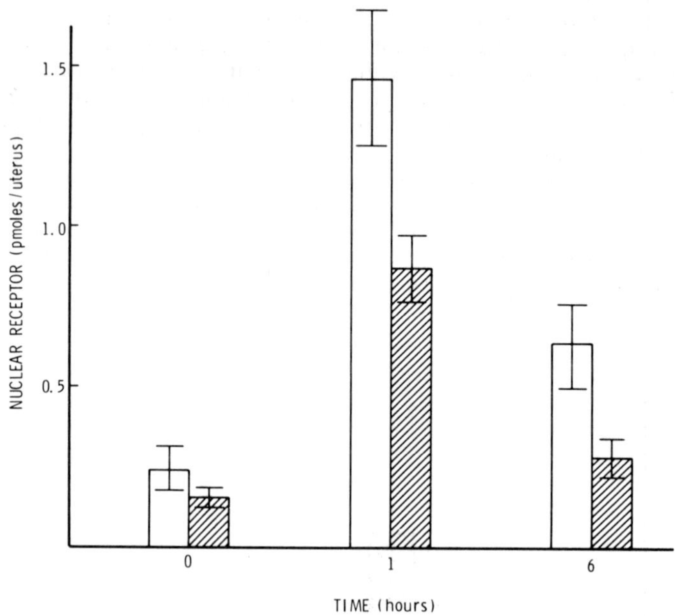

FIGURE 6. Nuclear accumulation and retention of receptor-estrogen complex in estradiol or estradiol plus progesterone-treated animals on Day 4. Immature female rats were treated with estradiol (□) or estradiol plus progesterone (▨) as described in the text. On Day 4, they were injected with 2.5 μg of estradiol, and the nuclear level of the complex was measured 0, 1, and 6 hr after treatment.

uterine luminal fluid weight was also observed, which appears to be responsible for the reduction in whole uterine weight. Slight reductions in empty uterine and dry weights were observed on Day 3. Estradiol injection on Day 3 further increased the difference in whole uterine and luminal fluid weights between the two groups on Day 4. Estradiol treatment on Day 3 did not increase the uterine weight responses in the E + P pretreatment group but increased significantly that of the E pretreatment group, thus indicating a decreased responsiveness of the E + P pretreatment group to further estrogen treatment.

No appreciable difference among treatment groups was observed when empty uterine weights were compared to those of saline-injected controls (TABLE 1).

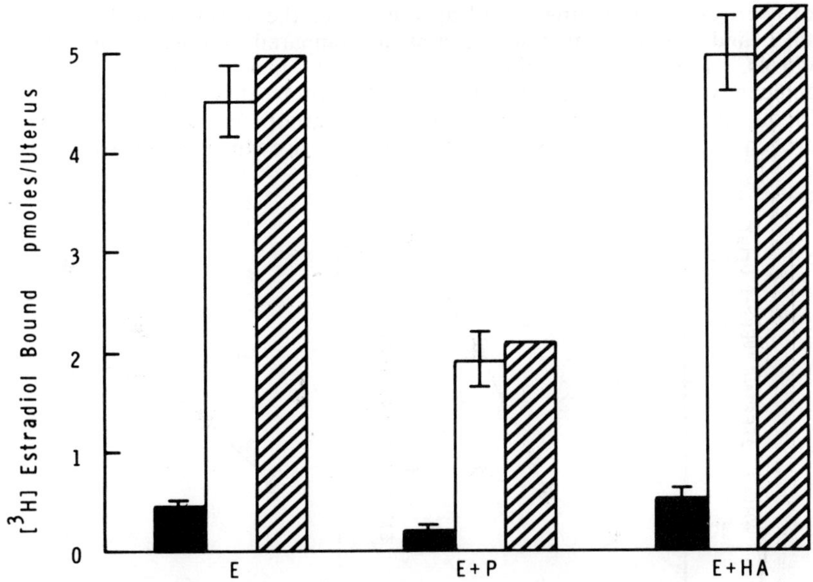

FIGURE 7. The effect of progesterone and hydrocortisone acetate on the quantity of estrogen receptor in the uteri of adult castrate rats. Three groups of castrate rats were given 10 μg of estradiol. Twenty-four hours later, the animals were injected with 10 μg of estradiol (E), 10 μg of estradiol plus 6.5 mg of progesterone (E + P), or 10 μg of estradiol plus 5 mg of hydrocortisone acetate (E + HA). Twenty-four hours later, the animals were sacrificed, and their uteri were analyzed for cytoplasmic (□), nuclear (■), and total (▨) estrogen receptor contents by the [^{3}H]estradiol exchange assay. The data represent the mean ± SE from six to eight experiments with three or four animals per experiment.

TABLE 1

PROGESTERONE ANTAGONISM OF ESTROGEN-INDUCED UTERINE GROWTH*

Pre-treatment (Day 2)	Treatment (Day 3)	Whole Uterine Weight (mg)	Percent of Saline Control	Empty Uterine Weight (mg)	Percent of Saline Control	Dry Weight (mg)	Percent of Saline Control
E	E (10)†	528.0 ± 51.0	187	237.0 ± 6.4	157	47.1 ± 1.8	144
	S (6)	282.0 ± 51.8	100	151.0 ± 9.6	100	32.6 ± 3.2	100
E + P	E (9)	176.0 ± 3.7	114	163.0 ± 3.6	116	32.9 ± 1.1	109
	S (6)	155.5 ± 11.8	100	141.8 ± 8.8	100	30.3 ± 1.6	100

*All animals were injected with 10 μg of 17β-estradiol on Day 1. Twenty-four hours later (Day 2), they were divided into two groups. Animals in the E pretreatment group were injected with 10 μg of estradiol plus 0.5 ml of sesame oil. Animals in the E + P pretreatment group were injected with 10 μg of estradiol plus 6.5 mg of progesterone dissolved in 0.5 ml of sesame oil. On Day 3, animals in both groups were injected with either 1 ml of saline (S) or 10 μg of estradiol dissolved in 1 ml of saline (E). All animals were sacrificed 24 hr after the last injection, and uterine weights were determined.

†Numbers in parentheses represent the numbers of animals used for each determination.

However, estradiol treatment on Day 3 increased the uterine weight responses in both E and E + P pretreatment groups, as compared to those of saline-injected controls. However, the ability of estradiol to increase uterine weight was significantly depressed ($p < 0.01$) in the E + P pretreatment group, as compared with its effect on the estrogen pretreatment group. Estradiol treatment after estrogen pretreatment caused dramatic uterine growth over the saline control

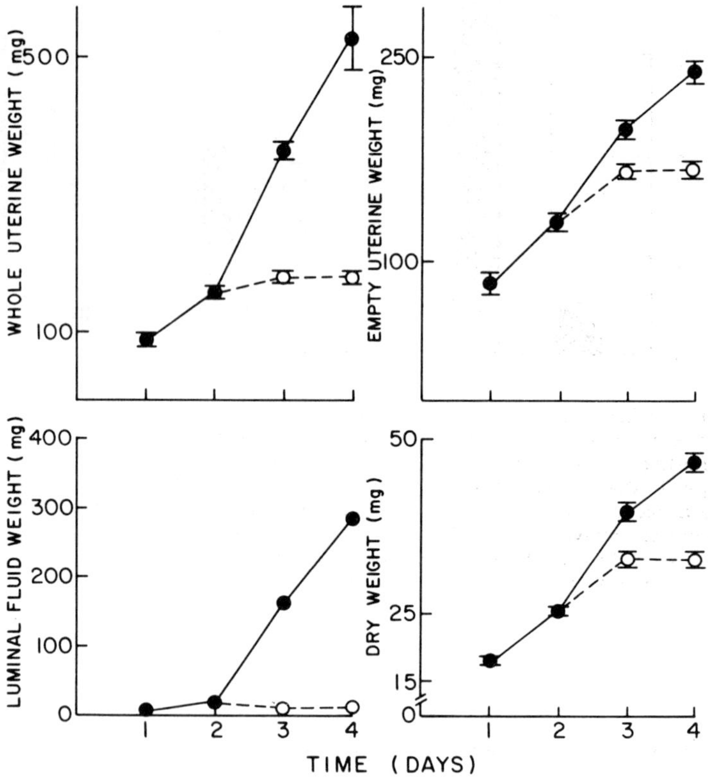

FIGURE 8. The effect of progesterone on uterine weight response in adult castrate rats. All animals were injected with 10 μg of 17β-estradiol on Day 1. Twenty-four hours later (Day 2), they were divided into two groups. The animals were injected with either 10 μg of estradiol plus 0.5 ml of sesame oil (●) or with 10 μg of estradiol plus 6.5 mg of progesterone dissolved in 0.5 ml sesame oil (○). On Day 3, the animals in both groups were injected with 10 μg of estradiol. Animals were sacrificed at various days of the experiment, and their uterine weights (whole, empty, and dry) and luminal fluid weights were determined, as described in MATERIALS AND METHODS. The data represent the mean ± SE from at least 10 animals in each group.

group, whereas estradiol treatment in the E + P pretreatment group caused only very slight stimulation. These data indicate that the antagonistic effect of progesterone on uterine growth response correlates with its depressive effect on the quantity of estrogen receptor (FIGURE 7).

The possible influence of progesterone on uterine DNA content was examined because it has been shown that progesterone antagonizes estrogen-induced cell division in the chick oviduct.[24] On Day 3, uterine DNA content was not significantly different between the two pretreatment groups (1.39 ± 0.10 mg/uterus in the E pretreatment group; 1.33 ± 0.12 in the E + P pretreatment group). Twenty-four hours after injection of estradiol on Day 3, uterine DNA content increased in both the E + P pretreatment group (1.67 ± 0.15 mg/uterus) and the E pretreatment group (1.51 ± 0.11 mg/uterus). Thus, no antagonistic effect of progesterone on uterine DNA synthesis was demonstrated.

The effect of hydrocortisone 21-acetate (HA) on uterine responsiveness was also tested. Animals in the E + HA pretreatment group were injected with estrogen on Day 3, and the uterine weights were measured 24 hr later. Hydrocortisone 21-acetate did not cause any appreciable change in any of the uterine growth parameters when compared to those in the estrogen pretreatment group (FIGURE 7).

Measurement of Estrogen Receptor Content in Myometrial and Enriched Endometrial Fractions of E- and E + P-Treated Animals

To establish that receptor replenishment is similar both in endometrium and in myometrium, the endometrium and myometrium from adult castrate rats were carefully separated, as described under MATERIALS AND METHODS. On Day 3 of treatment, estrogen receptor content was measured in nuclear and cytoplasmic fractions of these two uterine components (FIGURE 9). A significant inhibition of cytoplasmic receptor content in E + P-treated animals was observed in both myometrium and enriched endometrium. In addition, a similar decrease was also demonstrated in nuclear fractions of both tissue types.

Cyclic Fluctuation of Estrogen Receptor Content During the Estrous Cycle

The concentration of estrogen receptor in the cytoplasmic fraction of the uterus was measured during different stages of the estrous cycle. As shown in FIGURE 10, no significant difference in R_c content could be found during diestrus, proestrus, and estrus, whereas a significant decrease was observed at metestrus. To rule out the possibility that the observed reduction in R_c was due to a decreased affinity of R_c for estrogen, the dissociation constant of the receptor-estrogen complex was determined for each stage of the cycle: metestrus, 0.87 ± 0.11 nM; diestrus, 0.97 ± 0.11 nM; proestrus, 0.97 ± 0.15 nM; and estrus, 1.21 ± 0.20 nM. None of these values is significantly different ($p < 0.01$).

As we have shown in previous work, the nuclear level of estrogen receptor varies with the blood level of estrogen[16] and constitutes a significant amount of total uterine receptor. These nuclear values have been included in FIGURE 10 to show the variation in total receptor content during the estrous cycle. Total uterine receptor content or receptor content per milligram of DNA reached high levels during diestrus and proestrus and decreased to the lowest level at metestrus (FIGURE 10).

DISCUSSION

The results of this study demonstrate that progesterone interferes with the replenishment of the cytoplasmic estrogen receptor, R_c, in the estrogenized immature rat uterus. In addition, this reduction is correlated with a reduced sensitivity

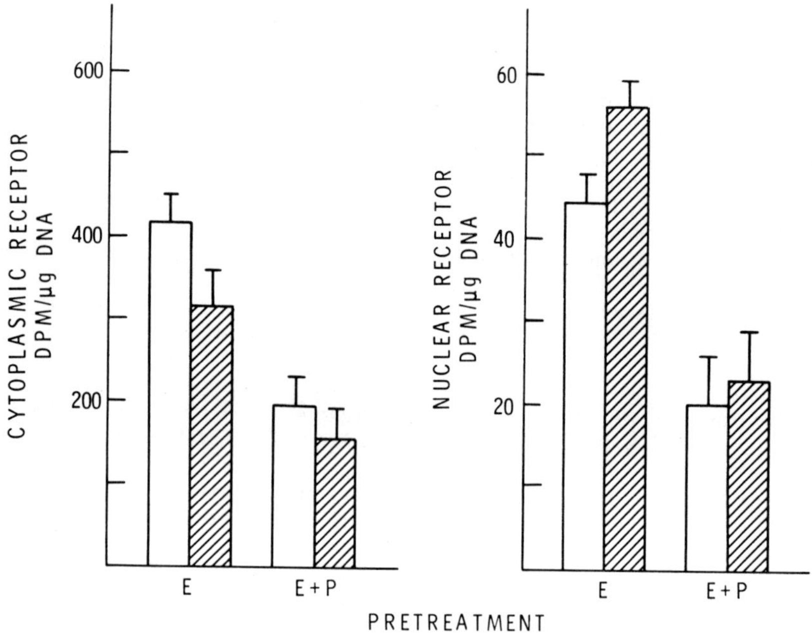

FIGURE 9. Concentration of cytoplasmic and nuclear estrogen receptor in the endometrium (□) and myometrium (▨) of the adult rat uterus. Ovariectomized adult rats were pretreated with estrogen or estrogen plus progesterone as described in text, and the quantity of estrogen receptor was measured in the endometrium and myometrium on Day 3.

of the uterus to the action of estrogen.[6,17] Cytoplasmic receptor replenishment appears to involve two phases. The first phase, which occurs 4–8 hr after injection, may represent a recycling of R_c that is not blocked by progesterone (FIGURES 1 & 2). The quantity of R_c that is replenished equals that which was depleted, and therefore recycling through some deactivation-reactivation mechanism could exist to account for this phase of replenishment. The second phase, which occurs 8–24 hr after injection, may involve synthesis of R_c that is blocked by progesterone treatment. The quantity of R_c that is *replenished* during phase 2 is approximately twofold greater than that which was initially present (FIGURES 1 & 2). The increase in R_c was inhibited by progesterone, even when the injection of progesterone was delayed 8 hr (FIGURE 2). This finding implies that progesterone may act on some late event in the sequence that leads to new R_c synthesis. These data suggest that R_c replenishment in estrogen-primed animals may be accomplished by two mechanisms: a recycling of existing R_c after nuclear accumulation, which is not blocked by the presence of progesterone, and a synthesis of new R_c, which is blocked by progesterone.

The replenishment of cytoplasmic receptors for glucocorticoids by a process that does not depend on protein and RNA syntheses has been proposed by Ishii *et al.*[18,19] and Rousseau *et al.*[20] It is possible that the first phase of replenishment that was observed in this report is of this type. The second phase of R_c replenishment may result from cellular hypertrophy induced by estrogen. The involvement of protein synthesis in the replenishment process has been suggested by Gorski *et al.*[21] and Cidlowski and Muldoon.[22] Recently, Mester and Baulieu[23] suggested that the replenishment of R_c in uteri of immature rats involves two separate processes. The first process, which occurs 0–6 hr after injection, could not be blocked by cycloheximide, whereas the second process, which occurs 6–11 hr after injection, was dependent on protein synthesis. Thus, in cell types that grow in size or number in response to a steroid hormone, R_c replenishment may involve both recycling and synthesis of new receptor, whereas in cells that do not grow in response to their target steroid, R_c replenishment may involve only recycling.

The reduction in estrogen binding by R_c that occurs after progesterone treatment could have resulted from changes in the steroid binding specificity and/or the binding affinity of R_c (FIGURES 3 & 4). However, these parameters appear to be unchanged by progesterone treatment. The effect of progesterone on decreased R_c does not appear to be a pharmacologic one, because the half-maximal dose of 0.5 mg of progesterone is well within the generally accepted "physiologic" ranges for the hormone.[17,28]

If reduced R_c on Day 4 is related to the reduced uterine growth that is observed 24 hr later,[6,17] the quantity of R_c that is translocatable to the nucleus and/or the re-

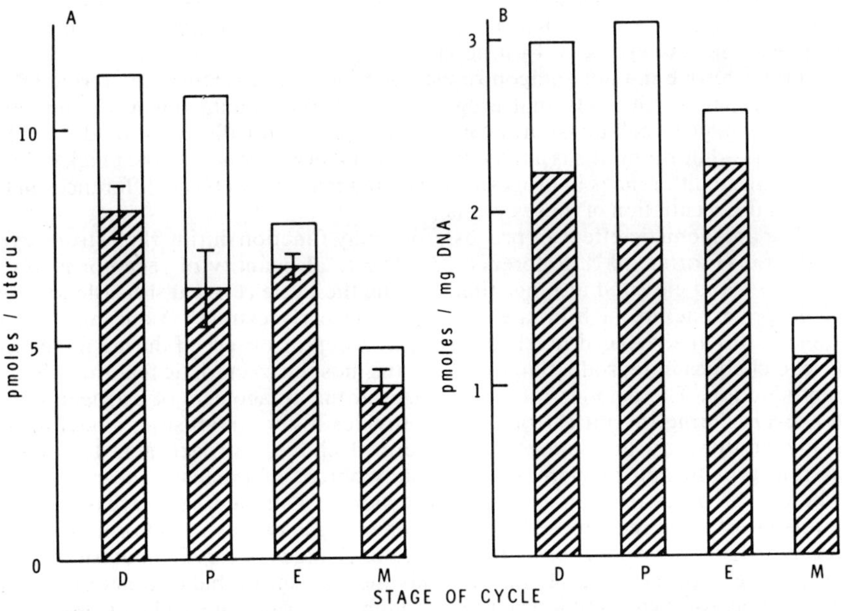

FIGURE 10. Concentration of estrogen receptor in cytoplasmic and nuclear fractions of rat uterus during the estrous cycle. Uterine tissues were taken from rats on the days of proestrus (P), estrus (E), metestrus (M), or diestrus (D). Cytoplasmic (▨) and nuclear (□) fractions were prepared, and the [^{3}H]estradiol exchange assay was used to measure the estrogen receptor concentrations in both fractions. Tissue fractions were incubated with various concentrations of either [^{3}H]estradiol alone or [^{3}H]estradiol plus diethylstilbestrol (DES). Specific binding was obtained by subtracting the amount of [^{3}H]estradiol bound in the presence of DES from total binding in the absence of DES. The quantity of estradiol receptor at various stages of the cycle was obtained from double-reciprocal plots. The $K_d{}^r$ values were also determined for the various stages: metestrus, 0.98 nM; diestrus, 0.97 nM; proestrus, 0.97 nM; and estrus, 1.21 nM.

tention time for nucleus-bound acceptor, R_n, should be reduced. As shown in FIGURE 6, the level of R_n 1 and 6 hr after injection of estradiol is significantly lower in progesterone-pretreated animals. We have shown that long-term nuclear retention of R_nE correlates with the stimulation of true uterine growth.[13–15] Therefore, any circumstance that results in diminished nuclear retention time or number of R_nE is likely to cause reduced uterine growth.

Progesterone also causes a significant decrease in the number of cytoplasmic estrogen receptors, R_c, in the adult rat uterus (FIGURE 7). This decrease is correlated with a reduced uterine sensitivity to estrogen (FIGURE 8). As discussed earlier, cytoplasmic receptor replenishment may involve both recycling and *de novo* synthesis of R_c, and progesterone may have a preferential inhibitory effect on synthesis alone. The possibility that these processes occur in an independent manner in different uterine cell types cannot be ruled out; however, the demonstration that receptor replenishment occurs both in endometrium and in myometrium makes this hypothesis unlikely (FIGURE 1).

The depressive effect of progesterone on levels of R_c appears to be specific for estrogen antagonists. We have shown that nonsteroidal estrogen antagonists, such as nafoxidine hydrochloride (Upjohn 11,000-A) and testosterone propionate, antagonize receptor replenishment and estrogen responsiveness.[4,5,17] In contrast, hydrocortisone 21-acetate had no effect on either receptor level or on uterine responsiveness to estrogen (FIGURE 7).

Progesterone did not antagonize estrogen-induced elevations in uterine DNA. Therefore, it is not likely that progesterone exerts its antagonism by inhibiting estrogen-induced cell division, as has been reported for the chick oviduct.[24] Because the adult rat uterus is a fully differentiated organ, whereas the chick oviduct is not, these differences in progesterone action may reflect basic differences in the state of differentiation of these organs.

The antagonistic effect of progesterone may function during the estrous cycle in the rat (FIGURE 10 & Reference 23). The total quantity of receptor is low at metestrus and elevated at other times during the cycle (FIGURE 10). Blood levels of progesterone are high in late proestrus and early estrus[26–29] and may be the stimulus for the reduced levels of estrogen receptor observed during metestrus. Cyclic changes in reproductive tracts are the most characteristic feature of female reproduction. The demonstration of progesterone antagonism of estrogen receptor levels during the rat estrous cycle provides a very interesting model for the study of these cyclic changes. As described above, estrogen acts to promote uterine growth and to increase the tissue content of progesterone receptor,[7,8] whereas progesterone antagonizes the action of estrogen by decreasing tissue levels of estrogen receptor. The interaction of these two ovarian hormones at the receptor level provides a basis for the cyclic changes observed in uterine tissues during the estrous cycle of the rat. This mechanism probably functions in primates, because cytoplasmic fractions of human uterus and monkey oviduct bind less estrogen during the luteal phase than during the follicular phase of the menstrual cycle.[30–33]

The ability of progesterone to antagonize and/or modify the action of estrogen may form a basis for interhormonal control mechanisms. This interplay between estrogen and progesterone may be considered in the following way (FIGURE 11). Estrogen, E, binds to the cytoplasmic estrogen receptor, R^e_c, to form a complex $R^e_c \cdot E$ that translocates to the nucleus, $R^e_n \cdot E$. This complex is responsible for the stimulation of events that lead to an increase in both R^e_c and the cytoplasmic progesterone receptor, R^p_c. Estrogen also stimulates uterine hypertrophy and hyperplasia (FIGURE 4). The elevated levels of R_c^p augment the ability of the uterus to respond to progesterone. Progesterone binds to its cytoplasmic receptor to form $R_c^p \cdot P$, which undergoes translocation to the nucleus to form $R_n^p \cdot P$, and elicits the characteristic progestational responses that prepare the uterus for implantation. Progesterone also reduces R_c^e and the nuclear retention time for $R_n^e \cdot E$, thereby decreasing the ability of the uterus to respond in a totally estrogen-directed fashion. Thus, progesterone reduces and/or redirects the ability of the uterine cells to respond to estrogen in such a way as to produce an appropriate uterine environment for implantation and pregnancy. This scheme does not rule out other possible interactional and control points, such as membrane effects, events not mediated by receptors, and steroid effects on pituitary hormone secretion. It is presented as a model that may provide a framework for testing ideas.

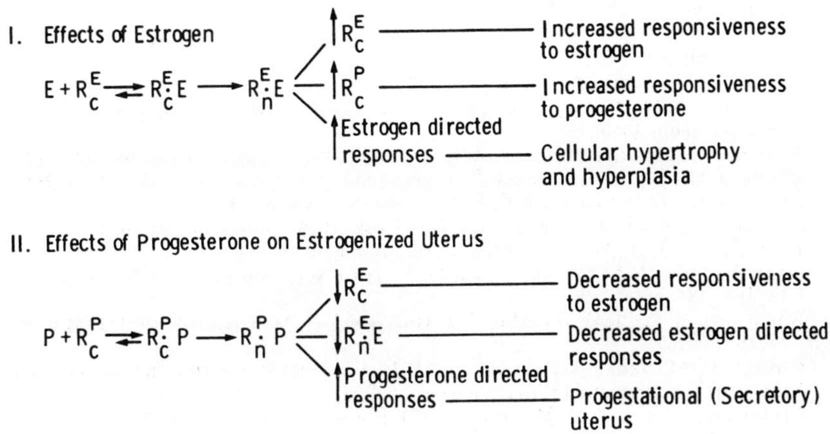

FIGURE 11. Interaction of estrogen and progesterone in the control of receptor level and uterine growth. See DISCUSSION for details of this Figure. Abbreviations: E, estrogen; R_c^e, cytoplasmic estrogen receptor; $R_c^e \cdot E$, nuclear receptor-estrogen complex; P, progesterone; R_c^p, cytoplasmic progesterone receptor; $R_c^p \cdot P$, cytoplasmic receptor-progesterone complex; $R_n^p \cdot P$, nuclear receptor-progesterone complex.

We conclude that progesterone antagonizes and redirects the ability of uterine cells to respond to estradiol by decreasing the quantity of R_c. This reduction of R_c decreases the number of receptor-estrogen complexes that are translocated and retained in uterine nuclei. Thus, the ability of estrogen to stimulate uterine growth is altered and greatly reduced. These interactions may occur during the estrous cycle of the rat and probably form a basic control mechanism by which the reproductive tract oscillates each cycle. These studies indicate that the traditional measurement of hormone levels in the blood offers an incomplete picture for understanding the action of steroid hormones under various physiologic states. Responsiveness of target organs may vary as the result of changes in receptor concentration, an important variable in the control of reproductive function that can be evaluated only by measurement of tissue levels of hormone receptors.

References

1. Leung, B. S. & G. H. Sasaki. 1973. Biochem. Biophys. Res. Commun. **55:** 1180–1185.
2. Brenner, R. M., J. A. Resko & N. B. West. 1974. Endocrinology **95:** 1094–1099.
3. Mester, J., D. Martel, A. Psychoyos & E.-E. Baulieu. 1974. Nature (London) **250:** 766, 767.
4. Clark, J. H., J. N. Anderson & E. J. Peck, Jr. 1973. Steroids **22:** 707–718.
5. Clark, J. H., J. N. Anderson & E. J. Peck, Jr. 1974. Nature (London) **251:** 446, 447.
6. Hsueh, A. J. W., E. J. Peck & J. H. Clark. 1975. Nature (London) **254:** 337, 338.
7. Milgrom, E., L. Thi, M. Atger & E.-E. Baulieu. 1973. J. Biol. Chem. **248:** 6366–6371.
8. Leavitt, W., D. O. Toft, C. A. Strott & B. W. O'Malley. 1974. Endocrinology **94:** 1041–1047.
9. Anderson, J., J. H. Clark & E. J. Peck, Jr. 1972. Biochem. J. **126:** 561–567.
10. Katzenellenbogen, J. A., H. J. Johnson & K. E. Carlson. 1973. Biochemistry **12:** 4091–4096.
11. Lowry, O. H., N. J. Rosebrough, A. L. Farr & R. J. Randall. 1951. J. Biol. Chem. **193:** 265–269.
12. Burton, K. 1966. Biochem. J. **62:** 315–318.
13. Anderson, J. N., J. H. Clark & E. J. Peck, Jr. 1972. Biochem. Biophys. Res. Commun. **48:** 1460–1468.
14. Anderson, J. N., E. J. Peck, Jr. & J. H. Clark. 1975. Endocrinology **96:** 160–167.
15. Clark, J. H., J. N. Anderson & E. J. Peck, Jr. 1973. Advan. Exp. Med. Biol. **36:** 15.
16. Clark, J. H., J. Anderson & E. J. Peck, Jr. 1973. Science **176:** 528, 529.
17. Hsueh, A. J. W., E. J. Peck, Jr. & J. H. Clark. 1976. Endocrinology **98:** 438.
18. Ishii, D. N. & L. J. Aronow. 1974. Steroid Biochem. **4:** 593–599.
19. Middlebrook, J. L., M. D. Wong, D. N. Ishii & L. Aronow. 1975. Biochemistry **14:** 180–185.
20. Rousseau, G. G., J. D. Baxter, S. J. Higgins & G. M. Tomkins. 1973. J. Mol. Biol. **79:** 593–601.
21. Gorski, J., M. Sarff & J. Clark. 1971. *In* Advances in the Biosciences. G. Raspé, Ed. Vol. 7: 6. Pergamon Press, Vieweg.
22. Cidlowski, J. A. & T. G. Muldoon. 1974. Endocrinology **95:** 1621–1627.
23. Mester, J. & E.-E. Baulieu. 1975. Biochem. J. **146:** 617–623.
24. Oka, T. & R. T. Schimke. 1969. Science **163:** 83, 84.
25. Van Brunt, L. A. 1972. M. S. Thesis. Purdue University. Lafayette, Ind.
26. Hori, T., M. Ide & T. Miyake. 1968. Endocrinol. Japon. **15:** 215–219.
27. Hashimoto, I., D. M. Henricks, L. L. Anderson & R. M. Melampy. 1968. Endocrinology **82:** 333–340.
28. Shaikh, A. A. 1971. Biol. Reprod. **5:** 297–301.
29. Butcher, R. L., W. E. Collins & N. W. Fugo. 1974. Endocrinology **94:** 1704–1711.
30. Brush, M. G., R. W. Taylor & R. J. B. King. 1967. J. Endocrinol. **39:** 599–605.
31. Evans, L. H. & P. Hahnell. 1971. J. Endocrinol. **50:** 209–218.
32. Brenner, R. M., J. A. Resko & N. B. West. 1974. J. Endocrinol. **95:** 1094–1101.
33. Tseng, L. & E. Gurpide. 1975. J. Clin. Endocrinol. Metab. **41:** 402.

Discussion

Dr. C. A. B. Clemetson (*Methodist Hospital of Brooklyn, Brooklyn, N.Y.*): In our studies of the rat uterus, we also observed secretion of water, sodium, and potassium after treatment with estrogens for 3 days. When we give progesterone, we get an immediate and almost total reabsorption of water, sodium, and potassium (Clemetson, C. A. B., U. L. Verma & S. J. DeCarlo. Unpublished results).

Dr. Clark: I agree with you. In the mature animal, if you give progesterone, you immediately see a loss of luminal fluid. Luminal fluid is, however, quite different from the secretory products that progesterone induces.

Dr. Clemetson: I have been studying rats with ligatures on alternate horns.

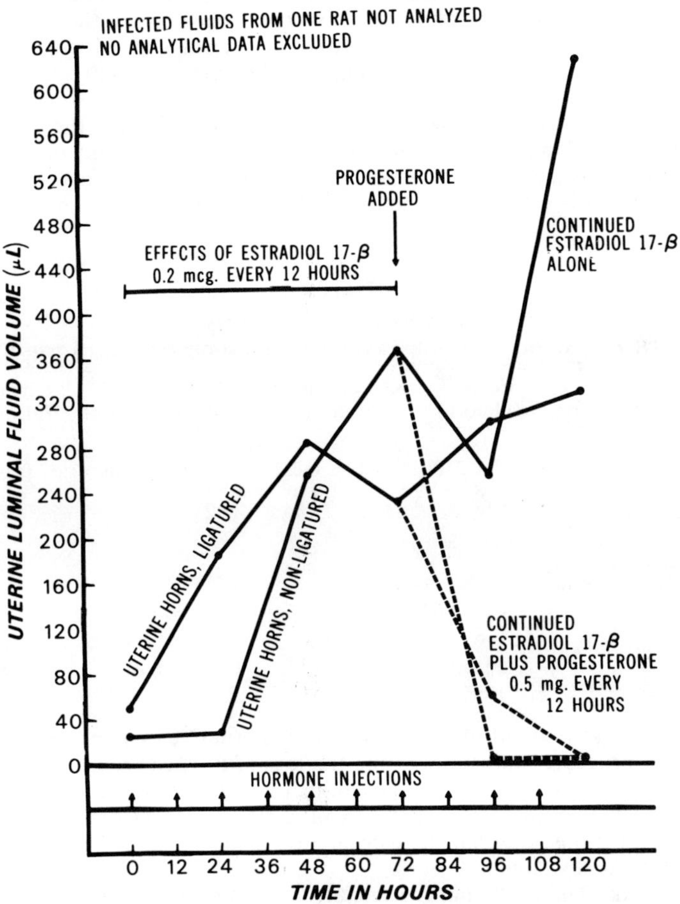

Figure D1. Effects of administration of continued doses of estradiol versus estradiol initially and estradiol plus progesterone thereafter in the rat.

One horn is ligatured top and bottom, and the other horn is not ligatured, so that any fluid that accumulates in the ligatured horn presumably is a secretion from the endometrial cells. This fluid is completely reabsorbed with progesterone; what puzzles me is why I'm getting complete abolition of the estrogen secretory effect and reabsorption by progesterone, while you are getting a partial blocking effect. Our treatment consists of estrogen alone, and we then continue estrogen in one group and add progesterone in the other group. With the continued estrogen plus progesterone, we get total reabsorption of the fluid (FIGURE D1). TABLE D1 shows the total potassium and total sodium per luminal fluid washing in the same experiments. The total sodium value, in nanoequivalents per uterine horn, is 37,000 with estradiol alone in 10 injections, whereas after estradiol treatment, six injections, and treatment with estradiol and progesterone, four injections, there are dramatic decreases in sodium, potassium, and water. I submit that this action is one of the main functions of progesterone in mammals, because it holds the membranes up against the uterine wall. If you didn't have the progesterone, the estrogen secretion would blow the membranes away from the uterine wall. However, I'm still a little puzzled as to why I'm getting complete blocking and you're getting a partial effect.

DR. CLARK: It is well known that progesterone causes the resorption of estrogen-induced luminal fluid. This effect of progesterone is only one of the many possible points of antagonism of estrogen action. Our experiments on response also show dramatic effects on luminal fluid (see FIGURE 8) and do not conflict with your data.

TABLE D1

TOTAL POTASSIUM AND SODIUM VALUES PER LUMINAL WASHING IN EXPERIMENTS WITH ESTRADIOL VERSUS ESTRADIOL PLUS PROGESTERONE IN THE RAT

Hormonal Injection	Volume (μl/horn)	K^+ Concentration (mEquiv/liter)	Total K^+ (nEquiv/horn)	Total Na^+ (nEquiv/horn)
Estradiol, 10 injections	327 ± 210	19 ± 6.23	6590 ± 5460	37,000 ± 21,100
n	8	8	8	8
Estradiol, six injections, then estradiol plus progesterone, four injections	3.4 ± 0.86	25.5 ± 9.76	90 ± 45	354 ± 72
n	8	8	8	8
p	<0.001	ns	<0.01	<0.001

DR. WALTER: I would like to put another alternative explanation to your suggestion that progesterone is increasing the loss of estrogen receptor from the nucleus. With the hormone regimen you're using, somewhere between 6 and 24 hr after you have given the progesterone, you're making the stromal cell go into cell division. Isn't it possible that the estrogen receptor just can't stay in the nucleus that is going into division?

DR. CLARK: The loss from the nucleus could be the result of cell division as you describe. Unfortunately, we have been unable to test this idea.

QUESTION: An injection of progesterone alone does not cause a decrease in the concentration of estrogen receptor. In fact, you get the slight increase.

DR. CLARK: In an estrogen-primed animal?

QUESTION: No, in animals devoid of estrogen.

DR. CLARK: Nonestrogen-primed animals have very low quantities of progesterone receptor. Therefore, no effect on estrogen receptor replenishment should be observed.

QUESTION: Yes, but you still can get an effect.

DR. CLARK: The problem is that you may be doing something totally abnormal and nonphysiologic, because the only time the uterus is exposed to progesterone to any significant degree is after it has been primed with estrogen.

DR. M. LIPPMAN: Have you performed experiments in which you primed the animal with estrogen and then simply either let the estrogen cytoplasmic receptor decay alone or administered progesterone alone, in other words, not estrogen plus progesterone, just progesterone?

DR. CLARK: Yes, we have done this experiment. Progesterone alone will cause a more rapid decrease in the amount of estrogen receptor. This decrease probably occurs because progesterone is more effective in the absence of estrogen.

ESTROGEN AND PROGESTERONE RECEPTORS IN THE FEMALE GENITAL TRACT OF HUMANS AND MONKEYS*

George L. Flickinger, Carlene Elsner, Doreen V. Illingworth, Eberhard K. Muechler, and George Mikhail

Department of Obstetrics and Gynecology
University of Pennsylvania School of Medicine
Philadelphia, Pennsylvania 19104

Studies in laboratory animals have shown that responses of target organs to ovarian hormones are influenced by the levels and intracellular location of specific steroid-binding proteins.[1,2] The cellular content of estrogen and progesterone receptors seems to be primarily regulated by the magnitude and duration of exposure of the tissues to circulating hormones. We have assessed endocrine regulation of human female genital tissues by measuring estrogen and progesterone receptors in different areas of the genital tract during the menstrual cycle, during administration of progestins and estrogens, and in some pathologic states. Other studies were performed on the genital tract of rhesus monkeys. In this primate model, the circulating levels of progesterone and estradiol were controlled by administration of hormones to castrated animals.

Estrogen Receptor

Human Fallopian Tube

The estradiol receptor of the human fallopian tube sediments as an 8S protein on sucrose gradients, and it has an equilibrium dissociation constant of 10^{-9}M.[3] Because the fallopian tube has segmental differences in terms of function and cell composition, the estradiol receptor was measured in the cytosol of the three anatomic portions (Figure 1). During the proliferative phase of the cycle, the ampullary region of the fallopian tube had significantly higher ($p < 0.05$) levels of receptor than did either the infundibulum or isthmus. A similar anatomic distribution of receptor concentration was found during the secretory phase. These differences may be related to variations in the cellular components; the ampulla is rich in endosalpinx, while the isthmus is mostly myosalpinx. In contrast to our findings with human uterine tissues, the levels of receptor in the fallopian tube did not differ between the two phases of the cycle. Fallopian tubes obtained from patients on oral contraceptives had significantly lower ($p < 0.05$) levels of cytosol receptor in the ampulla; in this group, the binding protein concentration did not differ between the anatomic segments.

Robertson *et al.* have recently confirmed the differences in anatomic distribution of the estradiol cytosol receptor of the human fallopian tube. In this study, higher levels of binding protein during the proliferative phase were attributed primarily to receptor in a subcellular organelle fraction.[4] Brenner *et al.* have found

*Supported by National Institutes of Health Grant HD0-6274-05.

that administration of progesterone to estrogen-treated monkeys resulted in a lowering of tubal cytosol receptor.[5]

Five fallopian tubes obtained during the secretory phase were studied for bilateral differences in receptor levels (FIGURE 2). The fimbria of the fallopian tube adjacent to the active corpus luteum had significantly lower ($p < 0.05$) levels of receptor than did the contralateral fimbria. Bilateral differences of receptor levels were not seen in the ampulla or isthmus. This finding suggests that progesterone may have locally suppressed the receptor of the fimbria. A local effect of this nature could influence the function of the tube at the time of ovulation and ovum pickup.

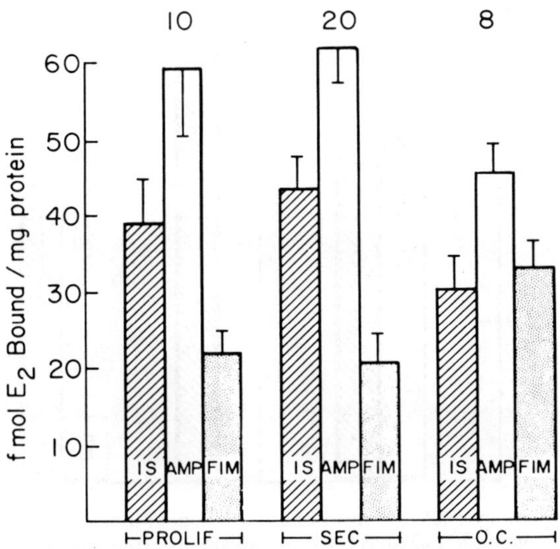

FIGURE 1. Estradiol cytosol receptor of human fallopian tubes. Is, isthmus; amp, ampulla; fim, infundibulum; prolif, proliferative phase; sec, secretory phase; O.C., oral contraceptives. Bars show means ± SEM with *n* above.

Human Endometrium

The endometrium undergoes cellular changes that are known to be caused by the cyclicity of ovarian function. Our studies[6] demonstrated that proliferative endometrium contained significantly higher ($p < 0.05$) levels of cytosol receptor for estradiol than did secretory endometrium (FIGURE 3). Similar findings have also been reported by other investigators.[7,8] Receptor levels in endometrium exposed to oral contraceptives for several months were similar to those of secretory endometrium. In these three groups of patients, similar changes in receptor concentration occurred when the results were based either on cytosol protein or on tissue DNA. Because the protein and DNA contents of the endometrium did not differ during the three hormonal states, it would appear that progestins resulted in a cellular reduction of the estradiol cytosol receptor. Atrophic endometrium from menopausal women contained the lowest levels of receptor per milligram of cytosol protein. When calculated on the basis of DNA, however, the

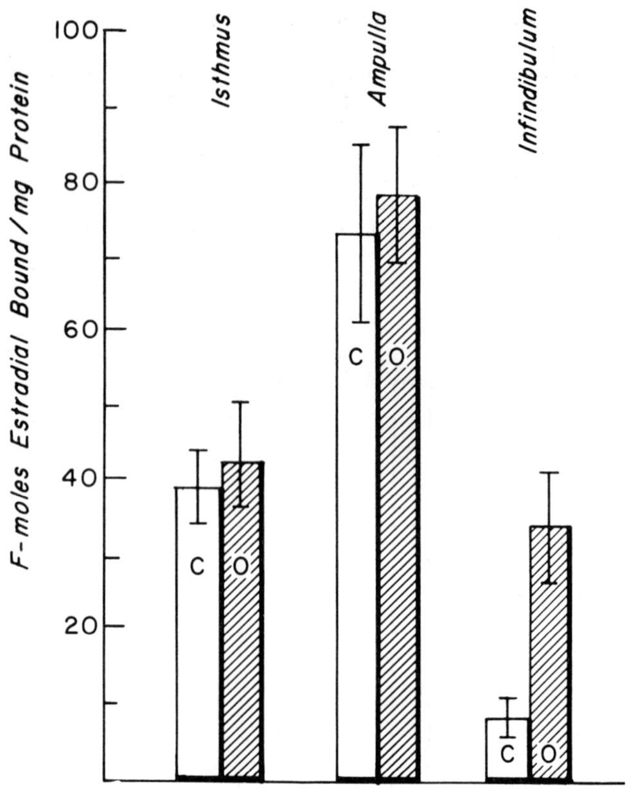

FIGURE 2. Estradiol cytosol receptor of human fallopian tubes during secretory phase of cycle. C, tubal segments ipsilateral to the ovary bearing active corpus luteum; 0, contralateral tissues. Bars show means ± SEM.

amounts of cytosol receptor were similar to those of secretory endometrium. The DNA and protein concentrations of atrophic endometrium were lower than those of proliferative or secretory endometrium. Areas of adenomatous hyperplasia from menopausal patients had amounts of estradiol receptor per milligram of cytosol protein that were significantly lower ($p < 0.05$) than those of the proliferative phase. The receptor level per microgram of DNA showed large variation and did not differ from that of either proliferative or secretory endometrium.

Endometrial Carcinoma

Because some cases of endometrial cancer respond to therapy with progestational agents, it appears that this lesion may be hormonally dependent. The well-established hormonal dependence of breast carcinoma has been associated with the presence of steroid receptors in the cancerous tissue.[9] Several studies have described the levels of estrogen receptor in endometrial lesions.[10–12]

In studies of estradiol receptor in endometrial carcinoma from 18 postmenopausal patients,[6] we found that seven cases had nondetectable levels of cytosol-binding protein (FIGURE 4). None of the patients in this group had received estrogen therapy, and the plasma levels of estrogens (estrone and estradiol) were all below 30 pg/ml, except for one case of a clear-cell adenocarcinoma, in which the plasma estrogen was 60 pg/ml.

The remaining cases could arbitrarily be divided into two categories. Six lesions had levels of estrogen receptor similar to those found in normal secretory endometrium. In this group, one patient had received estrogen therapy for menopausal symptoms. The plasma levels of estrogens were low and ranged from 18 to 30 pg/ml. The remaining five cases of carcinoma had receptor levels similar to those of proliferative endometrium. Two of the patients in this group were on estrogen replacement therapy. With the exception of one, the plasma estrogen levels were high, ranging from 80 to 180 pg/ml. In contrast to other reports,[13,14] there was no correlation of the estrogen receptor levels with the degree of differentiation of the lesions. These findings suggest that measurable amounts of estradiol receptor are present in approximately 60% of the cases of endometrial carcinoma. Higher levels of the receptor appear to be related to estrogen exposure either from therapy or high endogenous plasma estrogens.

In six postmenopausal patients bearing endometrial lesions, a comparison of estradiol receptor concentration was made on two different areas of endometrium (TABLE 1). In patient A, an area of adenomatous hyperplasia in an endometrial polyp was found to have more receptor than did the adjacent atrophic endometrium. Patient B, who was on estrogen therapy, had high levels of receptor in the atrophic endometrium and endometrial polyp. Patient C had low but measurable

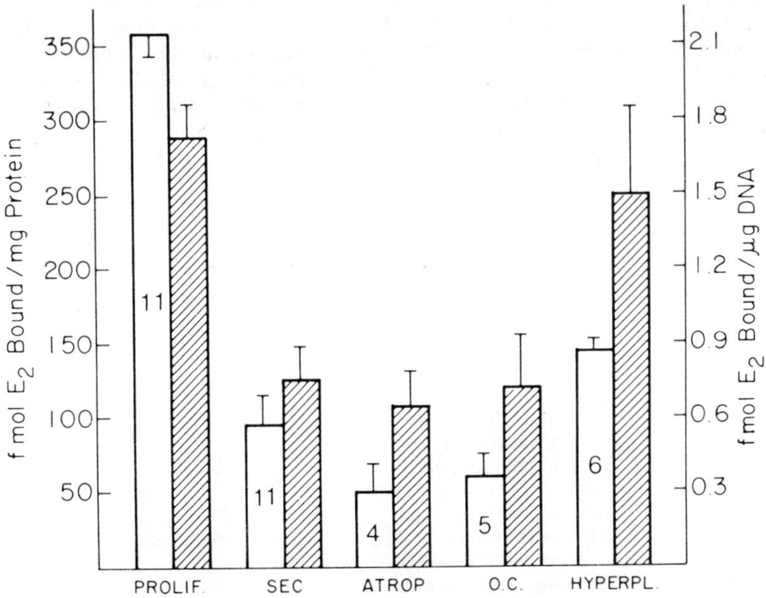

FIGURE 3. Estradiol cytosol receptor of human endometrium. Prolif, proliferative; sec, secretory; atrop, atrophic; O.C., oral contraceptives; hyperpl, hyperplastic. Bars show means ± SEM. Open bar, fmol of estradiol bound/mg of protein; hatched bars, fmol of estradiol bound/μg of DNA.

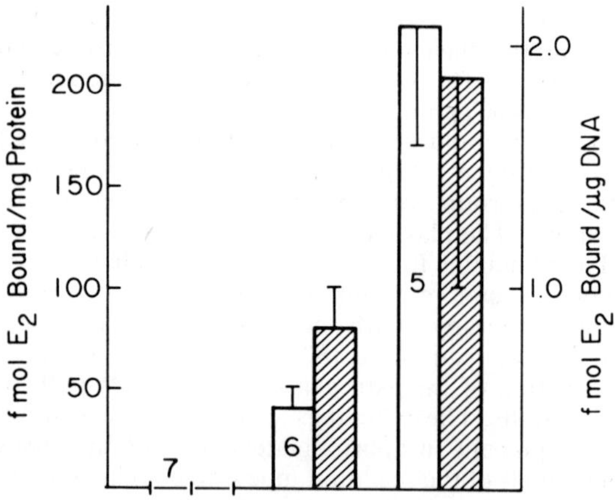

FIGURE 4. Estradiol cytosol receptor in human endometrial carcinoma. For details, see FIGURE 3.

levels of receptor in her atrophic endometrium, whereas receptor was not found in a cancerous lesion. Patients D and E were both on estrogen therapy. In patient D, the endometrial polyp had high levels of estrogen-binding protein, while an area of well-differentiated carcinoma contained much less receptor. An endometrial polyp in patient E contained a high amount of cytosol receptor; the area of carcinoma also had high levels of receptor. Two different areas of moderately well-differentiated carcinoma from patient F were used for measurement of estradiol receptor. In one area, which consisted almost exclusively of glandular malignant cells, receptor was not detectable. In the other area, which consisted of approximately one-third glandular cancer cells and two-thirds stromal cells, very high levels of receptor were detected. These results show that the cellular

TABLE 1

ESTRADIOL RECEPTOR IN DIFFERENT SEGMENTS OF ENDOMETRIUM

Patient	Tissue	Receptor Concentration (fmol/mg of protein)	Receptor Concentration (fmol/µg of DNA)
A	Atrophic endometrium,	48	—
	endometrial polyp	135	—
B*	Atrophic endometrium,	187	0.6
	endometrial polyp	240	1.1
C	Atrophic endometrium,	31	0.8
	endometrial cancer	ND	ND
D*	Endometrial polyp,	140	2.4
	endometrial cancer	32	0.7
E*	Endometrial polyp,	460	1.1
	endometrial cancer	140	1.6
F	Endometrial cancer,	340	2.5
	endometrial cancer	ND	ND

*Estrogen therapy.

response to the same hormonal environment can differ within the endometrium from the same patient.

Estradiol Receptor in the Genital Tract of the Monkey

As a complement to the studies with human tissues, the rhesus monkey has been used as a model to assess the influence of estrogen and progesterone on the distribution of estradiol receptor in the cytoplasm and nuclei of the genital tract.

Fifteen sexually mature rhesus monkeys were ovariectomized 60 days prior to hormone administration. Ten animals received Silastic® capsules that contained estradiol. The plasma level of estradiol reached 80–100 pg/ml on the day after treatment and remained at this concentration throughout the study. Five of these

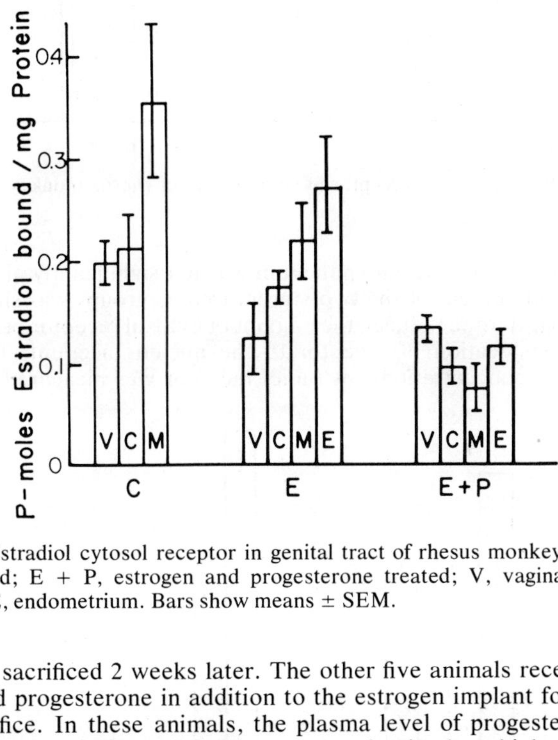

FIGURE 5. Estradiol cytosol receptor in genital tract of rhesus monkey. C, castrate; E, estrogen treated; E + P, estrogen and progesterone treated; V, vagina; C, cervix; M, myometrium; E, endometrium. Bars show means ± SEM.

animals were sacrificed 2 weeks later. The other five animals received a capsule that contained progesterone in addition to the estrogen implant for 1 more week prior to sacrifice. In these animals, the plasma level of progesterone remained constant at a level of 4–5 ng/ml. Five castrated animals, which received empty capsules, served as controls.

The estrogen receptor levels in the cytosol of the vagina, cervix, and myometrium from nontreated animals were similar to those of the animals treated with estrogen (FIGURE 5). The high amount of receptor in the atrophic tissues of castrates was probably a reflection of the low protein content of the tissues. In the estrogen-treated group, the cytosol receptor was present in larger amounts in the endometrium and myometrium than in the vaginal epithelium or cervix. When estrogenized animals received progesterone for 1 week, the cytosol level of receptor was significantly lowered ($p < 0.05$) in the endometrium, myometrium, and

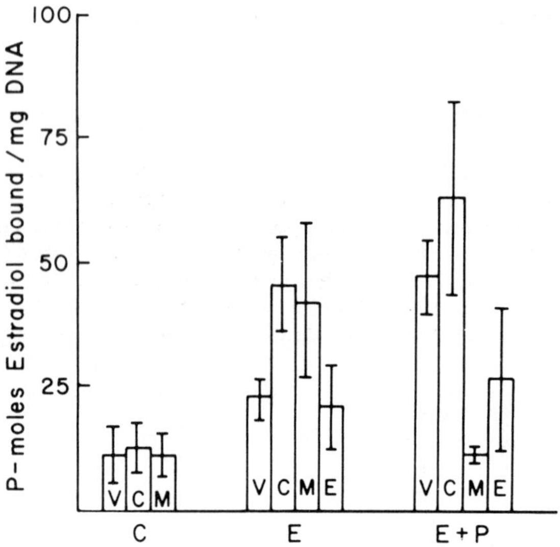

FIGURE 6. Estradiol nuclear receptor in genital tract of rhesus monkey. For details, see FIGURE 5.

cervix. The level in the vaginal epithelium was not significantly altered. Because the tissue protein content of the two steroid-treated groups was similar, it would appear that progesterone reduced the amount of cytosol receptor per cell.

Because translocation of receptor to the nucleus accounts for changes in cytosol receptor concentrations, estradiol receptor was measured in the nuclear

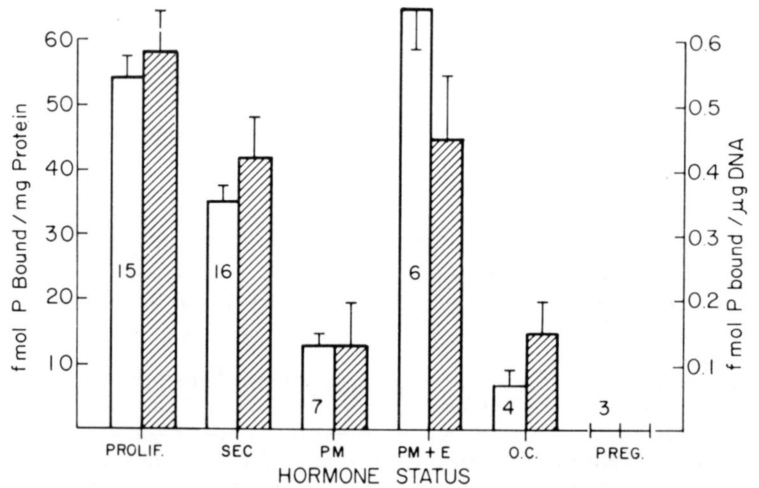

FIGURE 7. Progesterone receptor in human myometrial cytosol. PM, postmenopausal; PM + E, postmenopausal treated with estrogens; Preg, pregnancy. For further details, see FIGURE 3.

fraction of the genital tissues by an exchange assay. In the castrated animals, either very low or nondetectable amounts of binding protein were found associated with the nuclei. Estrogen treatment of the animals resulted in a significant increase ($p < 0.01$) in the nuclear receptor in all tissues. When these animals were further treated with progesterone, the amounts of receptor in the nuclear fraction did not change in the endometrium, vagina, or cervix. In the myometrium, progesterone administration was associated with a significant decrease ($p < 0.05$) of nuclear receptor (FIGURE 6).

Therefore, the lower level of estradiol receptor in the cytosol of the genital tissues can not be attributed to nuclear translocation. It would appear, therefore, that progesterone resulted in a cellular loss of the estrogen-binding protein.

PROGESTERONE RECEPTOR

Human and Monkey Myometrium

Although progesterone receptors have been identified in target organs of several species, including humans,[15–18] the relationship between this binding protein and progesterone's effects is not as well understood as that for the estrogen receptor. In our laboratory, we have characterized a progesterone receptor in

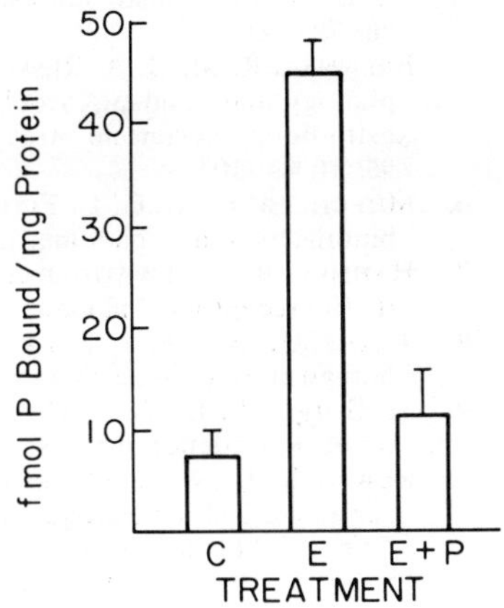

FIGURE 8. Progesterone receptor in monkey myometrial cytosol. For details, see FIGURE 5.

human cytosol and monkey myometrial cytosol that was distinct from circulating corticosteroid-binding globulin.[19] When this receptor was measured in different hormonal states, it appeared that the level of progesterone receptor was regulated in a manner similar to that for the estradiol receptor (FIGURE 7). In tissues exposed predominantly to estrogen during the proliferative phase of the cycle, significantly higher ($p < 0.05$) concentrations of progesterone receptor were found than during the secretory phase. Myometrium obtained from patients taking oral contraceptives had receptor levels lower than those of the secretory phase, and during the second trimester of pregnancy, receptor was not detectable in the myometrial cytosol. The myometrium of postmenopausal patients also had lower levels of binding protein. When such patients were treated for menopausal symptoms with low doses of estrogen, the amounts of progesterone receptor were significantly increased ($p < 0.01$) to levels similar to those found during the proliferative phases.

In the monkey model described above, very low or nondetectable levels of myometrial progesterone receptor were found in the nontreated castrates and in the animals treated with estrogen plus progesterone. The myometrium from monkeys that received only estrogen had significantly higher ($p < 0.05$) concentrations of cytosol receptor (FIGURE 8).

In summary, our findings and those of others have shown that the receptors for ovarian hormones in the primate genital tract seem to be regulated by the hormonal environment of the tissues. This information should provide a basis for further understanding of the pathophysiologic and therapeutic control of reproductive tract functions.

REFERENCES

1. O'MALLEY, B. W. & A. R. MEANS. 1974. Female steroid hormones and target cell nuclei. Science **183:** 610–620.
2. JENSEN, E. V. & E. R. DESOMBRE. 1971. Mechanism of action of the female sex hormones. Annu. Rev. Biochem. **41:** 203–230.
3. FLICKINGER, G. L., E. K. MUECHLER & G. MIKHAIL. 1974. Estradiol receptor in the human fallopian tube. Fertil. Steril. **25:** 900–903.
4. ROBERTSON, D. M., B. M. LANDGREN & R. GUERRERO. 1975. Oestradiol receptor levels in the human fallopian tube during the menstrual cycle. Acta Endocrinol. **80:** 705–718.
5. BRENNER, R. M., J. A. RESKO & N. B. WEST. 1974. Cyclic changes in oviductal morphology and residual cytoplasmic estradiol binding capacity induced by sequential estradiol-progesterone treatment of spayed rhesus monkeys. Endocrinology **95:** 1094–1104.
6. MUECHLER, E. K., G. L. FLICKINGER, C. E. MANGAN & G. MIKHAIL. 1975. Estradiol binding by human endometrial tissue. Gynecol. Oncol. **3:** 244–250.
7. HAHNEL, R., E. TWADDLE & L. BRINDLE. 1974. The influence of enzymes on the estradiol receptors of human uterus and breast carcinoma. Steroids **24:** 489–506.
8. TRAMS, G., B. ENGEL, F. LEHMAN & H. MAASS. 1973. Specific binding of oestradiol in human uterine tissue. Acta Endocrinol. **72:** 351–360.
9. MCGUIRE, W. L., G. C. CHAMNESS, M. E. CASTLOW & R. E. SHEPHERD. 1974. Hormone dependence in breast cancer. Metabolism **23:** 75–100.
10. RUBIN, B. L., S. B. GUSBERG, J. BUTTERLY, T. C. HAN & M. MARALIT. 1972. A screening test for estrogen dependence of endometrial carcinoma. Amer. J. Obstet. Gynecol. **114:** 660–669.
11. EVANS, L. H., J. D. MARTIN & R. HAHNEL. 1974. Estrogen receptor concentration in normal and pathological human uterine tissue. J. Clin. Endocrinol. Metab. **38:** 23–32.
12. KING, R. J. B., M. G. BRUSH & R. W. TAYLOR. 1973. Estradiol binding in human endometrium. *In* Endometrial Cancer. M. G. Brush, R. W. Taylor & D. Williams, Eds.: 165. Heinmann. London, England.
13. HENDERSON, S. R. & D. S. SCHALCH. 1972. Estrogen receptors in the human uterus. Amer. J. Obstet. Gynecol. **112:** 762–771.
14. TERENIUS, L., A. LINDELL & B. H. PERSSON. 1971. Binding of estradiol-17β to human cancer tissue of the female genital tract. Cancer Res. **31:** 1895–1898.
15. WIEST, W. G. & B. R. RAO. 1971. Progesterone binding proteins in rabbit uterus and human endometrium. *In* Advances in the Biosciences. G. Raspé, Ed.: 251. Pergamon Press, Vieweg.
16. VERMA, V. & K. R. LAUMAS. 1973. In vitro binding of progesterone to receptors in the human endometrium and the myometrium. Biochim. Biophys. Acta **317:** 403–419.
17. KONTULA, K., O. JANNE, T. LUUKKAINEN & R. VIHKO. 1973. Progesterone binding

protein in human myometrium. Ligand specificity and some physicochemical characteristics. Biochim. Biophys. Acta **328:** 145–153.
18. YOUNG, P. C. M. & R. E. CLEARY. 1974. Characterization and properties of progesterone binding, components in human endometrium. J. Clin. Endocrinol. Metab. **39:** 425–439.
19. ILLINGWORTH, D. V., G. P. WOOD, G. L. FLICKINGER & G. MIKHAIL. 1975. Progesterone receptor of the human myometrium. J. Clin. Endocrinol. Metab. **40:** 1001–1008.

DISCUSSION

DR. R. J. B. KING: Was there any relationship of your estrogen or progesterone receptors in carcinoma to the histologic picture?

DR. FLICKINGER: There was no relationship between the degree of differentiation of the tissue and the amount of receptor found in the lesions. Examples of well-differentiated and highly undifferentiated tumors were found with detectable, secretory phase levels and with high levels of estrogen receptor.

ESTRADIOL RECEPTOR AND 17β-DEHYDROGENASE IN NORMAL AND ABNORMAL HUMAN ENDOMETRIUM*

Linda Tseng,† Saul B. Gusberg, and Erlio Gurpide

Departments of Obstetrics and Gynecology and of Biochemistry
Mount Sinai School of Medicine
New York, New York 10029

Introduction

Previously reported work performed in our laboratories has demonstrated that the level of estradiol receptor (E_2R) and the activity of estradiol 17β-dehydrogenase (E_2DH) in human endometrium change during the menstrual cycle.[1-4] Evidence that the progesterone secreted during the luteal phase is responsible for these changes has also been presented.[2,5] Thus, administration of oral Provera® prior to endometrial curettage during the follicular phase of the cycle lowered the levels of E_2R and increased the E_2DH activity, in relation to the values found in proliferative endometrium from untreated patients. Furthermore, induction of E_2DH by progesterone and norgestrel was achieved *in vitro* during 1–3-day incubations of proliferative endometrium.[5]

A reduction of the concentration of E_2R in human endometrium during the luteal phase of the menstrual cycle has been observed by other investigators[6-13] with a variety of methods, some measuring nuclear binding and others only cytoplasmic binding. Involvement of progestins in the reduction of E_2R levels has been recently demonstrated by Brenner *et al.*[14] and by Elsner *et al.*[15] on the genital tract of the rhesus monkey and by Hsueh *et al.*[16] in rat uterus.

The increase of endometrial E_2DH activity during the luteal phase of the menstrual cycle has been confirmed by Pollow *et al.*,[17] who further demonstrated cyclicity of the enzymatic activity in subcellular fractions of the tissue.

The purpose of our more recent work has been to compare the levels of E_2R and E_2DH in normal, hyperplastic, and neoplastic endometrium and to study the control of these levels by estrogens and progestins. It is currently accepted that chronic estrogenic stimulation of the endometrium, in the absence of progesterone, favors the development of endometrial hyperplasia. This concept is supported by the high incidence of this abnormality in perimenopausal women, in patients with estrogen-secreting ovarian tumors, and in subjects who receive exogenous estrogens.[18] It is estimated that a significant fraction of these patients will develop, if untreated, endometrial carcinoma.[19] Studies on the effects of hormones on abnormal endometrium are further justified by reports that indicate that progestins are effective in the treatment of a considerable fraction of patients with endometrial adenocarcinoma.[20,21]

*Supported by National Cancer Institute Grant CA 15648 and by Ford Foundation Grant 680-0798A.

†Present address: Department of Obstetrics and Gynecology, School of Medicine, Health Sciences Center, State University of New York at Stony Brook, Stony Brook, N.Y. 11794.

Estradiol Receptor Levels

Several groups of investigators have measured E_2R levels in endometrial carcinoma by use of a variety of methods that estimate levels of receptor, either available or total, with different degrees of accuracy.[9,12,22,23] The number of specimens in each study is small, and the overall results are still inconclusive. We have attempted to contribute to this pool of information by measuring E_2R by a method that provides an estimation of total number of high-affinity estradiol-binding sites, utilized in our previous studies on normal human endometrium.

The method used to measure E_2R levels involves incubation of slices of endometrial tissue with excess $[^3H]E_2$ at 37°C, isolation and repeated washing of the nuclei to remove the nonspecifically bound $[^3H]E_2$, and measurement of the amounts of labeled hormone and DNA in the final pellet. Concentrations of E_2R are expressed as nanomoles of E_2 per milligram of DNA. This method is based on saturation of available receptor sites, on replacement of endogenous estradiol by the exogenous $[^3H]E_2$, and on translocation of all cytoplasmic estradiol receptors to the nucleus. That saturation of the receptor is achieved with this procedure is indicated by the constancy of E_2R values obtained during incubations of different portions of the same endometrial specimen with $[^3H]E_2$ at various concentrations and for different periods of time (1–3 hr). Table 1 shows that the saturation levels of estrogen receptor complex in the nucleus were not significantly different when either estradiol, ethynylestradiol, or estriol was used in this test. The absence of nonspecifically bound estradiol in the washed nuclei is evident from the total displacement of labeled estradiol during incubations with excess diethylstilbestrol.

Table 1

Measurement of Estrogen Receptors

Experiment*	Compound	Intracellular Concentration (pmol/mg of DNA)	Estradiol Receptor Concentration in Nuclei (pmol/mg of DNA)
1	estradiol	470	3.6
	estradiol	4600	3.4
2	estradiol	81	3.7
	estradiol + diethylstilbestrol (100 ×)	85	0.08
3	estradiol	37	2.5
	estriol	61	2.7
4	estradiol	90	2.9
	ethynylestradiol	1910	3.0
5	estradiol	480	1.6
	estetrol	310	1.1

*In each experiment, a specimen of proliferative endometrium was divided into two portions and incubated with the radioactive steroids for 2 hr at 37°C. Concentrations of labeled steroids in tissue and in washed nuclear pellet were measured as previously described.[1]

Figure 1 shows average values for E_2R in normal endometrium at different phases of the menstrual cycle, in hyperplastic endometrium, and in endometrial adenocarcinoma from postmenopausal patients. It is clear that the concentration of E_2R is not very different in postmenopausal hyperplastic or carcinomatous endometrium and in normal proliferative endometrium.

These results are in general agreement with those reported in the references

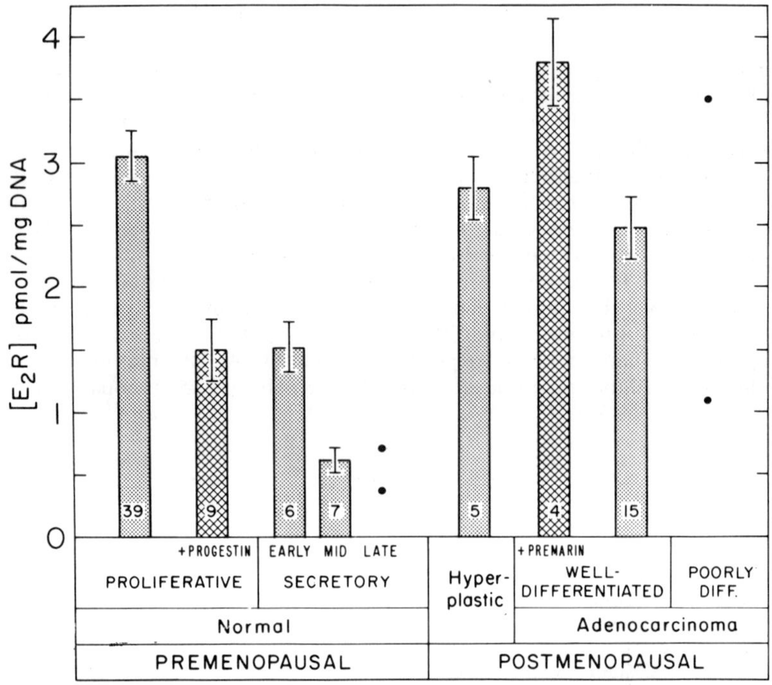

FIGURE 1. Mean values and standard errors of E_2R levels in normal and abnormal endometrium. The number of subjects studied in each group is indicated inside the bars.

given above. The E_2R levels in postmenopausal adenocarcinoma have been found by Pollow *et al.*[12] to be higher in the less differentiated forms. King *et al.*[11] did not see such differences, and one of our poorly differentiated specimens had an E_2R value below the average for well-differentiated adenocarcinoma. Rubin *et al.*,[23] who used a sucrose gradient ultracentrifugation method applied to cytosol preparations, and other investigators[9,22] have found that some specimens of endometrial adenocarcinoma had no detectable receptors. We have also observed that four of the 19 specimens of endometrial carcinoma studied had E_2R levels as low as those found in late secretory endometrium. Due to the small number of subjects in each of the groups studied by different laboratories, the diversity of methodologies applied, the dispersion of values in each group, problems of preservation of receptors, and inhomogeneity of the specimens, it does not seem justified at the moment to propose intrinsic differences in E_2R levels that could characterize endometrial hyperplasia or carcinoma of various degrees of differentiation. Because most of the specimens of abnormal endometrium studied are from postmenopausal patients, not exposed to progestins, it is not surprising, although still interesting, that E_2R levels in these tissues resemble those of normal proliferative endometrium.

FIGURE 1 shows the effects of intake of Premarin® or Provera on E_2R concentrations.

The E_2R levels in well-differentiated adenocarcinoma of patients taking Premarin for prolonged periods of time were higher than those in similar specimens from patients, also postmenopausal, who were not receiving estrogens.

As previously reported,[2] the E_2R levels in proliferative endometrium from patients taking about 30 mg/day of Provera for 2–4 days during the follicular phase were lower than those found in proliferative endometrium of untreated subjects.

Some patients with endometrial adenocarcinoma were treated with oral Provera (about 60 mg/day for 6 days), and E_2R levels were measured in samples of endometrium taken before and after the treatment with progestins. In three of eight patients, a significant reduction in E_2R levels was noted.

Estradiol 17β-Dehydrogenase

The method used to measure this enzymatic activity, described in detail elsewhere,[4] involves incubation of an 800*g* supernatant from tissue homogenates with an excess of $[^3H]E_2$ and NAD and measurement of the tritiated estrone

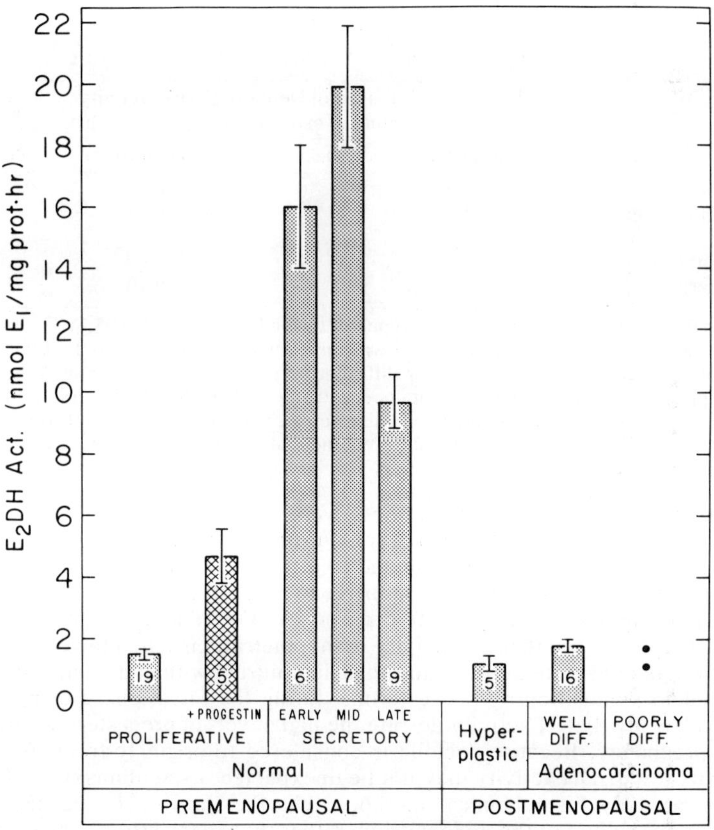

Figure 2. Mean values and standard errors of E_2DH activity in normal and abnormal endometrium. The number of subjects studied in each group is indicated inside the bars.

formed at various times of incubation. The enzymatic activity in the sample is expressed as nanomoles of estrone formed per milligram of protein per hour.

FIGURE 2 shows the levels of E_2DH found in normal endometrium at various phases of the menstrual cycle, in hyperplastic endometrium, and in well-differentiated and poorly differentiated adenocarcinoma specimens from postmenopausal patients. The results obtained with normally cycling patients illustrate the drastic rise in E_2DH activity during the secretory phase and the fact that administration of oral Provera during the follicular phase results in an increase of the activity. The levels of E_2DH in postmenopausal and abnormal endometrium correspond to those in proliferative endometrium, as would be expected from an absence of stimulation of E_2DH by progesterone.

Oral administration of Provera led to an increase in the level of E_2DH in five of eight postmenopausal patients with well-differentiated endometrial adenocarcinoma. The maximum stimulation observed was fourfold, in agreement with the results reported by Pollow *et al.*[24] These results indicate that, at least in some patients, endometrial adenocarcinoma is responsive to progestins. It should be

TABLE 2

ESTRADIOL DEHYDROGENASE ACTIVITY IN VARIOUS TISSUES*

	Estradiol Dehydrogenase Activity (nmol of estrone/mg of protein × hr)			
	Endometrium	Decidua	Myometrium	Placenta
Follicular phase	1.4	—	0.15	—
Midluteal phase	13	—	0.11	—
Pregnancy				
First trimester	—	4	0.09	360
Term	—	—	0.10	340

*The 800*g* supernatant from various types of tissue homogenate [0.05 M Tris buffer (pH 8.0) approximately 0.8 mg of protein/ml] was mixed with NAD^+ (1.4 μmol/ml) and $[^3H]E_2$ (37 nmol/ml) and incubated at 37°C for different periods of time (1–10 min). The reaction was stopped with methanol that contained estrone and estradiol carriers. Estrone was isolated by thin-layer chromatography. The rate of conversion of estradiol to estrone was estimated from five values obtained at different incubation times, as described previously.[4,5]

noted that in these cases, no attempts were made to prime the patients with estrogens before treatment with Provera. Further work is necessary to document the importance of estradiol priming and to attempt to conclude that some of the adenocarcinomas are, indeed, unresponsive to progestins.

TABLE 2 shows, for comparative purposes, E_2DH levels in various human tissues. It can be seen that the activity in myometrium is much lower than that in the corresponding endometrium and that, in contrast with endometrium, it is not subjected to stimulation by progesterone during the luteal phase or pregnancy. Decidua has low E_2DH activity despite the high levels of progesterone circulating during pregnancy. Because decidua is considered to originate from stromal elements, its low E_2DH activity may not be unexpected, as Scublinsky *et al.*[25] have demonstrated by histochemical methods that the enzyme is localized in the glandular epithelium of the endometrium rather than in the stroma. The extremely high E_2DH activity in placenta, both in early pregnancy and at term, is shown in the Table.

TABLE 3

EFFECT OF PLACENTAL ESTRADIOL DEHYDROGENASE ANTISERUM ON ENDOMETRIAL E_2DH ACTIVITY*

Source	E_2DH Activity (nmol/hr) Control	After Incubation with Placental E_2DH Antiserum	Inhibition of E_2DH Activity (%)
Placenta, cytosol $(NH_4)_2SO_4$ precipitate	67	1.5	98
Endometrium, microsomal plus mitochondrial extract $(NH_4)_2SO_4$ precipitate	36	36	0

*Crude preparations of E_2DH from placental cytosol and E_2DH solubilized from microsomal and mitochondrial fractions of endometrium (0.4 mg of protein) were incubated with placental E_2DH antiserum (0.5 mg of protein) in 0.05 ml of 0.05 M Tris buffer that contained 20% of glycerol for 2 days at 4°C. The enzyme was assayed as previously described in the footnote to TABLE 2.

The endometrial E_2DH appears to be different from the placental enzyme. First, their subcellûlar localization is not the same. Whereas in placenta the bulk of the enzyme is found in the cytosol fraction, most of the endometrial E_2DH is membrane bound.[26,27] The placental enzymes can work almost equally well with NAD or NADP, whereas the activity of the endometrial enzyme is much greater when NAD is used. We had an opportunity to compare more directly the placental and endometrial dehydrogenases when Dr. L. Engel and Dr. F. Naftolin kindly supplied to us antiserum from rabbits they had injected with the purified human placental enzyme. As shown in TABLE 3, we used a placental preparation obtained by ammonium sulfate precipitation of the enzyme in the cytosol fraction and an endometrial preparation obtained by ammonium sulfate precipitation of the enzyme solubilized by repeated sonication of microsomal and mitochondrial frac-

TABLE 4

STEROID SPECIFICITY OF INDUCTION OF ENDOMETRIAL E_2DH *in Vitro*

Compound	Induction*
Progesterone	+
17α-Hydroxyprogesterone	+
Medroxyprogesterone	+
Medroxyprogesterone acetate	+
R 5020	+
Norgestrel	+
Norethynodrel	+
Estradiol	−
Testosterone	−
Cortisol	−

*Proliferative endometrium was incubated with each of the steroids listed (1 μg/ml) for 2 days. Plus signs indicate at least onefold increases in E_2DH activity over the control; minus signs indicate no effect on enzymatic activity.

tions suspended in detergent solutions. Aliquots of these preparations, which contained similar enzymatic activities, were incubated with the placental E_2DH antiserum. The antiserum completely neutralized the placental enzyme but did not inhibit the activity of the endometrial E_2DH. It can be concluded from these results that the E_2DH in these two human tissues are immunologically different.

Another important aspect of the study of the endometrial enzyme concerns the steroid specificity of its induction. Previously, we have observed induction of the enzyme *in vitro* during incubations with progesterone. Because 20α-dihydroprogesterone dehydrogenase could be identical to E_2DH, it was important to show that norgestrel was also an inducer of the enzyme, thus eliminating the possibility of substrate induction.[5] We have extended these studies to the examination of other progestational agents and obtained clear responses with all of those tested. As shown in TABLE 4, 17α-hydroxyprogesterone, medroxyprogesterone, Provera, R 5020 (Roussel-UCLAF), and norethynodrel were effective inducers. In contrast, estradiol, testosterone, and cortisol were not. Preliminary results indicate that corticosterone is able to induce the enzyme.

The antiestrogenic effect of progesterone, evident from physiologic observations, such as the decline in mitosis in the glandular epithelium of the endometrium after ovulation, may be related to two of the phenomena described here: reduction in E_2R levels and increase in E_2DH activity. This enzyme accelerates the conversion of estradiol to estrone, a compound that may not be effective per se in altering transcription.[28] Whether any, one, or both of these mechanisms is of crucial physiologic importance is still unclear. Endogenous levels of estradiol in endometrium are lower in the luteal phase, as reported by Guerrero *et al.*[29] It is obvious from the data on endogenous concentration of estradiol in endometrium that the levels of E_2R in the proliferative phase are in excess to the amount of estradiol present in the tissue, but they may become rate limiting during the luteal phase. The lowering of concentrations of estradiol in endometrium, relative to the plasma concentrations of the hormone, is the likely result of its increased metabolism and reduced binding.

Acknowledgments

We are grateful to the physicians of the Department of Obstetrics and Gynecology, particularly Drs. G. Deppe and H. Hagens, for their collaboration in these studies and to Miss Cynthia Namit for skillful technical assistance.

References

1. Tseng, L. & E. Gurpide. 1972. Nuclear concentration of estradiol in superfused slices of human endometrium. Amer. J. Obstet. Gynecol. **114:** 995–1001.
2. Tseng, L. & E. Gurpide. 1975. Effect of progestins on estradiol receptor levels in human endometrium. J. Clin. Endocrinol. Metab. **41:** 402–404.
3. Tseng, L. & E. Gurpide. 1972. Changes in the in vitro metabolism of estradiol during the menstrual cycle. Amer. J. Obstet. Gynecol. **114:** 1002–1011.
4. Tseng, L. & E. Gurpide. 1974. Estradiol and 20α-dihydroprogesterone dehydrogenase activity in human endometrium during the menstrual cycle. Endocrinology **94:** 419–423.
5. Tseng, L. & E. Gurpide. 1975. Induction of human endometrial estradiol dehydrogenase by progestins. Endocrinology **97:** 825–833.

6. BRUSH, M. G., R. W. TAYLOR & R. J. B. KING. 1967. The uptake of [6,7-^{3}H] oestradiol by the normal human reproductive tract. J. Endocrinol. **39:** 599–607.
7. ROBERTSON, D. M., J. MESTER, J. BEILBY, S. J. STEELE & A. E. KELLIE. 1971. The measurement of high affinity oestradiol receptors in human uterine endometrium and myometrium. Acta Endocrinol. **68:** 534–542.
8. LIMPAPHAYOM, K., C. LEE, H. I. JACOBSON & T. H. KING. 1971. Estrogen receptor in human endometrium during the menstrual cycle and early pregnancy. Amer. J. Obstet. Gynecol. **111:** 1064–1067.
9. TRAMS, G., B. ENGEL, F. LEHMAN & H. MAASS. 1973. Specific binding of oestradiol in human uterine tissue. Acta Endocrinol. **72:** 351–360.
10. EVANS, L. H., G. D. MARTIN & R. HÄHNEL. 1974. Estrogen receptor concentration in normal and pathological human uterine tissues. J. Clin. Endocrinol. Metab. **38:** 23–32.
11. CROCKER, S. G., P. J. D. MILTON & R. J. B. KING. 1974. Uptake of [6,7-^{3}H]oestradiol-17β by normal and abnormal human endometrium. J. Endocrinol. **62:** 145–152.
12. POLLOW, K., H. LUBBERT, E. BOQUOI, G. KREUZER & B. POLLOW. 1975. Characterization and comparison of receptors for 17β estradiol and progesterone in human proliferative endometrium and endometrial carcinoma. Endocrinology **96:** 319–328.
13. BAYARD, F., S. DAMILANO, P. ROBEL & E. E. BAULIEU. 1975. Recepteurs de l'oestradiol et de la progesterone dans l'endometre humain au cours du cycle menstruel. Compt. Rend. Acad. Sci. Paris Ser. D **281:** 1341–1344.
14. BRENNER, R. M., J. A. RESKO & N. B. WEST. 1974. Cyclic changes in oviductal morphology and residual cytoplasmic estradiol binding capacity induced by sequential estradiol-progesterone treatment of spayed rhesus monkeys. Endocrinology **95:** 1094–1104.
15. ELSNER, C. W., D. V. ILLINGWORTH, K. DE LA CRUZ, G. L. FLICKINGER & G. MIKHAIL. 1975. Estradiol receptors in the genital tract of rhesus monkeys. Abs. 22nd Meet. Soc. Gynecol. Invest. **6:** 22.
16. HSUEH, A. J., E. J. PECK & J. H. CLARK. 1975. Progesterone antagonism of the oestrogen receptor and oestrogen-induced uterine growth. Nature (London) **254:** 337–339.
17. POLLOW, K., H. LUBBERT, E. BOQUOI, G. KREUZER, R. JESKE & B. POLLOW. 1975. Studies on 17β-hydroxysteroid dehydrogenase in human endometrium and endometrial carcinoma. Acta Endocrinol. **79:** 134–145.
18. GUSBERG, S. B. 1967. Hormone-dependence of endometrial cancer. Obstet. Gynecol. **30:** 287–293.
19. GUSBERG, S. B. & A. L. KAPLAN. 1963. Precursors of corpus cancer IV: Adenomatous hyperplasia as stage 0 carcinoma of the endometrium. Amer. J. Obstet. Gynecol. **87:** 662–678.
20. KELLY, R. M. & W. H. BAKER. 1965. The role of progesterone in human endometrial cancer. Cancer Res. **25:** 1190–1192.
21. REIFENSTEIN, E. C., JR. 1974. The treatment of advanced endometrial cancer with hydroxyprogesterone caproate. Gynecol. Oncol. **2:** 377–414.
22. TERENIUS, L., A. LINDELL & B. H. PERSSON. 1971. Binding of estradiol-17β to human cancer tissue of the female genital tract. Cancer Res. **31:** 1895–1898.
23. RUBIN, B., S. B. GUSBERG, J. BUTTERLY, T. C. HAN & M. MARALIT. 1972. A screening test for estrogen dependence of endometrial carcinoma. Amer. J. Obstet. Gynecol. **114:** 660–669.
24. POLLOW, K., E. BOQUOI, H. LUBBERT & B. POLLOW. 1975. Effect of gestagen therapy upon 17β-hydroxysteroid dehydrogenase in human endometrial adenocarcinoma. J. Endocrinol. **67:** 131, 132.
25. SCUBLINSKY, A., C. MARIN & E. GURPIDE. 1976. Localization of estradiol 17β dehydrogenase in human endometrium. J. Steroid Biochem. **7:** 745–748.
26. ENGEL, L. L. & E. V. GROMAN. 1974. Human placental 17β-estradiol dehydrogenase; characterization and structural studies. Rec. Progr. Hormone Res. **30:** 139–169.
27. POLLOW, K., H. LUBBERT & B. POLLOW. 1975. On the mitochondrial 17β-hydroxysteroid dehydrogenase from human endometrium and endometrial carci-

noma: characterization and intra-mitochondrial distribution. J. Steroid Biochem. **7:** 45–50.
28. TSENG, L. & E. GURPIDE. 1973. Effect of estrone and progesterone on the nuclear uptake of estradiol by slices of human endometrium. Endocrinology **93:** 245–247.
29. GUERRERO, R. B., M. LANDGREN, R. MONTIEL, Z. CEKAN & E. DICZFALUSY. 1975. Unconjugated steroids in the human endometrium. Contraception **11:** 169–177.

DISCUSSION

DR. G. MIKHAIL: Have you found specimens of endometrial adenocarcinoma with no estradiol receptors?

DR. TSENG: In four of the 15 specimens studied, the estradiol receptor levels were as low as those characteristic of secretory endometrium. The lowest value obtained was 0.5 pmol/mg of DNA.

DR. MIKHAIL: Were the doses of medroxyprogesterone acetate used in your *in vivo* experiments similar to those used for the treatment of endometrial carcinoma?

DR. TSENG: The subjects in our studies were given 60 mg of Provera/day, orally. Usual therapeutic doses (e.g., Bonte *et al., In* Recent Progress in Obstetrics and Gynecology, Excerpta Medica, Amsterdam, 1974) are about 150 mg/day.

HORMONAL CONTROL OF PROGESTERONE RECEPTORS*

M. T. Vu Hai,† F. Logeat,† M. Warembourg,‡ and E. Milgrom†§

†*Research Group on Endocrine Biochemistry and Reproduction (INSERM U135)*
Faculty of Medicine
University of Paris-Sud
94270 Bicêtre, France
‡*Laboratory of Histology*
Faculty of Medicine
59045 Lille Cedex, France

It is now well established, in various models, that the action of a hormone on a target cell is modulated not only by the blood level of the hormone but also by the concentration of receptor in the target cell. Uterine progesterone receptor variations under hormonal stimuli were one of the first known examples of such regulation. This paper will describe the mechanisms by which estrogen and progesterone itself control progesterone receptor concentration. The variations of receptor concentration and of its intracellular compartmentalization during the estrous cycle and pregnancy will also be discussed.

Uterine Progesterone Receptor Concentration Is under the Control of Estrogen and Progesterone [1-10]

When guinea pigs are ovariectomized at diestrus, during the following weeks they maintain a low and stable level of progesterone receptors. This situation enables the use of such animals for the study of receptor hormonal control.[5] A single injection of estradiol was administered at time 0 (Figure 1). During the first day, the concentration of receptor rose progressively and attained eightfold higher values. Then, a slow decrease (half-life of 5 days) was observed during the following days. Only the concentration of receptor varied; no differences were observed in affinity for the hormone. However, sedimentation properties of the receptor also changed. After an initial increase in the light form (4.5S), the heavier form (6.7S) became largely predominant 1 or 3 days after estradiol administration. It then decreased faster than did the 4.5S form: 7 days after estrogen injection, equal amounts of both forms were present. The physiologic significance of these variations, also observed during the estrous cycle, is not understood.

The effect of estradiol can be abolished when protein or RNA synthesis inhibitors are injected at the same time (Figure 2), which suggests that receptor (or an hypothetical activator of receptor) is synthesized under the effect of estrogen. When the inhibitors are injected 1 day or more after estradiol, there is no decrease in receptor concentration. This finding probably means that receptor synthesis has become negligible at this time. Thus, the decrease in receptor that begins 1 day

*Supported by INSERM Grant 25.75.48, the National Center of Scientific Research (CNRS), and the Foundation for French Medical Research (FRMF).

§Correspondence should be addressed to this author.

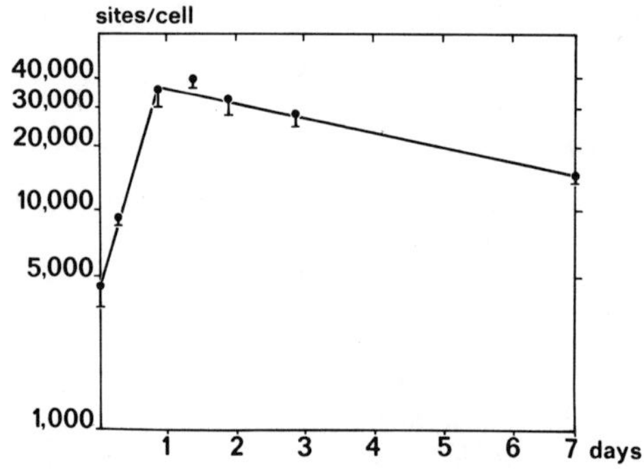

FIGURE 1. Effect of estradiol on progesterone receptor concentration in guinea pig uterus. Mature guinea pigs were castrated at diestrus. Two weeks later, they were injected (at time 0) with estradiol (10 μg/100 g). Cellular concentration of receptor was calculated on the basis of 5.9 pg of DNA per cell.

after estradiol injection probably reflects its turnover, and in this respect, the receptor is a stable molecule (half-life of about 5 days).

Progesterone was administered 1 day after estradiol. One, 2, and 6 days later, progesterone receptor concentration was measured. It was verified that the amounts of hormone still present at this time in the uteri were too low to interfere with the accurate measurement of progesterone receptor. Under the influence of progesterone, a very marked decrease in its receptor concentration was observed (FIGURE 3). This decrease could not be ascribed to an inhibition of receptor synthesis, because the latter has been shown to be negligible at this time. Therefore, progesterone probably exerts its effect through an enhancement of receptor inactivation rate, although the mechanism of this inactivation is not known. Protein synthesis inhibitors could not abolish the effect of progesterone. Because the nuclear receptor is markedly less stable than is the cytosol receptor,[5] it is possible that progesterone enhances receptor inactivation by promoting its translocation to the nucleus. It may thus be considered that there is an autolimitation of

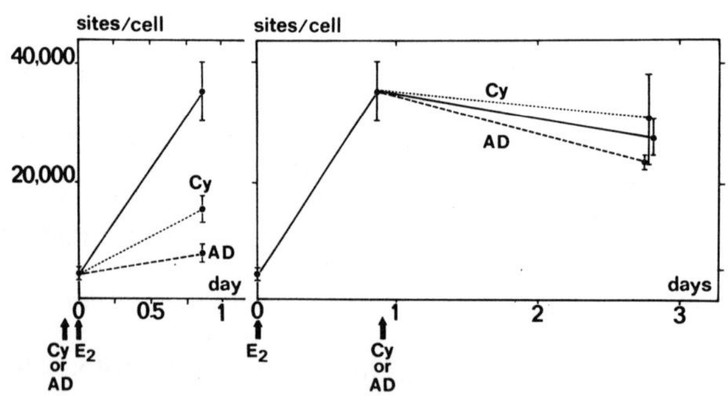

FIGURE 2. RNA and protein synthesis inhibitors and effect of estrogen on progesterone receptors. Conditions were the same as in FIGURE 1. Cycloheximide (400 μg/100 g) or actinomycin D (200 μg/100 g) was injected either 15 min before estradiol or 20.5 hr after estradiol.

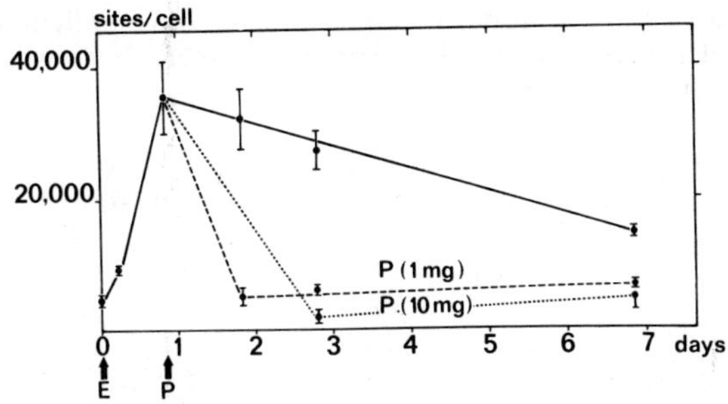

FIGURE 3. Effect of progesterone on uterine progesterone receptor concentration. Animals received estradiol (10 μg/100 g) at time 0 and progesterone (1 or 10 mg/animal) at 20.5 hr.

progesterone action, because as it exerts its biologic effect, the hormone decreases the concentration of its own receptor.[11]

VARIATIONS OF PROGESTERONE RECEPTORS DURING THE ESTROUS CYCLE

In the Guinea Pig

An exchange method was devised[12] that allowed measurement of the total concentration (hormone bound or free) of cytosol receptor in guinea pig uterus. It was observed[13] that the affinity constant of receptor for progesterone did not change during the estrous cycle. There were, however, marked variations in binding site concentration (FIGURE 4). Receptor peaked at proestrus (~40,000 binding sites per cell) and decreased rapidly during estrus and postestrus to attain 16-fold lower values at diestrus. In parallel, sedimentation coefficient variations were observed: heavy receptor (6.7S) was present at proestrus, and an equal mixture of heavy (6.7S) and light (4.5S) receptor was detected at estrus, whereas 4.5S receptor predominated at postestrus and was the only species detected at diestrus.

In the Rat

In the experiments reported above, only cytosol receptors were measured. Even if various experiments (castration of animals, distribution of radioactive hor-

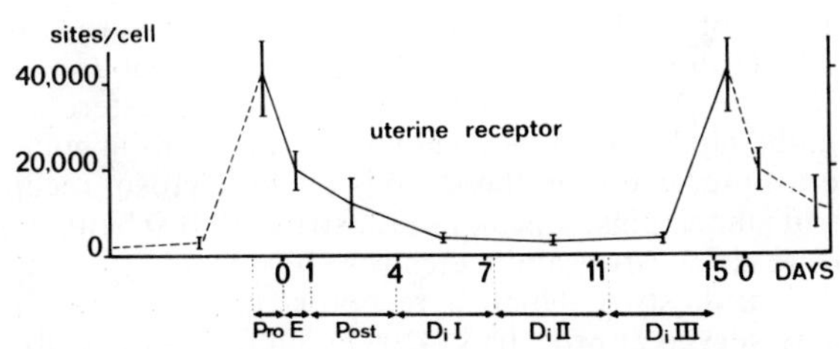

FIGURE 4. Variations of cytosol progesterone receptor during the estrous cycle in guinea pig uterus. Total receptor (hormone bound and free) was measured in the cytosol.[12,13]

mone after injection at different periods of the cycle) have indicated that the total cellular content of receptor varied in a similar manner, there was no direct evidence for this result. To solve this problem, we have recently devised a technique that permits measurement of receptor in both nuclei and cytosol of rat uterus. This method is based on the use of R 5020 (17,21-dimethyl-19-norpregna-4,9-diene-3,-20-dione), a synthetic progestational agent that has been shown by Philibert and Raynaud[14] to have a high affinity for progesterone receptor and not to be bound by corticosteroid-binding globulin (CBG). The details of the exchange techniques and of the appropriate controls will be published elsewhere.[17] In brief, endogenous hormone is removed from the cytosol by dextran-coated charcoal under conditions that have been shown not to harm the receptor. [^{3}H]R 5020 is then added to

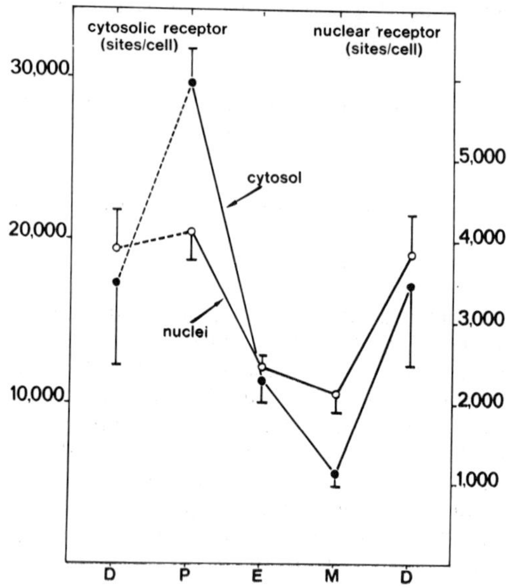

FIGURE 5. Variations of cytosol and nuclear progesterone receptors during the estrous cycle in the rat uterus. Total receptor (hormone bound and free) was measured in the cytosol and the nuclei. Cellular concentration of receptor was calculated on the basis of 6.5 pg of DNA per cell.

the cytosol, and receptor-[^{3}H]R 5020 complexes are measured. In the nuclei, a 6-hr incubation at 0°C allows complete exchange of endogenous progesterone with added [^{3}H]R 5020, and thus it is possible to measure progesterone-receptor complexes present in the nuclei. FIGURE 5 shows the variations in nuclear and cytosol receptors in the rat uterus during the estrous cycle. Cytosol receptors show the same pattern as in guinea pigs: a peak at proestrus (30,000 binding sites per cell), followed by a decrease at estrus and metestrus (5600 binding sites per cell), and an increase beginning at diestrus. Nuclear receptors have a very similar pattern: a maximum is also observed at proestrus (4100 binding sites per cell). However, the highest nuclear to cytosol receptor ratio is seen at metestrus. This ratio is very low in the rat in all physiologic situations, including pregnancy. This phenomenon is perhaps related to the strikingly low affinity of receptor for its physiologic ligand (K_d for progesterone ~10 nM), as compared to that of other receptors in other target organs. The concentration of nuclear receptor depends, as expected, on both the concentration of cytosol receptor and on plasma progesterone concentration. A correlation coefficient, r, of 0.78 was obtained when comparing nuclear receptor concentration with the product of cytosol receptor concentration times the plasma progesterone concentration.

Autoradiographic Studies

All of the experiments reported above measured the concentration of receptor in total uteri. However, because this organ contains many different cell types, one could ask if the observed receptor variations were due to molecular changes in individual cells or to cell population variations. We have isolated endometrial and myometrial parts of guinea pig uterus and have shown that although some differences could be observed, the overall mechanisms that control receptor concentration were identical.[10] However, because these tissues are still very heterogeneous, autoradiographic studies were undertaken to obtain a clear answer. Guinea pigs were injected with [^{3}H]progesterone at various periods of the estrous cycle, and autoradiograms of uterine horns, cervix, and vagina were obtained. Previous studies[15,16] have shown that the labeling observed has the characteristics of hormone interaction with receptor: saturability (abolished by excess unlabeled progesterone), hormone specificity (not inhibited by excess unlabeled cortisol), tissue specificity (absence in nontarget organs), and nuclear localization.

A very dense labeling was observed in uterine horns, cervix, and vagina at proestrus and estrus. It decreased at postestrus, and only a few silver grains were observed at diestrus. In all cell types of these three target organs, the same pattern was observed during the cycle. As an example, FIGURE 6 shows labeling variations in the endometrium. Because it could be argued that the decrease in labeling observed at diestrus was due to occupation of receptor sites by endogenous hormone, the following experiment was undertaken. The guinea pigs were ovariectomized at diestrus, and [^{3}H]progesterone was injected 24 hr after castration. This injection did not change the pattern observed (FIGURE 6,d) indicating that the decreased labeling was probably due to a low concentration of intracellular binding sites.

These experiments suggest that similar mechanisms probably regulate progesterone receptor concentration in the various cell types of uterine horn, cervix, and vagina.

VARIATIONS IN PROGESTERONE RECEPTORS DURING PREGNANCY IN THE RAT (FIGURE 7)

Cytosol receptor concentration was very low at the beginning of pregnancy (6000 binding sites per cell at Day 3), especially at the time of implantation, confirming results previously obtained in the guinea pig.[13] This concentration increased progressively during the entire duration of pregnancy, attaining 26,000 binding sites per cell by the 22nd day. In the nucleus, the concentration was also low at the beginning of pregnancy (1200 binding sites per cell at Day 3). It then increased to attain its highest values between Days 9 and 15 (~2600 binding sites

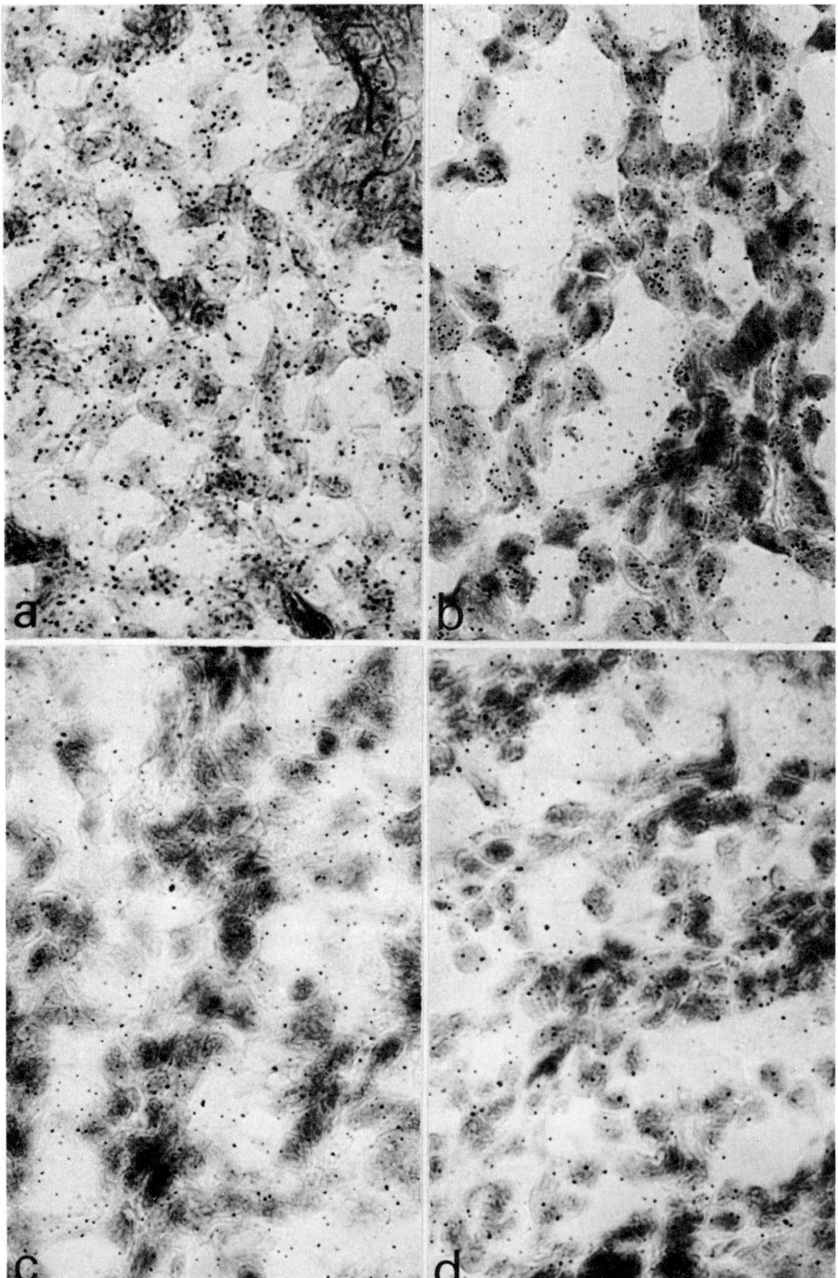

FIGURE 6. Autoradiography of the endometrium (uterine horn) after [^{3}H]progesterone injection in guinea pigs at various periods of the estrous cycle. a, Proestrus; b, estrus; c, diestrus; d, diestrus. [^{3}H]Progesterone was injected 24 hr after ovariectomy. ×530.

per cell). After this plateau, a decrease was observed. On Day 22, the mean concentration was 700 binding sites per cell; however, there were wide individual variations. In some animals, probably on the verge of parturition, no nuclear receptor could be detected.

Discussion

Uterine progesterone receptor concentration is under double hormonal control (estrogen and progesterone). This duality explains receptor concentration variations during the estrous cycle and pregnancy. The concentration of nuclear receptor is controlled by the plasma concentration of progesterone and also by the concentration of cytosol receptor. It is usually assumed that the concentration of

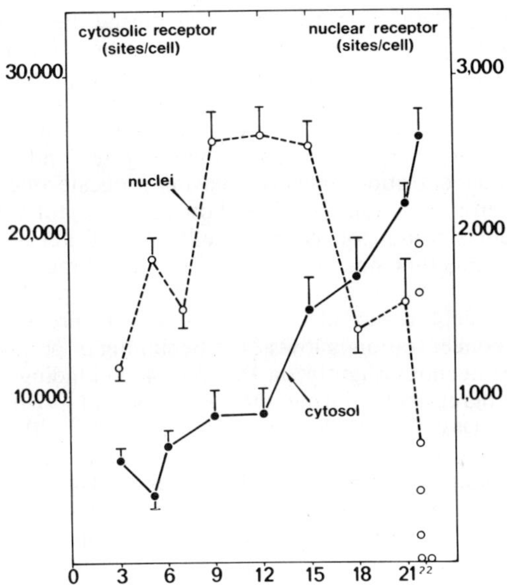

FIGURE 7. Variations of cytosol and nuclear progesterone receptors in the rat uterus during pregnancy. Total receptor was measured in uteri after excision of placentas and fetuses.

nuclear receptor determines the magnitude of the biologic response to the hormone. In this respect, it is not sufficient to consider, as is usually done, only plasma levels of progesterone to determine at which periods of the cycle or pregnancy the hormone exerts its greatest effects. Relatively low hormonal concentrations may determine quantitatively important effects at periods when receptor concentration is high, for instance, at proestrus or during the second half of pregnancy.

It may also be of interest to mention that (as has already been reported for guinea pigs[13]) a low level of progesterone receptor is found at implantation.

The onset of parturition seems to be correlated with the reduction in nuclear receptor concentration. However, this decrease, at least in the rat, is not explained by a lowering of cytosol receptor but by a fall of hormonal concentration in the plasma. It is possible that the increase in cytosol receptor during the second half of pregnancy compensates for the fall in progesterone concentration, thus preventing a premature onset of parturition. It will be interesting to compare the rat with other species (man, for instance) in which no clear-cut decrease in progesterone is observed at the end of pregnancy. The possibility remains that in these species, the "progesterone block" is removed, not by a decrease in hormone but in its receptor concentration.

Summary

Uterine progesterone receptors are under dual hormonal control. Estrogen increases the concentration of receptor through a mechanism that depends on synthesis of both RNA and protein. Progesterone decreases the concentration of its own receptor, probably by enhancing its inactivation rate.

This regulation explains receptor variations during the estrous cycle. In both guinea pig and rat uteri, cytosol receptor concentration is maximal at the preovulatory period and decreases after ovulation. Nuclear receptor was measured in the rat. Its concentration is also maximal at proestrus, but the higher nuclear to cytosol receptor ratio was observed at metestrus. There is a good correlation (r = 0.78) between nuclear receptor concentration, on one hand, and the product of cytosol receptor concentration times the plasma progesterone concentration, on the other hand. Autoradiographic studies show that receptor variations during the estrous cycle occur simultaneously in all cell types of uterine horn, cervix, and vagina, which suggests that similar mechanisms control receptor concentration in all of these cells.

Progesterone receptor was also measured during pregnancy in rat uterus. Cytosol receptor concentration is low at the beginning of pregnancy (~6000 binding sites per cell), declines slightly on Day 5 (~4000 binding sites per cell), and then increases progressively during the remainder of pregnancy to attain its highest value on Day 22 (26,000 binding sites per cell). Nuclear receptor concentration is very low on Day 3 (1200 binding sites per cell), increases slightly on Day 5 (1900 binding sites per cell), decreases on Day 6, and then increases again to attain a plateau between Days 9 and 15 (~2600 binding sites per cell). Thereafter, its concentration begins to decrease rapidly. On Day 22, the mean concentration is very low (700 binding sites per cell); in some animals (probably on the verge of parturition), no nuclear receptor can be detected.

Acknowledgments

We thank J. P. Raynaud and D. Philibert (Roussel UCLAF) for the gift of [^{3}H]R 5020 and J. Fontaine for secretarial assistance.

References

1. Milgrom, E., M. Atger & E.-E. Baulieu. 1970. Progesterone in uterus and plasma. IV—Progesterone receptor(s) in guinea pig uterus cytosol. Steroids **16:** 741–754.
2. Leavitt, W. W. & G. C. Blaha. 1972. An estrogen-stimulated, progesterone-binding system in the hamster uterus and vagina. Steroids **19:** 263–274.
3. Rao, B. R., W. G. Wiest & W. B. Allen. 1973. Progesterone receptor in rabbit uterus. I—Characterization and estradiol 17β augmentation. Endocrinology **92:** 1229–1240.

4. MILGROM, E., M. LUU THI & E.-E. BAULIEU. 1973. Control mechanisms of steroid hormone *receptors* in the reproductive tract. Acta Endocrinol. Suppl. **180:** 380–403.
5. MILGROM, E., M. LUU THI, M. ATGER & E.-E. BAULIEU. 1973. Mechanisms regulating the concentration and the conformation of progesterone *receptor(s)* in the uterus. J. Biol. Chem. **248:** 6366–6374.
6. LEAVITT, W. W., D. O. TOFT, C. H. STROTT & B. W. O'MALLEY. 1974. A specific progesterone receptor in the hamster uterus: physiological properties and regulation during the estrous cycle. Endocrinology **94:** 1041–1053.
7. FREIFELD, M. L., P. D. FEIL & C. W. BARDIN. 1974. The *in vivo* regulation of the progesterone receptor in guinea pig uterus: dependence on estrogen and progesterone. Steroids **23:** 93–103.
8. ATGER, M., E.-E. BAULIEU & E. MILGROM. 1974. An investigation of progesterone receptors in guinea pig vagina, uterine cervix, mammary glands, pituitary and hypothalamus. Endocrinology **94:** 161–167.
9. KONTULA, K., O. JÄNNE, T. LUUKKAINEN & R. VIHKO. 1975. Steroidal regulation of the progesterone receptor in human myometrium. Acta Endocrinol. Suppl. **199:** 215.
10. LUU THI, M., E.-E. BAULIEU & E. MILGROM. 1975. Comparison of the characteristics and of the hormonal control of endometrial and myometrial progesterone receptors. J. Endocrinol. **66:** 349–356.
11. MILGROM, E. 1975. Le paradoxal effet antiprogestatif de la progestérone. Recherche **6:** 877–879.
12. MILGROM, E., M. PERROT, M. ATGER & E.-E. BAULIEU. 1972. Progesterone in uterus and plasma: V—An assay of the progesterone cytosol *receptor* of the guinea pig uterus. Endocrinology **90:** 1064–1070.
13. MILGROM, E., M. ATGER, M. PERROT & E.-E. BAULIEU. 1972. Progesterone in uterus and plasma: VI—Uterine progesterone *receptors* during the estrous cycle and implantation in the guinea pig. Endocrinology **90:** 1071–1078.
14. PHILIBERT, D. & J. P. RAYNAUD. 1973. Progesterone binding in the immature mouse and rat uterus. Steroids **22:** 89–98.
15. WAREMBOURG, M. 1974. Radioautographic study of the guinea pig uterus after injection and incubation with [^{3}H]progesterone. Endocrinology **94:** 665–670.
16. SAR, M. & W. E. STUMPF. 1974. Cellular and subcellular localization of [^{3}H]progesterone or its metabolites in the oviduct, uterus, vagina and liver of the guinea pig. Endocrinology **94:** 1116–1125.
17. VU HAI, M. T. & E. MILGROM. 1976. In preparation.

DISCUSSION

DR. C. W. BARDIN: I know of two published exchange methods for nuclear progesterone receptors, one from Clark's laboratory that uses whole nuclei and one from our laboratory that uses an extraction procedure, followed by exchange. Both of these procedures involve a lot of problems, especially in relation to nonspecific binding, and they are not nearly as satisfactory as the original exchange assay for estradiol.

Could you tell us a little bit more about your assay? Have you overcome some of the problems that we all have faced in this kind of technology?

DR. MILGROM: We have used [^{3}H]R 5020, which has a high affinity for the receptor and which can thus be used at lower concentrations than can progesterone. This diminishes the nonspecific binding. Then, the time of exchange is very important, because if the exchange is prolonged, we have observed that whereas specific binding does not change, nonspecific binding still increases. So we use a 6-hr exchange, which allows us to totally exchange the endogenous hormone in the nuclei but does not give a too important increase in the concentration of nonspecific binding. We have also used albumin for washing the nuclei to decrease the amount of nonspecific binding. With all of these small improvements, we have achieved an exchange assay that seems to be about as good as the estrogen receptor exchange assay, which has been published by Anderson, Clark, and Peck (1974. Biochem. J. **126:** 561).

DR. BARDIN: What percentage of total receptor do you measure? In other words, the problem is exchange versus degradation. Do you have any idea of how much of the endogenous receptor you can measure?

DR. MILGROM: At 0°C in this exchange, there is no degradation of receptor. In the rat, the receptor affinity constant for progesterone is rather low, and you can achieve perfect exchange at 0°C.

DR. J. H. CLARK: We have obtained exactly the same data. We have also learned that at 0°C, these experiments can be performed very beautifully, with no degradation.

DR. W. W. LEAVITT: I would like to compliment you on your very fine studies. We have made similar measurements of progesterone receptor in the golden hamster and have been interested in changes in receptor levels during pseudopregnancy and pregnancy. There is a cytosol receptor in the decidual tissue and a receptor in myometrium that we can follow during pregnancy, and we find a pattern similar to what you are describing in the rat. We have also found a CBG-like material in the tissue, and we feel that it may be involved in the mechanism that stimulates delivery. Would you care to comment on that?

DR. MILGROM: In our assay with R 5020, we do not measure the CBG-like protein. But you are aware that Davis and Ryan (1972. Endocrinology **90:** 507; 1974. **95:** 165) have measured a binding protein in the pregnant rabbit and rat myometrium. I think what they have measured is at least in part CBG-like protein. They have also described variations of this protein in relation to parturition.

COMMENT: We find a great increase in the CBG-like protein in myometrial cytosol at the end of pregnancy. We think that it is an extracellular protein and may, in fact, be plasma CBG. We speculate that perhaps this protein is keeping progesterone out of the target cell or having some effect on the distribution of progesterone within the tissue.

DR. MILGROM: We have some evidence that the CBG-like protein may be intracellular.

DR. T. C. SPELSBERG: Dr. Milgrom, your differing changes in nuclear to cytosol receptor ratios are intriguing. Do you have any comments on why these changes occur, such as a possible masking of nuclear acceptor sites? Is there a possible defective or different type of receptor that has a site in the cell other than the nucleus?

DR. MILGROM: With the data we have obtained so far, we do not find any evidence for such a mechanism. We can totally explain the concentration of the complexes present in the nuclei on the basis of the blood level of progesterone and of the cytosol concentration of receptor. Therefore, receptor obviously increases in the nuclei during the first half of pregnancy due to the fact that there is more and more progesterone in the blood. It decreases thereafter because the concentration of progesterone is decreasing; the fall is less steep than it should be because receptor in the cytosol increases at the same time. So we have no evidence for any mechanism that regulates binding of receptor-steroid complexes at the nuclear level.

DR. SPELSBERG: How about doing some recombination studies with the nuclei and receptor from the pregnant animal?

DR. MILGROM: *In vitro* experiments? We haven't done such studies.

DR. ENGLE: Is there a similar rapid response in human breast cancer tissue to estrogen in terms of an increase in progesterone-binding sites?

DR. MILGROM: I do not see how, from an ethical point of view, this experiment could be done. The only indirect way of obtaining such information is to have many specimens at various periods of the menstrual cycle and determine if there is some kind of statistically significant variation. We have measured the progesterone receptor in human breast cancer, but we don't have enough patients who still have normal cycles to examine for such a correlation.

DR. ENGLE: I asked this question regarding the clinical evaluation of progesterone receptor to determine which patients may respond to endocrine or ablative therapy. Do you suppose that it would be helpful to administer estradiol, for instance, 24 or 48 hr prior to breast biopsy, to stimulate breast progesterone receptor?

DR. MILGROM: I can't answer this question.

DR. W. T. SCHRADER: Dr. Milgrom, I was curious about the work you did on the changes in the apparent molecular structure of the receptor during the estrous cycle. Did you ever take some of the receptor from proestrus and simply dilute it out to the same apparent concentration as in diestrus and run that?

DR. MILGROM: These experiments were performed a few years ago; they were published in *Endocrinology* (**90:** 1071, 1972), and some controls were included. One of the controls was the dilution experiment. With dilution, we observed a decrease in the sedimentation coefficient of the receptor at proestrus, but it never approached the S value observed at diestrus. We have also suspected that there could be some kind of proteolytic activity that would explain the changeover from an 8S to a 4S receptor. We have mixed proestrus and diestrus cytosols, but this mixture did not modify the sedimentation coefficients. So we think that these S variations are true. I don't know what they mean. Perhaps some kind of variation in the concentration of subunits is regulated in a slightly different manner.

REGULATION OF PROGESTERONE RECEPTOR FORMATION BY ESTROGEN ACTION*

Wendell W. Leavitt, Tong J. Chen, and Thomas C. Allen

Department of Physiology
College of Medicine
University of Cincinnati
Cincinnati, Ohio 45267

J. O'Neal Johnston

Merrell National Laboratories
Cincinnati, Ohio 45215

INTRODUCTION

A cytoplasmic progesterone receptor (Rp) protein has been characterized in avian and mammalian reproductive tissues, and there is ample evidence for Rp participation in the mechanism of progesterone action.[1] During the follicular phase of the female reproductive cycle, ovarian estrogen secretion stimulates the uterine progesterone-binding capacity,[2,3] and estrogen priming of the immature or ovariectomized animal augments Rp titers in uterine and vaginal cytosol.[3-6] Thus, estrogen stimulation of Rp formation would seem to provide a basis for the priming effect of estrogen in the preparation of target tissues for subsequent progestational response.

Although Rp has been identified in the reproductive tract, a cytoplasmic receptor has not been detected in other progesterone-sensitive tissues, such as brain and anterior pituitary gland.[6,7] New evidence to be presented in this paper will provide support for the existence of an estrogen-inducible Rp in the pituitary and hypothalamus. Studies of Rp regulation in the uterus and vagina indicate that Rp is produced by estrogen target cells, and binding and biologic activity data demonstrate that estrogen-induced Rp formation is mediated by the estrogen receptor system. Finally, *in vitro* experiments with a uterine strip system establish that Rp formation is controlled by RNA and protein synthesis.

METHODS AND MATERIALS

Animal Preparation

Adult female golden hamsters (Engles Laboratory, Farmersburg, Ind.) were ovariectomized 10 days before use. For *in vivo* experiments, animals were primed by subcutaneous administration of estrogen or antiestrogen for 3 days, and autopsies were performed 24 hr after the last injection of compound. Estradiol, diethylstilbestrol (DES), estrone, and estriol (Sigma) were administered in an oil vehicle (0.3 cm^3/animal). Antiestrogens were suspended in Tween® 80-saline vehicle (3% Tween 80 in 0.15 M NaCl). Cisclomiphene, transclomiphene, Tace®,

*Supported by Population Council Grant M74.113, National Science Foundation Grant PCM 75-16135, and by Merrell National Laboratories.

and MER-25 were obtained from Merrell National Laboratories; nafoxidine (U11,100A) was from Upjohn Co., and CI-628 (CN55,945) was supplied by Parke-Davis Co.

Buffers

Buffer A contained 50 mM Tris-HCl, 1 mM EDTA, and 12 mM thioglycerol (pH 7.5). Buffer B was the same as the above, except for Tris-HCl (10 mM). Glycerol was added to buffers A and B at 10% (v/v) or 30% (v/v) as indicated.

Sucrose-Glycerol Gradient Centrifugation

Linear sucrose-glycerol gradients and cytosol fractions were prepared as previously described.[3] Cytosol fractions, diluted 1/4 (w/v) in buffer A plus 10% glycerol, were labeled with either 2×10^{-8} M [1, 2-^{3}H]progesterone (sp act 48 Ci/mmol) or 5α-[1, 2-^{3}H]dihydroprogesterone (sp act 48 Ci/mmol) before being layered on gradients.[8] After centrifugation in the cold for 19 hr at 202,000*g*, gradients were fractionated from the bottom, and each gradient fraction was treated with 0.5 ml of dextran-charcoal solution (0.5% dextran 70 in buffer B) to remove free or loosely bound [^{3}H]steroid. Receptor-bound radioactivity was measured by scintillation counting, and sedimentation coefficients were estimated by use of bovine serum albumin (BSA) as the standard (4.6S).

Receptor Measurement

Cytosol was diluted with buffer A plus 30% glycerol, and Rp was determined as described elsewhere.[3,8] The same procedure was used for estimation of estrogen receptor (Re) with the following modifications: 17β-[6, 7-^{3}H]estradiol (sp act 45 Ci/mmol) was used as the radioactive ligand, and samples were treated with dextran-charcoal solution for 10 min before counting.

Competition Assay

The competitive binding activity of estrogens and antiestrogens for hamster uterine Re was determined according to the method of Korenman.[9] The molar concentration of competitor needed to reduce specific [^{3}H]estradiol binding by 50% was used to calculate the relative binding affinity (RBA) of each compound. The RBA of estradiol was arbitrarily set at 100.

Incubation System

An *in vitro* system was developed by use of uterine tissue derived from 10-day ovariectomized hamsters.[10,11] Uterine strips were placed in sterile 25-ml flasks, each containing 4 ml of medium 199 (Gibco). Paired flasks contained an equivalent amount (110–120 mg) of tissue from each donor animal. Flask pairs were preincubated with hormone or ethanol vehicle (3 μl/4 ml of medium 199) at 25°C for 1 hr. Then, the strips were rinsed and incubated in hormone-free medium at 37°C

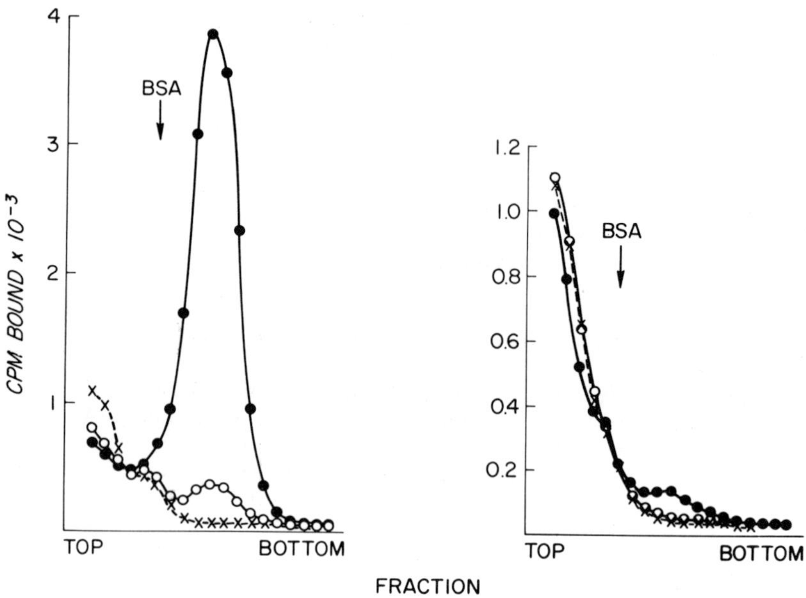

FIGURE 1. Sucrose-glycerol gradient centrifugation of pituitary (left) and hypothalamic (*right*) cytosol. Cytosol was labeled with ([^{3}H]P; ○) or [^{3}H]P plus a 250-fold excess of unlabeled progesterone (×) before centrifugation for 19 hr at 202,000g and at 2°C. Gradient fractions were treated with dextran-coated charcoal to remove free or low-affinity bound [^{3}H]steroid. The sedimentation peak of the BSA standard (4.6S) is indicated by the arrow. A presumptive Rp with a 6S to 7S sedimentation coefficient was resolved in the pituitary but not the hypothalamus of the ovariectomized animal. Estrogen priming caused Rp to increase in both pituitary and hypothalamic cytosols (●).

under an atmosphere of 95% O_2 and 5% CO_2. At the end of incubation, uterine strips were removed, chilled, and the cytosol fraction was prepared. The Rp or Re concentration (pmol/g of tissue) was measured in the cytosol as described above.

Results and Discussion

Pituitary and Hypothalamic Rp

The mechanism of progesterone action in the brain and anterior pituitary remains to be clarified. Although previous studies did not detect Rp in these target tissues,[6,7] we have been able to identify a presumptive Rp macromolecule in hamster pituitary and hypothalamus.

When the cytosol fraction of anterior pituitary tissue from ovariectomized hamsters was subjected to sucrose-glycerol gradient centrifugation, there was evidence of a specific progesterone-binding component with a 6S to 7S sedimentation coefficient (FIGURE 1). However, this component was not detectable in hypothalamic cytosol derived from the ovariectomized animal (FIGURE 1). After estrogen priming (100 μg of estradiol/day for 3 days), pituitary cytosol contained more of this binding component, and a similar substance was resolved in hypothalamic cytosol (FIGURE 1). Labeling of pituitary cytosol with [^{3}H]dihydroprogesterone resulted in less binding than with [^{3}H]progesterone (FIGURE 2), indicating that the 6S to 7S component had a higher binding affinity for progesterone. These results demonstrate the existence of an estrogen-inducible progesterone binder in the pituitary and hypothalamus that has sedimentation and binding properties similar to those previously established for uterine and vaginal Rp.[3,5,8]

Sensitivity of Vaginal and Uterine Rp to Estrogen Action

The temporal pattern of uterine Rp production during estrogen stimulation has been established.[3] In the present study, the responsiveness of two different target organs, uterus and vagina, was evaluated in terms of estradiol-induced Rp formation. Ovariectomized hamsters were primed with different doses of estradiol (0.1, 1, 10, or 100 μg) or oil vehicle (control) for 3 days. In the control preparation, measurable amounts of Rp were present in uterine and vaginal cytosol (FIGURE 3). The control Rp level is referred to as estrogen independent because it is maintained in the absence of ovarian estrogen.[3] The concentration of estrogen-independent Rp in uterus (35 pmol/g of tissue) was four times greater than the vaginal level (8 pmol/g of tissue).

A significant increase in Rp concentration was obtained with 0.1 μg of estradiol per day in both uterus and vagina, and maximal stimulation of estrogen-dependent Rp was achieved with the 1-μg dose in both organs (FIGURE 3). However, the magnitude of the uterine response was fourfold greater than the vaginal response. These results suggested that the magnitude of the estrogen-induced Rp response was related to the estrogen-independent Rp level. Additional support for this idea was provided by the dose-response relationship observed for uterine and vaginal Rp content (FIGURE 4). In the control, uterine Rp content was higher than vaginal Rp content, and estrogen treatment was more effective in raising the uterine Rp content. However, the uterine Rp content relative to vaginal Rp content remained constant in each treatment group (FIGURE 5). When estrogen-induced RP levels were expressed relative to control values (estrogen-independent Rp content), no difference was observed between the relative responses of uterus and vagina (FIGURE 5). These results show that uterus and vagina are equally

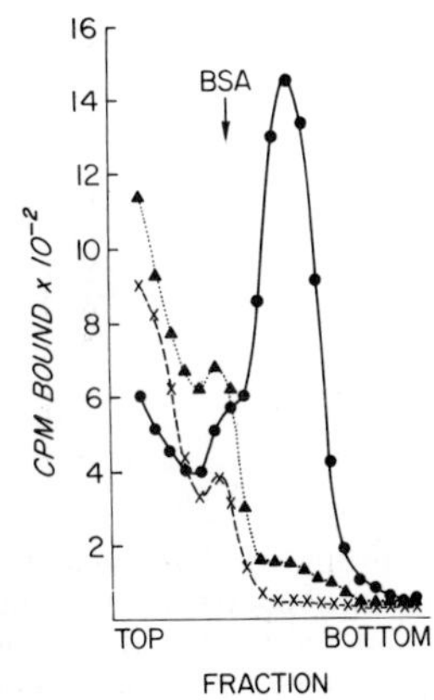

FIGURE 2. Binding specificity of pituitary Rp for progesterone (P) and 5α-dihydroprogesterone (DHP). Pituitary cytosol (estrogen-primed animal) was labeled with [^{3}H]P (●), [^{3}H]DHP (▲), or [^{3}H]P plus a 250-fold excess of unlabeled P (×) before sucrose-glycerol gradient centrifugation. Other conditions were the same as described in FIGURE 1. Pituitary Rp bound [^{3}H]P to a greater extent than [^{3}H]DHP.

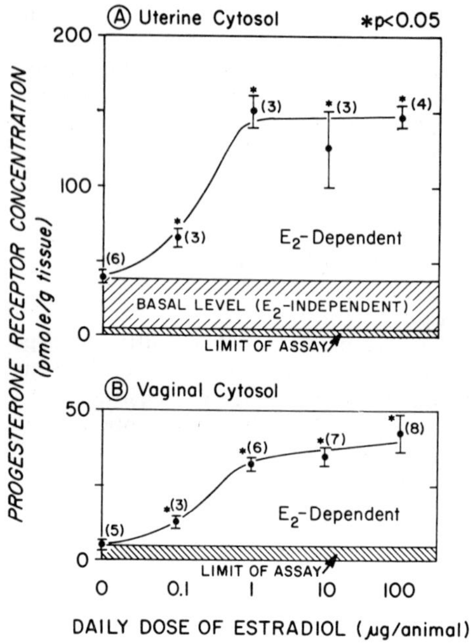

FIGURE 3. Uterine and vaginal Rp concentration in response to estradiol (E_2) action. Ovariectomized animals were primed for 3 days with various doses of E_2 or oil vehicle (control). The control Rp concentration (E_2 independent) was higher in uterus than in vagina, and E_2 treatment increased the uterine Rp level to a higher maximum value as compared to the vaginal Rp level. The limit of the Rp assay is indicated by the hatched area below each curve. Each point represents the mean ± SEM. Significant responses are indicated by the asterisks ($p < 0.05$).

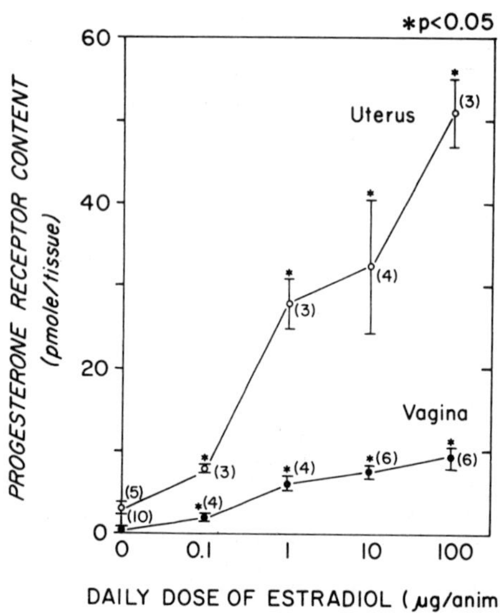

FIGURE 4. Uterine and vaginal Rp content in response to estradiol action. In the ovariectomized control animal, the uterine Rp content was higher than the vaginal Rp content, and estradiol treatment was more effective in raising the uterine Rp content. Each point represents the mean ± SEM. Significant responses are indicated by the asterisks ($p < 0.05$).

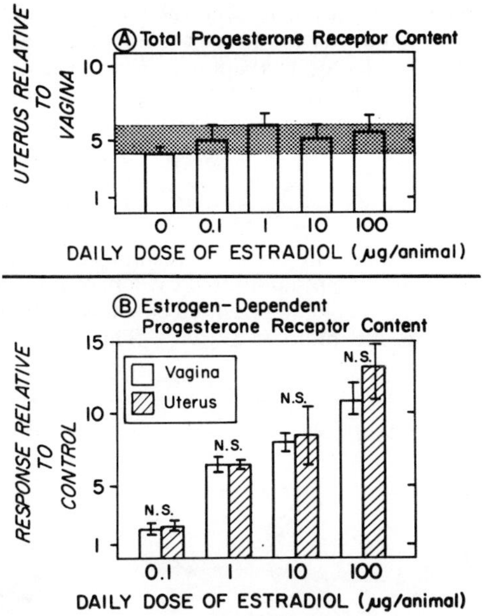

FIGURE 5. Constancy of uterine Rp content relative to vaginal Rp content. A: Uterine Rp content was four to six times higher than vaginal Rp content, and this ratio (shaded area) remained nearly constant in each estradiol treatment. B: The relative estrogen-induced Rp responses of uterus and vagina were not different.

sensitive to estrogen action but that uterus has a greater capacity to produce Rp in response to a given dose of estrogen. On the basis of this evidence, the following hypothesis is proposed. Estrogen-independent Rp (RpI) exists in estrogen target cells, and the RpI concentration is a function of the relative concentration of estrogen target cells. Each target cell has the same sensitivity to estrogen action, and a similar number of Rp molecules is produced per cell in response to estrogen action. According to this hypothesis, the magnitude of estrogen-induced Rp formation would depend primarily on the number of estrogen target cells present

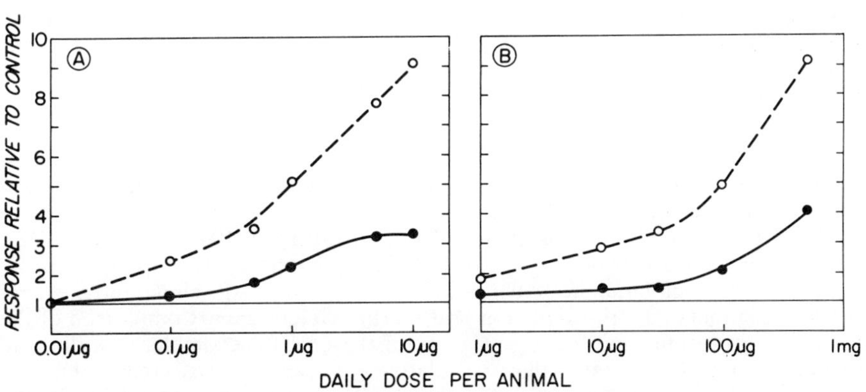

FIGURE 6. Relative uterotrophic and Rp responses induced by estrogens. Estradiol (A) and estriol (B) increased uterine weight (●) three- to fourfold and Rp content (○) eight- to 10-fold. Each point represents the mean of five or more observations.

in each target tissue. The relative concentration of estrogen target cells in uterus and vagina was estimated by measurement of Re concentration in tissue obtained from ovariectomized animals. Comparison of Re titers in uterine cytosol (9 pmol/g of tissue) and vaginal cytosol (3 pmol/g of tissue) verified that uterus had a higher concentration of estrogen target cells.

Activity of Estrogens and Antiestrogens

Although the previous results suggest an involvement of the Re system in the induction of Rp, additional evidence was needed to confirm this hypothesis. Such evidence would be provided by showing that a correlation exists between receptor binding and biologic activity. Thus, different estrogens and antiestrogens were

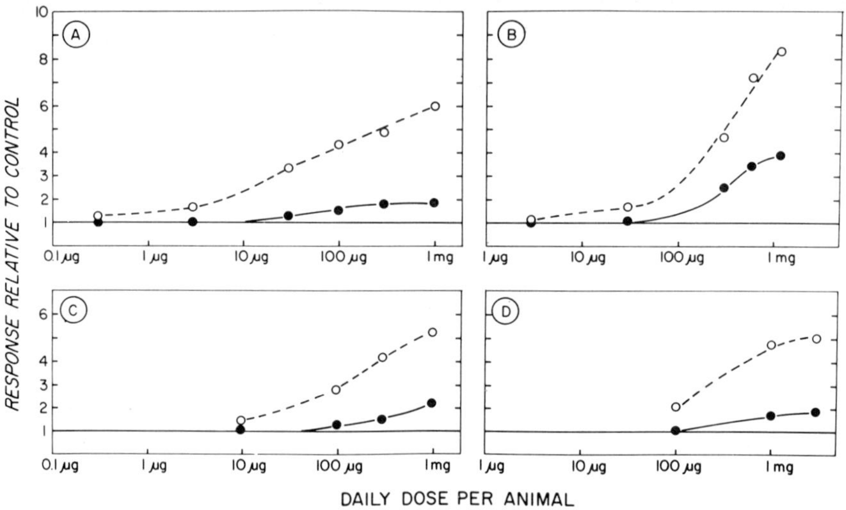

FIGURE 7. Relative uterotrophic and Rp responses induced by antiestrogens. Transclomiphene (B) stimulated uterine weight (●) and Rp content (○) to the same extent as with estrogen (see FIGURE 6). Cisclomiphene (A), nafoxidine (C), and CI-628 (D) increased uterine weight only two-fold and Rp content five- to sixfold.

tested for their ability to promote formation of uterine Rp in the ovariectomized hamster, and the relative binding affinity of each compound for uterine Re was measured by a competitive binding assay.

Hamster uterine Re had the highest RBA for estradiol (100), followed by DES (50), estrone (24), estriol (10), CI-628 (2), cisclomiphene (1), nafoxidine (0.2), Tace (0.1), transclomiphene (0.08), and MER-25 (0.01). All compounds, except MER-25, stimulated Rp production and uterine weight gain. Comparison of the relative uterotrophic and Rp responses for estrogens, for example, estradiol and estriol (FIGURE 6), revealed that the relative Rp response was greater than the relative uterotrophic response in all cases. Similar findings were obtained with the antiestrogens (FIGURE 7). Thus, it can be concluded that the Rp response is a more sensitive end point of estrogen action than is the uterine weight response. With the antiestrogens, it was possible to show that an Rp response could be obtained with doses lower than those needed to significantly increase uterine weight. Transclomiphene produced a full uterotrophic response (400–500 mg), and it increased Rp eight- to ninefold. In contrast, cisclomiphene, nafoxidine, and CI-628 produced incomplete uterine weight responses (200–250 mg), and the Rp response was correspondingly less than that produced by the estrogens.

Correlation of binding and biologic activity data (FIGURE 8) revealed good agreement between the binding affinity for Re and biologic activity (uterotrophic and Rp responses), particularly for estradiol, DES, estrone, cisclomiphene, and nafoxidine. With estriol and CI-628, the binding affinity for Re exceeded biologic activity, and binding activity was lower than biologic activity with transclomiphene and Tace. These discrepancies may be accounted for by various factors such as drug metabolism (e.g., Tace), biologic half-life (e.g., transclomiphene), or nuclear Re retention (e.g., estriol), and additional studies are required to explain the deviations observed.

The present results establish that a variety of estrogenic compounds can stimulate Rp production and provide evidence for the participation of the Re system in the induction of Rp. Several antiestrogens were found to stimulate uterine Rp formation, indicating that these compounds are weak estrogens that possess the ability to increase the target cell responsiveness to progestin action.

Rp Synthesis by Uterine Strips in Vitro

Recent results suggested that estrogen action might increase Rp production by stimulation of RNA and protein synthesis.[10,12] To study Rp synthesis under controlled conditions, an *in vitro* uterine strip system was developed. The rationale for the experimental design was as follows. Uterine tissue was exposed to estradiol during preincubation for 1 hr at 25°C to permit formation of an estradiol-Re complex and translocation of the complex to nuclear acceptor sites.[13] After these steps had been accomplished, hormone was removed from the medium during incubation at 37°C to prevent further activation of nuclear binding sites.

In a time course study performed with control and estradiol-treated uterine strips, it was established that Rp production could be measured with the *in vitro* system (FIGURE 9). The initial Rp concentration in fresh uterine tissue at the time of autopsy was 30 ± 2.1 pmol per gram of tissue, and after 0.5 hr of incubation at 37°C, less than 50% of the initial Rp level was recovered in either control or estrogen-treated strips. Although a substantial amount of Rp appeared to be lost during preparation and preincubation of the strips, Rp levels increased significantly in control strips during incubation from 0.5 to 24 hr (FIGURE 9). Furthermore, Rp production by estradiol-treated strips was significantly enhanced at 6, 12, and 24 hr, as compared to Rp production by control strips.

The responsiveness of the *in vitro* system to estrogen action was evaluated in a dose-response study performed with uterine strips that had been exposed to different doses of estradiol (concentration range, 3×10^{-6} to 3×10^{-12} M) during preincubation at 25°C. Paired tissues (estradiol vs vehicle treatment) were incubated subsequently at 37°C in estrogen-free medium 199 for 24 hr. The estrogen-dependent Rp response was the increment of Rp production observed between paired strips, that is, the difference between estradiol and control treatments, respectively (FIGURE 10). A significant Rp response was obtained with 3×10^{-11} M estradiol, and a maximum Rp response occurred after treatment with 3×10^{-8} M estradiol.

If the estrogen-induced Rp response was mediated by Re, it was reasoned that

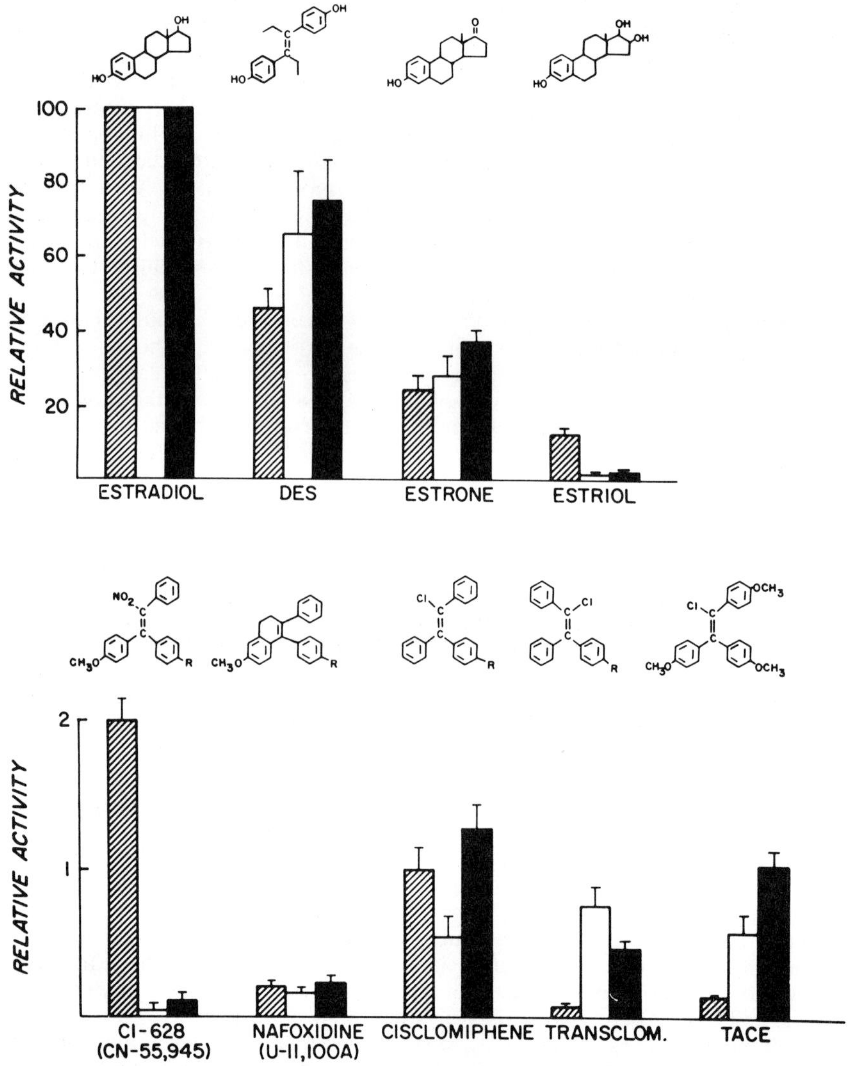

FIGURE 8. Correlation between binding affinity for Re and biologic activity. The binding and biologic activities are expressed on a molar basis relative to the activity of estradiol, which was arbitrarily set at 100. The RBA for hamster uterine Re ( ) was determined by competitive binding assay. Relative uterotrophic activity (□) was calculated from the amount of compound needed to elicit a half-maximal response. The relative Rp induction activity (■) was calculated from the amount of compound required to produce a four-fold increase in Rp content. Each bar represents the mean ± SEM of four or more determinations.

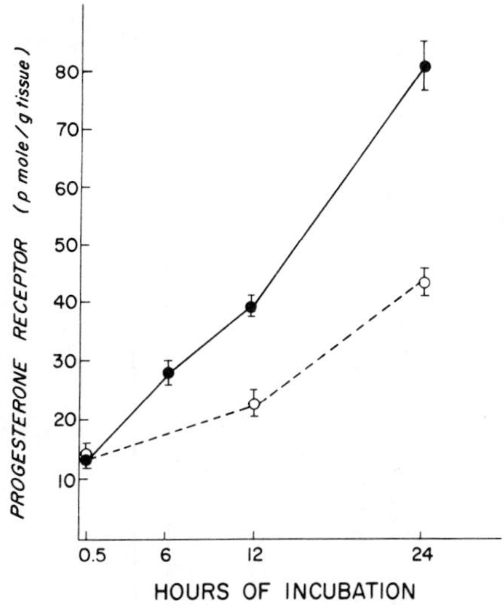

FIGURE 9. Rp production by hamster uterine strips during incubation at 37°C. Control strips (○) were exposed to ethanol vehicle (3 μl/4 ml of medium 199) during preincubation. Estradiol-treated strips (●) were preincubated with 17β-estradiol (3 X 10^{-8} M) for 1 hr at 25°C. Each point represents the mean ± SEM of three or more observations.

the amount of estrogen needed to produce an Rp response should approximate the amount of Re available for binding and that the Rp response should be specific for estrogen. Information bearing on the first point was obtained by measurement of Re in cytosol from untreated uterine strips. Uterine strips before incubation contained 7.1 ± 0.3 pmol of Re per gram of tissue, or about 0.8 pmol of Re per flask. A half-maximal Rp response was achieved with somewhat less than 3 × 10^{-10} M estradiol (1.2 pmol of estradiol/flask; FIGURE 10). Thus, there was reasonable agreement between the dose of estradiol needed for an Rp response and the amount of Re available for binding with hormone. The specificity of the

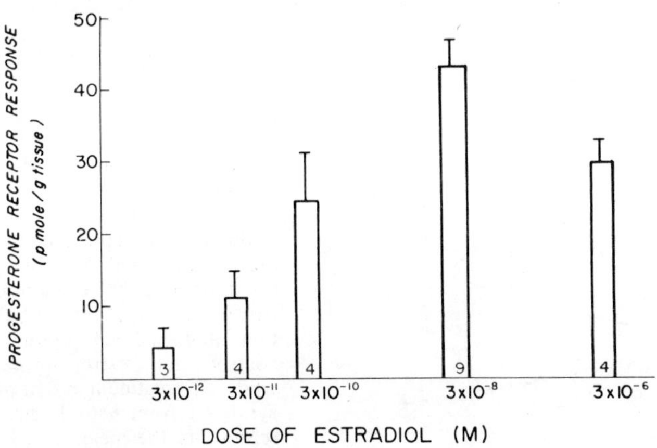

FIGURE 10. Responsiveness of hamster uterine strips to estrogen action *in vitro*. Uterine strips were exposed to different concentrations of estradiol during preincubation. Each bar represents the mean (±SEM) increment of Rp production comparing estradiol-treated (E_2Rx) and control strips at 24 hr of incubation.

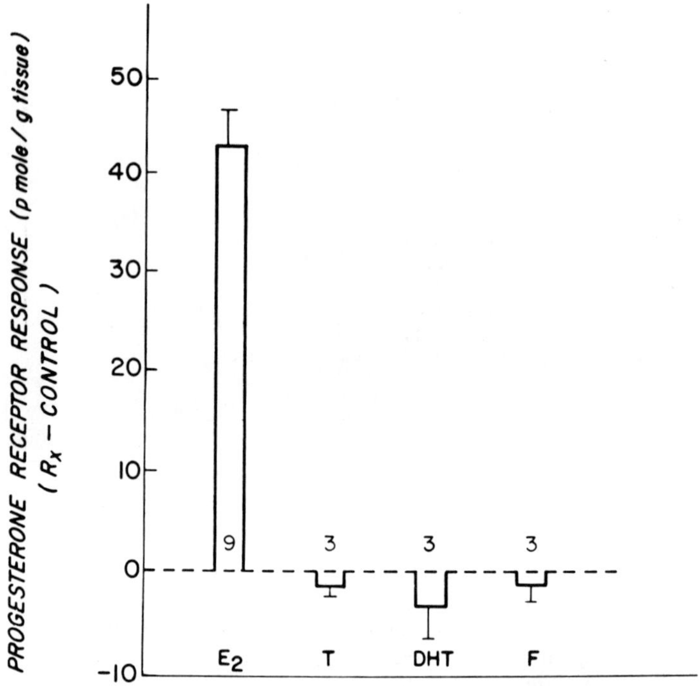

FIGURE 11. Specificity of Rp response to estrogen action *in vitro*. Uterine strips were preincubated with 3×10^{-8} M estradiol (E_2), testosterone (T), 5α-dihydrotestosterone (DHT), or cortisol (F). Each bar represents the mean (±SEM) increment of Rp production comparing hormone-treated and control strips.

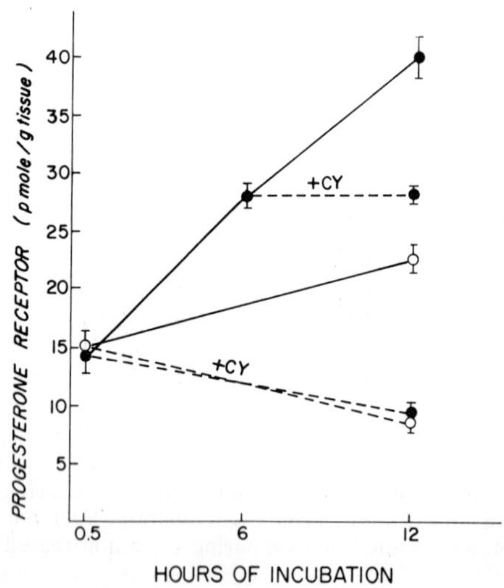

FIGURE 12. Dependence of Rp production on protein synthesis. Control uterine strips (○) were exposed to ethanol vehicle during preincubation. Solid circles represent uterine strips preincubated with 3×10^{-8} M estradiol for 1 hr at 25°C. Cycloheximide (CY) treatment (10 μg/ml; ---) before incubation abolished Rp production in both control and estrogen-treated strips, while CY treatment at 6 hr prevented Rp synthesis from 6 to 12 hr. Each point represents the mean ± S.E.M. of 3 or more observations.

response was evaluated by use of uterine strips exposed to different hormonal steroids (3×10^{-8} M) during preincubation at 25°C. Subsequent incubation of paired strips (hormone vs vehicle) for 24 hr at 37°C in hormone-free medium 199 revealed that Rp synthesis was increased only by estradiol and that Rp production was unaffected by treatment with testosterone, 5α-dihydrotestosterone, or cortisol (FIGURE 11).

The sedimentation properties of Rp produced during incubation of control and estrogen-treated uterine strips were determined. The Rp synthesized by both control and estrogen-treated strips had a 6S to 7S sedimentation coefficient in low-ionic-strength medium. In addition, the size of the Rp peak increased with time of incubation in both groups, and this finding was consistent with the results obtained by measurement of Rp binding capacity (FIGURE 9).

A protein synthesis inhibitor, cycloheximide, was used to study the involvement of protein synthesis in Rp production. The efficacy of cycloheximide inhibition of protein synthesis was evaluated, and 10 μg of cycloheximide per milliliter of medium inhibited protein synthesis by 98%, as measured by [^{14}C]leucine incorporation into trichloroacetic acid-precipitated protein. When uterine strips were exposed to cycloheximide (10 μg/ml) at time 0, Rp synthesis was blocked in both control strips and in estrogen-treated strips when measured after 12 hr of incubation (FIGURE 12). This finding indicated that Rp production was dependent on protein synthesis in both the control and estrogen-stimulated preparations. When estrogen-treated strips were exposed to cycloheximide (10 μg/ml) at 6 hr of incubation, Rp synthesis was inhibited from 6 to 12 hr. Thus, estrogen-stimulated Rp production appears to be dependent on continued protein synthesis throughout the time course of the response.

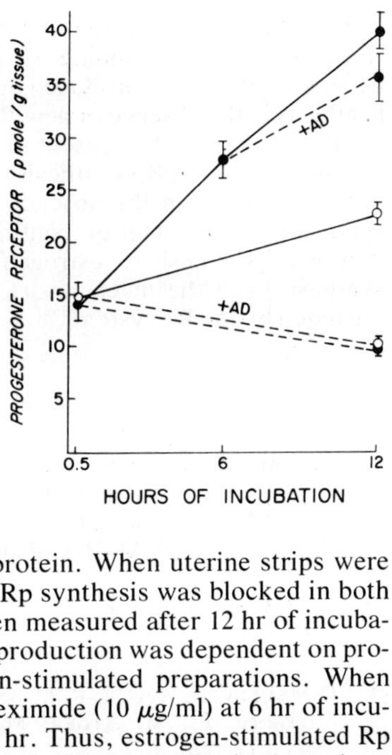

FIGURE 13. Dependence of Rp production on RNA synthesis. Actinomycin D (AD) treatment (10 μg/ml; ---) before incubation blocked Rp production in both control (○) and estrogen-treated (●) uterine strips. However, AD given at 6 hr to estrogen-treated strips failed to inhibit subsequent Rp synthesis. Each point represents the mean ± SEM of three or more observations.

Similar studies were performed with actinomycin D to determine whether Rp synthesis was dependent on RNA. Actinomycin D (10 μg/ml of medium) was found to decrease [^{3}H]uridine incorporation into RNA by 98%. As was the case with cycloheximide, application of actinomycin D (10 μg/ml) at time 0 blocked subsequent Rp production in both control and estrogen-treated strips (FIGURE 13). Thus, Rp synthesis in both preparations appeared to be dependent on nuclear RNA synthesis. However, when estrogen-treated strips were exposed to

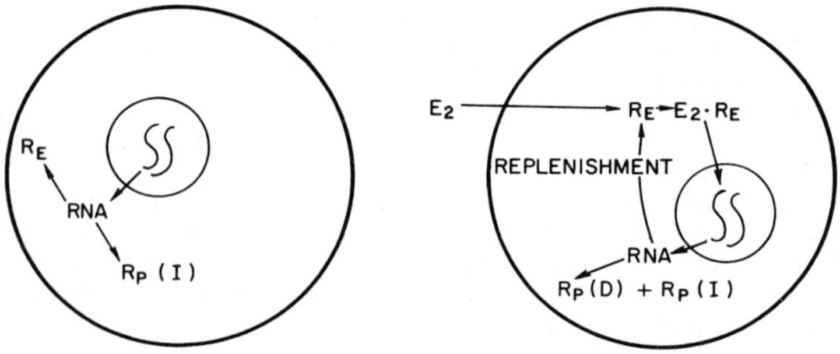

FIGURE 14. Proposed mechanism of Rp synthesis. See text for details. R_E, estrogen receptor; Rp (I), estrogen-independent progesterone receptor; Rp (D), estrogen-dependent progesterone receptor.

actinomycin D at 6 hr, Rp synthesis was not inhibited when measured at 12 hr (FIGURE 13). This finding is interpreted to indicate that enough estrogen-dependent RNA was produced during the first 6 hr of estrogen action to sustain Rp synthesis in the absence of new RNA synthesis from 6 to 12 hr of incubation.

The results of the present *in vivo* and *in vitro* studies are consistent with the following model of Rp synthesis (FIGURE 14). The estrogen target cell is capable of synthesizing Rp in the absence of estrogen support, and this basal level of Rp synthesis is dependent on continued RNA and protein synthesis. The augmentation of Rp synthesis by estrogen action involves stimulation of RNA and protein synthesis, and the mechanism of estrogen-induced Rp synthesis appears to be regulated by the Re system.

ACKNOWLEDGMENTS

We appreciate the excellent technical assistance of Christine M. Eldon, Barbara J. Reuss, and Nancy Roberts. The antiestrogens were generously supplied by Dr. A. L. Richardson, Merrell National Laboratories; Dr. J. C. Babcock, The Upjohn Co.; and Dr. M. R. Callantine, Parke-Davis Co.

REFERENCES

1. O'MALLEY, B. W. & A. R. MEANS. 1974. Science **183:** 610.
2. MILGROM, E., M. ATGER, M. PERROT & E.-E. BAULIEU. 1972. Endocrinology **90:** 1071.
3. LEAVITT, W. W., D. O. TOFT, C. A. STROTT & B. W. O'MALLEY. 1974. Endocrinology **94:** 1041.
4. FEIL, P. D., S. R. GLASSER, D. O. TOFT & B. W. O'MALLEY. 1972. Endocrinology **91:** 738.
5. ALLEN, T. C. & W. W. LEAVITT. 1975. Fed. Proc. **34:** 279.
6. REEL, J. R. & Y. SHIH. 1975. Acta Endocrinol. **80:** 344.
7. ATGER, M., E.-E. BAULIEU & E. MILGROM. 1974. Endocrinology **94:** 161.
8. LEAVITT, W. W. & C. J. GROSSMAN. 1974. Proc. Nat. Acad. Sci. USA **71:** 4341.
9. KORENMAN, S. G. 1970. Endocrinology **87:** 1119.

10. CHEN, T. J. & W. W. LEAVITT. 1975. Physiologist **18:** 166.
11. FABER, L. E., J. SAFFRAN, T. J. CHEN & W. W. LEAVITT. 1976. *In* Steroid Hormone Action and Cancer. K.M.J. Menon & J.R. Reel, Eds.: 68. Plenum Publishing Corporation. New York, N.Y.
12. MILGROM, E., L. THI, M. ATGER & E.-E. BAULIEU. 1973. J. Biol. Chem. **248:** 6366.
13. JENSEN, E. V. & E. R. DESOMBRE. 1973. Science **182:** 126.

DISCUSSION

QUESTION: I'm interested in your results that showed that several antiestrogens were able to stimulate progesterone receptor synthesis. During stimulation of uterine progesterone receptor levels, do the antiestrogens at the same time fail to replenish estradiol receptor?

DR. LEAVITT: Estrogen receptor replenishment was not measured in our studies. However, in studies done with the rat, estrogen receptor replenishment was reduced during antiestrogen action [1973. Clark *et al.*, Steroids **22:** 707; 1974. Nature (London) **251:** 446].

QUESTION: So the antiestrogens are really acting by different mechanisms to prevent replenishment of estrogen receptor and increase progesterone receptor production.

DR. LEAVITT: No, the antiestrogens are not acting by different mechanisms. As shown in my FIGURE 14, estrogen receptor replenishment and progesterone receptor synthesis are different end points of the estrogenic response. The antiestrogens are weak or incomplete agonists (estrogens) that act by the estrogen receptor system to increase progesterone receptor formation. Since these agents do not stimulate estrogen receptor replenishment to the same extent as do more potent estrogens, such as estradiol, I proposed that antiestrogens may preferentially increase progesterone receptor titers in the target cell. This action would render the target cell more responsive to progestin action. Progesterone has been shown to inhibit estrogen receptor replenishment (1976. Hsueh *et al.*, Endocrinology **98:** 438). Therefore, exposure of the antiestrogen-primed target cell to progestin derived from either ovarian or adrenal sources would be expected to reduce estrogen receptor levels and blunt the target cell response to estrogen action. Our results suggest that regulation of progesterone receptor levels could be an important part of antiestrogen action in the target cell, and this hypothesis should be tested in future experiments with these agents.

DR. D. W. BULLOCK: In the hamster, estrogen does not seem to be required for implantation. If one removes the ovary shortly after mating, progesterone alone will sustain endometrial development. Similarly, in the guinea pig, neither estrogen nor progesterone seems to be required at the time of implantation. At 3 days after mating, one can ovariectomize the guinea pig, and implantation will occur, indicating that endometrial sensitivity is not dependent on the presence of progesterone. In both of these species, could there be very long-lived progesterone receptors, either in the cytoplasm or in the nucleus, that maintain the progestational endometrium in the absence of circulating steroids?

DR. LEAVITT: I don't have data pertinent to the point you raised regarding the half-life of progesterone receptor in the progestational endometrium. Although estrogen is not required for implantation in the hamster (1960. Prasad *et al.*, Proc.

Soc. Exp. Biol. Med. **104:** 48), prior estrogen action during the estrous cycle causes proliferation and differentiation of endometrial target cells. Apparently, these cells persist in the ovariectomized hamster under progesterone support. It may be pertinent that a significant amount of progesterone receptor is produced by the target cell without estrogen support. We have referred to this amount as the estrogen-independent progesterone receptor level (see my FIGURE 14). This level could be the source of progesterone receptor needed to maintain progesterone action in the ovariectomized animal prior to implantation. Progesterone receptor has been identified in the preimplantation endometrium and in deciduomal tissue after implantation (Leavitt & Reuss, Program 57th Meeting, Endocrine Soc., p. 273; Do *et al.*, Program 9th Meeting, Soc. Study Reprod., p. 61). Presumably, progesterone receptor is necessary for the development of endometrial sensitivity and for deciduomal growth. However, the exact role the receptor plays in these processes is not known at the present time.

DR. C. W. BARDIN: In some tissues, progesterone action influences the androgen receptor, and we have some evidence that this may be true for some synthetic progestins in the central nervous system and the pituitary. On the slides that you presented that showed progestin receptor in the pituitary, you don't show us the specificity of that binding protein for androgens. Have you done that?

DR. LEAVITT: No. Since a large number of hamster pituitaries are required for each gradient study, we were limited as to the number of experiments that could be performed. We are in the process of accumulating this information. Although the competition experiment with androgen has not been done, glucocorticoids, such as cortisol, do not compete for the pituitary progesterone receptor.

DR. BARDIN: It is probably a key experiment, because an androgen receptor is known to be present in the pituitary.

DR. LEAVITT: I agree. We recently studied the regulation of androgen receptor levels in the rat pituitary, hypothalamus, and ventral prostate [1976. Leavitt & Sholiton, Andrologia (Suppl. 1) **8:** 112]. In comparing data from the rat and hamster, the sedimentation coefficient of rat pituitary dihydrotestosterone receptor (8S) is greater than that of hamster pituitary progesterone receptor (6S to 7S), as determined by identical analytic procedures. The difference in sedimentation properties suggests that the pituitary androgen and progesterone receptors are different proteins.

DR. B. W. O'MALLEY: You showed that the concentration of progesterone receptor in uterus and vagina was related to the mass of target cells that respond to estrogen. Would you amplify on that?

DR. LEAVITT: The estrogen receptor concentration in uterus and vagina of the ovariectomized animal provided an estimate of the relative concentration of estrogen target cells. Comparison of estrogen and progesterone receptor levels in the ovariectomized preparation revealed a quantitative relationship between those two receptors. This finding suggested that the estrogen target cell might contain the progesterone receptor that was produced in the absence of estrogen action. Analysis of the estrogen-induced progesterone receptor response in uterus and vagina revealed that the magnitude of the response was correlated with estrogen target cell numbers in each organ. This evidence provided support for the hypothesis that progesterone receptor exists in the estrogen target cell. Thus, the progesterone receptor response to estrogen action appeared to be a function of the number of estrogen target cells responding per organ. This hypothesis predicts that the estrogen target cell produces a certain ratio of estrogen receptor and progesterone receptor. Exposure of the target cell to estrogen alters this ratio during translocation of estrogen receptor and induction of the estrogen response. A new receptor ratio is established as progesterone receptor synthesis and estrogen receptor replenishment occur. It seems likely that changes in the receptor ratio would be important in terms of regulating the target cell's responsiveness to estrogen and progestin action.

DR. M. LIPPMAN: There may be very important species differences in terms of both uterotrophic and progesterone receptor induction effects of antiestrogens. Antiestrogens do not stimulate a weight response of the oviduct in the chicken (J. Clark, personal communication). We have studied the regulation of progesterone receptors in human breast cancer cells in tissue culture. In this system, antiestrogens inhibit cell growth and macromolecular synthesis, and they induce a very prompt fall in the level of progesterone receptor, both on a per cell basis and on a per milligram of protein basis.

DR. LEAVITT: It is certainly possible that species differences exist in antiestrogen action. It is also possible that antiestrogen effects vary in the different target tissues within the same animal.

LOCAL TREATMENT OF THE ENDOMETRIUM WITH PROGESTERONE

Bruce B. Pharriss

ALZA Research
Palo Alto, California 94304

In working with intact animals, the endocrinologist must deal with an environment that is ever changing, difficult to control, and impossible to quantify. Administering a hormone to study its effect on a given tissue *in situ* produces a transient concentration of the substance, with an unknown amount reaching the tissue under study. Moreover, it is not simple to sort out the direct effect of the hormone on the target tissue from secondary effects caused by physiologic responses of the nontarget tissues to the administered hormone.

During the last 5 years, we have been working on methods to deliver substances to animals and humans at fixed rates for specific time periods, that is, 20 μg/hr for 7 days or 65 μg/day for 1 year.[1-3] In some instances, the purpose is the specific treatment of given tissues. To accomplish this goal, we have utilized systems that provide three types of controlled drug release: a polymer that erodes by hydrolysis, an osmotic pumping system, and a solution-diffusion system.

Bioerodible delivery systems for local or systemic drug delivery are composed of solid polymeric material admixed with hormone or drug (FIGURE 1). The polymer is biodegradable by hydrolytic cleavage of its bonds at a constant rate, controlled by variation in pH, which can be adjusted by incorporating buffer substances in the drug system. The drug is delivered at the same rate that the polymer erodes, and the drug and erosion products are absorbed and carried away from the implant site, leaving no residue. One such system[4] has been designed to release a progestin for 1–6 months from an implant 6 mm in diameter. Studies in rabbits, rats, and baboons have shown that systems of this type, implanted intramuscularly or subcutaneously, can reliably release progestins at constant rates, depending on drug concentration, without toxic responses at the local site.

Small implantable osmotic pumping systems (FIGURE 2) have also been developed to deliver a continuous, precisely controlled flow of almost any biologically active agent into laboratory animals, including those as small as mice, for up to 7 days.[5] The unit can be placed subcutaneously or intraperitoneally, and by attaching a catheter to the end of the implanted pump, the flow of drug or hormone solution can be directed to precise target areas. The potential applications of such a delivery system in endocrinology are quite extensive.

The solution-diffusion method of delivery[6] utilizes a polymer membrane that encloses a reservoir of drug crystals suspended in an inert vehicle (FIGURE 3). The vehicle is compatible with, and insoluble in, the membrane. Hormone or drug solubility is low in the vehicle and even lower in the membrane. A large excess of hormone in the reservoir maintains a constant thermodynamic activity that generates zero-order release of the agent from the reservoir. The energy for diffusion is the chemical concentration difference across the polymeric membrane, which is constant, because concentration outside is at infinite dilution. Such modules can be used for systemic (subcutaneous) or localized (intraocular, intrauterine) delivery of active substances.

The solution-diffusion method has provided considerable data on the biochemical and physiologic effects of delivering constant doses of progesterone to the human endometrium. Following the pioneering effort of Scommegna *et al.*,[7] we designed the intrauterine progesterone contraceptive system (IPCS), which could be placed in the human uterus to deliver a predictable daily dose of progesterone for 1 year. FIGURE 4 shows the release rate curve obtained during exposure *in utero* for 400 days.[8] The average release rate for the system depicted is 65 ± 10 μg per day, but other systems have been designed to reliably produce higher or lower rates. This system produces considerable contraceptive protection without measurable alterations in systemic endocrinary functions. Detailed studies on pituitary gonadotropins, ovarian steroid and relaxin production, and lipid and carbohydrate metabolic indicators have shown normal patterns.[9–12] Because no systemic alterations were measurable, the contraceptive action by exclusion resided completely within the uterus, and our attention thus shifted to alterations that occurred in the endometrium.

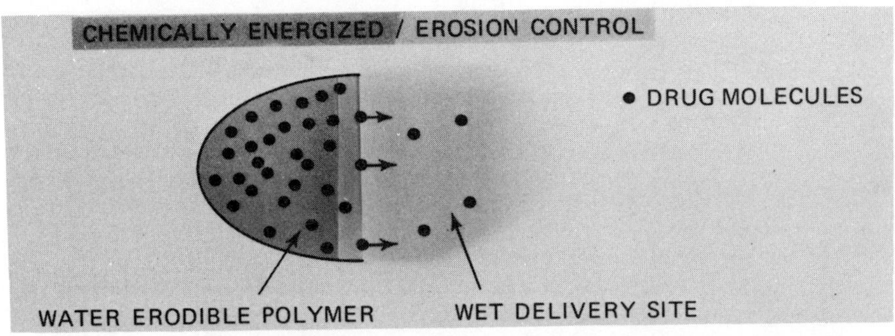

FIGURE 1. Schematic diagram of bioerodible delivery system for local or systemic drug delivery.

ENDOMETRIAL HISTOLOGY

Histologic examination of more than 400 biopsy or hysterectomy specimens from women wearing the IPCS indicate that the response to progesterone is decidual in nature and, initially, is most intense immediately adjacent to the delivery system; later, it tends to spread to distal endometrium.[13,14] The glands are small and few, while the cells are cuboidal rather than columnar, and show little evidence of secretion or other biochemical activity. The stroma becomes lacy and edematous. The reaction is greatest in the functionalis; the basalis shows little or no alteration. After 2–3 months of exposure, proliferation during the follicular stage decreases, and the endometrium generally becomes thinner.

The decidualization occurs early in the cycle, with the result that dating of the endometrium is impossible. The proliferative and secretory endometria are histologically similar, yet regular menstruation continues, which indicates that the ovarian hormones are still exerting control.

ALTERATIONS IN CHEMICAL CONSTITUENTS

Alterations occur in chemical constituents of the endometrium during the release of exogenous progesterone to that tissue.[15,16] Biopsies on fertile women who used uterine systems that release 10, 65, or 120 μg of progesterone per day

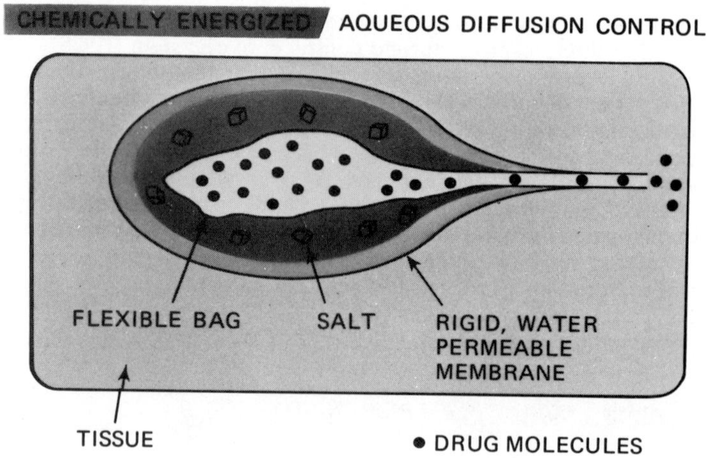

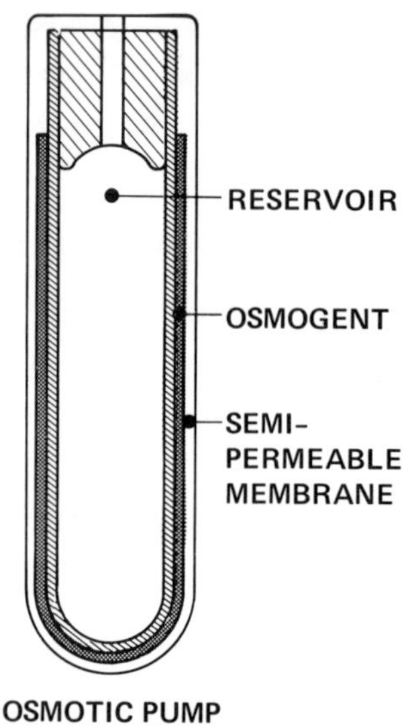

FIGURE 2. Schematic diagram (*top*) and photograph (*bottom*) of implantable osmotic pumping system.

and on an equal number who received no hormonal treatment showed that those who received the hormone had significant reductions in the concentrations of fucose, sialic acid, and the fucose to sialic acid ratio throughout the cycle. Zinc and calcium concentrations were increased during the proliferative phase. Sodium, potassium, and manganese concentrations rose during the secretory phase, whereas zinc concentrations were lower than in controls. None of the groups showed statistically significant changes in proteins, DNA, RNA, and total hexoses. No differences were apparent in the endometrial response of groups that received 10, 65, or 120 μg of progesterone per day.

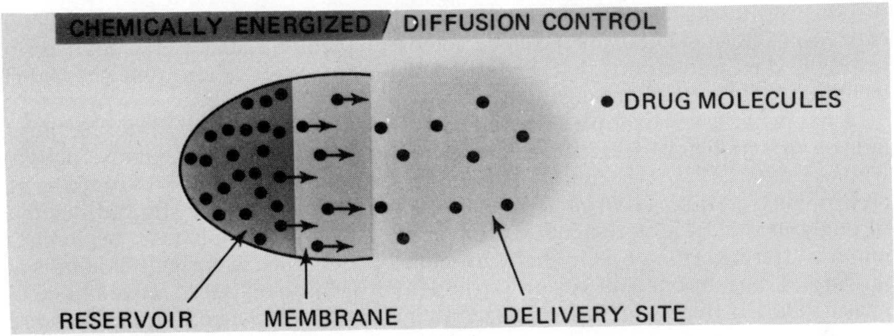

FIGURE 3. Schematic diagram of solution-diffusion method of drug delivery.

BIOCHEMICAL ACTIVITY

Depression of biochemical activity of the endometrium accompanies its morphologic suppression. To investigate the effect of exogenous progesterone on the tissue's metabolic capacity, biopsies were taken from women who used systems that had the same three hormone release rates listed above.[17] The systems had been placed 6 months prior to the study. Utilization of [U$-^{14}$C]glucose by endometrial tissue was determined by a radiorespirometry system, in which the production of $^{14}CO_2$ and of [^{14}C]lactate was measured, as was the incorporation of ^{14}C into proteins and lipids. Compared with control groups that did not receive any hormone, biopsies from the groups that used progesterone systems exhibited a decrease in the production of [^{14}C]lactate and in the incorporation of ^{14}C into protein and lipids during the proliferative phase. In the secretory phase, no statistically significant changes were apparent between the progesterone groups and the control group. This finding was interpreted as an indication that the endometrial

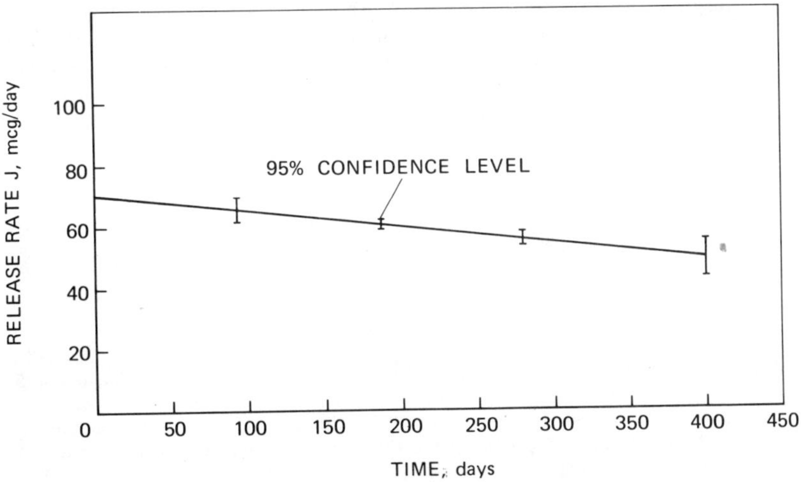

FIGURE 4. *In vivo* release rate of progesterone from the PROGESTASERT® system.

response to intrinsic progesterone is of such a magnitude that the low levels of exogenous hormone do not produce major metabolic changes. Comparison of results in the three groups that received different amounts of hormone showed no meaningful differences among them in either phase of the cycle.

Enzymatic assays showed that progesterone released directly into the uterus induces a significant decrease in the endometrial alkaline phosphatase activity within 2 months.[17] At 6 months, this reduction was apparent only during the secretory phase. Biopsies from women wearing the system also showed declines throughout the cycle in the endometrial activity of acid phosphatase, beginning 6 months after insertion, and in β-glucuronidase, beginning as early as 2 months afterward. Progesterone's effect on lactic dehydrogenase activity appears to be biphasic. During the proliferative phase, an increase is observed; during the secretory phase, there is a decrease.

Steroid analyses of endometrial specimens taken from women who used systems that released 65 μg of progesterone per day indicated five- to 10-fold increases in progesterone, compared with specimens from women who used identical nonhormonal units.[16] These higher progesterone levels were characteristic of both the proliferative and the secretory endometria. Estradiol levels, on the other hand, were significantly depressed (50–75%) among women who used progesterone systems. Circulating levels of both steroids, however, failed to reflect the changes observed in the endometrium. Preliminary evidence indicates that the decrease in estradiol concentration is associated with a decline in estradiol receptors, observed in women undergoing treatment with either progesterone from the IPCS or with oral medroxyprogesterone acetate.[18] Similar parallels are suggested in estradiol 17β-hydrogenase, the estradiol-metabolizing enzyme in the endometrium.[19]

Conclusions

Results of studies where single tissues are exposed to predictable constant levels of progesterone *in situ* by use of hormonal delivery systems will help to unravel the effect of this hormone and of others on target tissues. By elimination of cyclic concentrations and recruitment of other organs of the body that could impact on the tissue under study, we can approach *in situ* the experimental control we exert *in vitro*. These small delivery systems with predictable delivery rates also have the advantage that constant levels of hormones can be administered to animals without the use of anesthetics or restrictions on physical activity, both of which can alter hypothalamic physiology. In addition to providing assistance in unraveling the endocrinology of various control systems, these delivery systems may play an important role in pharmacology and the development of new approaches to drug therapy.[20]

References

1. Urquhart, J. 1975. Novel methods of ocular drug delivery. Clin. Pharmacol. **5:** 63–72.
2. Place, V. A. & B. B. Pharriss. 1974. Progress in the development of the PROGESTASERT® 65 progesterone therapeutic system for contraception. J. Reprod. Med. **13:** 66–68.
3. Pharriss, B. B. 1974. Uterine progesterone system. *In* Intrauterine Devices; Development, Evaluation and Program Implementation. R. G. Wheeler, G. W. Duncan & J. J. Speidel, Eds.: 203–210. Academic Press, Inc. San Francisco, Calif.

4. PHARRISS, B. B., V. A. PLACE, L. SENDELBECK & E. SCHMITT. 1976. Steroid delivery system for contraception. J. Reprod. Med. In press.
5. AMKRAUT, A., S. I. YUM & M. B. RITTENBERG. 1976. Specific suppression of IgG plaque forming cells (PFC) by continuous administration of antigen from implantable delivery system. Fed. Proc. **35:** 675.
6. SWANSON, D., P. WONG & B. B. PHARRISS. 1975. Drug Delivery Systems in Contraception. The Contribution of the Pharmaceutical Sciences.: 45–52. Excerpta Medica. Amsterdam, The Netherlands.
7. SCOMMEGNA, A., G. N. PANDYA, M. CHRIST, A. W. LEE & M. R. COHEN. 1970. Intrauterine administration of progesterone by a slow-releasing device. Fertil. Steril. **21:** 201–210.
8. PHARRISS, B. B., R. ERICKSON, J. BASHAW, S. HOFF, V. A. PLACE & A. ZAFFARONI. 1974. PROGESTASERT®: a uterine therapeutic system for long-term contraception: I. Philosophy and clinical efficacy. Fertil. Steril. **25:** 915–921.
9. TILLSON, S. A., B. B. PHARRISS & J. D. NEILL. 1974. The effect of intrauterine progesterone on the hypothalamic-pituitary-ovarian axis in baboons. J. Steroid Biochem. **5:** 376.
10. TILLSON, S. A., M. MARIAN, R. HUDSON, P. WONG, B. PHARRISS, R. AZNAR & J. MARTINEZ-MANAUTOU. 1975. The effect of intrauterine progesterone on the hypothalamic-hypophyseal-ovarian axis in humans. Contraception **11:** 179–192.
11. BRYANT, G. D., F. C. GREENWOOD, R. W. HALE & W. K. MORISHIGE. 1977. Hormonal evaluation of the intrauterine contraceptive system. J. Clin. Endocrinol. Metabol. In press.
12. SPELLACY, W. 1976. Personal communication.
13. MARTINEZ-MANAUTOU, J., M. MAQUEO, R. AZNAR, B. B. PHARRISS & A. ZAFFARONI. 1975. Endometrial morphology in women exposed to uterine systems releasing progesterone. Amer. J. Obstet. Gynecol. **121:** 175–179.
14. MARTINEZ-MANAUTOU, J. 1975. Contraception by intrauterine release of progesterone: clinical results. J. Steroid Biochem. **6:** 889–894.
15. HICKS, J. J., R. AZNAR, P. LEROY & A. ROSADO. 1975. Comparative effect of different concentrations of progesterone (IUD) on the biochemical composition of the human endometrium. Rev. Invest. Clin. **27:** 83, 84.
16. HAGENFELDT, K. & B.-M. LANDGREN. 1975. Contraception by intrauterine release of progesterone—effects on endometrial trace elements, enzymes and steroids. J. Steroid Biochem. **6:** 895–898.
17. ROSADO, A., R. AZNAR, P. LEROY & J. J. HICKS. 1975. Effect of the progesterone-releasing intrauterine system on the utilization of glucose by the human endometrium. Rev. Invest. Clin. **27:** 83.
18. TSENG, L. & E. GURPIDE. 1975. Effects of progestins on estradiol receptor levels in human endometrium. J. Clin. Endocrinol. Metab. **41:** 402–404.
19. TSENG, L. & E. GURPIDE. 1975. Induction of human endometrial estradiol dehydrogenase by progestins. Endocrinology **97:** 825–833.
20. ZAFFARONI, A. 1975. Therapeutic implications of controlled drug delivery. Clin. Pharmacol. **5:** 53–61.

DISCUSSION

DR. W. G. WIEST: Dr. Pharriss, in view of the relatively high concentration of tissue progesterone that was measured in the presence of the implants, do you postulate effects not mediated by cytosol or nuclear receptors?

DR. PHARRISS: Quite possible. Progesterone has very many nonspecific binding sites in the membranes, for example. We are attempting to get around this high concentration by building systems that deliver as low as 5 μg per day and in which we have deployed the delivery more equally throughout the uterus to see if we obtain the same biologic end points. We indeed can, at 5 μg per day, bring about the same histologic patterns, but as of yet we don't have any biochemical data.

DR. RICHARDSON: I'm a little puzzled by a clinical problem. I thought you said that the endometrium did not cycle, and yet these women menstruate. Is that correct? Does the basal layer cycle, while the portion of the endometrium that is proximate to the insert does not cycle?

DR. PHARRISS: It's a mystery to us. The people who have read the slide blindly for us have said that in all likelihood, these women are not cycling, and yet they do menstruate regularly. Some of them tend to have much lighter cycles than do others as the amount of blood lost decreases. We're not exactly sure where the menstruating is occurring, because the basilar layer is essentially unchanged between control and treated situations.

PROTEIN COMPOSITION OF HUMAN ENDOMETRIUM AND ITS SECRETION AT DIFFERENT STAGES OF THE MENSTRUAL CYCLE

P. J. Hirsch,*† I. L. C. Fergusson,‡ and R. J. B. King*

Hormone Biochemistry Department
Imperial Cancer Research Fund Laboratories
Lincoln's Inn Fields
London WC2A 3PX, England
and ‡Department of Obstetrics and Gynaecology
St. Thomas Hospital
London SE1 7EH, England

Introduction

The changes that occur in human endometrium under the influence of estrogen plus progesterone during the secretory phase of the menstrual cycle are largely related to the nurturing of the fertilized human egg followed by its implantation. Endometrial secretion starts on about Day 18 and is maximal by Days 20–22 of a normal cycle. If fertilization has occurred, the blastocyst attaches to the endometrium on Days 19–20 and is completely implanted by Day 25. Histologic characterization of these progesterone-induced events is well documented,[1–3] but biochemical information on endometrium is more sparse[4–6] and includes virtually no data on protein composition. More information is available for other species, and, in particular, the composition of rabbit uterine secretions is eliciting much interest because of the presence of a progesterone-induced protein called blastokinin or uteroglobin.[7,8] This protein is secreted just prior to implantation and may play an important role in the development and implantation of the blastocyst.[7] The applicability of the rabbit data to humans is dubious, and it is noteworthy that there is no convincing evidence for the existence of a specific progesterone-sensitive protein in human luminal fluid.[9,10] Indeed, the data quoted in References 9 and 10 suggest that the proteins of human luminal fluid are derived mainly from plasma.

This paper describes experiments undertaken to determine if progesterone can affect the protein composition of human endometrium and uterine flushings in a manner that might be related to the presence of a blastocyst. The experiments fall into two categories: electrophoretic analysis of endometrium and flushings throughout the menstrual cycle, and maintenance of endometrium in organ culture in the presence and absence of progesterone accompanied by incorporation of isotopically labeled leucine into the cell proteins.

Materials and Methods

Endometrium was obtained at curettage or hysterectomy, mainly from patients with regular menstrual cycles, the dates of which were checked histologically. Occasional samples were obtained from patients with cystic hyperplasia.

†Present address: Department of Obstetrics and Gynaecology, Hope Hospital, Salford 6, Lancashire, England.

Uterine flushings were obtained at different stages of the cycle from two premenopausal women who had undergone voluntary sterilization by tubal diathermy at least 1 year earlier. These flushings were obtained by injecting 20 ml of physiologic saline through the cervix by means of a Gravlee jet washer.[11] Approximately 18 ml of fluid were recovered in both cases. Endometrium was homogenized by hand in 10 mM tris, 1 mM EDTA (pH 7.4, 1:5 w/v), and the cytosol was obtained by centrifugation for 1 hr at $10^5 g$ at 4°C. The cytosol or uterine flushings were dialyzed overnight at room temperature against 0.1% sodium dodecyl sulfate (SDS) in 10 mM sodium phosphate buffer (pH 7.5) that contained 0.1% β-mercaptoethanol. Where necessary, the dialyzed fractions were concentrated by immersing the dialysis sacs in powdered Aquacide® (Calbiochem Ltd.) The proteins were then separated according to molecular weight by electrophoresis in 10% (w/v) polyacrylamide gels.[12] The gels were run for 5 hr at 8 mA per gel. Gels were fixed overnight in 10% (w/v) sulfosalicylic acid, stained with Coomassie blue (Coomassie blue 125 mg per liter of methanol:water:glacial acetic acid:glycerol, 403:520:53:24) and destained in 7.5% (v/v) glacial acetic acid. The optical density profile at 550 nm was recorded automatically with a Gilford spectrophotometer. When [^{3}H/^{14}C]leucine-labeled proteins had been electrophoresed, the gels were cut into 1-mm slices without prior fixation. Two slices were put into each scintillation vial and incubated for 2 hr at 60°C with 0.5 ml of Soluene® (Packard Instrument Co.), followed by another incubation for at least 1 hr at room temperature with 5 ml of phosphor (5 g of PPO per liter of toluene). Radioactivity was measured after at least 2 hr of cooling.

For organ culture, fresh endometrium was cut into 1-mm square pieces and placed on 1-cm^2 stainless steel grids in the compartments of a Repli dish (Sterilin Ltd., Teddington). Medium 199 supplemented with 10% (v/v) calf serum and 10 μg of insulin per milliliter was routinely used. The gas phase was 95% air, 5% carbon dioxide. Cultures were maintained for 48 hr. In the [^{3}H/^{14}C]leucine experiments, the [^{3}H]leucine (L-[4,5-^{3}H]leucine, 50 Ci/mmol, 25 μCi/ml; Radiochemical Centre, Amersham) or [^{14}C]leucine (L-[U-^{14}C]leucine, 270 mCi/mmol, 5 μCi/ml; Radiochemical Centre, Amersham) was added 24 hr after starting the culture and was present throughout the subsequent 24-hr period. Routinely, [^{3}H]leucine was added to the progesterone plus estradiol-treated cultures, and [^{14}C]leucine was added to the control incubations. At the end of the 48-hr culture period, the endometrial explants were removed, blotted dry, homogenized, and processed as described above.

Protease activity was measured by the method of Notides *et al.*[13] by use of benzoyl-DL-arginine *p*-nitroanilide as the substrate. Glycogen was assayed by the method of Montgomery,[14] and protein was determined by the method of Lowry *et al.*[15]

Plasma was obtained from a premenopausal woman who was regularly taking Norinyl®-1 (1 mg of norethisterone plus 50 μg of mestranol; Syntex).

Results

Electrophoretic Profiles of Endometrial Proteins

Endometrial proteins give SDS-polyacrylamide gel profiles of the type shown in Figure 1. We have selected and numbered 13 major peaks by virtue of their easy visual identity; these 13 peaks in no way represent the total number of proteins present in the extract. Rabbit uteroglobin has a molecular weight of 12,000 daltons in SDS[16] and in this gel system would run in the region of peak 12. In none of our experiments has a major protein been identified in this region. To determine whether the proportions of these proteins changed throughout the cycle, we took the peak height of the Coomassie blue-stained proteins as a measure of the amount of protein in the band. Because the amount of stain taken up is not constant for all proteins, this amount cannot be taken as an absolute measure of the protein, but it is satisfactory as an index of how a given protein band changes throughout the cycle. However, if one wants to know how endogenous hormones affect endometrial proteins, such a relative comparison is only valid if one knows how much endometrium is present in the uterus and that proteins from a known amount of endometrium are being applied to the gels. The latter, but not the former, parameter can be controlled; even standardization of protein content does not circumvent the problem of variation in proportions of stromal and epithelial cells between specimens. As a less than ideal, but "best under the circum-

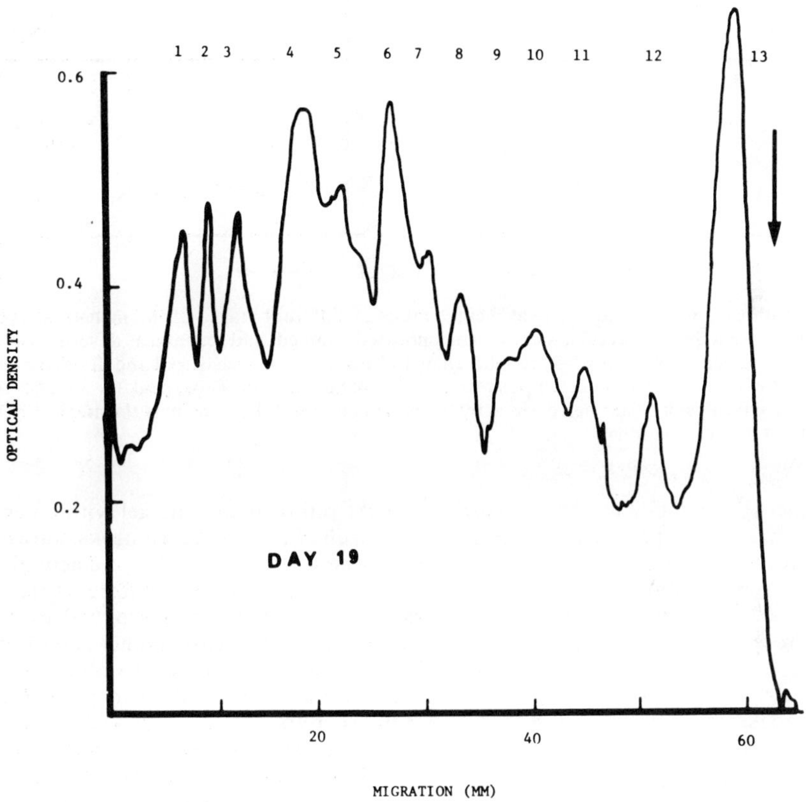

FIGURE 1. SDS-polyacrylamide gel electrophoretic profile of soluble proteins from Day-19 endometrium. The bromphenol blue marker is designated by the arrow. Proteins were stained with Coomassie blue.

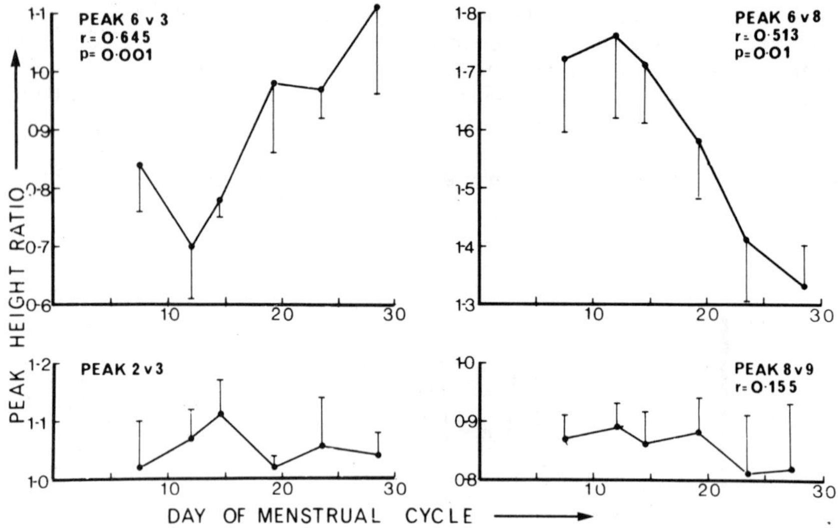

FIGURE 2. Comparison of peak height ratios at different stages of the menstrual cycle. Soluble endometrial proteins were electrophoresed, stained, and scanned as described in the text. The height of each peak, numbered as in FIGURE 1, was measured and divided by the height of an arbitrarily selected peak to give a peak height ratio. Thus, peak 6 v 3 means that the height of peak 6 has been divided by the height of peak 3. Each point is the mean ± SD of at least four estimations.

stances,'' method, we compared peak height ratios in any one gel with an arbitrarily selected peak used as the standard. Each of the numbered peaks shown in FIGURE 1 was quantitated as a proportion of one selected peak. These calculations were repeated both with different endometrial samples and with different selected peaks as the denominator. In this way, we obtained a series of values that represented the proportion of a given stained band relative to another band at different stages of the menstrual cycle. Four examples of the results obtained are shown in FIGURE 2. It is clear that peak 6 increases relative to peak 3 but decreases relative to peak 8 throughout the secretory stage of the cycle. On the other hand, peaks 2 and 8 do not change relative to peaks 3 and 9, respectively. In the context of how progesterone influences these protein profiles, attention can be confined to samples obtained after Day 10, and one can ask if there is a statistically significant increase or decrease in ratio as the progestational stage of the cycle progresses. The results of this type of calculation are shown in FIGURE 3 for each of the protein bands numbered in FIGURE 1. The calculations have been repeated for peak heights relative to four different bands. It is clear that peaks 6–11 change (all increase) relative to both peaks 1 and 3. Peaks 1–4 and 6 change (all decrease) relative to peak 8. With the possible exceptions of peaks 1 and 3, there are no significant changes relative to peak 9.

These data indicate that several low-molecular-weight proteins (<60,000 daltons) progressively increase relative to two large proteins during the secretory phase of the cycle. Conversely, several high-molecular-weight proteins decrease relative to peak 8. These data could be explained by hormonally induced changes in either cellular protein synthesis/degradation or tissue content of plasma proteins. Alternatively, the rather general increase in small, as compared to large, proteins could be explained by a progesterone-induced increase or estrogen-induced inhibition of protease activity. Analysis of protease activity of both endometrial homogenates and of high-speed supernatants did not support the protease idea but did not rule out a contribution from other proteases not measured by our assay.

The endometrial proteins just described could be cellular and/or extracellular (plasma). Distinction between cellular and plasma proteins is difficult, and plasma proteins cannot be ignored, because they comprise a sizable proportion of soluble uterine proteins[17] and because their tissue content can be hormonally regulated.[18] Immunologic methods have been used to demonstrate the presence of specific

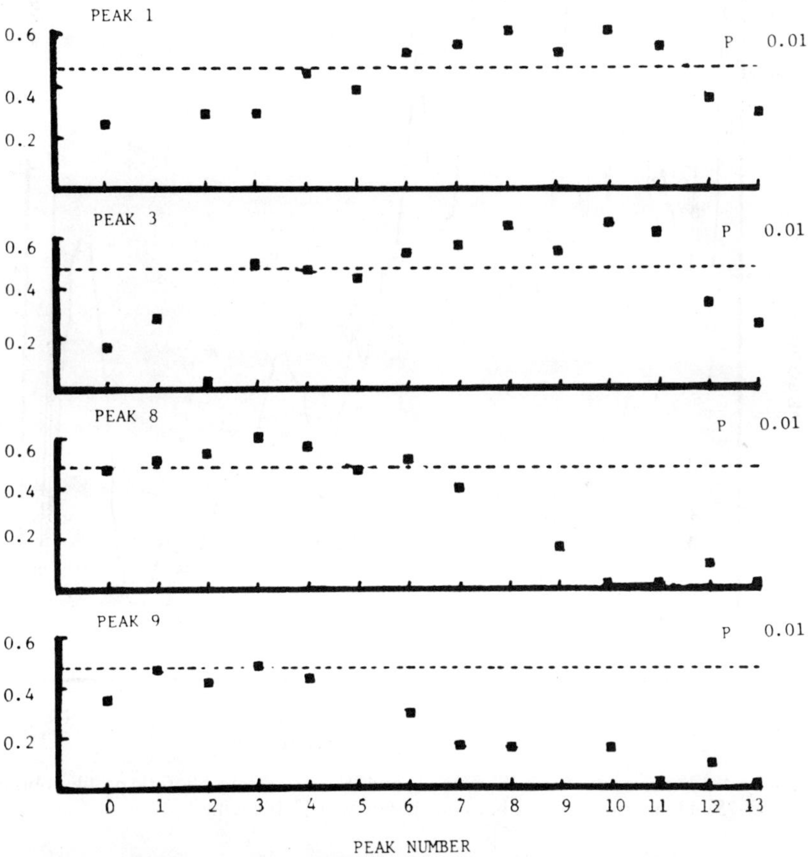

FIGURE 3. Significance of linear regression coefficient for peak height ratio against time of the menstrual cycle. Peak height ratios throughout the cycle were calculated as described in FIGURE 2 with either peak 1, 3, 8, or 9 used as the denominator and with each of the remaining peaks used as the numerator. The linear regression coefficient for each peak number has been calculated from plots of the type shown in FIGURE 2. The dashed line indicates the level above which the linear regression coefficient for peak height ratio against time of menstrual cycle is statistically significant at $p < 0.01$.

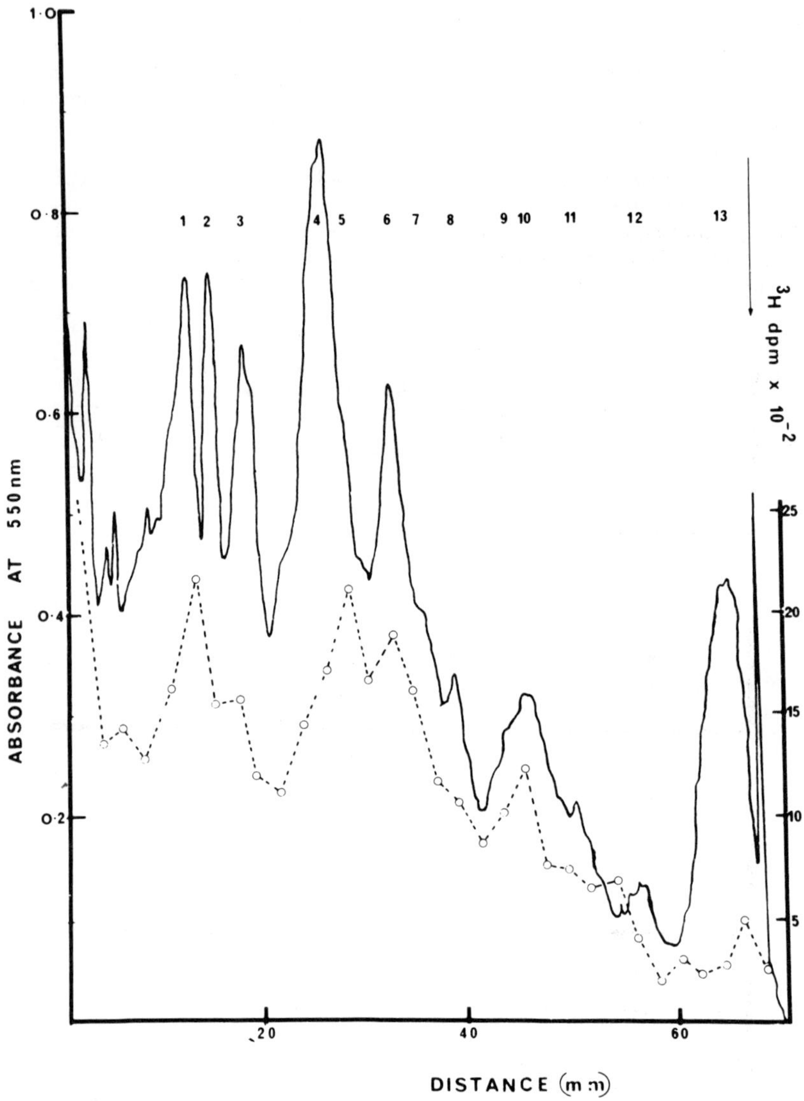

FIGURE 4. Comparison of absorbance (—) and ^{3}H (- - -) electrophoretic profiles obtained from Day-25 endometrium after 24 hr of incubation with [^{3}H]leucine.

plasma proteins in luminal fluid[9,10] but not to identify specific electrophoretic bands. We have tried an alternative approach to locate the cellular proteins.

Because plasma proteins within the endometrium would not be labeled with [^{3}H]leucine during an *in vitro* incubation, we compared the electrophoretic profiles of ^{3}H-labeled proteins with stained bands (FIGURE 4). The resolution of the ^{3}H-labeled peaks is inferior to that of the absorbancy profile, but it seems that at least part of peaks 3, 5, 6, and 10 is due to tissue protein. We are not certain if peaks 1 and 2 represent the other labeled entity. It would thus seem that the absorbancy profiles represent a contribution from both plasma and tissue proteins. Comparison of the data shown in FIGURE 4 with the changes noted during the cycle (FIGURE 3) suggests that both plasma and tissue protein contents are hormonally sensitive.

Effect of Progesterone in Vitro

The foregoing data do not distinguish among protein changes due to estrogen withdrawal, progesterone inhibition of estrogen stimulation, or progesterone stimulation. Microexplants of human endometrium retain their sensitivity to both estrogens[19] and progestins[2,5] in organ culture, and we have used this technique to determine if any of the endometrial proteins are progesterone sensitive. The system we used (see MATERIALS AND METHODS) exhibited progesterone sensitivity at both biochemical and histologic levels. A 48-hr culture in the presence of 1 μg/ml of progesterone plus 0.01 μg/ml of estradiol increased the glycogen content of the explants by more than 20% relative to that of cultures with no added steroid. Lower concentrations (0.01 μg/ml) of progesterone were less efficacious than was 1 μg/ml, whereas inconsistent results were obtained in the absence of estradiol. Estradiol alone had no effect on either glycogen content or histology. Histologically, the progesterone-induced changes can be most marked; in the example shown in FIGURES 5a–5d, a Day-17 endometrium with little or no sign of secretion has been converted to approximately a Day-20 appearance, with luminal secretion and ragged luminal epithelial edges. These changes were not seen in the absence of progesterone.

Amino acid incorporation into proteins was performed by incubating endometrium in the presence or absence of 0.01 μg of estradiol plus 1 μg of progesterone per milliliter of medium. After 24 hr of culture, isotopically labeled leucine was added, and the culture was continued for a further 24 hr. Incorporation into soluble proteins was analyzed by SDS-polyacrylamide gel electrophoresis. In the initial experiments, [^{3}H]leucine was added to both hormone-treated and control cultures, and the cell extracts were electrophoresed on separate gels. These experiments indicated that progesterone was specifically increasing incorporation into a protein that migrated slightly faster than did albumin (mol wt 69,000; see FIGURE 6). A similar progesterone-sensitive protein appeared when different isotopes were used to label the proteins in hormone-treated and control cultures, respectively. In the experiment illustrated in FIGURE 7, [^{3}H]leucine was added to the treated cultures, and [^{14}C]leucine was added to the control cultures. A change in the ^{3}H/^{14}C ratio of a protein with a molecular weight of about 50,000 was regularly seen in this type of experiment. Reversal of the isotopes did not change the peak, but it was not present when progesterone was omitted from the culture medium. The other changes in the ^{3}H/^{14}C ratio noted in FIGURE 7 were not always seen.

Our conclusion from this series of experiments is that the soluble endometrial proteins represent a mixture of proteins made both within the endometrial cells and elsewhere, possibly derived from the bloodstream. Of particular interest was a cellular protein with a molecular weight of about 50,000 daltons (band 6) that was induced by progesterone. The proportions of endometrial proteins change with the menstrual cycle, but the function of none of these proteins is known.

An important question one might ask about these proteins, regardless of

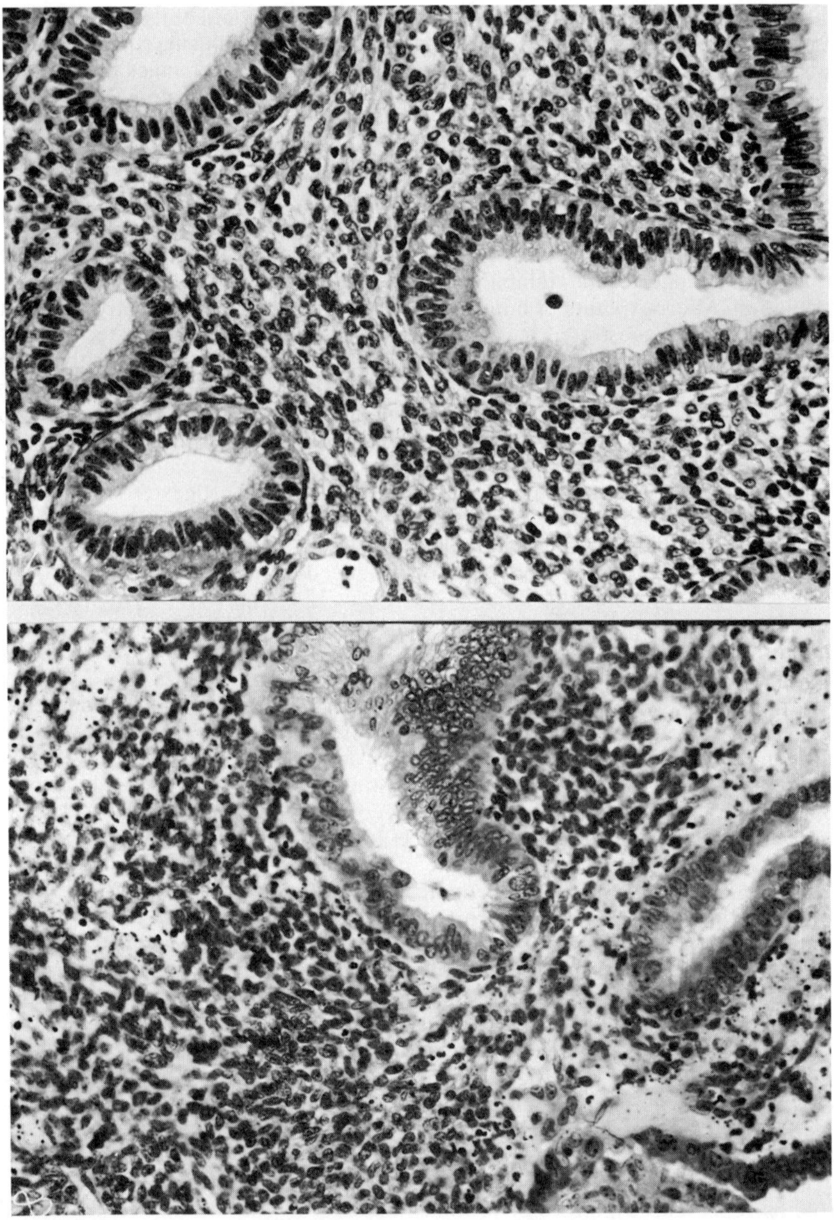

FIGURES 5a & 5b. Histologic appearance of Day-17 endometrium before (a, *top*) and after (b, *bottom*; c, *top* facing page; d, *bottom* facing page) a 48-hr culture. b, No steroids added; c, 1 μg of progesterone per milliliter of medium; d, 0.01 μg of estradiol plus 1 μg of progesterone per milliliter of medium. $\times$280.

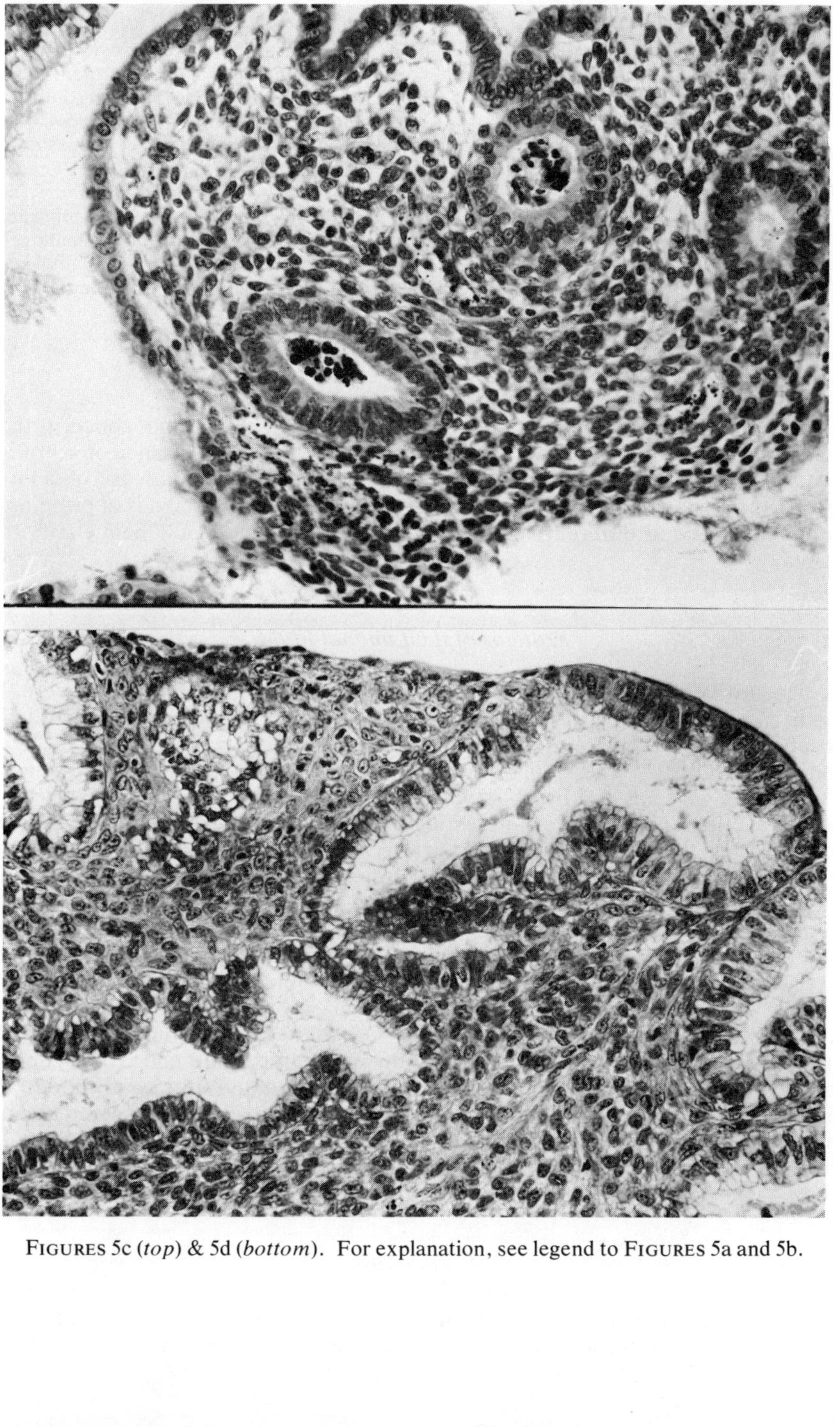

FIGURES 5c (*top*) & 5d (*bottom*). For explanation, see legend to FIGURES 5a and 5b.

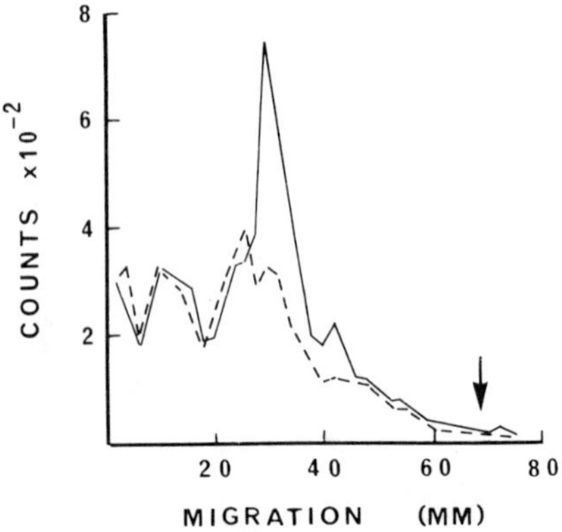

FIGURE 6. Incorporation of [^{3}H]leucine into soluble proteins from Day-8 endometrium. Endometrium was cultured for 48 hr in the presence (—) or absence (- - -) of 1 μg of progesterone per milliliter of medium. [^{3}H]Leucine was added for the final 24-hr culture. The soluble proteins were electrophoresed separately on SDS-polyacrylamide gels, as described in the text. Arrow indicates migration of the bromphenol blue marker.

whether made by the endometrial cells or derived from the plasma, concerns their relationship to the luminal secretion. Does the histologic appearance of secretion into the lumen seen from Day 21 onward represent a general release of cellular proteins, or is it a very specific release of certain proteins? Analysis of proteins in the luminal fluid at different stages of the menstrual cycle would help clarify this point.

Proteins of the Luminal Fluid

Qualitatively, the electrophoretic profiles obtained with luminal fluid were the same as those derived from serum (FIGURE 8). This finding agrees with the observations of Garcea *et al.*[10] and is similar, but not identical, to the data of Beier and Beier-Hellwig.[9] The similarity of profiles was evident both with Coomassie blue-stained gels and with gels stained for carbohydrate by the periodic acid-Schiff reaction. This result is interesting for several reasons. The histologic data suggest that the endometrial cells actively make and secrete proteins. Presumably, at least some of these proteins should exhibit electrophoretic behavior different from that of serum proteins. Second, the endometrial blood vessels do not penetrate the basal membrane between epithelium and stroma. Therefore, how do the serum proteins enter the lumen? Luminal injection of saline might artifactually release serum or intercellular proteins, but this possibility does not provide a complete answer, in view of the observation that uterine fluid obtained without washing also behaves like serum.[10] Our limited studies indicate that qualitative differences may exist between serum and luminal fluid and would support the idea that the luminal proteins represent a selective ultrafiltrate of blood.[9] As far as can be judged from our two patients, the relative amounts of some luminal proteins may change with the menstrual cycle (FIGURE 9). Particularly striking are the increases in bands 1, 5, and 6 relative to band 11 at about the time of implantation.

CONCLUSIONS

Our studies show that both cellular and extracellular proteins of the human endometrium change throughout the menstrual cycle, but the relationship of these

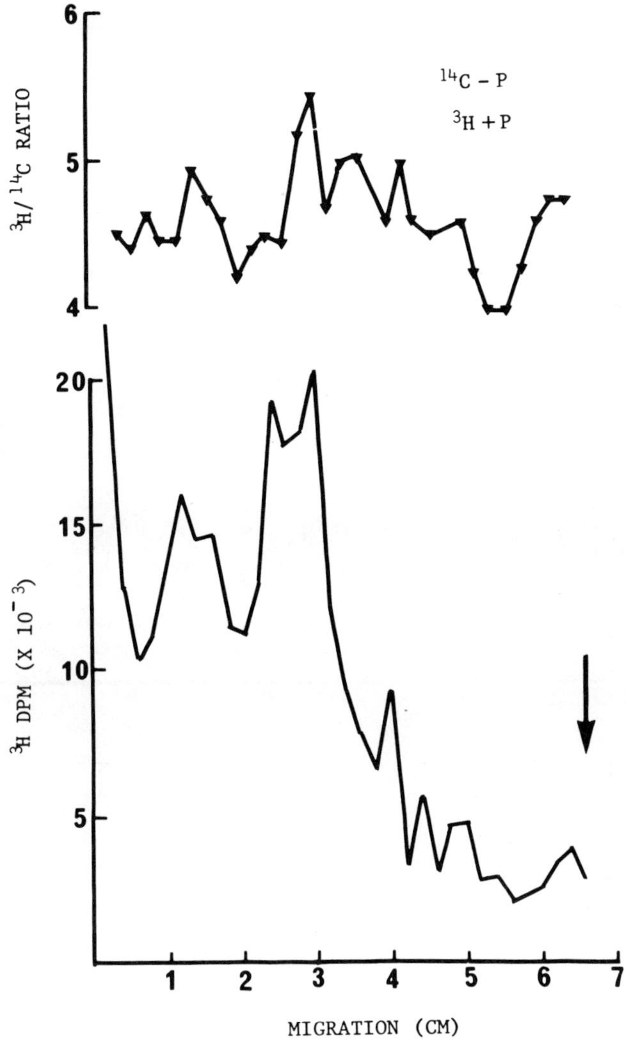

FIGURE 7. Incorporation of [^{3}H]- and [^{14}C]leucine into soluble proteins from secretory phase endometrium (exact date not known). The experiment was performed as described in the legend to FIGURE 6, except that 0.01 μg of estradiol per milliliter of medium was included with the progesterone. The samples cultured in the absence of steroid were incubated with [^{14}C]leucine, and the ^{3}H- and ^{14}C-labeled proteins were mixed prior to coelectrophoresis. Arrow indicates migration of the bromphenol blue marker.

two pools of proteins to the proteins that appear in the secretion is not clear. Superficially, our data suggest that luminal fluid is derived from blood; however, a single electrophoretic system is a poor basis on which to identify proteins from different sources. Therefore, it is quite possible that specific endometrial proteins do occur in the luminal fluid.

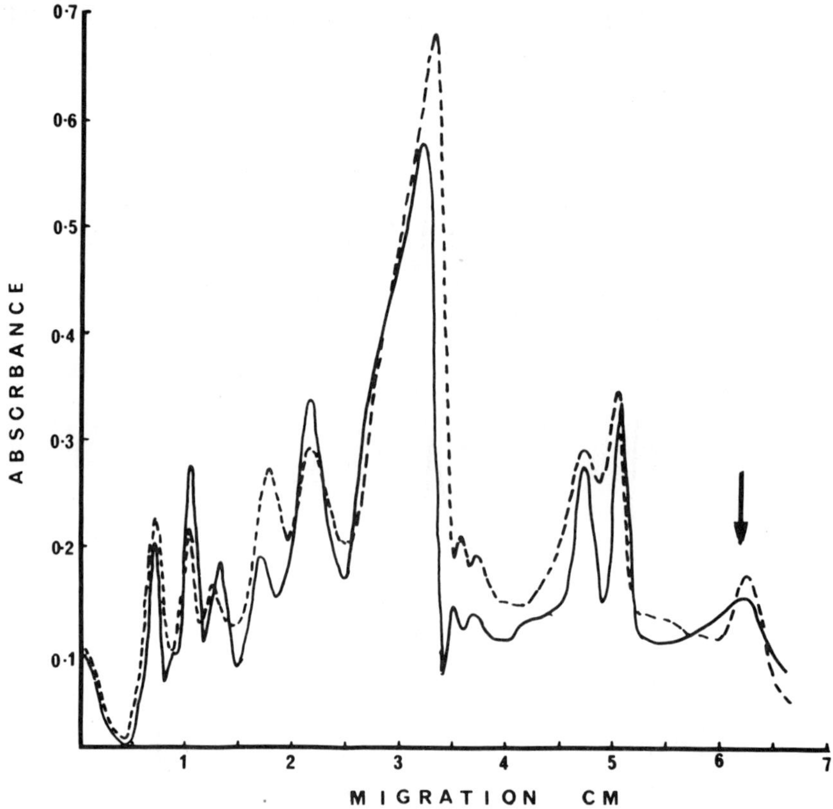

FIGURE 8. Electrophoretic profiles of serum (—) and luminal fluid (- - -) obtained on Day 18 of the cycle. Arrow indicates migration of the bromphenol blue marker.

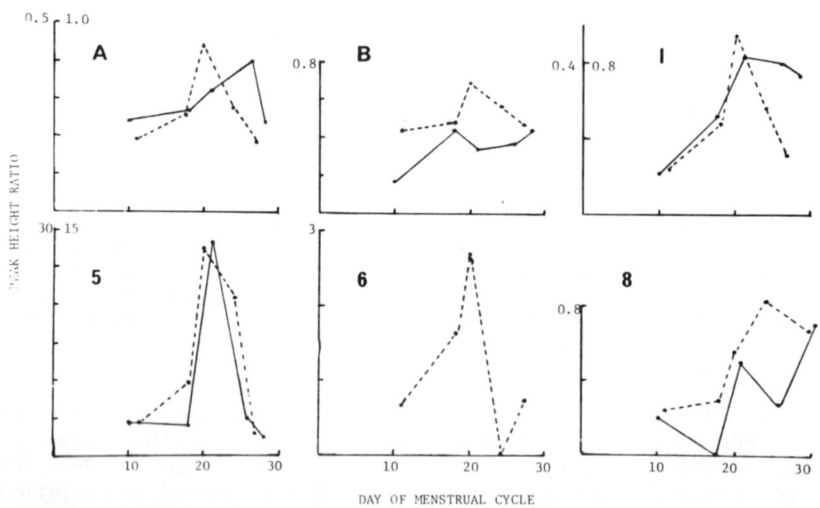

FIGURE 9. Changes in peak height ratios of proteins in the luminal fluid through the menstrual cycle for subject A (—) and subject B (- - -). Peak height ratios relative to peak 11 were calculated as described in FIGURE 2.

The coincidence of the relative change in content of certain luminal proteins with the potential time of blastocyst presence and implantation suggests a physiologic function for the proteins; although this function is not known.

References

1. Ferenczy, A. & R. M. Richart. 1974. Female reproductive system. *In* Dynamics of Scan and Transmission Electron Microscopy. John Wiley & Sons, Inc. New York, N.Y.
2. Kohorn, E. I., S. I. Rice, S. Hemperley & M. Gordon. 1972. The relation of the structure of progestational steroids to nucleolar differentiation in human endometrium. J. Clin. Endocrinol. **34:** 257–264.
3. Novak, E. R. & J. D. Woodruff. 1974. Gynecologic and Obstetric Pathology. 7th edit.: 155–168. W. B. Saunders Company. Philadelphia, Pa.
4. Downie, J., N. L. Poyser & M. Wunderlich. 1974. Levels of prostaglandins in human endometrium during the normal menstrual cycle. J. Physiol. (London) **236:** 465–472.
5. Hughes, E. C., T. V. Csermely, R. D. Jacobs & P. A. O'Hern. 1974. Biochemical parameters of abnormal endometrium. Gynecol. Oncol. **2:** 205–220.
6. Crocker, S. G., P. J. D. Milton, R. W. Taylor & R. J. B. King. 1975. In vitro studies on endometrium, endometrial and ovarian carcinoma. *In* Gynaecological Malignancy. M. G. Brush & R. W. Taylor, Eds.: 179–193. Baillière Tindall. London, England.
7. Beier, H. N. 1974. Ovarian steroids in embryonic development before nidation. *In* Advances in the Biosciences. G. Raspé, Ed. Vol. 13: 199–219.
8. Daniel, J. C. 1971. Uterine proteins and embryonic development. *In* Advances in the Biosciences. G. Raspé, Ed. Vol. 6: 191–203.
9. Beier, H. N. & K. Beier-Hellwig. 1973. Specific secretory protein of the female genital tract. Acta Endocrinol. Suppl. **180:** 404–425.
10. Garcea, N., A. Caruso & A. Bompiani. 1973. Proteic content of human uterine secretion. Acta Eur. Fertil. **4:** 11–22.
11. Gravlee, L. C. 1969. Jet-irrigation method for the diagnosis of endometrial adenocarcinoma. Obstet. Gynecol. **34:** 168–173.
12. Weber, K. & M. Osborn. 1969. The reliability of molecular weight determinations by dodecyl sulphate-polyacrylamide gel electrophoresis. J. Biol. Chem. **244:** 4406–4412.
13. Notides, A. C., D. E. Hamilton & J. H. Rudolph. 1973. The action of a human uterine protease on the estrogen receptor. Endocrinology **93:** 210–216.
14. Montgomery, R. 1957. Determination of glycogen. Arch. Biochem. **67:** 378–386.
15. Lowry, O. H., N. J. Rosebrough, A. L. Farr & R. J. Randall. 1971. Protein measurements with the Folin phenol reagent. J. Biol. Chem. **193:** 265–276.
16. Levey, I. L. & J. C. Daniel. 1976. Isolation and translation of blastokinin mRNA. Biol. Reprod. **14:** 163–174.
17. Wagner, R. K. & P. W. Jungblut. 1976. Differentiation between steroid hormone receptors, CBG and SHBG in human target organ extracts by a single-step assay. Mol. Cell. Endocrinol. **4:** 13–24.
18. Peterson, R. P. & E. Spaziani. 1969. Cycloheximide and cortisol inhibition of estradiol-stimulated uterine uptake and distribution of homologous serum albumin and alphaglobulin in the rat. Endocrinology **85:** 932–940.
19. Wilson, E. W. 1969. The effect of oestradiol-17β on enzymes concerned with metabolism of carbohydrate in human endometrium *in vitro*. J. Endocrinol. **44:** 63–68.

Discussion

Dr. Joshi: It may be pertinent to discuss here our recent work on the synthesis of specific proteins in the human endometrium. We have identified two antigenic proteins, tentatively designated as antigens A and B, in progestational phase endometria by immunologic methods, by use of antisera generated against soluble antigens of decidual phase endometrium of tubal pregnancy. Immunoelectrophoretic analysis of 84 endometrial specimens (Table D1) has revealed the presence of antigens A and B in all decidualized endometria (DE) of uterine or tubal pregnancy and in eight of 31 samples of secretory phase endometrium (SE). Antigen A alone was encountered in three specimens of SE. However, none of the 32 proliferative phase endometria (PE) or 20 samples of SE contained detectable amounts of antigen A or B. In subsequent studies, the conventional double-labeling technique was employed to determine whether the progestational phase endometrium was the site of synthesis of the two antigens. In each of the six experiments performed, soluble proteins in PE and DE were labeled *in vitro* with [^{14}C]- and [^{3}H]leucine (311 mCi/mmol), respectively. Duplicate aliquots of the mixture of ^{14}C- and ^{3}H-labeled soluble proteins were subjected to sodium dodecyl sulfate-gel electrophoresis (1969. J. Biol. Chem. **244:** 4406–4412) on two separate 1% acrylamide gels. After electrophoresis, one gel was utilized for the localization of antigens A and B by immunodiffusion (1976. Fertil. Steril. **27:** 730–739), by use of an antiserum that was absorbed with normal male serum and cytosol of human term placenta. The other gel was sectioned into about 1.2-mm thick slices, and ratios of ^{3}H/^{14}C in the slices were determined by liquid scintillation spectrometry. The results of a typical experiment, presented in Figure D1 demonstrate that the ratios (1.75–3.07) of ^{3}H/^{14}C in the protein fractions that contained both antigens A and B (fractions 23–25) were significantly higher than that (1.21) in the original mixture. In other studies, the mixtures of tissue cytosol proteins, which contained ^{14}C- and ^{3}H-labeled proteins derived from PE and DE, respectively, were supplemented with partially pure preparations of antigens A and B (nonradioactive carrier antigen). A predetermined amount of absorbed antiserum was added to precipitate antigens A and B from the mixture. Analysis of radioactivity in the immunoprecipitate showed that ^{3}H/^{14}C ratios in the precipitates were two- to sixfold higher than those in the original mixtures used for immunoprecipitation. These studies suggest that the development of the progestin-dominated human endometrium during early pregnancy is associated with induction or stimulation of the synthesis of at least two specific antigenic proteins. Antigens A and B have now

Table D1

Analysis of Antigenic Components in Human Endometria

Tissue	Source of Tissue	Total Number	Number of Tissues Containing Antigens: A + B	A	B	Nil
Decidualized endometrium	early (5–7 weeks) pregnancy	20	20	0	0	—
Decidualized endometrium	tubal pregnancy	1	1	0	0	—
Proliferative phase endometrium	postmenopausal, infertility, or menstrual disorders	32	—	0	0	32
Secretory phase endometrium	infertility or menstrual disorders	31	8	3	0	20

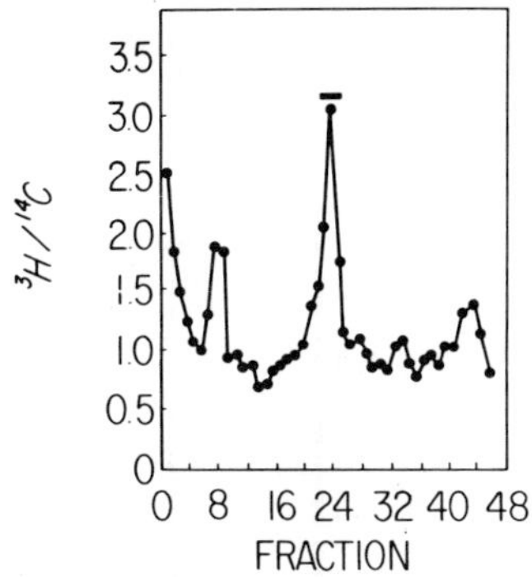

FIGURE D1. Fractionation of soluble leucine-labeled endometrial proteins by SDS-gel electrophoresis. $^{3}H^{14}C$ ratios were determined in fractions that contained ^{3}H- and ^{14}C-labeled proteins synthesized by DE and PE, respectively. The solid bar represents the location of antigens A and B in the fractions. Fractions 43–45 contained the tracking dye. (From Joshi *et al.* By permission of *Fertility and Sterility*.)

been partially purified and characterized. However, their role in early pregnancy is not known.

DR. L. M. DEMERS: Dr. King, I have looked at the Gravlee wash of endometrium in the same way that you have, and I also don't see any difference in the protein profile between serum and the material in the wash.

Have you performed the organ culture experiments for periods longer than 40 hr? Have you measured progesterone receptors in the tissues in culture?

DR. KING: Tissue morphology is not maintained well after 48 hr in culture. Therefore, we have confined our experiments to 48-hr incubations. In answer to your question about the progesterone receptors, we suspect that the addition of estrogen helps to maintain progesterone receptor levels. I would, however, stress that our results on this point are not conclusive. Second, we did control experiments in which tritiated amino acids were added to unlabeled proteins and electrophoresis was then performed. Virtually no tritium was associated with the various protein bands, with the majority of the tritium running at the front of the gel.

DR. M. FEIGELSON: You mentioned at the beginning of your talk that you did not find uteroglobin in these human secretions. Was that by molecular weight determination? Did you not find a 15,000 molecular weight peak?

DR. KING: My conclusion about not finding uteroglobin was based purely on the absence of a peak on the SDS gels at 15,000 molecular weight.

DR. FEIGELSON: We do see antigenic material in human endometrium and uterine and tubal flushings, which cross-reacts with antibodies to rabbit uteroglobin. This cross-reaction may mean that there is a protein in the human with antigenic sites similar to that of rabbit uteroglobin but possibly of a different molecular weight.

DR. P. BECK: Dr. King, you mentioned that you used insulin in your incubation media for the culture. Can you see any synthesis of peak 6 in the absence of any insulin in your medium? I raised the question because, as I'll show in my talk tomorrow, there is a fairly consistent increase in insulin production in various species given large doses of progesterone at the level comparable to that found in pregnancy. This would seem to be a natural enhancing effect of this kind of protein synthesis in cells. There is a lot of evidence that certain kinds of protein synthesis may be enhanced by insulin secretion.

DR. KING: I cannot answer you directly, because we have not carried out a comparison of protein profiles in the presence or absence of insulin. Insulin was added because it increased the morphologic integrity of the explants.

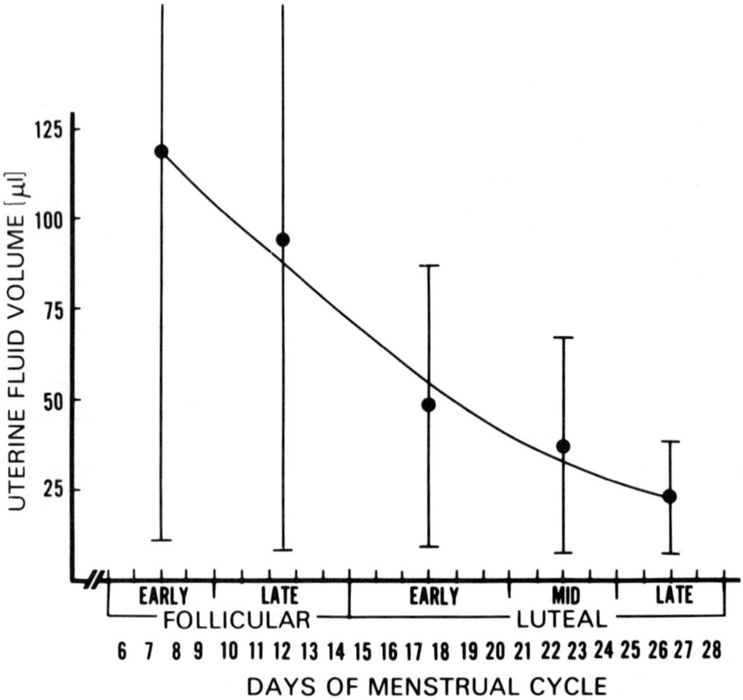

FIGURE D2. (From Clemetson *et al.* By permission of *Journal of Obstetrics and Gynaecology of the British Commonwealth.*)

DR. C. A. B. CLEMETSON *(Methodist Hospital of Brooklyn, Brooklyn, N.Y.):* Dr. King, in your first slide, you showed a very conventional view of secretion, an increase in fluid volume in the human uterus during the luteal phase. What was that increase based on? I have measured uterine fluid volume in humans (FIGURE D2) and found a decrease in the luteal phase (1973. Clemetson *et al.*, J. Obstet. Gynaecol. Brit. Commonwealth **80:** 553). Were those proteins in the glandular lumen not inspissated as a result of reabsorption of water? I think the luteal phase is the resorptive phase. Now, maybe there is secretion of proteins, but the volume is actually less in the luteal phase according to my findings.

DR. KING: I have no other information on whether the luminal material is a secretion. My graph was taken from the standard textbook *Gynecologic and Obstetric Pathology* by E. R. Novak and J. D. Woodruff (1974).

DR. CLEMETSON: Have you measured total protein washings in the proliferative and luteal phases? Is there any increase of protein in the luteal phase?

DR. KING: Our measurements on these two patients indicate no significant differences in protein content as one passes through the cycle.

FACTORS THAT INFLUENCE STEROID INDUCTION OF ENDOMETRIAL GLYCOGENESIS IN ORGAN CULTURE*

Laurence M. Demers, Peter D. Feil, and C. Wayne Bardin

Departments of Pathology, Medicine, and Biological Chemistry
The Milton S. Hershey Medical Center
The Pennsylvania State University
Hershey, Pennsylvania 17033

Introduction

Studies of progesterone action on chick oviduct have suggested that hormone-stimulated differentiation is mediated via steroid receptor interaction with the genome.[1] The mechanism of action of progesterone on the mammalian uterus, however, is less well understood, due in part to its broad spectrum of activities. Progesterone can stimulate uterine growth,[2] inhibit contraction,[3,4] potentiate[5] or inhibit actions of estrogen,[6,7] and increase specific uterine proteins, such as blastokinin.[8,9] In addition, progestins promote the formation of a secretory endometrium, an event required for ovum implantation and pregnancy.[10-12] One of the features of the latter steroid-mediated response is the accumulation of endometrial glycogen.[13] The specificity of this effect suggested that it might be used to study the action of progesterone on the uterus.

Experiments with fragments of human endometrium indicated that progesterone-induced glycogenesis can be studied *in vitro*.[14,15] There are several reasons, however, that make the use of human material inconvenient. First, the tissue supply is unpredictable. Second, the hormonal milieu of the tissue donors is variable, which alters both the endogenous glycogen levels and the amount of glycogen that endometrial explants will accumulate in culture. For studies on the mechanism of hormone-stimulated glycogenesis, it was important, therefore, to find an animal that could provide uniform endometrial fragments for *in vitro* experiments. The present study defines some of the factors that influence this response in guinea pig uterus. The results indicate that this *in vitro* system will provide both insight into the mechanism of steroid action and a simple bioassay of progestational activity.

Materials and Methods

Animals

Female guinea pigs were treated with diethylstilbestrol† (DES, 20 μg/day) not sooner than 10 days after castration. Tissue was usually removed 18–24 hr after the last injection.

*Supported by Contract NO1-HD-1-2228 from the National Institutes of Health.

†Chemical names of the steroids used are as follows: diethylstilbestrol, 3,4-bis(*p*-hydroxyphenyl)-3-hexene; progesterone, Δ^4-pregnene-3,20-dione; medroxyprogesterone acetate, 6α-methyl-17α-hydroxy-4-pregnene-3,20-dione acetate; 6α-methylprogesterone, 6α-methyl-4-pregnene-3,20-dione; 16α-hydroxyprogesterone, 16α-hydroxy-4-pregnene-3,-20-dione; 17α-hydroxyprogesterone, 17α-hydroxy-4-pregnene-3,20-dione.

Chemicals

[1,2-^{3}H]Progesterone (57.4 Ci/mmol) and [4-^{14}C]progesterone (52.8 mCi/mmol) were purchased from New England Nuclear. [1,2-^{3}H]Medroxyprogesterone acetate (MPA, 58 Ci/mmol) and [^{14}C]medroxyprogesterone acetate were synthesized in this laboratory, as described previously.[16] Unlabeled steroids were obtained from various sources. The remaining chemicals were purchased from the following companies: actinomycin D and α-amanitine, Calbiochem; cycloheximide, Sigma Chemical Company; regular insulin, Squibb; and Trowell's T8 medium, fetal calf serum, and antibiotic-antimycotic solution (no. 524), Grand Island Biological Company. Glass-distilled solvents used for thin-layer chromatography were obtained from Burdick and Jackson.

Organ Culture

The animals were killed, and the excised uteri were immediately placed in a glass container of ice cold medium. The endometrium was separated from myometrium by use of fine scissors. Organ culture was performed in siliconized glass dishes that contained a steel grid and sufficient medium (ca. 2 ml) to adequately wet the top of the grid. Endometrial explants (20–40 mg, total wet weight) were placed symmetrically on the grid in contact with culture medium. The cultures were maintained at 37°C in a mixture of air and 5% CO_2. Steroid stock solutions (1 mg/ml in ethanol) were diluted with culture medium immediately prior to use and were added dropwise to the culture. The final ethanol concentration in the culture medium was maintained at 0.4%. In each experiment, the control culture contained the tissue and ethanol vehicle without steroids. All other compounds added to the culture medium were dissolved in distilled water. All cultures were performed in duplicate. The results of each assay were compared to the control culture (absence of steroid).

Glycogen Assay

At the termination of the culture period, the explants were removed from the grid and immediately frozen on dry ice and weighed. One explant from each culture dish was removed to fixative for histologic (hematoxylin and eosin) and histochemical (periodic acid-Schiff) analysis. In cell experiments, histology and histochemistry confirmed the biochemical results. Glycogen content was determined colorimetrically, as previously described.[17]

Thin-Layer Chromatography

In some experiments, culture was performed supplemented with ^{3}H-labeled steroid (ca. 50,000 cpm), with incubation conducted as described above. Medium was decanted into an extraction tube. The culture dishes and grids were then rinsed successively with medium and ethanol to assure quantitative recovery of steroid. The medium and washes were pooled and extracted with 7 vol of dichloromethane after addition of 50 μg of the appropriate unlabeled steroid and ^{14}C-labeled steroids (500–1000 cpm). The extracts were washed, dried, and fractionated by thin-layer chromatography, as described previously.[16] After correcting for procedural losses, the extent of metabolism was calculated from the original tritium added to the culture and the amount recovered as unmetabolized steroid.

Results

Effect of Steroid Dose and Incubation Time on Endometrial Glycogen Synthesis

An increase in uterine glycogen deposition occurred *in vivo* in response to progestins, as shown in Figure 1. MPA was more effective than progesterone in stimulating a glycogenic response at 6 hr.

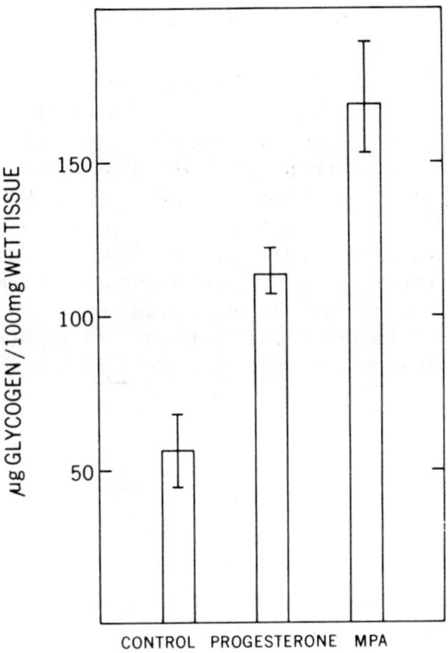

Figure 1. Effect of progestins on endometrial glycogen accumulation *in vivo*. Two-day estrogen-primed guinea pigs were injected intravenously with vehicle, progesterone (1 mg), or MPA (1 mg) and sacrificed after 6 hr. Glycogen was determined as described in Materials and Methods. Each group contained at least three animals, and the results show the mean and range of the glycogen measurements.

The ability of progestins to induce glycogen synthesis *in vitro* was then examined. A positive dose-response relationship between the concentration of progesterone and MPA in the culture medium and glycogen synthesis could also be demonstrated *in vitro* (Figure 2). A two- to fivefold increase in glycogen deposition was observed in endometrial explants cultured for 48 hr in the presence of the highest dose of progestins. Again, MPA was more potent than progesterone at all doses tested. That this *in vitro* response was specific for the uterus was suggested by the observations that MPA and progesterone had no dose-dependent effect on glycogen synthesis in liver and spleen cultured under similar culture conditions.

The time course of progestin-induced glycogen synthesis was studied next. The effect of two doses of progesterone and MPA are shown in Figure 3A and

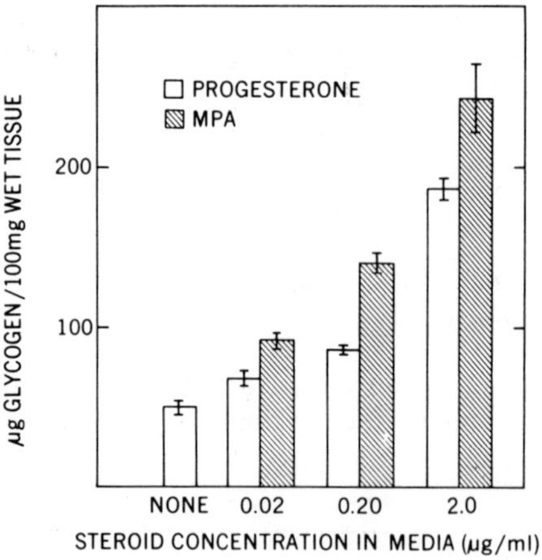

FIGURE 2. Dose-dependent progestin-induced glycogen response *in vitro*. Guinea pig endometrial fragments were cultured for 48 hr in the presence of increasing concentrations of steroid, and glycogen was measured as described in MATERIALS AND METHODS. The results show the average and range of duplicate determinations.

3B, respectively. The glycogen content of endometrium cultured in the absence of progestin remained relatively constant for 72 hr; however, glycogen accumulation was increased significantly ($p < 0.05$) by 12 hr in response to 1.0 μg/per milliliter of progesterone and MPA. In cultures treated with a low dose of progesterone (0.1 μg/ml), glycogen synthesis appeared to plateau after 48 hr. By contrast, the large dose of progesterone (1.0 μg/ml) and both doses of MPA produced a steady increase in glycogen for 72 hr. That the response appeared to plateau with the lowest dose of progesterone raised the possibility that steroid metabolism could limit the biologic response in this system.

To test this hypothesis, ^{3}H-labeled steroids were added to the cultures, and recovery studies were performed to determine the extent of metabolism at 48 hr.

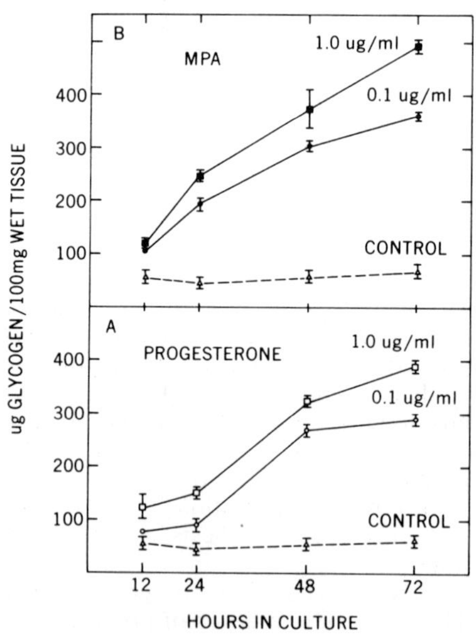

FIGURE 3. Accumulation of glycogen with incubation time. Guinea pig endometrial fragments were placed in culture for various times along with progesterone (open symbols) or MPA (solid symbols) and assayed for glycogen as described in MATERIALS AND METHODS. Controls (△) in the absence of steroid are shown for comparison. Each point represents the average and range of duplicate determinations.

Complete recovery of added tritium was achieved, and chromatographic analysis revealed that 50 and 25% of progesterone and MPA, respectively, were metabolized.

Effect of Prior Hormone Treatment on Endometrial Glycogen Synthesis

Estrogen treatment of guinea pigs and other mammals increases uterine progesterone receptor content and potentiates the action of progesterone *in vivo*.[5,18] The effect of *in vivo* estrogen administration on the *in vitro* response to progesterone was investigated next. Endometrial fragments were removed from castrate guinea pigs (treated for 0–4 days with estrogen) and cultured with progesterone for 48 hr. The results shown in FIGURE 4 indicate that estrogen is required to maximize the sensitivity of the uterine endometrium to progestin action. Two days of *in vivo* estrogen priming were selected for routine use in the organ culture assay.

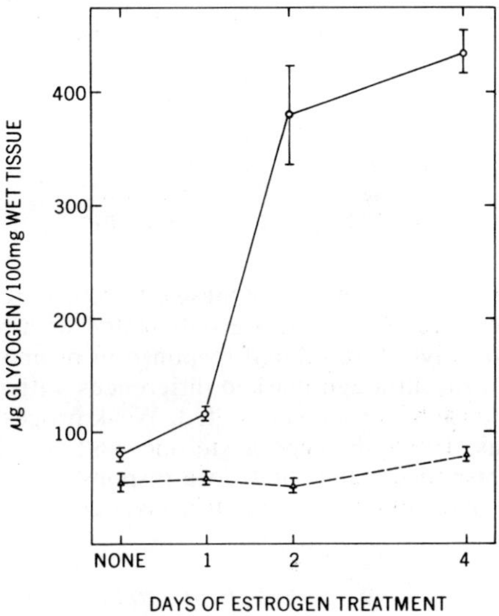

FIGURE 4. Effects of *in vivo* estrogen treatment on progestin-induced *in vitro* glycogen response. Guinea pigs were injected subcutaneously with DES as indicated, and endometrium was then cultured for 48 hr with (○) or without (△) progesterone (2 µg/ml), as described in MATERIALS AND METHODS. Each point represents the average and range of duplicate determinations.

The effect of *in vivo* administration of progesterone on endometrial glycogenesis was investigated next. Animals were estrogen primed for 2 days and then given a single injection of progesterone (1 mg, iv) on the third day. After 24 hr, uteri were removed and placed in culture. The results of this study (FIGURE 5) indicate that *in vivo* administration of progesterone potentiates the action of this steroid *in vitro*. *In vivo* administration of MPA also potentiates subsequent progestin action on cultured endometrium.

Steroid Specificity of Endometrial Glycogenesis in Organ Culture

Having maximized conditions with respect to the medium, time, and estrogen priming, the comparative effects of several steroids were then tested to determine their ability to induce endometrial glycogenesis in organ culture. TABLE 1 depicts

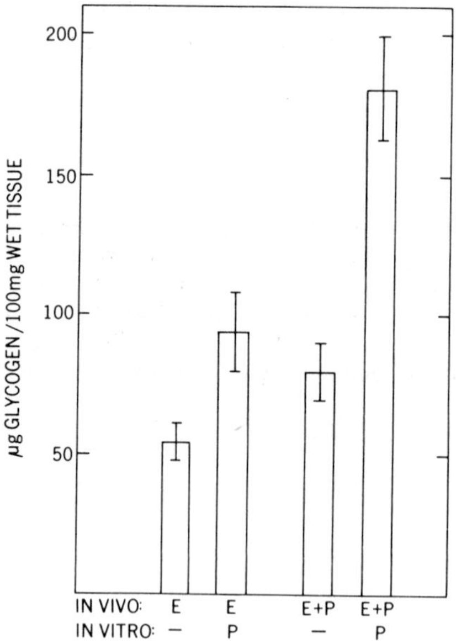

FIGURE 5. Effect of *in vivo* progesterone treatment on progestin-induced *in vitro* glycogen response. Two-day estrogen-primed guinea pigs were injected intravenously with vehicle or progesterone (1 mg). After 24 hr, endometrium was placed in culture for 48 hr with or without progesterone supplementation. The results show the average and range of duplicate determinations.

the relative effects of these different steroids on endometrial glycogen synthesis in culture. All of the steroids tested with reputed progestational activity showed a positive dose-related response in promoting endometrial glycogen deposition *in vitro*, although marked differences with respect to the magnitude of the response to each steroid were noted. Weak progestins that were possible metabolites, such as 16α-hydroxyprogesterone and 17α-hydroxyprogesterone, produced minor responses, and their dose-response curves were flat. Testosterone and cortisol, while inducing endometrial glycogenesis, also yielded flat dose-response curves.

Effects of Fetal Calf Serum (FCS) and Insulin on Endometrial Glycogen Synthesis

Because 10% FCS was used in the studies described above, the requirement for this component was next assessed. Endometrial explants were cultured in Trowell's T8 medium supplemented with 0–20% FCS and progesterone (FIGURE

TABLE 1

PROGESTIN INDUCTION OF ENDOMETRIAL GLYCOGEN ACCUMULATION*

Steroid	Micrograms of Glycogen/100 mg of Wet Tissue
Progesterone	238
Medroxyprogesterone acetate	299
6α-Methylprogesterone	375
17α-Hydroxyprogesterone	70

*Guinea pig endometrium was cultured 48 hr in the presence of steroid (2 µg/ml) and then assayed for glycogen, as described in MATERIALS AND METHODS.

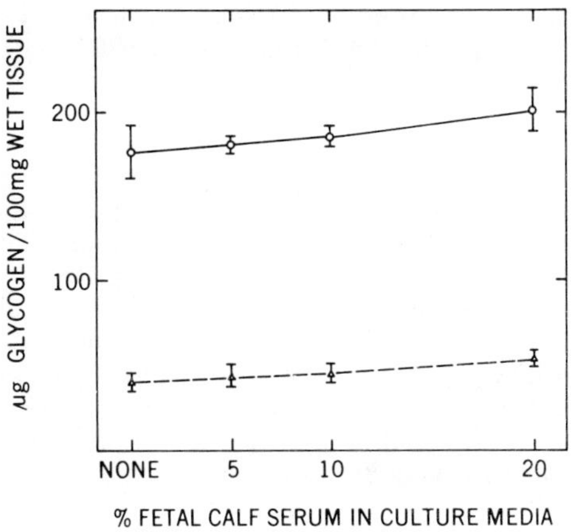

FIGURE 6. Effect of FCS on *in vitro* glycogen response to progestin. Endometrial fragments were incubated for 48 hr with (○) or without (△) progesterone (2 µg/ml) in media supplemented with FCS. Each point shows the average and range of duplicate determinations.

6). The addition of FCS produced no further enhancement of progestin-induced glycogen response that could be dose related to the amount of serum in the culture. These observations indicate that glycogen synthesis can be studied in Trowell's chemically defined medium.

Because insulin (50 µg/ml) is a component of Trowell's T8 medium, it was important to determine the role of this hormone on the progesterone response. Accordingly, endometrial explants were cultured in complete Trowell's T8 medium and in incomplete medium with various concentrations of added insulin. The results of this study are shown in FIGURE 7. Progesterone produced no increase in endometrial glycogen synthesis in the incomplete Trowell's T8 medium (without insulin). This requirement for insulin could not be overcome by increasing the progesterone concentration 10-fold (not shown). The sensitivity of the endometrium

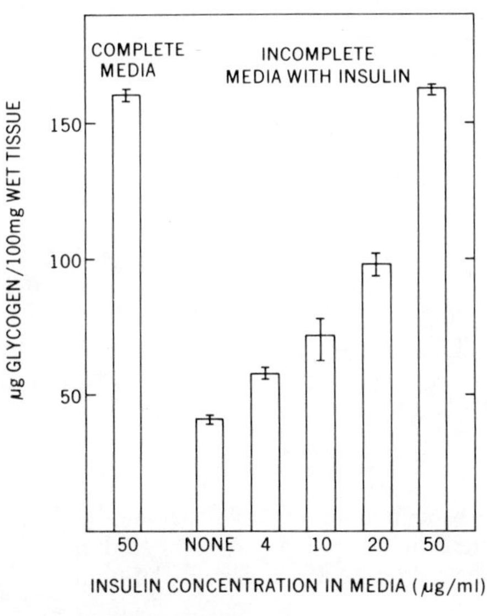

FIGURE 7. Effect of insulin on endometrial glycogen response. Endometrial fragments were incubated with progesterone (1 µg/ml) for 48 hr in complete media or in media supplemented with increasing concentrations of insulin and then were assayed for glycogen as described in MATERIALS AND METHODS. The results show the average and range of duplicate determinations.

to progesterone was partially restored by as little as 4 μg per milliliter of insulin and was completely restored with 20–50 μg per milliliter (FIGURE 7).

Inhibition of Endometrial Glycogen Synthesis

To determine whether progesterone-induced glycogenesis was dependent on RNA and protein synthesis, several inhibitors of transcription and translation were added to the medium. As shown in FIGURE 8, addition of actinomycin D, α-amanitine, or cycloheximide to the medium completely inhibited the glycogen response. In another study (not shown), endometrial fragments were cultured with progesterone for 24 hr to initiate glycogen synthesis. This tissue was then cultured for an additional 24 hr in the presence of inhibitors (1 μg/ml of actinomycin D or α-amanitine or 10 μg/ml of cycloheximide) plus progesterone. Each of the inhibitors blocked further glycogen synthesis.

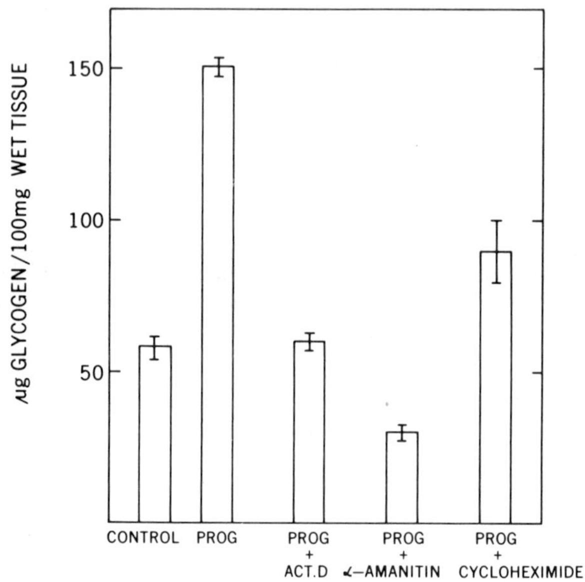

FIGURE 8. Effect of inhibitors of RNA and protein synthesis on *in vitro* glycogen response. Endometrial fragments were incubated with progesterone (1 μg/ml) for 48 hr in the presence of actinomycin D (1 μg/ml), α-amanitine (1 μg/ml), or cycloheximide (1 μg/ml) and then assayed for glycogen as described in MATERIALS AND METHODS. The results show the average and range of duplicate determinations.

DISCUSSION

In recent years, the molecular events associated with steroid-mediated cellular responses have been studied with a variety of techniques. Several studies have shown that the initial step of progesterone action on the uterus is the binding of steroid by a specific receptor protein.[1,19] From these experiments, a correlation was established between *in vitro* binding and *in vivo* biologic activity of some progestins. Before these studies could be extended, it was necessary to establish a sensitive system in which progestational activity could be assayed *in vitro*. The results of the present study demonstrate that endometrial organ culture provides such a system in which both the potency relationship of different synthetic progestins and the mechanism of steroid hormone action can be studied.

The precise requirements for *in vitro* endometrial glycogen synthesis were established in tissue explants. A dose-related response to progestins was demonstrated. In the culture system, as *in vivo*, MPA was more potent than progesterone in promoting glycogen deposition. Furthermore, other potent progestins also were able to promote a dose-related increase in glycogen synthesis. Although testosterone and cortisol are known to induce glycogen synthesis in other tissues, in the present study, these steroids did not produce a dose-related response, which suggests that they affect carbohydrate metabolism at a control point different from that of progestins.

In vivo estrogen administration for at least 2 days was essential for maximum response to progestin. That there was some increase in glycogen in untreated animals was most likely due to a response by the myometrium. The response by the myometrium to progestin, however, does not seem to be as dependent on estrogen sensitization as that of the endometrium, because the response in 2-day estrogen-primed animals was only about one-third of that in endometrium.[23]

Exposure of the uterus to progesterone *in vivo* resulted in an augmented *in vitro* response. Previous studies have shown that *in vivo* tissue and blood levels of progesterone at 24 hr after its administration are sufficiently low as to preclude the involvement of residual progesterone in the glycogen response in culture.[16] In addition, the control levels from the *in vivo* progesterone-treated animals are only slightly higher than the controls from untreated animals, indicating that organ culture in the presence of progesterone does not release stored glycogen that had been formed in the *in vivo* response.

Two components of the culture medium (FCS and insulin) were investigated to determine their role in the glycogen response. Although FCS contributed little to glycogen synthesis, it was usually added to the culture medium because it helped maintain progestins in solution. By contrast, the presence of insulin was found to be an obligatory requirement for glycogen synthesis, and this requirement could not be overcome by increasing the progesterone content 10-fold. Whether insulin promotes glucose entry into endometrial tissue or stimulates the enzymes that control glycogen synthesis cannot be determined from these experiments. Further studies are underway to define the role of insulin in this system.

The control of glycogen metabolism has been shown to occur both hormonally and nonhormonally (substrate, product, or cofactor inhibition) at the level of the enzymes glycogen synthetase and glycogen phosphorylase. Both cortisol and insulin promote liver glycogen synthesis through either activation or induction of the glycogen synthetase enzyme system.[20,21] Whether progesterone acts in a similar fashion on this enzyme in endometrial tissue remains to be established. The complete inhibition of progestin-induced glycogenesis in our system by inhibitors of RNA and protein synthesis suggests that progesterone may be causing this response by induction of the enzymes that control glycogen metabolism. Recent evidence in the rat indicates that both actinomycin D and cycloheximide can completely block estrogen-directed synthesis of new synthetase enzyme.[22] Mechanisms by which progestins and insulin affect glycogen metabolism in the guinea pig endometrium remain to be elucidated.

Acknowledgments

The authors thank Miss Naomi R. Cole for her expert technical assistance and Marlene Brinser and Susan Keller for their help in typing the manuscript.

References

1. O'Malley, B. W. & A. R. Means. 1974. Science **183:** 610.
2. Telfer, M. A. & F. L. Hisaw. 1957. Acta Endocrinol. **25:** 390.
3. Csapo, A. I. & H. Takeda. 1965. Amer. J. Obstet. Gynecol. **91:** 221.
4. Ichikawa, S. & A. Bortoff. Amer. J. Physiol. **219:** 1763.
5. Zarrow, H. X., F. L. Hisaw & H. A. Salhanick. 1954. Amer. J. Obstet. Gynecol. **67:** 1139.
6. Singhal, R. L., J. R. E. Valadares & G. M. Ling. 1967. Metabolism **16:** 271.
7. Oka, T. & R. T. Schimke. 1969. Science **163:** 83.
8. Arthur, A. T. & J. C. Daniel, Jr. 1972. Fertil. Steril. **23:** 115.
9. Bullock, D. W. & G. F. Willen. 1974. Proc. Soc. Exp. Biol. Med. **146:** 294.
10. Boyd, J. D. 1957. Men. Soc. Endocrinol. **6:** 26.
11. Allen, W. M. & G. W. Corner. 1930. Proc. Soc. Exp. Biol. Med. **27:** 403.
12. Connolly, M. R., J. Bitman, H. C. Cecil & T. R. Wrenn. 1962. Amer. J. Physiol. **203:**717.
13. Noyes, R. W., A. T. Hertig & J. Rock. 1950. Fertil. Steril. **1:** 3.
14. Hughes, E. C., L. M. Demers, T. Csermely & D. B. Jones. 1969. Amer. J. Obstet. Gynecol. **105:** 707.
15. Csermely, T., L. M. Demers & E. C. Hughes. 1969. Obstet. Gynecol. **34:** 252.
16. Feil, P. D., M. Miljković & C. W. Bardin. 1976. Endocrinology **98:** 1508.
17. Demers, L. M., S. G. Gabbe, C. A. Villee & R. O. Greep. 1972. Endocrinology **91:** 270.
18. Freifeld, M. L., P. D. Feil & C. W. Bardin. 1974. Steroids **23:** 93.
19. Kontula, K., O. Jänne, R. Vihko, E. deJager, J. deVisser & F. Zeelen. 1975. Acta Endocrinol. **78:** 574.
20. Hers, H. G. & H. deWulf. 1968. *In* Control of Glycogen Metabolism. W. J. Whelan, Ed. Academic Press, Inc. New York, N.Y.
21. Larner, J., C. Villar-Palasi, N. D. Goldberg, J. S. Bishop, F. Huijing, J. I. Wenger, H. Sasko & N. B. Brown. 1968. *In* Control of Glycogen Metabolism. W. J. Whelan, Ed. Academic Press, Inc. New York, N.Y.
22. Demers, L. M. 1974. J. Steroid Biochem. **5:** 343.
23. Feil, P. D. & L. M. Demers. 1976. Unpublished observations.

Discussion

Dr. P. Beck: Do you have any idea as to whether progesterone may have some effect on the speed at which insulin gets into these cells? I ask that question because Srivastava *et al.* (1975, Eur. J. Clin. Invest. **5:** 425) and others within the last year have published some data that suggest that women on contraceptive steroids have an increase in the space of distribution of insulin and a prolongation of the half-life of insulin. This finding suggests that perhaps the insulin is going into bigger spaces, including cells.

Dr. Feil: There are several possible points, including the one you mention, where insulin may be affecting glycogen metabolism, such as substrate levels or enzyme activities. At this time, we have not examined any of these possibilities.

DR. P. K. SIITERI: I was intrigued with the observation that you can block the progesterone effect with 16α-hydroxyprogesterone. Do you have any information concerning its ability to block progesterone binding in uterine or other systems? Do you believe your effect is mediated by receptors?

DR. FEIL: We have information on the affinity of 16α-hydroxyprogesterone for the receptor, and it is only about 2%, with progesterone being 100%. It does not block cytosolic progesterone binding. We are presently open-minded as to whether this effect is mediated via the receptor.

DR. L. TSENG: Have you studied the effect of cortisol *in vitro* at various concentrations?

DR. FEIL: Yes, we had a dose response for cortisol over the same dose range that we used for progesterone. Cortisol was in the physiologic range, as reported by Diamond *et al.* (1969. Endocrinology **84:** 1143).

DR. J. H. CLARK: How are you going to use glycogen deposition as a specific assay for progestational activity?

DR. FEIL: We hope to use this system as an *in vitro* assay for progestational activity. It may be that the response to estrogen is another peculiarity of the guinea pig, because human endometrium apparently does not respond to estrogen with increased glycogen deposition (1971. Csermely *et al.* Amer. J. Obstet. Gynecol. **109:** 1066; 1974. Shapiro & Hagerman, J. Endocrinol. **62:** 663). There may also be different steroid effects on the various enzymes involved in the glycogen metabolic pathway.

DR. CLARK: Simple glycogen deposition could not be used, though.

DR. FEIL: With the guinea pig and the assay in its present form, that is correct. We hope that the combined use of inhibitors will enable us to determine specific progestational activity.

PROGESTERONE INDUCTION OF MESSENGER RNA AND PROTEIN SYNTHESIS IN RABBIT UTERUS*

D. W. Bullock

Department of Cell Biology
Baylor College of Medicine
Houston, Texas 77030

In all mammalian species, with the possible exception of the elephant, progesterone is essential for the maintenance of pregnancy. Together with estrogen, progesterone is also responsible for the endometrial changes that prepare the uterus for implantation. Yet, in contrast to estrogen, little is known of the biochemical events in the uterus that follow progesterone administration, and almost nothing is known about the molecular mechanisms by which progesterone acts on this tissue.

Part of the reason for this dearth of knowledge lies in the lack of a suitable biochemical marker in the uterus comparable to the secretion of avidin by the hen oviduct, which has allowed progress in understanding the mechanism of action of progesterone in a nonmammalian system.[1] The discovery, about 10 years ago, of uteroglobin, a major secretory protein of the preimplantation uterus in the rabbit,[2] provided a mammalian end point that we have begun to exploit as a model system for studying the mechanism of action of progesterone in the uterus.

The rabbit offers several advantages as a system for these investigations. Ovulation is induced by mating, so that the time of ovulation, and therefore the "age" of the endometrium, can be known precisely. Estrogen is not required for implantation in the rabbit, and the uterine changes in early pregnancy can be supported by progesterone alone.[3] Uteroglobin is induced by progesterone[4–7] and is a protein that has been fairly well characterized that provides a biochemical marker for progesterone action.

Regulation of Uteroglobin Secretion

Uteroglobin shows a characteristic pattern of secretion in early pregnancy, becoming detectable by gel electrophoresis on Day 3, reaching a peak at Days 5–6, and disappearing by Day 10[5,8,9] (Figure 1). The protein can be detected immunologically in uterine flushings from nonpregnant rabbits,[9] and measurable amounts are found by radioimmunoassay before Day 3 and as late as Day 12 of pregnancy.[10]

Several groups have shown that uteroglobin can be induced by treatment of ovariectomized rabbits with progesterone.[5–7] Pretreatment with estrogen is not necessary, although estrogen treatment may potentiate the stimulation achieved with progesterone.[11] The pattern of secretion induced by progesterone is similar to that seen in pregnancy or pseudopregnancy, where uteroglobin accounts for more than 40% of the total secreted protein. The tissue levels of uteroglobin have not been established.

The protein may be induced also by treatment of estrous rabbits with

*Supported by Ford Foundation Grants 68-900 and 680-0900, Rockefeller Foundation Grant 06976, and National Institutes of Health Grant HD 09378-01.

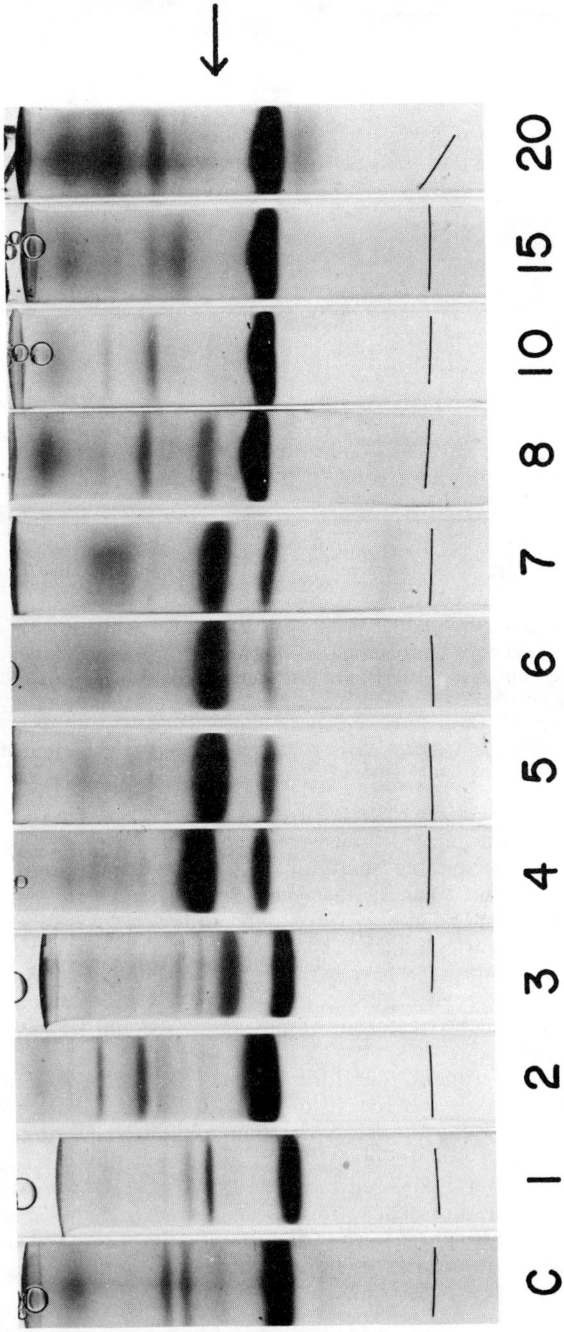

FIGURE 1. Electrophoresis of uterine flushings on 7% polyacrylamide gels in 0.02 M Tris-0.19 M glycine buffer (pH 8.4). C, control (nonpregnant); 1–20, day of pregnancy. The arrow marks the position of uteroglobin.

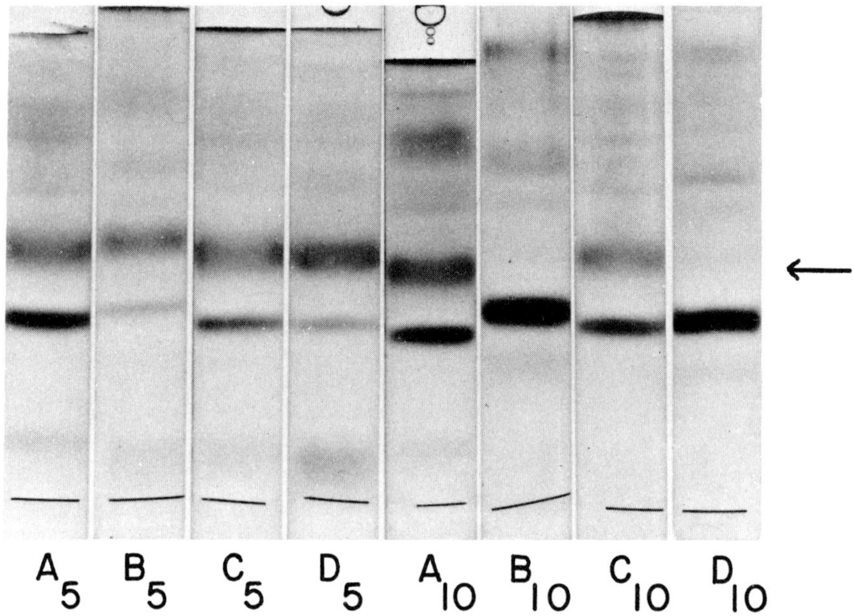

FIGURE 2. Electrophoresis of uterine flushings in 7% polyacrylamide gels in 0.02 M Tris-0.19 M glycine buffer (pH 8.4). Ovariectomized rabbits were treated with the following: A, progesterone (3 mg/kg) on Days 1–10; B, progesterone (3 mg/kg) on Days 1–10, plus estradiol benzoate (5 μg/kg) on Days 6–10; C, progesterone (1 mg/kg) on Days 1–10; D, progesterone (1 mg/kg) on Days 1–10, plus estradiol benzoate (5 μg/kg) on Days 6–10. Subscript 5 indicates collection after 5 days; subscript 10 refers to collection after 10 days. The arrow marks the position of uteroglobin.

progesterone[4] or gonadotropin.[12] When estrogen was administered during the first 3 days postcoitum, however, the secretion of uteroglobin was delayed.[12] This observation provided a clue to an anomaly in the pattern of uteroglobin secretion induced by progesterone. The anomaly arose from the fact that daily administration of progesterone to ovariectomized rabbits resulted in the persistence of uteroglobin secretion after 10 days,[6] whereas the protein has disappeared by this time in the pregnant animal. Because plasma progesterone is still rising at Day 10 of pregnancy,[13] regulation by progesterone alone cannot account for the normal pattern of uteroglobin secretion.

We performed an experiment, therefore, in which ovariectomized rabbits were treated daily with progesterone for 10 days, with estradiol superimposed on progesterone for the last 5 days in half of the animals.[7] Uterine flushings were obtained after 5 and 10 days of treatment. FIGURE 2 shows that uteroglobin was present in both groups after 5 days but that it had disappeared after 10 days in the animals treated with estradiol. These results suggested that the appearance of uteroglobin is stimulated by progesterone and that its disappearance is caused by estrogen, an interpretation not inconsistent with the reported changes in plasma estradiol in early pregnancy.[14]

The possibility that uteroglobin secretion is under dual hormonal control thus offers further inducement for its use as a model of steroid hormone action in the uterus.

Mechanism of Action of Progesterone

Detailed discussion of the molecular mechanism of action of progesterone is presented by other authors in this monograph. Our current understanding is that progesterone enters the cell by simple diffusion and binds in its target tissue to a specific cytoplasmic receptor. The progesterone receptor has been demonstrated in the rabbit uterus.[15] The progesterone-receptor complex migrates to the nucleus, where it modulates cell metabolism, principally by regulating protein synthesis.

There are three possible loci at which hormonal regulation of protein synthesis could occur: stimulation of specific messenger RNA (mRNA) synthesis by induction of specific gene transcription, posttranscriptional regulation of mRNA degra-

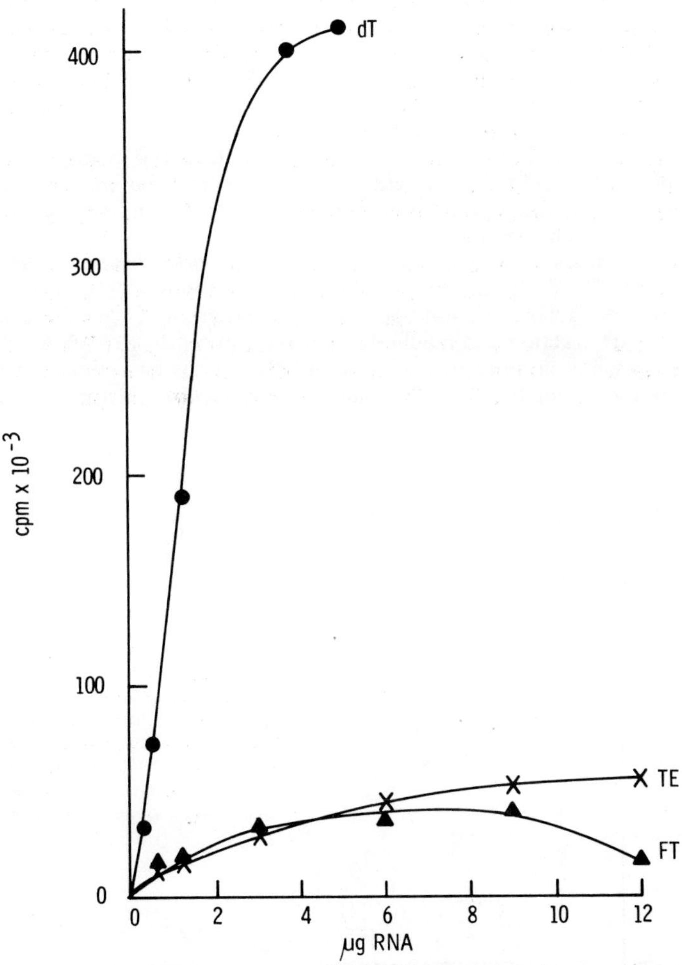

FIGURE 3. Total mRNA activity of 6-day pregnant endometrial RNA translated in a 50-μl wheat germ assay. TE, total RNA extract; dT, RNA bound to oligo-dT-cellulose; FT, RNA not bound to dT-cellulose (flow through).

dation, and stimulation of mRNA translation. To distinguish among transcriptional, posttranscriptional, and translational control, it is necessary to quantitate hormonally induced changes in specific mRNA by its extraction and translation *in vitro* in a cell-free heterologous protein-synthesizing system.

Translation *in vitro* of uteroglobin mRNA has been reported, by use of oocytes of *Xenopus laevis*[16] and a protein-synthesizing system based on a cell-free fraction of wheat germ.[17] We have also used the wheat germ system for the translation of uteroglobin mRNA and its quantitation under the different hormonal conditions of early pregnancy.

TRANSLATION *in Vitro* OF UTEROGLOBIN mRNA

Total RNA extracts were prepared from endometrium on Day 4 or 6 of pregnancy, as described previously,[18] by use of a phenol-sodium dodecyl sulfate buffer (pH 9.0) at 0°C, similar to that described by Brawerman.[19] Enrichment of mRNA was accomplished by binding to oligo-dT-cellulose,[20] and the activity of the mRNA was assessed by translation *in vitro* in a cell-free system derived from wheat germ,[21] under conditions published elsewhere.[18]

Total mRNA activity was measured by precipitation of synthesized radioactive peptides with trichloroacetic acid (TCA), and uteroglobin mRNA activity was determined by immunoprecipitation with monospecific uteroglobin antibodies purified by affinity chromatography.[18]

FIGURE 3 shows dose-response curves of total mRNA activity in the total RNA extract (TE), dT-bound RNA (dT), and non-dT-bound RNA (flow through, FT). The specific activity (counts per minute/microgram of RNA) was increased 10-fold in the dT fraction and reached a plateau at about 4 μg of RNA. Multiplication of the specific activity by the mass of RNA gives an estimate of the total mRNA activity of each fraction. This calculation revealed that approximately 10%

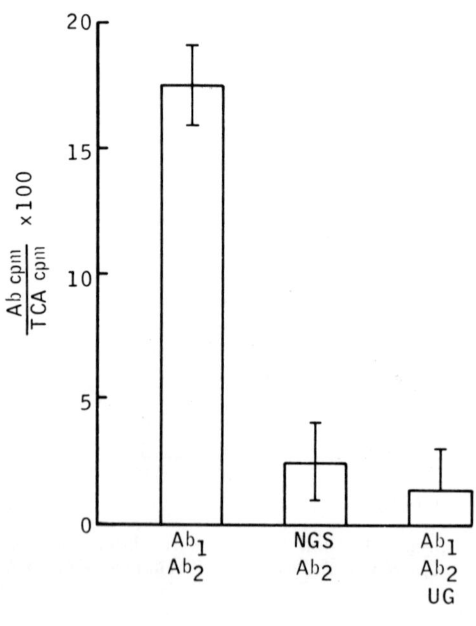

FIGURE 4. Immunoprecipitable translational products of 4-day pregnant endometrial dT-bound RNA. Ab$_1$, uteroglobin antibodies purified by affinity chromatography; Ab$_2$, rabbit antigoat IgG; NGS, normal goat serum; UG, excess nonradioactive uteroglobin. Vertical lines show ± SE of the mean (3 df).

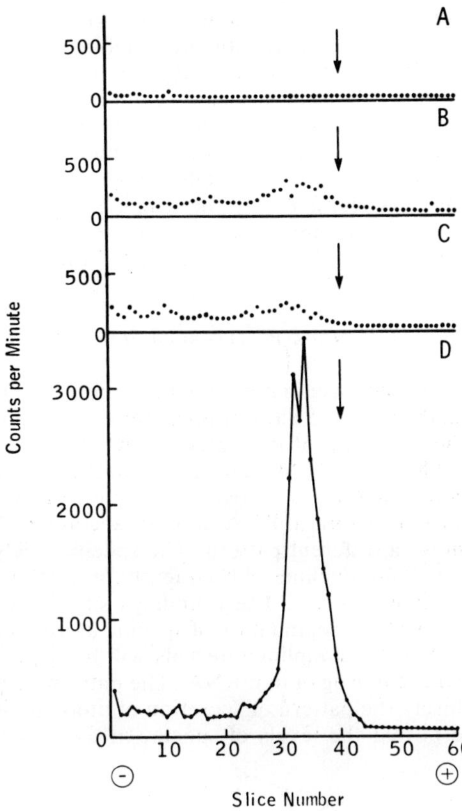

FIGURE 5. Immunoprecipitable translational products of 4-day pregnant endometrial dT-bound RNA analyzed by gel electrophoresis on 15% polyacrylamide gels that contained 0.1% sodium dodecyl sulfate, by the method of Laemmli.[24] The immunoprecipitates were dissolved in 80 μl of 1% SDS, 10 mM dithiothreitol, and 10 mM sodium phosphate (pH 7.5); 20 μl of authentic uteroglobin (1 mg/ml) were added, and the samples were heated at 90°C for 5 min before layering on the gels. Stained gels were sliced into 1-mm segments, which were dissolved in 15% H_2O_2, and the radioactivity was counted in a liquid scintillation fluid (ACS, Amersham-Searle). A, background (no added RNA), precipitated with purified antibodies against uteroglobin and anti-IgG; B, dT-RNA, precipitated with normal goat serum and anti-IgG; C, dT-RNA, precipitated with uteroglobin antibodies and anti-IgG in the presence of 20 μg of nonradioactive uteroglobin; D, dT-RNA, precipitated with uteroglobin antibodies and anti-IgG. The arrows mark the position of uteroglobin.

of the initial mRNA activity was recovered in the dT fraction and 75% in the FT fraction.

Binding to dT-cellulose is a property of the poly(A) tail of mRNA,[22] so that endometrial mRNA is unusual in the high proportion of its translatable message that lacks poly(A) sequences of sufficient length (>20 residues) to bind to oligo-dT-cellulose. This finding was substantiated by [^{3}H]poly(U) hybridization,[23] which showed no detectable poly(A) in the FT fraction under conditions sensitive to 0.01 μg of standard poly(A). Control experiments with rabbit liver RNA established that 69% of translatable mRNA activity in this tissue was bound to dT-cellulose.

The conditions used for immunoprecipitation have been shown previously to be specific for uteroglobin.[18] Double-antibody precipitation of the cell-free products of translation of Day-4 endometrial dT-RNA gave 17.5 ± 1.8% (mean ± SE, 3 df) of the total mRNA activity in the immunoprecipitate (FIGURE 4). In the absence of specific antibodies or on addition of excess nonradioactive uteroglobin, the immunoprecipitable radioactivity was reduced to 1–2%.

The immunoprecipitable translational products were examined further by electrophoresis on 15% polyacrylamide gels under denaturing conditions.[24] FIGURE 5 (D) shows a single peak of radioactivity, which was absent from translational products without added RNA (FIGURE 5, A). The peak was absent when uteroglobin antibodies were replaced by normal goat serum (FIGURE 5, B) and was completely displaced by the addition of nonradioactive uteroglobin to the immunoprecipitation reaction (FIGURE 5, C). The cell-free product migrated more slowly than did authentic uteroglobin.

These results indicate that the mRNA codes for a prouteroglobin about 4000 daltons larger in molecular weight than the native protein. It is not known whether uteroglobin *in vivo* is derived from a precursor molecule. Beato and Rungger[16] obtained an *in vitro* product that comigrated with uteroglobin, perhaps a reflection of the greater processing ability of the intact oocyte compared to the cell-free fraction of wheat germ. In the wheat germ assay, Levey and Daniel[17] also showed a product that appeared to comigrate with uteroglobin, but the translational assay was not quantitative, and the size of the product was not determined.

CHANGES IN UTEROGLOBIN mRNA DURING EARLY PREGNANCY

An increase in rapidly labeled polysomal RNA in the rabbit endometrium during the first 4–5 days of pregnancy was reported recently by Levey and Daniel.[17] The induction of uteroglobin mRNA by progesterone was also shown by Beato and Rungger.[16] Our data show that the total mRNA activity of the dT-bound endometrial RNA rises progressively up to Day 8 of pregnancy (FIGURE 6). The proportion of total mRNA activity accounted for by uteroglobin mRNA, however, shows a different pattern. The specific mRNA for uteroglobin reaches a peak on Day 4 and declines subsequently, even though endometrial total mRNA activity continues to rise. These findings suggest a selective control mechanism for the synthesis or degradation of specific uteroglobin mRNA.

Shorter sampling intervals will be required to establish more closely the peak level of uteroglobin mRNA. The pattern shown in FIGURE 6, however, resembles closely the pattern of secretion of uteroglobin during early pregnancy, which suggests that the levels of specific mRNA may be under hormonal control. Kinetic

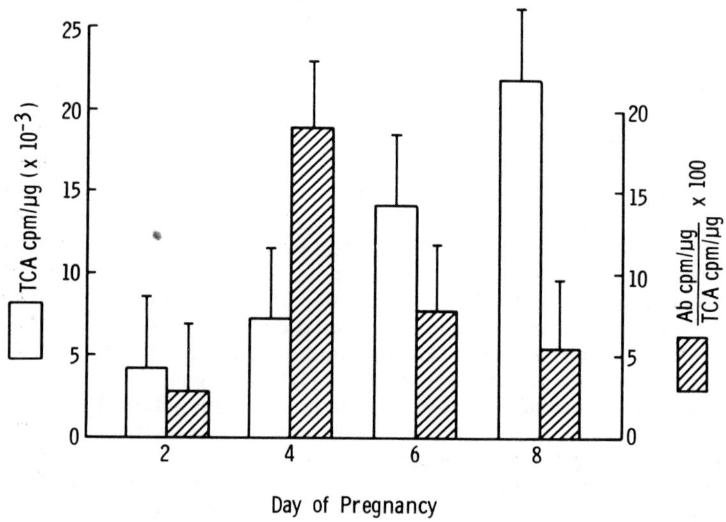

FIGURE 6. Changes in endometrial dT-RNA total mRNA activity (open bars) and specific uteroglobin mRNA activity (hatched bars) during early pregnancy. Vertical lines show ± SE of the mean (4 df).

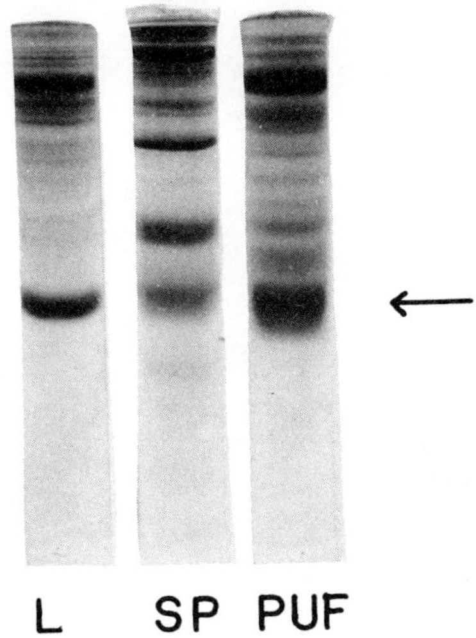

FIGURE 7. Electrophoresis of rabbit lung homogenate (L), seminal plasma (SP), and pregnant uterine flushings (PUF) on 15% polyacrylamide-SDS gels by the method of Laemmli.[24] The arrow marks the position of uteroglobin.

studies of the induction of uteroglobin mRNA and of uteroglobin will be required to establish whether the action of progesterone on these processes is directed toward specific gene expression.

TISSUE SPECIFICITY OF UTEROGLOBIN

Uteroglobin has been regarded as a uterus-specific protein, hence its name.[2] Recently, Feigelson *et al.* have found immunologically similar proteins in other tissues.[25] Beier *et al.* have also reported the presence of a uteroglobin-like protein in rabbit seminal plasma.[26] It now appears that the rabbit oviductal "cone" protein[27] is actually uteroglobin. Curiously, the protein in the oviduct is induced by estrogen rather than by progesterone.

Evidence for uteroglobin in rabbit lung is based on immunologic identity and in seminal plasma on immunologic identity and electrophoretic mobility in native gels. We have confirmed these findings and have extended them to show size identity of the lung and seminal protein with uteroglobin, by gel electrophoresis under denaturing conditions (FIGURE 7). The uteroglobin area was removed from the gel, and the protein was eluted in 10 mM Tris-HCl buffer (pH 7.5). After precipitation of sodium dodecyl sulfate (SDS) with potassium chloride, the eluates of both lung and seminal plasma gave precipitin lines on immunodiffusion against uteroglobin antibodies purified by affinity chromatography (FIGURE 8).

There arises the question of whether uteroglobin is synthesized in tissues other than the uterus. Although the protein has not been demonstrated unequivocally in blood,[10] the possibility exists that its presence in the lung, for example, could be the result of blood-borne contamination. We have examined this point directly by preparing dT-bound RNA from rabbit lung and investigating the wheat germ translational products for immunoprecipitable uteroglobin. On Day 6 of pregnancy, immunoprecipitable uteroglobin mRNA activity accounted for 4% of the lung total mRNA activity.

Analysis of the immunoprecipitable translational products of lung mRNA in SDS-polyacrylamide gels demonstrated a single peak of radioactivity (FIGURE 9,

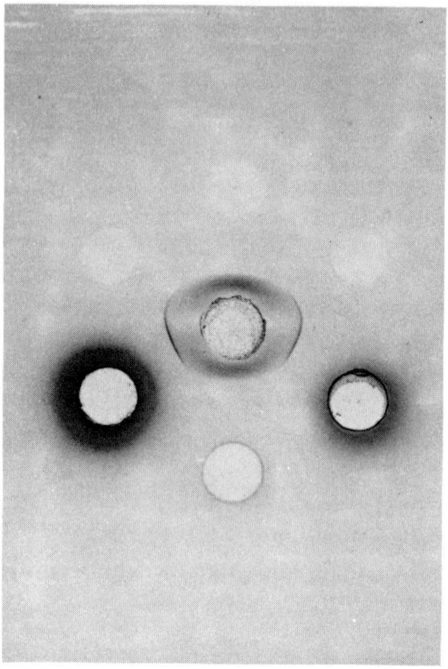

FIGURE 8. Immunodiffusion in 1% agar of lung, seminal plasma, and uterine antigens against uteroglobin antibodies purified by affinity chromatography (center well). Counting clockwise from the top, the outer wells contain uteroglobin, lung SDS-gel eluate, lung homogenate, pregnant uterine flushings, seminal plasma, and seminal plasma SDS-gel eluate.

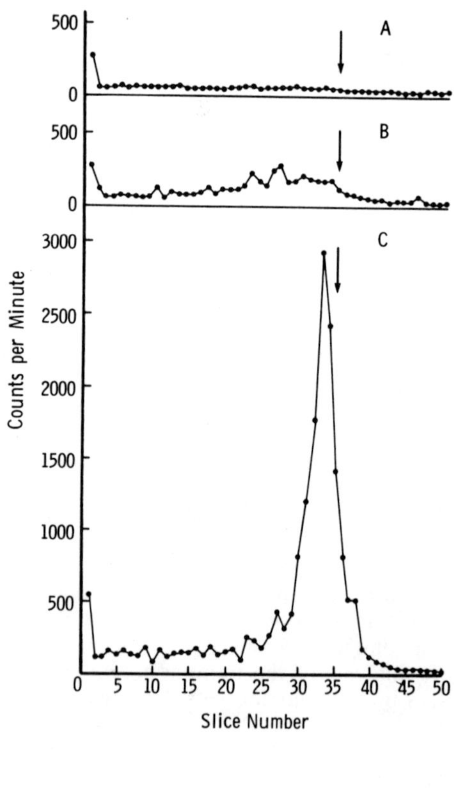

FIGURE 9. Analysis of immunoprecipitable translational products of lung dT-RNA in the wheat germ assay, by use of 15% polyacrylamide-SDS gel electrophoresis by the method of Laemmli.[24] The immunoprecipitates of 100-μl reaction mixtures were dissolved in 80 μl of 1% SDS, 10 mM dithiothreitol, and 10 mM sodium phosphate (pH 7.5); 20 μl of authentic uteroglobin (1 mg/ml) were added, and the solution was heated at 90°C for 5 min before layering on the gels. Stained gels were sliced into 1-mm segments, which were dissolved in 15% H_2O_2, and the radioactivity was counted in a liquid scintillation fluid (ACS, Amersham-Searle). A, background (no added RNA), precipitated with anti-uteroglobin antibodies and anti-IgG; B, dT-RNA, precipitated with anti-uteroglobin antibodies and anti-IgG, in the presence of excess nonradioactive uteroglobin; C, dT-RNA, precipitated with antiuteroglobin antibodies and anti-IgG. The arrows mark the position of uteroglobin.

C), which was absent from the products of translation without added RNA (FIGURE 9, A) and was completely displaced by nonradioactive uteroglobin (FIGURE 9, B). The lung product also migrated more slowly than did authentic uteroglobin, but the difference in molecular weight (about 2000) appeared to be smaller than the difference between that of uteroglobin and of the endometrial cell-free product. A system with greater resolution will be necessary to establish these size differences more precisely.

We have found no detectable uteroglobin mRNA in rabbit liver nor can the protein be found in this tissue.[10] The existence of uteroglobin in rabbit lung and seminal plasma, however, is now established by antigenic, charge, and size identity. The presence of uteroglobin mRNA in the lung proves that this tissue is an additional site of synthesis. It is not known whether uteroglobin in the lung is under hormonal regulation.

These findings prompt renewed speculation about the possible function of uteroglobin. A discussion of the biologic role of this protein is beyond the scope of this paper. Suffice it to say that initial claims of embryotrophic activity,[8] on the basis of which the protein was called "blastokinin," have not been confirmed.[28] Its presence in lung and semen suggests that uteroglobin may be a general product of secretory epithelium. One might argue that the name "uteroglobin" is now no more appropriate than "blastokinin."

Despite its sudden ubiquity, the possibility remains that uteroglobin may have a specific uterine function in reproduction. In the uterus, its hormonal regulation is firmly established, and the changes in specific uteroglobin mRNA in the endometrium show a relationship to the hormonal status of the animal. This enigmatic protein may thus continue to provide a useful model for studies of the mechanism of action of progesterone in the mammalian uterus.

ACKNOWLEDGMENTS

I thank Drs. S. L. C. Woo and B. W. O'Malley for their help and interest. Contributions to this work by Drs. B. M. Bhatt, K. M. Connell, G. F. Willen, Mr. Karl Ebert, Mrs. Sara Dinyari, and Ms. Rebecca Russell are acknowledged gratefully.

REFERENCES

1. O'MALLEY, B. W. & A. R. MEANS. 1974. Female steroid hormones and target cell nuclei. Science **183:** 610–620.
2. BEIER, H. M. 1968. Biochemisch-entwicklungsphysiologische untersuchungen am Proteinmilieu fur die Blastozystenentwicklung des Kaninchens (*Oryctolagus cuniculus*). Zool. Jahrb. Anat. **85:** 72–190.
3. WU, D. H. & W. M. ALLEN. 1959. Maintenance of pregnancy in castrated rabbits by 17-alpha-hydroxy-progesterone caproate and by progesterone. Fertil. Steril. **10:** 439–460.
4. BEIER, H. M. 1968. Uteroglobin: a hormone-sensitive endometrial protein involved in blastocyst development. Biochim. Biophys. Acta **160:** 289–291.
5. URZUA, M. A., R. STAMBAUGH, G. FLICKINGER & L. MASTROIANNI. 1970. Uterine and oviduct fluid protein patterns in the rabbit before and after ovulation. Fertil. Steril. **21:** 860–865.
6. ARTHUR, A. T. & J. C. DANIEL, JR. 1972. Progesterone regulation of blastokinin production and maintenance of rabbit blastocysts transferred into uteri of castrated recipients. Fertil. Steril. **23:** 115–122.

7. BULLOCK, D. W. & G. F. WILLEN. 1974. Regulation of a specific uterine protein by estrogen and progesterone in ovariectomized rabbits. Proc. Soc. Exp. Biol. Med. **146:** 294–298.
8. KRISHNAN, R. S. & J. C. DANIEL, JR. 1967. "Blastokinin": inducer and regulator of blastocyst development in the rabbit uterus. Science **158:** 490–492.
9. BULLOCK, D. W. & K. M. CONNELL. 1973. Occurrence and molecular weight of rabbit uterine "blastokinin." Biol. Reprod. **9:** 125–132.
10. MAYOL, R. F. & D. E. LONGENECKER. 1974. Development of a radioimmunoassay for blastokinin. Endocrinology **95:** 1534–1542.
11. RAHMAN, S. S. U., R. B. BILLIAR & B. LITTLE. 1975. Induction of uteroglobin in rabbits by progestogens, estradiol-17β and ACTH. Biol. Reprod. **12:** 305–314.
12. BEIER, H. M. 1970. Protein patterns of endometrial secretion in the rabbit. *In* Ovo-implantation, Human Gonadotropins and Prolactin. P. Hubinont, F. Leroy & C. Robyn, Eds.: 157–163. S. Karger. Basel, Switzerland.
13. HILLIARD, J. & L. W. EATON. 1971. Estradiol-17β, progesterone and 20α-hydroxy-pregn-4-ene-3-one in rabbit ovarian venous plasma. II. From mating through implantation. Endocrinology **89:** 522–527.
14. CHALLIS, J. R. G., I. J. DAVIES & K. J. RYAN. 1973. The concentrations of progesterone, estrone and estradiol-17β in the plasma of pregnant rabbits. Endocrinology **93:** 971–976.
15. FABER, L. E., M. L. SANDMANN & H. E. STAVELY. 1973. Progesterone and corticosterone binding in rabbit uterine cytosols. Endocrinology **93:** 74–80.
16. BEATO, M. & D. RUNGGER. 1975. Translation of the messenger RNA for rabbit uteroglobin in *Xenopus* oocytes. FEBS Lett. **59:** 305–309.
17. LEVEY, I. L. & J. C. DANIEL, JR. 1976. Isolation and translation of blastokinin mRNA. Biol. Reprod. **14:** 194–201.
18. BULLOCK, D. W., S. L. C. WOO & B. W. O'MALLEY. 1976. Uteroglobin messenger RNA: translation *in vitro*. Biol. Reprod. **15:** 435–443.
19. BRAWERMAN, G. 1973. The isolation of RNA from mammalian cells. *In* Methods in Cell Biology. D. M. Prescott, Ed. Vol. 7: 1–22. Academic Press, Inc. New York, N.Y.
20. AVIV, H. & LEDER, P. 1972. Purification of biologically active globin messenger RNA by chromatography on oligothymidilic acid cellulose. Proc. Nat. Acad. Sci. USA **69:** 1408–1412.
21. ROBERTS, B. W. & B. M. PATERSON. 1973. Efficient translation of tobacco mosaic virus RNA and rabbit globin 9S RNA in a cell-free system from commercial wheat germ. Proc. Nat. Acad. Sci. USA **70:** 2330–2334.
22. KATES, J. 1970. Transcription of the vaccinia virus genome and the occurrence of polyriboadenylic acid sequences in messenger RNA. Cold Spring Harbor Symp. Quant. Biol. **35:** 743–752.
23. GILLESPIE, D., S. MARSHALL & R. C. GALLO. 1972. RNA of RNA tumour viruses contains poly A. Nature [New Biol.] **146:** 294–298.
24. LAEMMLI, U. K. 1970. Cleavage of structural proteins during the assembly of the head of bacteriophage T4. Nature (London) **227:** 680–688.
25. FEIGELSON, M., I. G. NOSKE, A. K. GOSWAMI & E. KAY. This monograph.
26. BEIER, H. M., H. BOHN & W. MULLER. 1975. Uteroglobin-like antigen in the male genital tract secretions. Cell Tissue Res. **165:** 1–11.
27. KAY, E. & M. FEIGELSON. 1972. An estrogen modulated protein in rabbit oviducal fluid. Biochim. Biophys. Acta **271:** 436–441.
28. MAURER, R. R. & H. M. BEIER. 1976. Uterine proteins and development of preimplantation embryos of the rabbit. J. Reprod. Fertil. **48:** 33–41.

DISCUSSION

DR. P. K. SIITERI: Dr. Bullock, I noticed that you show a decline in both uteroglobin synthesis and in mRNA about Day 6 or 8 of pregnancy. Yet, if I remember correctly, the corpus luteum is still secreting progesterone at a high level. How can you account for this paradox. Is there a fall in uteroglobin when you continue to give progesterone?

DR. BULLOCK: The evidence from Daniel's group (Arthur, A. T. & J. C. Daniel, Jr. 1972. Fertil. Steril. **23:** 115) is that there is a slight fall as one continues to give progesterone, but uteroglobin stays up much longer than it does in pregnancy. The time when the protein and the messenger disappear in pregnancy coincides approximately with the beginning of the rise in estrogen levels in the plasma. Putting that together with our steroid injection experiment, which I showed, one might think that estrogen is responsible for the disappearance of uteroglobin, perhaps even by a mechanism that involves mRNA synthesis, but that's speculation.

DR. M. FEIGELSON: Have you done any experiments on the effect of estrogen on the mRNA level? In other words, the mRNA level drops after Day 4, shortly before the protein drops. Do you think that this phenomenon is controlled by estrogen?

DR. BULLOCK: We don't have direct evidence. This is, of course, one of the questions we want to answer. Before I do that experiment, I want to know the rate of synthesis of the protein, by radiolabeling experiments. I would then like to administer estradiol at the time of peak synthesis and determine whether synthesis can be curtailed and, if so, whether curtailment is mediated by a reduction in messenger synthesis. These experiments are in progress.

DR. R. M. ROBERTS (*University of Florida, Gainesville, Fla.*): I want to comment on the induction of the protein. The "purple" protein from the pig uterus is also a clear case of progesterone induction. On the other hand, cultured cells from the endometrium produce the protein apparently without the presence of progesterone in the medium, although I can't rule out progesterone in fetal calf serum. Induction appears to occur via the presence of iron in the medium; this protein contains iron. You may be dealing with a very complicated series of induction phenomena in the uterus, such as blood supply, nutrients, and several other factors, which may have nothing to do with the mRNA.

DR. BULLOCK: I hope I didn't give the impression that the data I presented indicate that progesterone is acting by inducing a specific mRNA. We do not yet have evidence, and it can't be obtained from the kind of study I presented. I just commented that I think it's encouraging that the changes in the messenger do appear to mimic the changes in the protein.

DR. C. A. VILLEE: I was interested in your comment that the uterine mRNA seems to have a smaller fraction of poly(A), or a smaller fraction of it has a poly(A) tail, than that from other tissues. Some of our experiments are consistent with that observation. We have isolated mRNA from rat uterus and liver, among other tissues, and less of the RNA is bound when the RNA comes from the uterus than from the liver. You made a statement in which you indicated a fraction. How did you estimate this fraction of your total mRNA?

DR. BULLOCK: I suppose it's an approximate estimation. One does the dose-response assay that I showed and calculates the specific activity in counts per minute per microgram of RNA added to the translational assay from the linear portion of the curve. One multiplies that by the mass of RNA in the fraction to obtain total mRNA activity. The bound and unbound fractions are expressed as a percentage of the total extract.

DR. W. S. KISTLER (*University of South Carolina, Columbia, S.C.*): In your initial gels, when you were looking at the appearance of uteroglobin as a function of day of pregnancy, there seemed to be a magical disappearance of albumin. Could you comment on that phenomenon?

Dr. Bullock: Yes, I don't think it is very mysterious. There is an inverse relationship between the proportion of total uterine protein represented by albumin and that represented by uteroglobin. However, the amount of uteroglobin increases during the first five days and declines subsequently, disappearing by Day 10. Albumin is a blood protein and is present in uterine secretions not as a secreted protein but as a transudated protein. I think progesterone interferes with this mechanism. Without wanting to reopen the discussion of this morning, the presence of water in the uterus has very little to do with secretion. I think progesterone affects permeability of capillaries and perhaps plasma membranes in a reverse way to estrogen, and I think this is why water and albumin disappear with progesterone. I don't think these phenomena have anything to do with uterine secretion.

Dr. Kistler: But didn't albumin reappear on your gels after uteroglobin disappears?

Dr. Bullock: Yes, and I think that's due to the rising estrogen levels in the plasma. What's important is the balance between estrogen and progesterone.

Dr. M. R. Sherman: With regard to the last comment, wasn't your total protein load on each gel kept the same? Therefore, if the proportion of one went up, the amount of the other, even if it was constant, would appear to be less because out of the total protein load the fraction was lower?

Dr. Bullock: Yes, that is true, but the absolute amounts of uteroglobin (per uterine horn) have also been measured during this period. These measurements were made by Mayol and Longenecker (1974. Endocrinology **95:** 1534) with radioimmunoassays, and the results show something like a 2000-fold increase in the amount of uteroglobin.

Dr. Sherman: Do you need other explanations for the changes in the albumin?

Dr. Bullock: Yes, I think that, because of the last point that was made, it does reappear later on.

REPRODUCTIVE TRACT FLUID PROTEINS AND THEIR HORMONAL CONTROL*

Muriel Feigelson, Ingrid G. Noske,† Ajit K. Goswami, and Ernest Kay‡

Departments of Biochemistry and of Obstetrics and Gynecology
College of Physicians and Surgeons
Columbia University
The Roosevelt Hospital
New York, New York 10019

Introduction

Oviductal and uterine fluids of the mammal constitute the immediate environment for early reproductive events. Preimplantation reproductive processes, such as sperm capacitation, the subsequent acrosome reaction, supernumerary sperm degeneration, cumulus cell dispersion, sperm penetration into the zona pellucida and vitellus, cleavage, blastulation, zona pellucida disintegration, and preparatory processes for nidation, all occur in the milieu of female genital tract secretions.

A protein present in rabbit uterine fluid, designated as "uteroglobin"[1,2] or "blastokinin,"[3] has been the subject of intensive study. Uteroglobin is a low-molecular-weight glycoprotein[3] that migrates to the postalbumin region during nondenaturing acrylamide gel electrophoresis.[1] This protein is observed in high concentration in uterine fluid of progesterone-treated ovariectomized rabbits and in animals 3–7 days postcoitus (representing 40–50% of the total uterine fluid protein at that time).[1,3–8] High concentrations are also found in blastocoelic fluid.[1,9] An endometrial origin for uterine uteroglobin is suggested by the observations that uteroglobin antigens are detected with fluorescent antibodies in the endometrium[10] and that radioactively labeled amino acids instilled *in vivo*[4,11,12] or perfused *in vitro*[13] through uterine lumina, or added to the media of *in vitro* endometrial cultures,[14] are rapidly incorporated into uteroglobin. In these systems, amino acid incorporation rates were considerably higher in uteri of pregnant or progesterone-treated rabbits than in nonpregnant untreated controls, indicating progesterone-induced increased rates of synthesis of this protein. Similar evidence of *de novo* synthesis of uteroglobin by blastocoelic cells has been obtained.[15] Both actinomycin D and puromycin block uteroglobin accumulation,[16] which implies that there is a requirement for ongoing RNA synthesis to effect progesterone induction of uteroglobin synthesis. Indeed, a translatable messenger RNA that codes for uteroglobin subunits[17,18] or a higher-molecular-weight subunit precursor,[18a,18b] has been prepared from progesterone-treated and pregnant rabbits and shown to be present at higher levels in uteri from pregnant than from nonpregnant animals.[18,18b]

The possible biologic function of uteroglobin has attracted considerable interest. Uteroglobin, as well as other equally effective uterine fluid protein

*Supported by National Institutes of Health Research Grant HD-05116.

†Present address: Max Planck Institute for Biochemistry, Munich, Federal Republic of Germany.

‡Present address: Laboratory of Nuclear Medicine and Radiation Biology, University of California, Los Angeles, Calif. 90024.

fractions, has been reported to enhance blastocyst development, in terms of promoting blastocyst expansion *in vitro*[3] and stimulating radioactive precursor incorporation into blastocyst RNA.[19,20] On the other hand, blastocyst protein synthetic patterns *in vitro* have been shown to be independent of such maternal factors.[21] Thus, whether blastulation processes are a specific and physiologically significant locus of action of uteroglobin is a moot point. Uteroglobin has been reported by some laboratories to bind progesterone and estrogen.[6,22] That this binding is very weak[23] and is dependent on exogenously supplied reductants[24] has been recently reported. Whether uterine fluid *in vivo* manifests appropriate reducing conditions is not known; therefore, progesterone binding as a significant biologic action of uteroglobin is also unclear at present. It has been reported that monospecific antibodies prepared against uteroglobin and administered to pregnant rabbits during the first 6 days of pregnancy proved to be an efficient preimplantation abortifacient,[25] indicating some significant reproductive role for this protein.

The possibility that a uteroglobin-like protein (same electrophoretic mobility as that of rabbit uteroglobin) is present in human uterine flushings during the progestational phase of the cycle has been suggested[26]; evidence of immunologic cross-reactivity of progestational human uterine fluid with monospecific antirabbit uteroglobin[27,28] strengthens the evidence for the existence of a human uteroglobin-like protein.

In an independent line of investigation, our laboratory has described a low-molecular-weight female genital tract protein, originally observed in oviductal, and subsequently in uterine, fluids of the estrous and estrogenized rabbit but not in serum.[29,30] At the inception of these studies, although certain properties of this protein were common to uteroglobin (e.g., electrophoretic mobility and progesterone induction in the uterus), several characteristics seemed dissimilar: the molecular weight of uteroglobin was originally reported as 30,000,[1] then approximately 27,000[3,6]; there appeared to be no evidence of its presence in uterine fluid of nonpregnant rabbits[3] or in oviductal fluid of rabbits in any endocrine state; and it was reported to bind progesterone with high affinity.[6,22] In contrast, the protein under study in our laboratory had a molecular weight of 16,000 daltons,[29] was detectable in nonpregnant estrous rabbit oviductal and uterine fluids,[29,30] and did not manifest progesterone binding.[30] Therefore, for some time, we believed that these two proteins might be distinct. However, many of the properties originally attributed to uteroglobin have since been modified, namely, its molecular weight has been revised to 15,000[31] and it has been subsequently observed in low quantities in estrous rabbit uterine[7] and oviductal[32] fluids. As cited above, recent studies with uteroglobin have indicated extremely weak steroid-binding activity[23] and a requirement for sulfhydryl reduction[24]; as our experiments indicated, in the absence of exogenous reductant, no significant progesterone binding occurs. Thus, with the passage of time and clarification of the properties of uteroglobin, discrepancies that distinguished uteroglobin from the reproductive tract protein under study in our laboratory have been eliminated.

The present communication reports studies on the molecular properties of a nonserum reproductive tract protein of the rabbit, establishes its immunologic identity with uteroglobin, demonstrates its presence both in male and in female productive tracts and in several nonreproductive tissues and their secretions, demonstrates differential steroidal hormone regulation of this protein in the oviduct, uterus, and at nongenital sites, and describes preliminary studies on a possible reproductive function of this protein.

CONE PROTEIN

During a study on protein patterns of estrous rabbit oviductal fluid, as evaluated by acrylamide gel electrophoresis, a protein was detected that migrates to the postalbumin region and is absent from serum electropherograms[33] (FIGURE 1). After electrophoresis of oviductal fluid, brief (30 min) denaturation and staining of the acrylamide gels with Amido black in 7% acetic acid, followed by immediate electrophoretic destaining, elicits a single conical configuration that points cathodally, which emanates from this postalbumin band[29] (FIGURE 2,a).

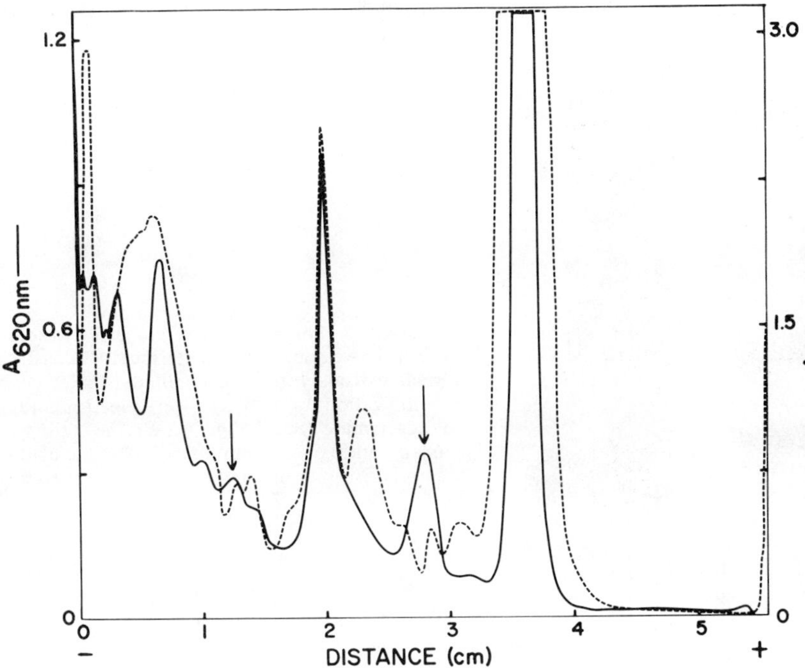

FIGURE 1. Protein patterns of rabbit oviductal fluid (—) and serum (- - - -). Densitometric tracings of polyacrylamide gels were taken after electrophoresis and Amido black (AB) staining. Arrows indicate oviductal fluid-specific bands.[33]

This conical formation was not observed in any other oviductal fluid protein band or in acrylamide gels of rabbit serum prepared in the same manner but was detectable at the same R_f in estrous rabbit uterine fluid[30] (FIGURE 2,b). Cone formation thus serves as a specific marker for this protein, which has been accordingly designated as "cone protein" (CP). Evidence suggests that brief exposure to 7% acetic acid after electrophoresis results in incomplete denaturation and precipitation of this low-molecular-weight (16,000)[29] protein at the core of the gel; during electrophoretic destaining in acid, the nonprecipitated core migrates cathodally along the longitudinal axis of the gel.[29]

Hormonal Control of Cone Protein in the Female Genital Tract

Ovarian hormones regulate CP levels in the oviduct and uterus differentially (Figure 3, a & b; Table 1). After ovariectomy, CP becomes undetectable on acrylamide gels of both oviductal and uterine fluids. A course of 17β-estradiol injections induces CP in oviductal fluid and to an even greater extent in the uterine fluid of ovariectomized rabbits. Progesterone elicits only negligible amounts of CP in oviductal fluid of ovariectomized rabbits but induces this protein in uterine fluid to a level almost 100-fold of that which is present in normal estrous uterine fluid (Table 1). CP levels in fluids retrieved from oviducts and uteri 3–5 days postcoitum were consistent with the endocrine state of the animals.[30] Thus, CP of oviductal and uterine fluids are differentially responsive to these two ovarian hor-

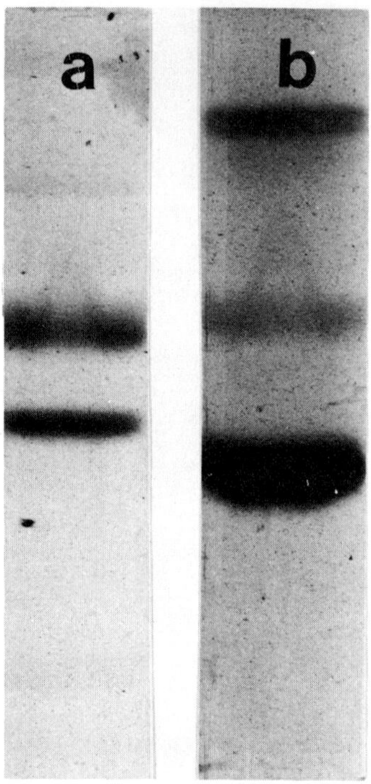

Figure 2. Polyacrylamide gel electrophoretic patterns of oviductal (a) and uterine (b) fluids of the normal estrous rabbit. Both fluids, collected by double ligation for 5 days,[30] were electrophoresed on acrylamide gels, after which the gels were stained with 0.5% Amido black-7% acetic acid for precisely 30 min and immediately destained electrophoretically.[29]

mones: estrogen, but not progesterone, induces this protein in oviductal fluid, and both steroids increase CP in uterine fluid, with progesterone being a particularly potent inducer of uterine fluid CP levels.[29,30]

Immunologic Identity of Cone Protein and Uteroglobin (Blastokinin)

As indicated above, some of the properties of CP under study in our laboratory and those reported for uteroglobin (UG) seemed discrepant during the early phases of this investigation. However, as further studies on UG led to revisions in several of these reported attributes (see above), the properties of these two pro-

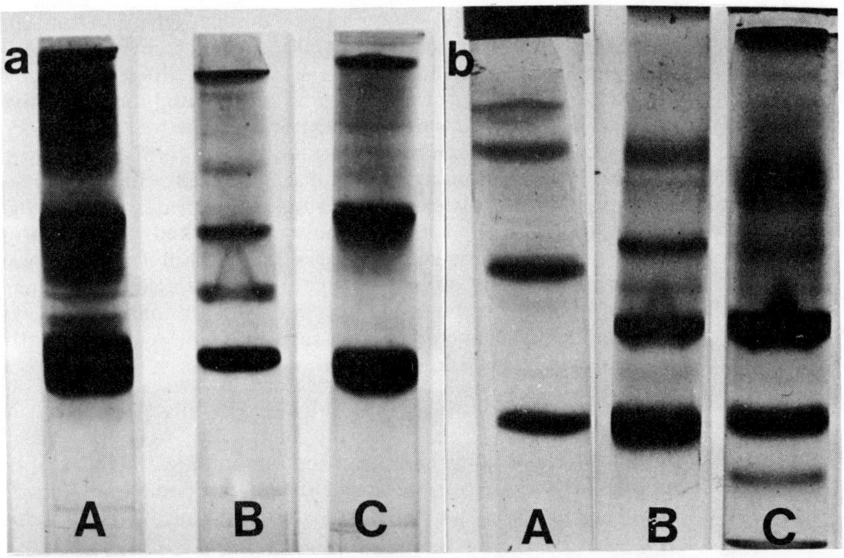

FIGURE 3. Polyacrylamide gel electrophoretic patterns of oviductal (a) and uterine (b) fluids from rabbits in various endocrine states. Ovariectomized (14–30 days) rabbits received 10–12 daily doses of: A, propylene glycol (PG); B, 5 μg of 17β-estradiol/kg/day in PG; and C, 1 mg of progesterone/kg/day in PG. Oviductal fluid was collected during the final 24 hr by means of an externalized cannula inserted into the fimbrium[29,33]; uterine fluid was collected by double ligation during the last 5 days.[30] Both fluids were electrophoresed on polyacrylamide gels, stained, and destained, as described for FIGURE 2.

teins began to converge. To further estabish the identity of these two female reproductive tract proteins, monospecific antisera were obtained against each protein. CP was purified from estrous rabbit uterine fluid by Sephadex® G-100 gel filtration, followed by preparative acrylamide gel electrophoresis. Antiserum to the purified CP was elicited on the goat and deemed monospecific by the criteria of

TABLE 1
EFFECT OF OVARIAN HORMONES ON CONE PROTEIN LEVELS IN OVIDUCTAL AND UTERINE FLUIDS

Endocrine State	Number of Rabbits	Cone Protein/Albumin × 10³*	
		Oviductal Fluid	Uterine Fluid
Intact estrous	5	42 ± 1.3	33 ± 0.8
Ovariectomized	5	0	0
Ovariectomized plus 17β-estradiol	4	37 ± 1.2	363 ± 13.0
Ovariectomized plus progesterone	4	3 ± 0.4	2975 ± 231.0

*Means ± SE of ratios of cone protein and albumin. Five days after ovariectomy, rabbits received 10 daily doses of propylene glycol, 5 μg/kg of 17β-estradiol or 1 mg/kg of progesterone. Fluids were collected by double ligation, electrophoresed on acrylamide gels, stained with Amido black, and quantitated densitometrically.[30]

single precipitin band formations on Ouchterlony double diffusion and immunoelectrophoresis.[28] An antiserum to UG, partially purified from pregnant rabbit uterine fluid, was kindly provided by Dr. D. W. Bullock, Baylor College of Medicine, Houston, Texas, and absorbed in our laboratory with lyophilized liver cytosol, which rendered it similarly monospecific monospecific by the above criteria. FIGURE 4(a) illustrates that pregnant rabbit uterine fluid forms single precipitin bands when diffusing versus both anti-CP and anti-UG. The complete fusion of the precipitin bands formed against each antiserum demonstrates immunologic identity between CP isolated from estrous rabbit uterine fluid and UG from pregnant fluid. Likewise, on immunoelectrophoresis, pregnant uterine fluid forms single precipitin arcs with identical mobilities when diffusing against both antibodies.[28] Either antiserum may thus be used interchangeably in immunologic test systems, CP and UG being terms for the same antigen, which will be hereafter referred to as "cone protein-uteroglobin" (CP-UG).

In Vivo Distribution of Cone Protein-Uteroglobin Antigen

FIGURE 4(b) provides further confirmation of the immunologic identity of the CP-UG antigen in pregnant and estrous uterine fluids and purified CP (pCP) from the latter secretion and of its presence in estrous and pregnant oviductal fluids;

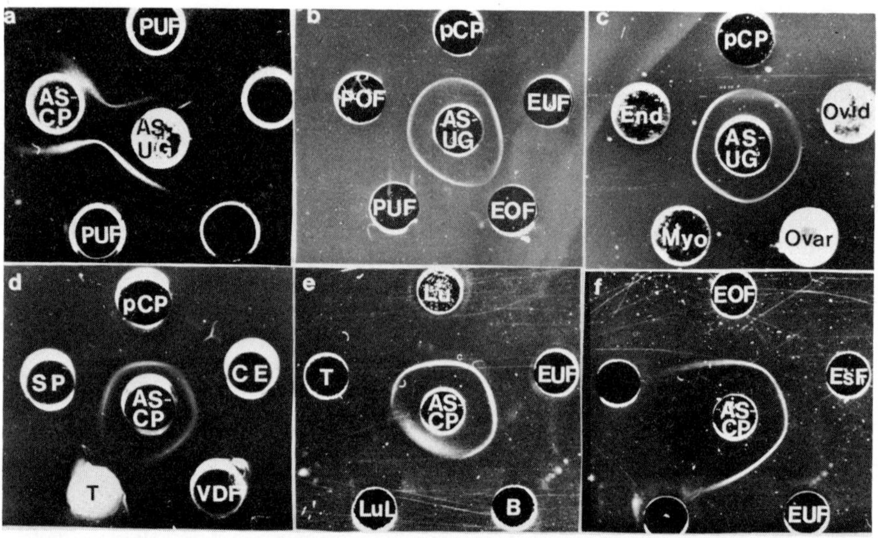

FIGURE 4. Immunologic identity of the CP and UG (a) and the presence of the CP-UG antigen in female genital tract secretions (b) and tissue extracts (c), male reproductive tract (d), respiratory tract (e), and esophageal secretions (f). Goat antiserum to rabbit CP purified from estrous rabbit uterine fluid (AS-CP)[28] absorbed goat antiserum to pregnant rabbit uteroglobin (AS-UG), and the following antigens were introduced into the indicated wells: purified CP from estrous rabbit uterine fluid (pCP); estrous uterine (EUF) and oviductal (EOF) fluids collected by double ligation; 3–5-day pregnant uterine (PUF) and oviductal (POF) flushings; phosphate-buffered saline (PBS) extracts of oviduct (Ovid), ovary (Ovar), myometrium (Myo), endometrium (End), cauda epididymis (CE), and testis (T, black type); vas deferens flushings (VDF); seminal plasma, concentrated 10-fold (SP); PBS extracts of lung (Lu), trachea (T, white type), and bronchus (B); lung lavage (LuL); and esophageal flushings (EsF).[28]

TABLE 2

DISTRIBUTION OF CONE PROTEIN-UTEROGLOBIN ANTIGEN IN TISSUES AND SECRETIONS OF THE RABBIT AND HUMAN

	Tissue	Secretion
Rabbit		
Reproductive tract		
Female	ovary	uterine fluid
	oviduct	oviductal fluid
	endometrium	
	myometrium	
	vagina	
Male	vas deferens	vas deferens flushings
	cauda epididymus	seminal plasma
Nonreproductive tract		
	lung	lung lavage
	bronchus	tracheal flushings
	trachea	esophageal flushings
	esophagus	jejunal flushings
Human		
Reproductive tract		
Female	endometrium	uterine flushings
		oviductal flushings
Male		seminal plasma

precipitin lines of identity are formed among all of these materials when diffusing in the Ouchterlony system against either antibody. CP-UG antigen, furthermore, is detectable in extracts of female genital tract tissues (FIGURE 4,c), the presumed synthetic sites of this secreted protein.[28] After ovariectomy, all immunologic evidence of CP-UG antigen disappeared from the female genital tract tissues and their secretions, corroborating results obtained by acrylamide gel electrophoresis of oviductal and uterine fluids of ovariectomized rabbits (FIGURE 3 & TABLE 1).

FIGURE 4 (d) depicts the presence of an antigen in various tissues and fluids of the male reproductive tract, namely, sperm-free flushings of vas deferens, extracts of caudae epididymides, and concentrated seminal plasma, which form precipitin lines of identity with that of CP purified from a female genital tract secretion.[28] CP-UG, therefore, is immunologically detectable both in male and in female reproductive tracts of the rabbit, a finding that may be relevant to its biologic action.

Human genital tract tissue extracts and secretions of both sexes, namely, endometrial extracts, uterine and oviductal flushings, and seminal plasma, also interact with antiserum against rabbit CP. Human endometrial extracts form a single line of identity with rabbit reproductive tract preparations, indicating similar antigenic sites on both human and rabbit proteins.[28]

Of particular interest is the finding that the CP-UG antigen is also present in at least two nonreproductive organ systems comprised of ductal structures. Extracts of respiratory tissues and their secretions (lung, bronchus, trachea) from male and intact and ovariectomized female rabbits demonstrate precipitin bands when migrating toward either anti-CP or anti-UG (FIGURE 4,e). Furthermore, preparations of digestive tract tissues and secretions [esophagus (FIGURE 4,f) and jejunum] from rabbits of either sex also cross-react with anti-CP. The precipitin

Ouchterlony plates all fused with those formed by female reproductive tract fluids and pCP, indicating the presence of a protein with antigenic sites similar or identical to those of CP-UG in the respiratory and digestive tracts of both sexes. Furthermore, the CP-UG antigen of lung tissue extracts coelutes with the uterine fluid antigen on gel filtration, forms a conical configuration at the same R_f on acrylamide gel electrophoresis, and completely absorbs genital tract fluid precipitating capabilities of both antisera. In contrast to tissues and fluids of the genital, respiratory, and digestive tracts, neither immunoprecipitin bands nor absorption of CP-UG antibodies is observed with highly concentrated rabbit sera or tissue extracts of liver, heart, spleen, or kidney.[28]

TABLE 2 summarizes our observations on the distribution of the CP-UG antigen in various tissues and secretions of the rabbit and human. All findings obtained with the Ouchterlony double-immunodiffusion system have been confirmed with radial immunodiffusion and with immunoelectrophoresis; in the latter test system, all precipitin arcs manifest identical electrophoretic mobilities, which further attests to the immunologic identity of this antigen at each locus cited in TABLE 2.

EFFECTS OF PREGNANCY AND STEROID HORMONES ON CP-UG LEVELS IN UTERINE FLUID AND LUNG

Since there is no known evidence that the lung is a target tissue for pregnancy hormones, it was of interest to compare the levels of CP-UG antigen in uterine fluid and in lung during the first week of pregnancy and under the influence of estrogen and progesterone. Quantitation of CP-UG antigen levels in uterine fluid and lung extracts by radial immunodiffusion[34] and immunoelectrophoretic[35] assays reveals that whereas uterine fluid CP-UG levels of the 6-day pregnant rabbit are elevated approximately 30-fold above those of estrous does, the level of this antigen in the lung is not significantly altered (TABLE 3). Thus, the increased progesterone levels of the pregnant rabbit, which induces CP-UG in uterine fluid (FIGURE 3, b & Reference 5) and is thereby responsible for its elevation at that site during pregnancy, is ineffective in inducing this antigen in the lung. That uteri and lung respond differentially to pregnancy steroids with respect to CP-UG induction is further corroborated by the results shown in TABLE 4. Quantitative immunologic determinations indicate that ovariectomized does manifest no uterine fluid CP-UG. Furthermore, a course of estradiol or progesterone treatment in these

TABLE 3

LEVELS OF CONE PROTEIN-UTEROGLOBIN ANTIGEN IN UTERINE FLUID AND LUNG IN ESTROUS AND PREGNANT RABBITS

	Cone Protein-Uteroglobin* (antigen units/μg of protein)	
	Uterine Flushings	Lung
Estrous	5.5 ± 1.8 (6)	1.00 ± 0.12 (7)
Pregnant	178.0 ± 23.0 (12)	0.74 ± 0.10 (8)
p Value	<0.01	>0.05

*Mean levels of CP-UG antigen per microgram of protein ± SE, as quantitatively estimated,[34,35] employing anti-CP. Numbers in parentheses represent numbers of samples.

TABLE 4

EFFECTS OF STEROID HORMONES ON CONE PROTEIN-UTEROGLOBIN ANTIGEN LEVELS OF UTERINE FLUID AND LUNG OF OVARIECTOMIZED RABBITS

Hormonal Treatment	Number of Rabbits	Cone Protein-Uteroglobin* (antigen units/μg of protein)		p Value
		Uterine Flushings	Lung	
Diluent	4	0	1.06 ± 0.15	
17β-Estradiol	4	5.7 ± 3.1	1.04 ± 0.24	
Progesterone	4	77.3 ± 9.6	0.97 ± 0.06	
Testosterone	4	76.9 ± 17.8	1.36 ± 0.36	>0.05
Cortisol	3	0	1.68 ± 0.10	<0.02

*Mean levels of CP-UG antigen per microgram of protein ± SE, as quantitatively estimated,[34,35] employing anti-CP. Five days after ovariectomy, rabbits received 10 daily doses of diluent, 5 μg/kg of 17β-estradiol, 1 mg/kg of progesterone, 25 mg/kg of testosterone propionate, or 20 mg/kg of cortisol acetate.

animals induces this antigen in uterine fluid to modest and marked extents, respectively, results compatible with those presented in TABLE 1, employing quantitative procedures based on densitometry of protein staining. In contrast, lung CP-UG antigen of 2-week ovariectomized does is distinctly measurable and remains unaltered when either estradiol or progesterone is administered (TABLE 4). Thus, CP-UG antigens of uterus and lung are differentially regulated by ovarian steroids; neither estrogen nor progesterone, both of which induce this protein in uterus, alters the CP-UG content of lung.

Since CP-UG antigen was detected in the male genital tract, the possibility that androgen may induce this protein was explored. TABLE 4 illustrates that testosterone administration to ovariectomized does markedly induces this protein in the uterus, with little effect in the lung. Analogous androgenic influences on other uterine parameters have been previously reported.[36–38]

Since pulmonary tissue is a known target tissue for glucocorticoids (lung possesses glucocorticoid receptors,[39] and glucocorticoids are capable of influencing lung phospholipid synthesis[40]), the effect of cortisol on CP-UG antigen was explored. TABLE 4 demonstrates that whereas no effect of cortisol on uterine CP-UG of ovariectomized rabbits is detectable, a 63% increment in pulmonary CP-UG antigen is observed. Thus, all four steroid hormones tested demonstrate differential regulation of CP-UG at its uterine and pulmonary sites: female and male gonadal hormones induce this uterine protein but are ineffective on the lung antigen; conversely, glucocorticoids increase CP-UG levels in the lung but not in the uterus.

BIOLOGIC ACTION OF CONE PROTEIN-UTEROGLOBIN; EFFECT ON ACROSOME LOSS *in Vitro*

As indicated above, the possible biologic roles of uteroglobin have long been under consideration in many laboratories. Although the effects of this protein on blastocyst development[1,3] and its progesterone-binding capabilities[6,22,24] have been proposed as primary physiologic actions of uteroglobin, the nonspecificity of the former action and the possible nonphysiologic requirement necessary for the latter (see above) leave the question of biologic action of uteroglobin essentially unresolved.

The presence of CP-UG antigen in the male and female reproductive tracts has suggested possible influences of this protein on sperm, which might occur in the reproductive tract of either or both sexes. TABLE 5 presents the effects of oviductal and uterine fluid fractions on acrosome loss *in vitro*. During 12–14 hr of incubation in unfortified Brackett's medium, a small proportion of ejaculated sperm undergoes acrosome loss. Supplementation of the medium with either total estrous oviductal or uterine fluids or a high-molecular-weight fraction of uterine fluid resulted in an acrosome loss that did not significantly differ from that of controls. However, fortification of the medium with the low-molecular-weight CP-UG-rich fraction of either fluid elicited a significantly greater acrosome loss *in vitro*. Whether this acrosome loss represents a "true" acrosome reaction[44] or a degradation phenomenon cannot be ascertained from phase microscopy assessment. These results suggest, however, that the CP-UG-enriched fractions derived from estrous rabbit uterine and oviductal fluids accelerate labilization of acrosome membranes. That this promotion of acrosome labilization by CP-UG may occur in the male and/or female genital tract remains a possibility.

TABLE 5
EFFECT OF FEMALE REPRODUCTIVE TRACT FLUID FRACTIONS ON SPERM ACROSOME LOSS *in Vitro**

	Percentage of Acrosome Loss	
	12 hr	14 hr
Brackett's medium	26	
Total estrous oviductal fluid	26.3 ± 6.2	
Low-molecular-weight oviductal fluid fraction (cone protein-uteroglobin-rich)	44.9 ± 2.7	
Brackett's medium		39.0 ± 2.5
Total estrous uterine fluid		37.1 ± 5.8
High-molecular-weight uterine fluid fraction		42.9 ± 14.9
Low-molecular-weight uterine fluid fraction (cone protein-uteroglobin-rich)		80.1 ± 1.2

*Test materials were total estrous rabbit oviductal or uterine fluids or various protein peaks eluted therefrom following fractionation on Sephadex G-100 and concentration. 100 μg of protein/ml of each test material were added to approximately 100,000 ejaculated washed sperm in 50 μl of Brackett's medium.[41] Incubation was performed at 37°C under 5% CO_2 in air at saturated humidity. Sperm samples were removed at the indicated times, stained,[42] and assessed for presence or absence of acrosomes under the phase microscope.[43]

SUMMARY AND CONCLUSIONS

CP-UG, a protein that reacts with immunologic identity to uteroglobin (blastokinin), a female reproductive tract protein, has been detected in male genital tract tissues and fluids and in several nonreproductive tract ductal tissues and their secretions, namely, those of various portions of the respiratory and digestive tracts. The tissue distribution of CP-UG antigen in reproductive and nonreproductive ductal structures and their secretions in both sexes suggests morphologic and functional common denominators. It is likely that this protein is synthesized in mucosal glandular cells present in all of these ducts and secreted into their respective lumina, where it may serve a related biologic function. Although uteroglobin has been implicated in the promotion of blastulation processes and/or progesterone binding in the female genital tract, oviductal and uterine fluid fractions rich in uteroglobin are preferentially capable of labilizing sperm acrosomes *in vitro*. A possible reproductive function for uteroglobin in both the male and female reproductive tracts is thus suggested. The presence of uteroglobin antigens at nongenital sites suggests, furthermore, that the physiologic action of uteroglobin is not limited to reproductive functions alone.

Uteroglobin is differentially regulated by various steroid hormones in oviduct, uterus, and lung. Estrogen is a relatively weak inducer of this protein in the oviduct and uterus. Although progesterone has little influence on this protein within the oviductal lumen, it is a potent inducer of the protein in uterine fluid, which is thereby present in high concentration in uterine secretions during the first week of pregnancy. Testosterone is also capable of marked uteroglobin induction in the uterus. In the lung, however, this protein is unresponsive to these gonadal steroids and thus is not elevated at the time of high progesterone levels during the first week of pregnancy. On the other hand, cortisol administration enhances pulmonary uteroglobin levels but has no influence on this protein in the uterus. Thus, the endocrinologic control of this protein in the oviduct and uterus of the female, in the male reproductive tract, and at nonreproductive tissue sites clearly differs, illustrating differential regulation of a given protein in different cell types. In some instances (e.g., lung), the possible absence of receptors for gonadal hormones may underlie the lack of response of the protein at that site. In the oviduct, progesterone receptors are present, but refractoriness of oviductal cells to progesterone induction of this protein may be due to the absence of some specific process distal to progesterone-receptor interactions.

Acknowledgment

The authors gratefully acknowledge the skilled technical assistance of Mrs. Emily Scott.

References

1. Beier, H. M. 1968. Uteroglobin—a hormone sensitive endometrial protein involved in blastocyst development. Biochim. Biophys. Acta **160:** 289–291.
2. Beier, H. M. 1974. Oviducal and uterine fluids. J. Reprod. Fertil. **37:** 221–237.
3. Krishnan, R. S. & J. C. Daniel. 1967. "Blastokinin": inducer and regulator of blastocyst development in the rabbit uterus. Science **158:** 490–492.
4. Daniel, J. C. 1971. Uterine proteins and embryonic development. *In* Advances in the Biosciences. G. Raspé, Ed. Vol. 6: 191–206. Pergamon Press Vieweg.
5. Arthur, A. T. & J. C. Daniel. 1972. Progesterone regulation of blastokinin production and maintenance of rabbit blastocysts transferred into uteri of castrate recipients. Fertil. Steril. **23:** 115–122.
6. Urzua, M., R. Stambaugh, C. Flickinger & L. Mastroianni. 1970. Uterine and oviduct fluid protein patterns in the rabbit before and after ovulation. Fertil. Steril. **21:** 860–865.
7. Bullock, D. W. & K. M. Connell. 1973. Occurrence and molecular weight of rabbit uterine "blastokinin." Biol. Reprod. **9:** 125–132.
8. Mayol, R. F. & D. E. Longenecker. 1974. Development of a radioimmunoassay for blastokinin. Endocrinology **95:** 1534–1542.
9. Hamana, K. & E. S. E. Hafez. 1970. Discelectrophoretic patterns of uteroglobin and serum proteins in rabbit blastocoelic fluid. J. Reprod. Fertil. **21:** 555–558.

10. KIRCHNER, C. 1972. Immune histologic studies on the synthesis of a uterine specific protein in the rabbit and its passage through the blastocyst coverings. Fertil. Steril. **23:** 131–136.
11. MURRAY, F. A. & J. C. DANIEL. 1973. Synthetic pattern of proteins in rabbit uterine flushings. Fertil. Steril. **24:** 692–697.
12. BULLOCK, D. W. & G. F. WILLEN. 1974. Regulation of a specific uterine protein by estrogen and progesterone in ovariectomized rabbits. Proc. Soc. Exp. Biol. Med. **146:** 294–298.
13. BEATO, M. & J. ARNEMANN. 1975. Hormone dependent synthesis and secretion of uteroglobin in isolated rabbit uterus. FEBS Lett. **58:** 126–129.
14. WHITSON, G. L. & F. A. MURRAY. 1974. Cell culture of mammalian endometrium and synthesis of blastokinin *in vitro*. Science **183:** 668–670.
15. PETZOLDT, U. 1974. Autoradiographic studies on the origin of the rabbit blastocyst fluids proteins. Cytobiologie **9:** 401–406.
16. MURRAY, F. A. & G. L. WHITSON. 1974. Effects of actinomycin-D and puromycin on blastokinin synthesis by rabbit uterus. Biol. Reprod. **11:** 421–428.
17. BEATO, M. & D. RUNGGER. 1975. Translation of messenger RNA for rabbit uteroglobin in xenopus oocytes. FEBS Lett. **59:** 305–309.
18. LEVEY, I. L. & J. C. DANIEL. 1976. Isolation and translation of blastokinin mRNA. Biol. Reprod. **14:** 163–174.
18a. BEATO, M. & A. NIETO. 1976. Translation of the mRNA for rabbit uteroglobin in cell-free systems. Eur. J. Biochem. **64:** 15–25.
18b. BULLOCK, D. W., L. C. WOO & B. W. O'MALLEY. 1976. Uteroglobin messenger RNA: translation *in vitro*. Biol. Reprod. **15:** 435–443.
19. GULYAS, B. J., J. C. DANIEL & R. S. KRISHNAN. 1969. Incorporation of labelled nucleosides *in vitro* by rabbit and mink blastocysts in the presence of blastokinin or serum. J. Reprod. Fertil. **20:** 255–262.
20. EL-BANNA, A. A. & J. C. DANIEL. 1972. The effect of protein fractions from rabbit fluids on embryo growth and uptake of nucleic acid and protein precursors. Fertil. Steril. **23:** 105–114.
21. VAN BLERKOM, J. & C. MANES. 1974. Development of preimplantation rabbit embryos *in vivo* and *in vitro*. Develop. Biol. **40:** 40–51.
22. ARTHUR, A. T., R. D. COWAN & J. C. DANIEL. 1972. Steroid binding to blastokinin. Fertil. Steril. **23:** 85–92.
23. RAHMAN, S. S. U., N. VELAYO, P. DOMRES & R. B. BILLIAR. 1975. Evaluation of progesterone binding to uteroglobin. Fertil. Steril. **26:** 991–995.
24. BEATO, M. & R. BAIER. 1975. Binding of progesterone to the proteins of the uterine luminal fluid. Identification of uteroglobin as the binding protein. Biochim. Biophys. Acta **392:** 346–356.
25. KRISHNAN, R. S. 1971. Effect of passive administration of antiblastokinin on blastocyst development and maintenance of pregnancy in rabbits. Experientia **27:** 955, 956.
26. SHIRAI, E., R. IIZUKA & Y. NOTAKE. 1972. Analysis of human uterine fluid protein. Fertil. Steril. **23:** 522–528.
27. DANIEL, J. C. 1973. A blastokinin-like component from the human uterus. Fertil. Steril. **24:** 326–328.
28. NOSKE, I. G. & M. FEIGELSON. 1976. Immunological evidence of uteroglobin (blastokinin) in the male reproductive tract and in nonreproductive ductal tissues and their secretions. Biol. Reprod. **15:** 704–713.
29. KAY, E. & M. FEIGELSON. 1972. Estrogen modulated protein in rabbit oviducal fluid. Biochim. Biophys. Acta **271:** 436–441.
30. GOSWAMI, A. & M. FEIGELSON. 1974. Differential regulation of a low molecular weight protein in oviductal and uterine fluids by ovarian hormones. Endocrinology **95:** 669–675.
31. MURRAY, F. A., R. W. MCGAUGHEY & M. J. YARUS. 1972. Blastokinin: its size and shape and an indication of the existence of subunits. Fertil. Steril. **23:** 69–77.
32. PETZOLDT, U., W. DAMES, G. H. M. GOTTSCHEWSKI & V. NEUHOFF. 1972. Protein patterns in early developmental stages of the rabbit. Cytobiologie **5:** 272–280.

33. Feigelson, M. & E. Kay. 1972. Protein patterns of rabbit oviducal fluid. Biol. Reprod. **6:** 244–252.
34. Mancini, G., A. Carbonara & J. F. Heremans. 1965. Immunochemical quantitation of antigens by single radial immunodiffusion. Int. J. Immunochem. **2:** 235–254.
35. Laurell, C. B. 1966. Quantitative estimation of proteins by electrophoresis in agarose gels containing antibodies. Anal. Biochem. **15:** 45–52.
36. Lerner, L. J. 1964. Hormone antagonists: inhibitors of specific activities of estrogen and androgen. Rec. Progr. Hormone Res. **20:** 435–490.
37. Lerner, L. J., R. Hilf, A. R. Turkheimer, I. Michel & S. L. Engel. 1966. Effects of hormone antagonists on morphological and biochemical changes induced by hormonal steroids in the immature rat uterus. Endocrinology **78:** 111–125.
38. Schmidt, W. N., M. Sadler & B. S. Katzenellenbogen. 1976. Androgen-uterine interactions: nuclear translocation of the estrogen receptor and induction of synthesis of the uterine induced protein (IP) by high concentrations of androgens *in vitro,* but not *in vivo*. Endocrinology **98:** 702–716.
39. Giannopoulos, G., M. Shree & S. Solomon. 1973. Glucocorticoid receptors in lung. II. Specific binding of glucocorticoids to nuclear components of rabbit fetal lung. J. Biol. Chem. **248:** 5016–5023.
40. Kotas, R. V. & M. E. Avery. 1971. Accelerated appearance of pulmonary surfactant in the fetal rabbit. J. Appl. Physiol. **30:** 358–361.
41. Brackett, B. B. & W. L. Williams. 1968. Fertilization of rabbit ova in a defined medium. Fertil. Steril. **19:** 144–155.
42. Wells, M. E. & O. A. Awa. 1970. New technique for assessing acrosomal characteristics of spermatozoa. J. Dairy Sci. **53:** 227–232.
43. Noske, I. G. & M. Feigelson. 1975. Unpublished observations.
44. Bedford, J. M. 1970. Sperm capacitation and fertilization in mammals. Biol. Reprod. Suppl. **2:** 128–158.

Discussion

Question: Could you give us some idea as to the dosage of testosterone, compared with that of progesterone, used for the induction of uterine fluid uteroglobin?

Dr. Feigelson: The dosage of testosterone is much higher than that of progesterone. We administered 1 mg/kg/day of progesterone and 25 mg/kg/day of testosterone, both for 10 consecutive days. These doses were chosen, as they are known replacement doses for each hormone in the rat. Dose-response curves for each hormone must be acquired to compare the inducing potency of the two steroids. The point I wish to emphasize, however, is that both testosterone and progesterone are capable of induction of uterine uteroglobin.

Dr. R. J. B. King: Do you know how much of the protein in human uterine fluid might be made up of uteroglobin from your data?

Dr. Feigelson: We have only qualitative identification of uteroglobin in human materials. We have not quantitatively estimated human uteroglobin, as yet.

Dr. King: At what times does the acrosome reaction occur, relative to the time of appearance of uteroglobin in the rabbit? Are their time courses comparable?

Dr. Feigelson: The acrosome reaction occurs just prior to fertilization. Capacitation, which is associated with labilization of acrosomal membranes, occurs prior to actual disintegration of those membranes and loss of the acrosome, during sperm transit through the uterus and oviduct. During this period of capacitation and acrosome reaction (between coitus and fertilization), both uterine and oviductal fluids contain basal levels of uteroglobin, due to estrogen domination of the animal at that time. Uterine fluid uteroglobin levels rise progressively from this basal estrous level during the first week of pregnancy, due to a corresponding rise in circulating progesterone levels during that period; maximum uteroglobin levels are attained just prior to implantation (Mayol, R. F. & D. E. Longenecker. 1974. Endocrinology **95:** 1534–1542). The time course of alterations in oviductal fluid uteroglobin during these periods in unknown. Because the respective roles of uterine and oviductal environments in capacitation and subsequent acrosome reaction are not, as yet, clearly understood, it is difficult at this time to relate uteroglobin levels with acrosome labilization. However, I do not wish to leave the impression that we believe that uteroglobin is necessarily involved in capacitation or the acrosome reaction. For example, uteroglobin may participate in degradation of supranumerary sperm, which may occur to a significant extent subsequent to fertilization, at a time when uteroglobin levels are reasonably high. On the other hand, this protein may be involved in some generalized hydrolytic action, concerned perhaps with cell membrane breakdown, for which acrosome loss *in vitro* serves as a model.

DR. D. W. BULLOCK: In the electrophoresis of estrous uterine fluids, was the uteroglobin band that you showed from a single animal or was that a pool of a large number of fluids?

DR. FEIGELSON: The figure depicted is an acrylamide gel of uterine fluid from a single animal, but we have, of course, many such gels. In these experiments, uterine fluid was collected by double ligation for 5 days. The relative concentrations of proteins in fluids obtained by double ligation may differ from those obtained by flushing. However, we also see a definite cone protein band in the postalbumin region by use of flushings from nonligated uteri from estrous animals. It is possible that cone formation serves as a sensitive marker, enabling detection of the low levels of uteroglobin present in the estrous animal more easily than with conventionally stained gels. Indeed, many workers in the field are able to detect uteroglobin immunologically in estrous animals.

DR. BULLOCK: What were the units of quantitative measurements of uteroglobin?

DR. FEIGELSON: We used the Laurell "rocket" technique as a quantitative immunologic measurement of the amount of uteroglobin antigen. The results are expressed as arbitrary units per milligram of total protein, based on a preparation of pregnant uterine fluid as an arbitrary standard.

DR. BULLOCK: Could you tell us, in nanograms of uteroglobin, what those numbers could be converted to?

DR. FEIGELSON: This is a problem. We have preparations of purified uteroglobin, which we have attempted to use as a primary standard and on which we have performed Lowry protein determinations. As you are aware from its amino acid analysis (Bullock, D. W. & K. M. Connell. 1973. Biol. Reprod. **9:** 125–132), uteroglobin contains relatively low concentrations of aromatic amino acids; thus, protein estimations by the Lowry method or absorbance at 280 nm may give aberrant results, values for purified uteroglobin that are too low. We thus felt that protein measurements of uteroglobin performed by these methods were invalid, and we therefore have thought it better to use arbitrary units at this time. We are planning to submit purified uteroglobin to a micro-Kjeldahl nitrogen determination, which we should be able to use to accurately convert our arbitrary units to amounts of protein nitrogen.

EFFECTS OF PROGESTERONE ON THE ADRENERGIC MECHANISMS OF THE GENITAL TRACT*

Atef H. Moawad, Moon H. Kim, Frederick P. Zuspan,
Rebecca Chagrasulis, Frederick T. Pishotta, and Kathryn J. Zuspan

Department of Obstetrics and Gynecology
Pritzker School of Medicine
The University of Chicago
Chicago, Illinois 60637

Brief Description of the Adrenergic Innervation of the Genital Tract

The organization of the sympathetic innervation of the genital tract is different from that of other regions of the body. The postganglionic neurons originate in ganglia located peripherally near the effector organs. Short adrenergic neurons have been found to innervate the accessory male organs,[1–3] the female reproductive tract,[4–6] and the trigonal area of the urinary bladder.[7] This phenomenon has been confirmed in various species, including the human, by demonstrating sympathetic ganglia formations in the immediate vicinity of the uterus.[8,9] Use of the histochemical fluorescence technique for cellular localization of catecholamines developed by Carlsson *et al.*,[10] Falck,[11] and Falck and Owman[12] has permitted direct determination of adrenergic innervation of various tissues.

The female genital tract of the rat, rabbit, cat, and man has been studied. These nerves are partly associated with the vascular system, but the majority of them have been shown to innervate the smooth muscle, except in the rat uterus,[13] which lacks such adrenergic innervation.

In man, both the area of the internal os of the uterine cervix and the regions around the isthmus of the two fallopian tubes are richly innervated with adrenergic neurons.[14–16] With this information, we chose to investigate the effects of various hormones on adrenergic neurons with the oviductal isthmic region used as the experimental model.

Effects of Hormones on the Adrenergic Neurotransmitters in the Genital Tract

Uterus

Norepinephrine (NE)

By use of the histochemical fluorescence technique and chemical determination of the norepinephrine content of the rabbit uterus, Sjöberg[15] found a marked increase in total content of norepinephrine in this tissue after daily injections of 17β-estradiol for 14 days. This rise in norepinephrine content was manifested by

*Supported by Biomedical Center for Population Research Grant PHS-HD-07110-04, Ford Foundation Grant 690-0108, and Rockefeller Foundation Grants RF 70097 and RF 72062.

an increased number of fluorescent nerves. On the other hand, Miller and Marshall[17] could not confirm this finding. Rosengren and Sjöberg[18] investigated the effect of pregnancy on this increase in the same species. They found that the norepinephrine (NE) concentration, expressed per unit weight, was significantly lower than in the nonpregnant state, a finding confirmed by Cha *et al.*[19] The decline in both the total content of NE and in fluorescence progressed in pregnancy until there were hardly any adrenergic nerves detected histochemically during the last days of pregnancy. In the guinea pig, Gardmark *et al.*[20] confirmed this finding and, moreover, demonstrated a return of the NE level to the nonpregnant (baseline) level within 1 month.

Epinephrine (E)

Rudzik and Miller[21] found that during estrus, the amount of epinephrine in rat uterine tissue is twice that which exists in diestrus. Wurtman *et al.*[22] suggested that epinephrine is probably removed from the circulation by the uterus. Green and Miller[23] measured the concentration of plasma epinephrine (E) and NE and found that E increases markedly in the plasma during estrus, whereas NE decreases. On the other hand, experiments performed in many species[6,15–18,24–29] failed to demonstrate any significant amounts of E in uterine tissues.

The marked decrease in the amount of neurotransmitter in uterine tissues of pregnant rabbits and guinea pigs might mean that, in this state, the function of the neurotransmitter is minimal.

Oviduct

Oviductal sympathetic innervation in the rabbit,[4,14,30] cat,[6] dog,[31] and primate and man[32,33] have been investigated mainly by fluorescence histochemistry. As mentioned earlier, the isthmic region is richly innervated by adrenergic short neurons.

Sex steroids have been claimed to alter both the fluorescence and the total NE content in this organ. In the rabbit, Owman and Sjöberg[34] found that treatment with 17β-estradiol benzoate doubles the level of NE, whereas addition of progesterone to this regimen in the latter period normalized the value.

Owman and Sjöberg,[34] in recent work on the monkey, have shown that the number of fluorescent axons present during the secretory phase of the estrous cycle is much higher than which exists during the proliferative phase. This finding was confirmed by these workers by means of chemical determination of oviductal NE content. These authors did not offer a satisfactory explanation for this unexpected result, as they did for earlier work with other species.

In view of these findings, we investigated the effect of estrogen and progesterone on adrenergic fluorescence and NE content in the rabbit and human oviductal isthmus.

Methods of Study of the Neurotransmitter Norepinephrine in the Oviductal Isthmus

Immature New Zealand white rabbits were divided into three groups: group I (35 animals), treated with 5 μg of ethynylestradiol daily for 12 days; group II (35 animals), treated with 5 μg of ethynylestradiol daily for 7 days, then with 5 μg of ethynylestradiol plus 5 mg of progesterone daily for 5 additional days; and group

III (25 animals), an immature control group treated only with the inert oil base for 12 days.

Human tissues were obtained from hysterectomy specimens of subjects whose peripheral plasma progesterone and serum estrone (E_1) and estradiol (E_2) levels were determined. Tissues were classified into three groups according to serum estrogen and progesterone values: group I, low-estrogen and low-progesterone tissues from 21 subjects; group II, high-estrogen and low-progesterone tissues from 11 subjects; and group III, high-estrogen and high progesterone tissues from 15 subjects.

In humans, we analyzed our data in terms of peripheral sex steroid levels. The estrogen values were expressed in picograms per milliliter as $E_1/10 + E_2$, because we considered estrone to be a weaker estrogen at the tissue level. Progesterone

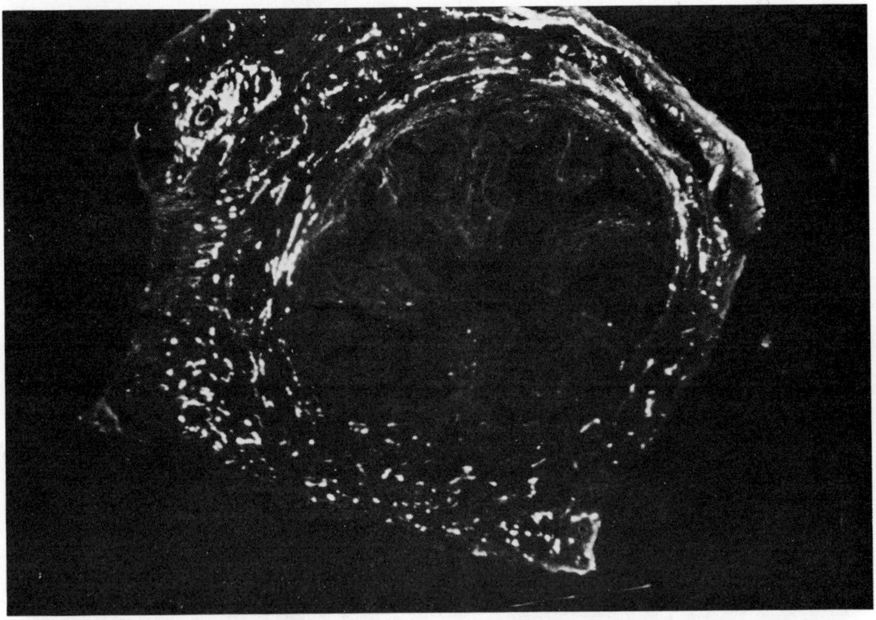

FIGURE 1. Photomicrograph of a cross-section of the isthmus from an immature rabbit (not injected with steroid hormones) that illustrates the fluorescent neurotransmitter, especially in the circular muscle layer.

was expressed in nanograms per milliliter. Estrogen levels ($E_1/10 + E_2$) less than 40 were considered low, and those of 40 or above were considered high. Progesterone values less than two were considered low, and those of two or more were considered high.

Fluorescence histochemistry was performed according to the method of Carlsson *et al.*[10] The tissues were coded and read under the fluorescence microscope without knowledge of the hormonal background of the animal or of the human subjects. Fluorescence was assigned values of one to four according to brightness and amount observed.

NE content was determined in human tissues fluorometrically, as modified from the technique of Zuspan and Cooley.[35]

Results

Effects of Progesterone Injections on Fluorescence

In the rabbit tissues, we were not able to visualize any significant differences between tissues from animals injected with estrogen and those injected with estrogen and progesterone (Figures 1–3). Therefore, we were not able to confirm the work reported by Owman and Sjöberg.[34]

In the human tissues, following the same procedure in reading the results of fluorescence histochemistry, we failed to demonstrate any significant difference in brightness or distribution of fluorescence between tissues associated with low or high progesterone levels (Figures 4 & 5).

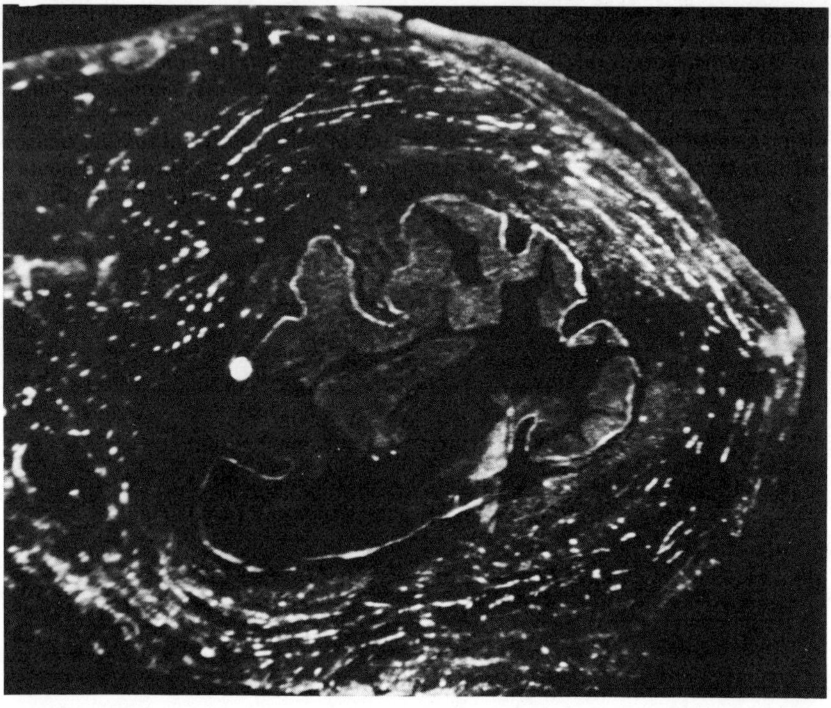

Figure 2. Photomicrograph of a cross-section of the oviductal isthmus from a rabbit injected with estrogen for 12 days that shows the fluorescent neurotransmitter in the region of the circular muscle layer.

Chemical Determination of NE Contents in the Isthmus of the Human Oviduct

Tissues from Subjects with Low Progesterone Values (<2, groups I and II)

The presence of low estrogen levels in peripheral blood was associated with a marked increase in NE content, as shown in Table 1 (group I). On the other hand, tissues from subjects with high estrogen levels were associated with significantly

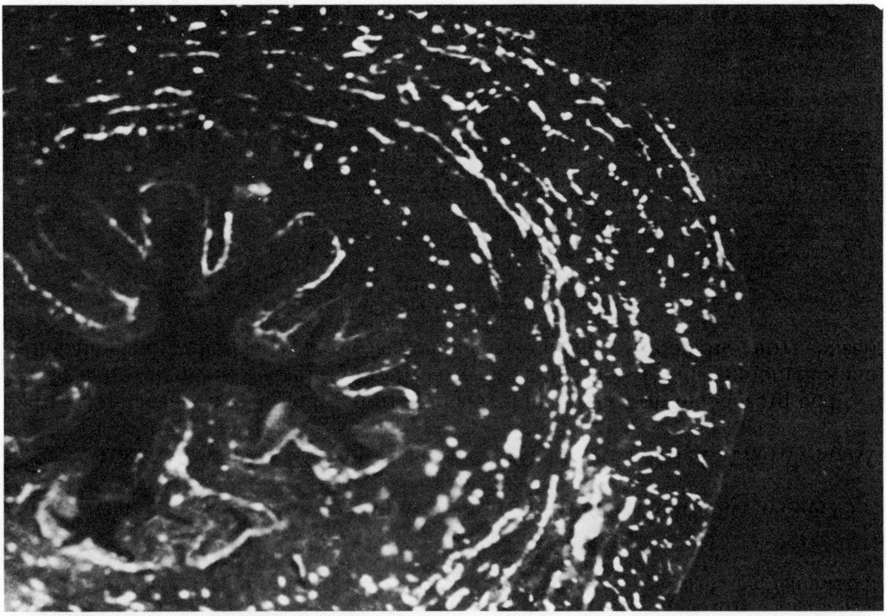

FIGURE 3. Photomicrograph of a cross-section of the oviductal isthmus from a rabbit injected with estrogen for 7 days and with estrogen plus progesterone for 5 additional days.

low tissue NE, as shown in TABLE 1 (group II). The difference in tissue NE between the two groups was statistically significant. In plotting the estrogen values against NE content, one finds a reciprocal relationship, as illustrated in FIGURE 6.

Tissues from Subjects with High Estrogen Values ($E_1/10 + E_2$, ≥40, groups II and III)

The presence of serum progesterone values equal to or higher than two (group III, TABLE 2) was associated with an increase in tissue NE content. If groups II and III are compared, the difference is statistically significant (TABLE 2). In other words, the presence of progesterone contributed to the elevation of tissue NE.

TABLE 1

NOREPINEPHRINE CONTENT IN THE OVIDUCTAL ISTHMUS OF HUMAN SUBJECTS WITH LOW PLASMA PROGESTERONE LEVELS

	$E_1/10 + E_2$ (pg/ml)	Progesterone (ng/ml)	Tissue Norepinephrine* (μg/g ± SEM)
Group I Low estrogen Low progesterone	< 40.0	< 2.0	0.3123 ± 0.0410
Group II High estrogen Low progesterone	≥ 40.0	< 2.0	0.1203 ± 0.0254

*Differences were significant at the 95% confidence limit.

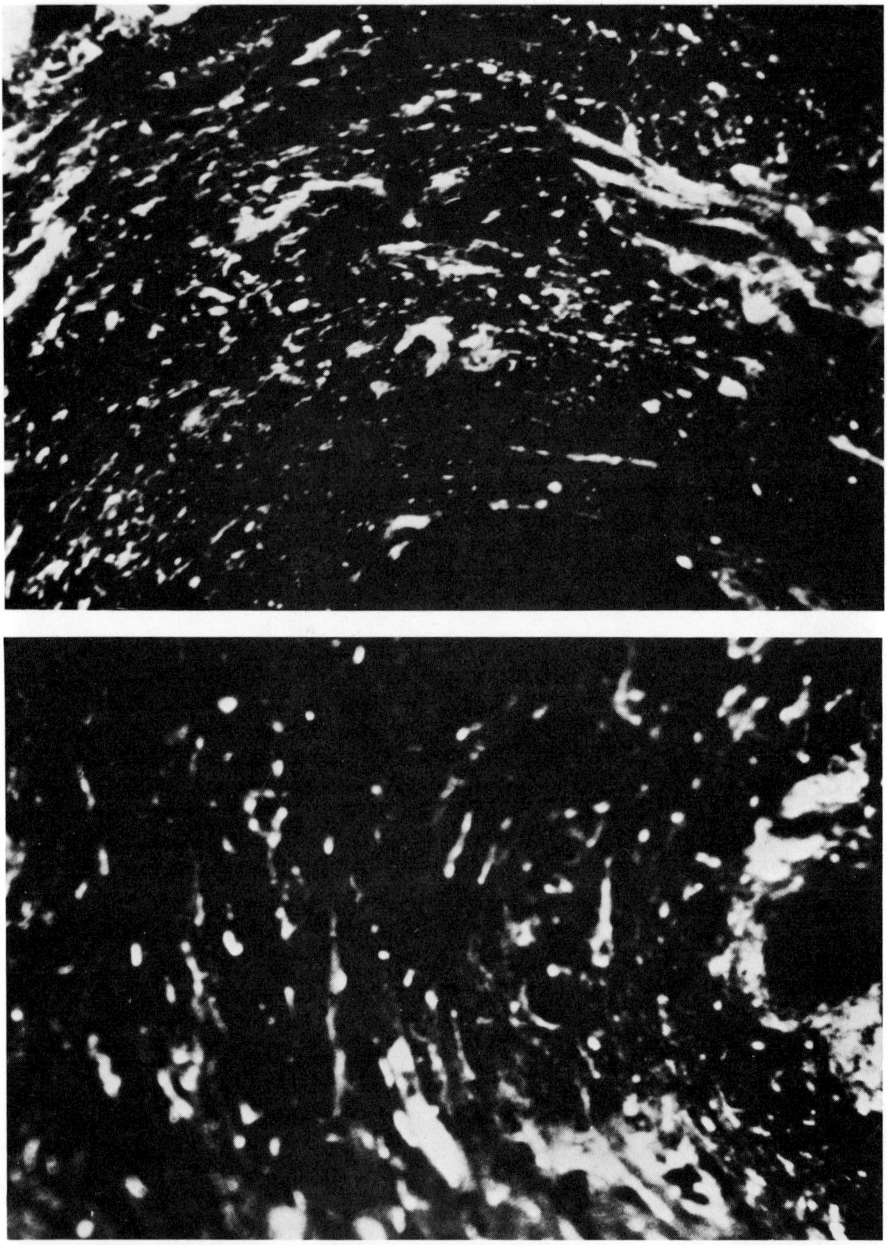

FIGURES 4 (*top*) and 5 (*bottom*). Photomicrographs of cross-sections of human oviductal isthmus from the follicular and luteal phases of the estrous cycle, respectively. These Figures illustrate the fluorescent neurotransmitter, especially in the region of the circular muscle layers. Note the difficulty in finding any significant differences between the fluorescence in both figures.

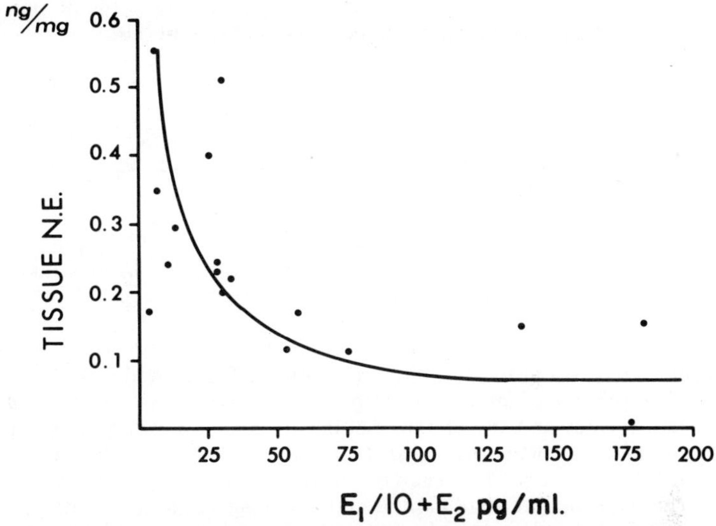

FIGURE 6. A graph that shows the correlation between estrogen levels from the peripheral blood of human subjects and NE content in the regions of the oviductal isthmus.

COMMENTS

These results show that in the human, serum estrogen levels can in some way be correlated with tissue NE content, wherein high estrogen levels are associated with low NE content and vice versa. These results also demonstrate that in the presence of physiologically high levels of progesterone, NE content increases significantly. Although we could not establish any relationship between sex steroids and fluorescence of the adrenergic neurotransmitter, we have at least shown that there are no differences in adrenergic neurotransmitters between follicular and luteal tissues in the human. Likewise, in the rabbit, there are no differences between the effects of estrogen and estrogen plus progesterone. A recent report by Dujovne *et al.*[36] indicated that NE content was either unchanged or

TABLE 2

NOREPINEPHRINE CONTENT IN THE OVIDUCTAL ISTHMUS OF HUMAN SUBJECTS WITH HIGH SERUM ESTROGEN LEVELS

	$E_1/10 + E_2$ (pg/ml)	Progesterone (ng/ml)	Tissue Norepinephrine* (μg/g ± SEM)
Group II High estrogen Low progesterone	⩾ 40.0	< 2.0	0.1203 ± 0.0254
Group III High estrogen High progesterone	⩾ 40.0	⩾ 2.0	0.2330 ± 0.0438

*Differences were significant at the 95% confidence limit.

significantly increased in this tissue during the luteal phase of the human estrous cycle. This finding is in agreement with the work reported herein.

Changes in NE content constitute the net result of many processes, namely, synthesis, release, breakdown, and turnover. Therefore, it is extremely difficult to explain the results based on determination of amine contents. Unless one determines the effect of sex steroids on each of these peripheral adrenergic mechanisms separately, results from these data cannot be satisfactorily interpreted.

Effect of Progesterone on the Pharmacology of Adrenoreceptors in the Genital Tract

In the genital tract, it is generally agreed that the contractile response is initiated through α receptors, while the relaxation effect is mediated through the β receptors. The relative dominance of either α or β adrenergic receptors in uterine and oviductal tissues and the effect of either or both sex steroidal hormones on these receptors have been the subject of many studies. In the many species studied, including man, the influence of pretreatment with progesterone is one of inhibition, in contrast to that exhibited by estrogen alone, namely, stimulation.[25,26,32,33,37,38]

This report will summarize the results we obtained from attempts to quantitate the effects of physiologic progesterone levels on adrenergic receptors of the human oviductal isthmus.

Materials and Methods

In 83 subjects, correlation of the peripheral plasma levels of estrone, estradiol, and progesterone (P) with the *in vitro* response of the human oviductal isthmus to transmural nerve stimulation was performed in circular preparations. Tissues were classified according to their plasma hormonal values into four groups: low estrogens and low progesterone, high estrogens and low progesterone, high progesterone, and pregnant values. The responses were observed by measuring the change in frequency (F), tone (T), and area under the contractility curve (A). Details of the procedures employed in this aspect of the study have been reported elsewhere.[32,33,39] Low progesterone values were defined as being less than 2.0 ng/ml of plasma.

Results

Figures 7–9 describe the relationship between hormonal levels and tissue response to nerve stimulation as measured by F, T, and A, respectively. A positive correlation was established between plasma estrogens and stimulation of the contractility parameters. An $E_1/10 + E_2$ value of approximately 48 pg/ml represents the turning point for the reversal of the response. In other words, a value higher than 48 is usually associated with stimulation of contractility rather than inhibition. On the other hand, the presence of progesterone in significant amounts prevents this reversal, regardless of the estrogen values. Figures 10–12 are illustrative examples of the typical responses.

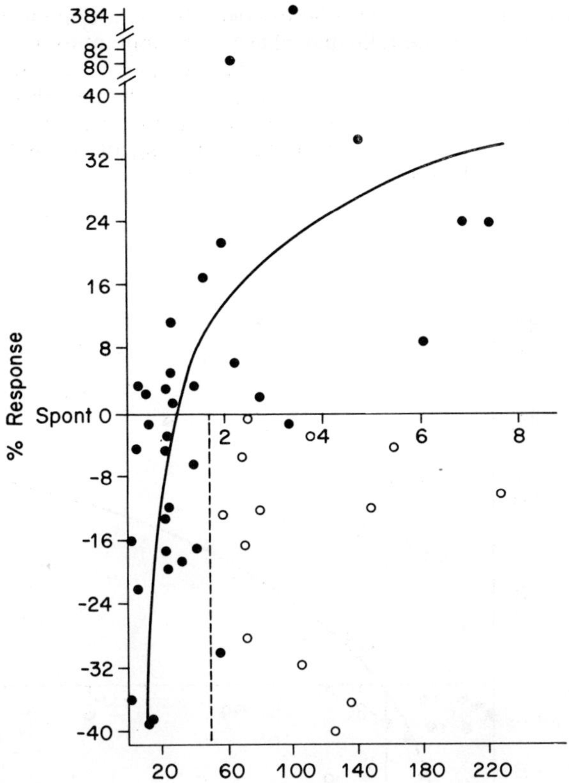

FIGURE 7. A graph that shows the correlation between plasma hormonal levels and percentage change in frequency of contractions after transmural field stimulation. Solid circles represent the tissue levels from the follicular phase [estrogen levels are represented as $E_1/10 + E_2$ (pg/ml) in the lower graph]. The broken line represents the estrogen level (48) beyond which stimulation rather than inhibition is expected. Tissues from the luteal phase with progesterone levels of 2.0 ng/ml or higher are shown as open circles. (The progesterone level scale is the upper one.) Notice the decrease in frequency after transmural nerve stimulation in all of the tissues tested. Each point in this figure and the next two figures represents the average of three observations in one subject.

In the same preparation, we constructed the E dose-response relationship by measuring A in tissue from either the follicular or luteal phase of the cycle (groups II and III). FIGURE 13 shows the stimulation obtained in follicular phase tissues as contrasted with the inhibition observed in the luteal group.

COMMENTS

To interpret these results, one must relate hormonal levels to a hypothetical model of the α and β adrenergic receptor activities in this tissue, as shown in FIGURE 14. We have shown that α-receptor activity is low near the beginning and end of the ovulatory cycle, when the estrogen levels are modest, and that this activity increased during the follicular phase, concomitant to the rise of estrogen levels. On the other hand, β-receptor activity becomes enhanced in the presence of significant progesterone levels in the luteal phase. Perhaps this pronounced effect of reversing the contractility response plays an important role in relaxation of the circular muscle and in the consequent opening of the isthmic lumen for passage of the fertilized ovum.

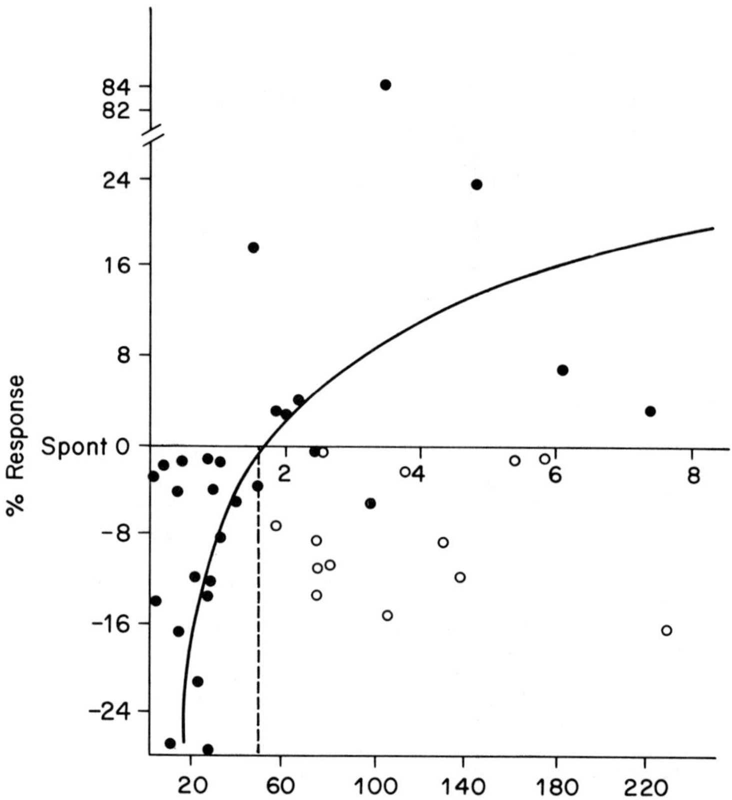

FIGURE 8. A graph that shows the correlation between plasma hormonal levels and percentage change in tone after transmural nerve stimulation, labeling. Symbols are the same as in FIGURE 7.

Although the effect of progesterone on the adrenergic receptor activity seems more clear, we have not yet identified the mechanisms involved (if any) in the processes of synthesis, release, breakdown, and reuptake of NE at the peripheral axons in the genital tract. Fluorescence histochemistry lacks quantitation, and chemical analysis of the tissue catecholamines cannot determine dynamic processes.

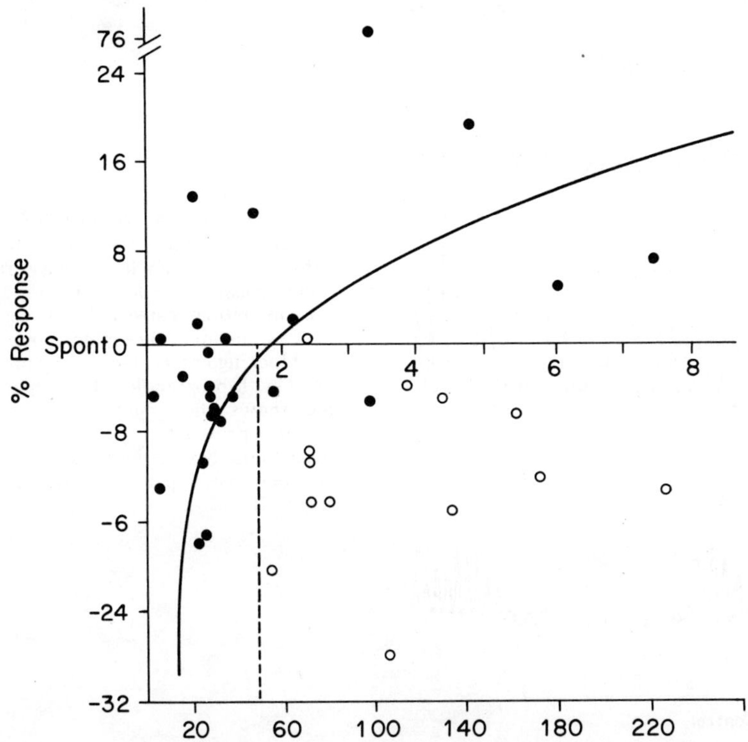

FIGURE 9. A graph that shows the correlation between plasma hormonal levels and percentage change in area under the contractility curve after transmural nerve stimulation, identification, and labeling. Symbols are the same as in FIGURE 7.

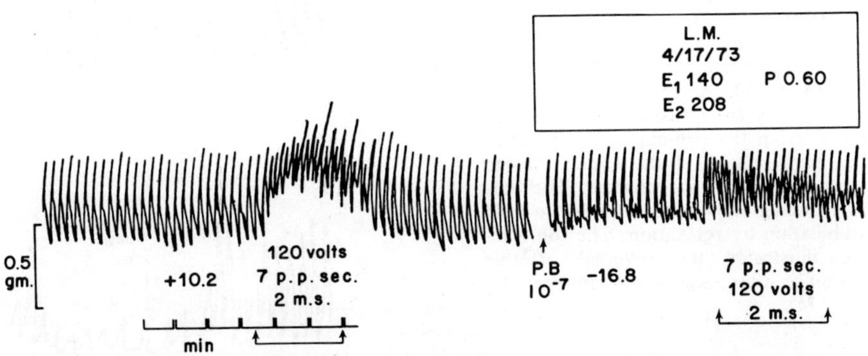

FIGURE 10. A record from a subject with very high estrogen and insignificant progesterone levels. Transmural nerve stimulation was applied before and after blocking with phenoxybenzamine (10^{-7} M).

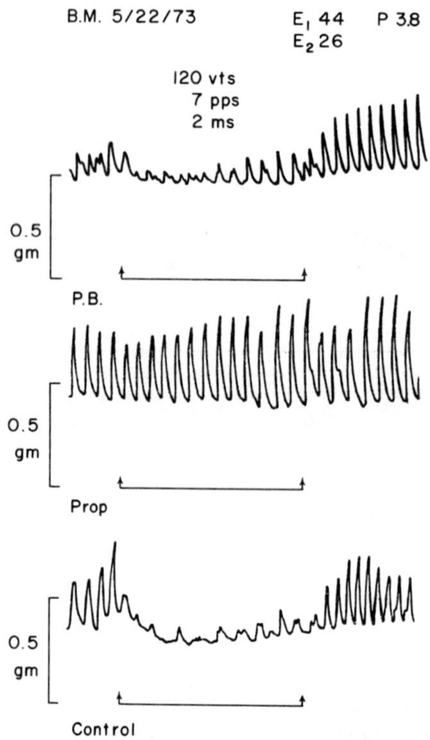

FIGURE 11. A record of three consecutive tissue specimens from a subject in the early luteal phase run simultaneously. The lower record shows the inhibition caused by transmural nerve stimulation. The middle one shows the blocking of this response by pretreatment with propranolol. The upper tracing shows the results obtained with tissue pretreated with phenoxybenzamine. Notice the marked similarity between the upper and lower records (control).

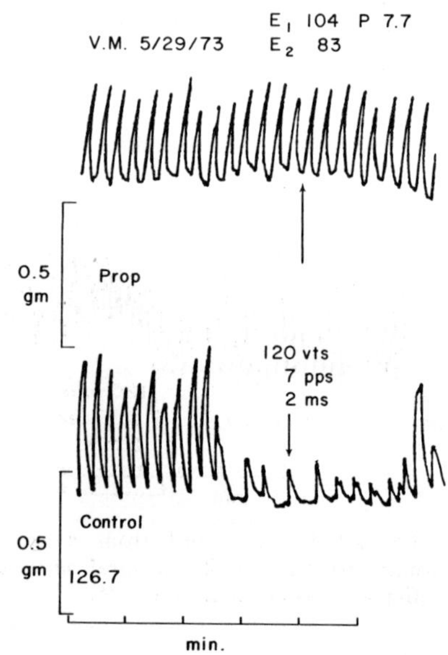

FIGURE 12. A record of *in vitro* contractility from two consecutive segments from the isthmus of a subject in the luteal phase of the cycle. Plasma hormonal values are charted. The bottom tracing shows the response to field stimulation by relaxation. The top tracing illustrates the reversal of this response after exposure to propranolol (10^{-7} M).

It has recently been shown that NE release from adrenergic terminals in many tissues may be subject to feedback control by prostaglandin E and by presynaptic α and β adrenergic receptors.[32,33,40–44] Hedqvist and Moawad[44] have shown that in the isthmic portion of the human oviduct, NE release from the adrenergic nerve terminals may be controlled by any one of these three mechanisms. Positive feedback operates through the activation of presynaptic β adrenergic receptors, leading to increased neurotransmitter release. On the other hand, activation of the presynaptic α adrenergic receptors results in decreased neurotransmitter release. The nature of the presynaptic and of the effector organ adrenergic receptors is

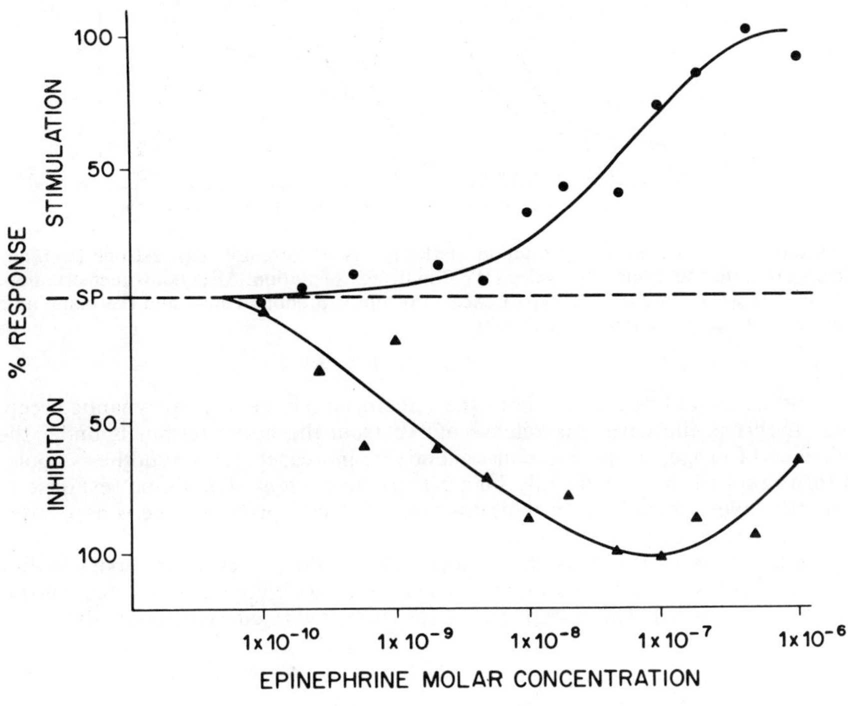

FIGURE 13. Comparison between the cumulative dose-response curves of follicular (●) and luteal (▲) phase tissues.

identical; that is, they are stimulated and blocked by the same pharmacologic agents.

PROPOSAL FOR A HYPOTHETICAL MODEL

At this point, there is a need for a model to explain the findings summarized in these studies as regards the action of progesterone on adrenergic mechanisms in the genital tract smooth muscle. FIGURE 15 graphically illustrates our hypothesis. In this report, we have shown that in the presence of both estrogen and significant concentrations of progesterone, there is a β-receptor predominance. Presumably,

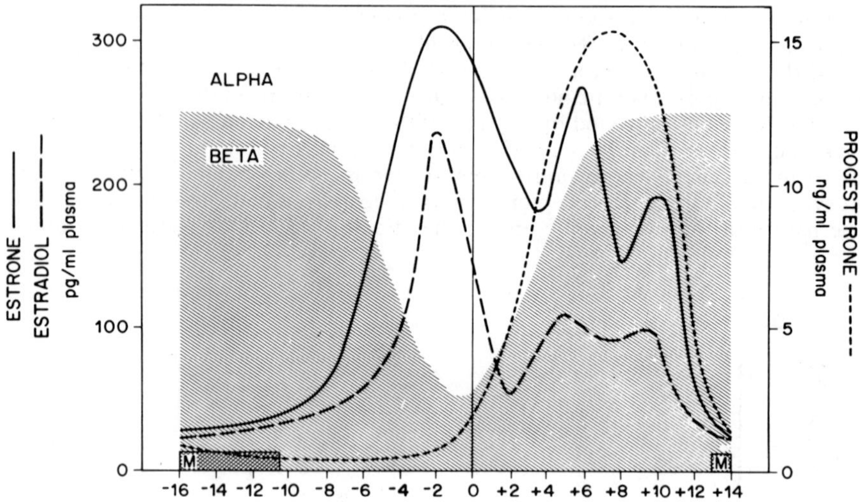

FIGURE 14. A graphic representation of the levels of estradiol (E_2), estrone (E_1), and progesterone in the ovulatory cycle. Day 0 indicates ovulation; M denotes menstruation. The shaded area represents a hypothetical β-receptor predominance, and the blank area represents the contribution of α receptors.

this finding should be true for both the effector organ and the presynaptic receptors. If this is the case, the release of NE from the nerve terminals under the influence of progesterone will consequently be increased. This hypothesis could, in turn, explain the significantly high NE tissue content. The tissue response to high NE levels should be an inhibitory one, because progesterone is associated with a β-adrenergic predominance.

Under the influence of estrogen alone, one would expect the reverse situation to exist, as illustrated in FIGURE 15. Various steps are involved in the mechanisms shown in this model. These steps have to be further verified experimentally.

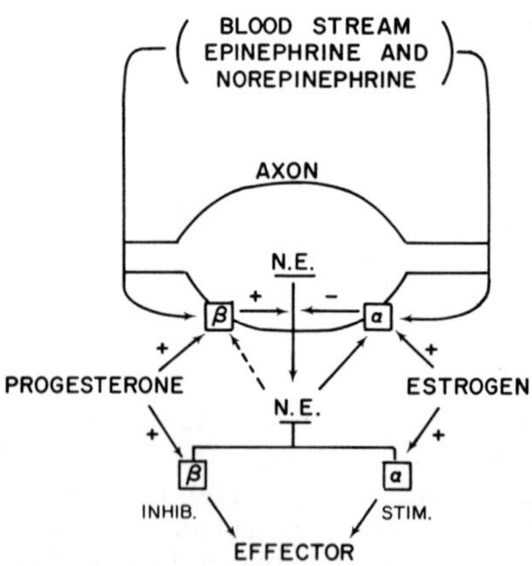

FIGURE 15. A graphic model that describes the possible relationship between sex steroids and the peripheral adrenergic nerve terminals and effector organs (NE is norepinephrine). Progesterone stimulates the presynaptic and effector organ β-adrenergic receptors. This stimulation results in an increased norepinephrine release and inhibition of the effector organ. On the other hand, estrogen activates the presynaptic and effector organ α-adrenergic receptors. This activation results in a decreased norepinephrine release and stimulation of the effector organ.

In summary, we have shown in a series of studies that:

There is no demonstrable difference between the adrenergic fluorescence of the isthmus from rabbits injected with estrogen alone and that of those injected with estrogen plus progesterone.

There is no difference between the adrenergic fluorescence of human tissues from the isthmus during the follicular phase of the cycle and that of similar tissues collected during the luteal phase.

Norepinephrine content in the human oviductal isthmus from subjects with low progesterone levels is decreased significantly in the presence of high estrogen content.

In the presence of high estrogen levels, the tissue content of norepinephrine is significantly increased with the rise of progesterone levels.

The α adrenergic receptors in the genetal tract tissues predominate in the presence of high, unopposed estrogen values.

The presence of plasma progesterone in quantities greater than or equal to 2.0 ng/ml is associated with a reversal of α adrenergic receptor predominance to β-receptor predominance.

Acknowledgment

The authors thank Miss Susan Vellner for her expert secretarial assistance.

References

1. Sjöstrand, N. O. 1962. Acta Physiol. Scand. **56.**
2. Sjöstrand, N. O. 1965. Acta Physiol. Scand. **65** (Suppl. 257).
3. Owman, C. & N. O. Sjöstrand. 1965. Z. Zellforsch. **66.**
4. Brundin, J. 1965. Acta Physiol. Scand. **66** (Suppl. 259).
5. Owman, C., E. Rosengren & N. O. Sjöberg. 1966. Life Sci. **5.**
6. Rosengren, E. & N. O. Sjöberg. 1967. Amer. J. Anat. **121.**
7. Hamberger, B. & K. A. Norberg. 1965. Acta Physiol. Scand. **65** (Suppl. 235).
8. Marshall, J. M. 1970. Ergeb. Physiol. 62: 1.
9. Sjöberg, N. O. 1967. Acta Physiol. Scand. (Suppl. 305).
10. Carlsson, A., B. Falck & N. A. Hillarp. 1962. Acta Physiol. Scand. **56** (Suppl. 196).
11. Falck, B. 1962. Acta Physiol. Scand. **56** (Suppl. 197): 1.
12. Falck, B. & C. Owman. 1966. *In* Mechanisms of Release of Biogenic Amines. U.S. von Euler, S. Rosell & B. Uvnas, Eds.: 59. Pergamon Press. Oxford, England.
13. Norberg, K. A. & B. Fredricsson. Acta Physiol. Scand. **68** (Suppl. 277): 149.
14. Owman, C. & N. O. Sjöberg. 1966. Z. Zellforsch. **74:** 182.
15. Sjöberg, N. O. 1968. Acta Endocrinol. **57:** 405.
16. Owman, C., E. Rosengren & N. O. Sjöberg. 1967. Obstet. Gynecol. **30:** 763.
17. Miller, M. D. & J. M. Marshall. 1965. Amer. J. Physiol. **209:** 859.
18. Rosengren, E. & N. O. Sjöberg. 1968. Acta Physiol. Scand. **72:** 412.
19. Cha, K. S., W. C. Lee, A. Rudzik & J. W. Miller. 1965. J. Pharmacol. Exp. Ther. **148:** 9.
20. Gardmark, S., C. Owman & N. O. Sjöberg. 1971. Amer. J. Obstet. Gynecol. **109:** 997.
21. Rudzik, A. D. & J. W. Miller. 1962. J. Pharmacol. Exp. Ther. **138:** 88.
22. Wurtman, R. J., J. Axelrod & I. J. Kopin. 1963. Endocrinology **73:** 501.
23. Green, R. D. & J. W. Miller. 1966. Science **151:** 825.
24. Gutman, Y. & H. Weil-Malherbe. 1967. Nature (London) **214:** 108.

25. DIAMOND, J. & T. M. BRODY. 1966a. J. Pharmacol. Exp. Ther. **152:** 202.
26. DIAMOND, J. & T. M. BRODY. 1966b. Life Sci. **5:** 2187.
27. OSKARSSON, V. 1960. Acta Endocrinol. **34:** 38.
28. SWEDIN, G. & J. O. BRUNDIN. 1968. Experientia **24:** 1015.
29. GAFFNEY, E., R. L. BURKET & S. WORONKOW. 1965. Obstet. Gynecol. **25:**340.
30. EDDY, C. A. & D. L. BLACK. 1973. J. Reprod. Fertil. **33:** 1.
31. OWMAN, C. & N. O. SJÖBERG. 1972. J. Reprod. Med. **3:** 63.
32. MOAWAD, A. H., P. HEDQVIST & M. BYGDEMAN. 1975a Acta Physiol. Scand. **95:** 142.
33. MOAWAD, A. H., P. HEDQVIST & M. H. KIM. 1975b. *In* Proceedings of the Symposium on Ovum Transport and Fertility Regulation, San Antonio, Texas.
34. OWMAN, C. & N. O. SJÖBERG. 1975. *In* Proceedings of the Symposium on Neuroendocrine Regulation of Fertility, Simla. In press.
35. ZUSPAN, F. P. & M. A. Cooley. 1970. Advan. Auto. Anal. **1:** 35.
36. DUJOVNE, A. R., N. P. D., LABORDE, L. M. CARRIL, S. CHEVIAKOFF, E. PEDROZA & J. M. ROSNER. 1976. Amer. J. Obstet. Gynecol. **124:** 229.
37. PATON, D. M. 1968. Eur. J. Pharmacol. **3:** 310.
38. TOTHILL, A. 1967. Brit. J. Pharmacol. Chemother. **29:** 291.
39. HIGGS, G. H. & A. H. MOAWAD. 1974. Can. J. Physiol. Pharmacol. **52:** 74.
40. STARKE, K. 1972. Naunyn-Schmiedeberg's Arch. Pharmakol. **275:** 11.
41. ENERO, M. A., S. Z. LANGER, R. P. ROTHLIN, & F. J. E. STEFANO. 1972. Brit. J. Pharmacol. **44:** 672.
42. LANGER, S. Z. 1975. *In* Chemical Tools in Catecholamine Research. T. Malmfors, Ed. North-Holland Publ. Co. Amsterdam, The Netherlands. In press.
43. STJÄRNE, L. & J. BRUNDIN. 1975. Acta Physiol. Scand. **94:** 139.
44. HEDQVIST, P. & A. H. MOAWAD. 1975 Acta Physiol. Scand. **95:** 494.

DISCUSSION

DR. F. A. KINCL *(Richmond College, City University of New York, Staten Island, N.Y.):* Have you thought of measuring the monoamine oxidase levels?

DR. MOAWAD: We have not made these measurements, although we may in the future. However, we are now also trying to determine the effect of progesterone on the actual secretion of norepinephrine from the terminals, because, as you know, when we measure only the total norepinephrine content of the tissue, we are measuring the total effect of the process of synthesis, release, reuptake, and degradation.

DR. SCHULMAN *(Albert Einstein College of Medicine, Bronx, N.Y.):* How big are the tissue strips in your stimulation studies?

DR. MOAWAD: The tissues are, of course, circular cross-sections of the oviduct, and they measure 2–3 mm in length. We do not have the exact length of each section, but we do restrict it to this range.

DR. SCHULMAN: I don't understand the stimulus of 120 V; this seems like an extraordinary stimulus to supply. When you are working with myometrium, this stimulation level bypasses membrane levels, so I am not quite sure what you are measuring with this system.

DR. MOAWAD: The 120 V specified is a somewhat misleading value. It is important to remember that this is a field stimulation procedure and that the 120 V only measures the potential across the platinum electrodes. The resistance of the space between these electrodes (which contains not only the tissue, but also the semiconductive physiologic salt solution) falls into the 40,000 Ω range, yielding a total current of only about 3 mA. It is also true that the potential developed across any individual membrane within the field would be considerably less than the 120-V potential that exists between the electrodes that establish the field. We determined that we did not get an optimal response from the tissue if a stimulus of less than 120 V was supplied to the primary electrodes, but we also established that the presence of tetrodotoxin eliminated the response of the tissue to field stimulation, while the subsequent addition of exogenous norepinephrine elicited a response that mimicked the response of tissue to field stimulation (FIGURE D1). Considered in this perspective, therefore, 120 V does not appear to be an excessive stimulus.

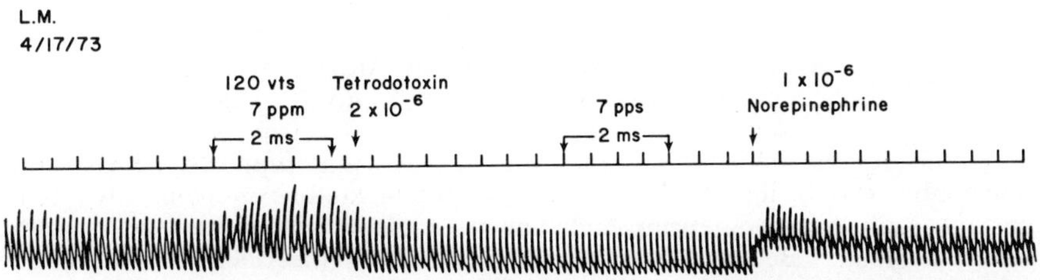

FIGURE D1. A record of the *in vitro* contractility of a tissue from the isthmic region. Transmural field stimulation resulted in an increased activity. This response was abolished when repeated after the application of tetrodotoxin (2×10^{-6} M). On the other hand, the tissue still responded by increased activity to subsequent treatment with norepinephrine (10^{-6} M).

PROGESTERONE BINDING AND METABOLISM IN HUMAN FETAL MEMBRANES*

Barry E. Schwarz, Leon Milewich, Norman F. Gant, John C. Porter, John M. Johnston, and Paul C. MacDonald

Cecil H. and Ida Green Center for Reproductive Biology Sciences and Departments of Obstetrics and Gynecology, Biochemistry, and Physiology University of Texas Southwestern Medical School Dallas, Texas 75235

Introduction: A Proposed Basic Model for the Initiation of Human Labor

A considerable body of evidence has accrued that supports the view that human labor may be initiated by the action of prostaglandins or chemically related substances on the myometrium and that prostaglandin synthesis occurs in the uterine decidua.[1] Because free arachidonic acid is the obligate biosynthetic precursor of both prostaglandin E_2 and $F_{2\alpha}$, we measured the arachidonic acid content of the human chorioamnion and found that arachidonic acid accounted for nearly 20% of the total fatty acid content.[2] This value is a remarkably high arachidonic acid content for a human tissue. For example, arachidonic acid comprises only 0.4% of the total fatty acids in maternal parietal peritoneum.[2] Thus, the fetal membranes may serve as a storage site for arachidonic acid, which is found in tissues in an esterified form primarily in the 2-position of glycerophospholipids or possibly in cholesterol esters. However, only free unesterified arachidonic acid may serve as a prostaglandin precursor.[3] The enzyme phospholipase A_2 (E.C.3.1.1.4) catalyzes the hydrolysis reaction that results in the release of free arachidonic acid from the 2-position of glycerophospholipids. We have identified a phospholipase in human chorioamnion and confirmed that it is a phospholipase A_2.[4] Moreover, we have demonstrated that at least a portion of this phospholipase A_2 activity is localized in lysosomes[5] and have provided preliminary evidence that the phospholipase A_2 of human chorioamnion has some specificity for arachidonyl esters.[6]

Based on these observations, we propose a model for the metabolic events that lead to the initiation of human labor, a model in which the fetal membranes play a central role. The metabolic reactions envisioned are diagrammatically illustrated in Figure 1. That phospholipase A_2 is sequestered in fetal membrane lysosomes is central to this hypothesis. At or near term, the lysosomes are perturbed, allowing accelerated expression of phospholipase A_2 activity and resulting in the hydrolysis of glycerophospholipids and the release of free arachidonic acid. Free arachidonic acid may diffuse to the decidua and therein be converted to prostaglandins or prostaglandin-like substances, for example, endoperoxides or thromboxanes, which, in turn, may diffuse to the myometrium and therein inhibit the ATP-dependent sequestration of calcium ions by the sarcoplasmic reticulum[7] and thus initiate the myometrial contractions of human labor. The model provides for the diffusion of both free arachidonic acid and prostaglandins into the amniotic

*Supported in part by United States Public Health Service Grant 5 PO1 HD 08672-03.

fluid, where the concentrations of both substances have been measured and found to be increased in laboring women.[8] An additional and important feature of the proposed model is that such a system could be self-perpetuating. One product of the hydrolysis reaction catalyzed by phospholipase A_2 is lysophospholipid, a substance known to perturb lysosomes, while the other product, free arachidonic acid, may be converted to prostaglandins, which are also known to affect lysosomal enzyme activity. Defining the events that cause the initial perturbation of the fetal membrane lysosomes becomes critical to our understanding of the initiation of labor.

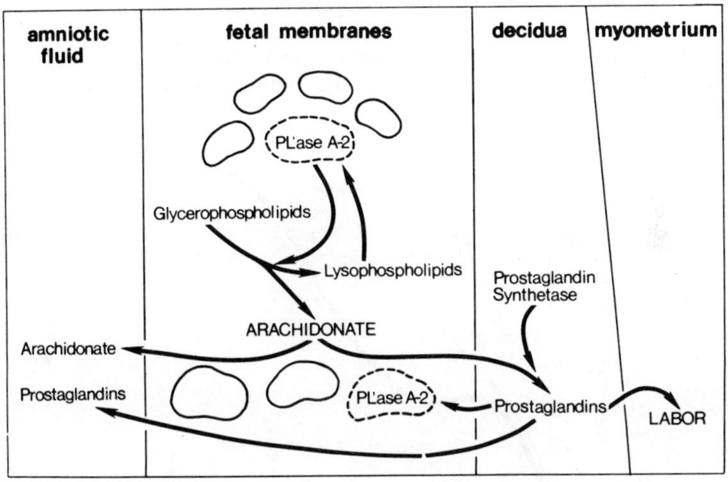

FIGURE 1. A proposed basic model for the initiation of human labor.

A Role for Progesterone in the Initiation of Human Labor

In considering the factors that may cause the initial perturbation of fetal membrane lysosomes, we have turned our attention to steroid hormones. The role of steroid hormones, particularly progesterone, in human parturition has long been considered and studied but as yet not clarified. In most animal species studied to date, there is a precipitous decline in maternal plasma progesterone concentration just prior to the onset of labor. This decline in progesterone concentration is illustrated in FIGURE 2 for the rat, the cow, and the sheep. This decline does not appear to occur in women. In fact, the preponderance of evidence is consistent with the pattern illustrated in FIGURE 2, in which maternal plasma progesterone concentrations in women reach a peak at 33–34 weeks of gestation and then remain essentially constant until after delivery. It is intriguing to note that progesterone withdrawal at the end of the human ovarian cycle is coincident with an increase in prostaglandin production in the endometrium and the onset of menstruation.[9]

It might be possible to effect a local, *in situ,* progesterone withdrawal at the level of the fetal membranes without significantly altering maternal plasma progesterone concentrations, which represent primarily placental progesterone production. Three mechanisms that act independently or in concert might accomplish this withdrawal: the fetal membranes may be capable of progesterone synthesis, and this capability may be altered as term approaches; the fetal membranes may be capable of progesterone metabolism, and this capability may be altered in late gestation; and progesterone action in the fetal membranes may be modulated by a progesterone-binding substance by any of several mechanisms, and the amount or character of such a substance may be altered with advancing gestation. We shall consider each of these possible mechanisms in turn.

Progesterone Synthesis in Human Fetal Membranes

We have measured progesterone synthesis in human amnion and chorion laeve from various stages of gestation by incubating whole tissue minces with

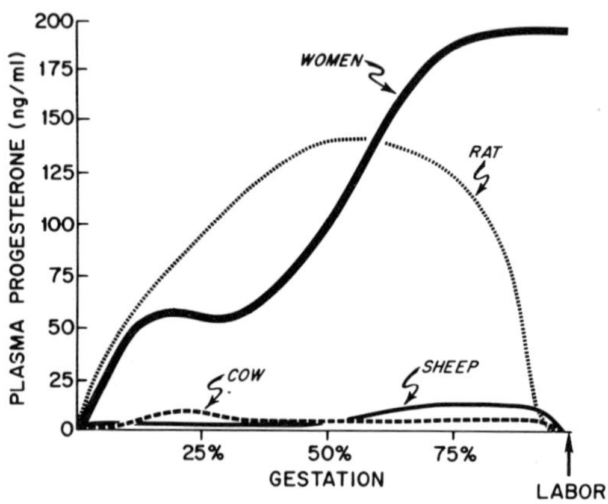

FIGURE 2. Maternal plasma progesterone concentration throughout gestation (after Bedford *et al.*)[16]

^{3}H-labeled cholesterol or pregnenolone. Chorion laeve is capable of progesterone synthesis of significant magnitude from pregnenolone, but progesterone formation was not demonstrated by use of cholesterol as the substrate. The mean rate of conversion of pregnenolone to progesterone in 11 specimens was 0.26 ± 0.03 (SEM) nmol per gram of tissue per hour, and in this limited sample, there was no significant difference in progesterone-synthesizing capability when chorion laeve tissues from term gestations were compared to those obtained from early gestations. No labeled progesterone was produced in incubation mixtures that contained minced amnion.

Progesterone Metabolism in Human Fetal Membranes

We have measured, *in vitro,* the ability of human fetal membranes to convert progesterone to other steroids. By careful product isolation and identification after incubation of whole homogenates with tritium-labeled progesterone, we have demonstrated two routes of progesterone metabolism that may occur in chorion and amnion, 5α reduction and 20α reduction. We have measured the activities of the two enzymes responsible for the observed progesterone metabolism, 5α-reductase and 20α-hydroxysteroid oxido-reductase, in whole homogenates of amnions and chorions obtained at various stages of gestation. The activities of both enzymes are relatively high in membranes obtained from early gestations but fall dramatically as gestation advances. In fact, the activity of 5α-reductase in term chorion approaches zero.[10]

It is possible that progesterone action in the fetal membranes actually represents the action of a major metabolite(s) of progesterone and that withdrawal of the metabolite(s) by the failure of its production initiates labor by a mechanism totally analogous to that envisioned for progesterone withdrawal. This possibility remains essentially unexplored to date. One may, however, interpret the data in a different way. The enzyme 5α-reductase appears to be substrate induced,[11] whereas 20α-hydroxysteroid oxido-reductase appears to be a progesterone- or progestin-induced enzyme.[12,13] The decline in enzymatic activity in late gestation could therefore represent a decline in progesterone action, that is, progesterone withdrawal, rather than a maturation or aging process that occurs within the fetal membranes. If this were the case, these data would be consistent with an interpretation of localized progesterone withdrawal but would offer no mechanism for the actual removal of progesterone from these tissues late in human pregnancy.

Progesterone Binding in Human Fetal Membranes

We have examined the ability of human fetal membranes to bind progesterone and observed that cytosols (105,000 *g* supernatant fractions) prepared with human chorion laeve and amnion contain a substance that binds progesterone and sediments in a sucrose density gradient at 4S. This substance loses its ability to bind progesterone when heated to 56°C for 15 min or when treated with pronase. RNase and DNase have no significant effect on the progesterone-binding substance. The substance also binds cortisol with essentially equal affinity.

The progesterone-binding substance will bind 5α-dihydroprogesterone but will not bind 20α-hydroxypregn-4-en-3-one. Transcortin and maternal serum bind 20α-hydroxypregn-4-en-3-one but do not bind 5α-dihydroprogesterone. Based on these observations, we conclude that the progesterone-binding substance of human fetal membranes is not transcortin, and we find no evidence that it circulates in maternal blood. In addition, the progesterone-binding substance of human fetal membranes will not bind R 5020, (17,21-dimethyl-19-norpregna-4,9-diene-3,-20-dione), a progestin that binds to human progesterone receptor proteins.[14] Based on these observations, we conclude that the progesterone-binding substance of human fetal membranes is not a typical progesterone "receptor." Furthermore, the progesterone-binding substance of human fetal membranes will not bind dexamethasone, a steroid that binds to glucocorticoid receptors. Based on these observations, we conclude that the progesterone-binding substance of human fetal membranes is unique: It is not transcortin. It is not a progesterone receptor. It is not a glucocorticoid receptor.

The progesterone-binding capacity of the chorioamnion has been measured at various stages of gestation. Prior to 20 weeks of gestation, little or no progesterone-binding capacity can be detected in the fetal membranes. After the 20th week and through the 37th week of gestation, a modest but detectable amount of progesterone-binding activity is present in the membranes. However, during the last 2–3 weeks of pregnancy, there is a dramatic increase in progesterone-binding capacity of the fetal membranes to a mean value of 450 *f*mol of progesterone bound per milligram of protein. This mean is statistically different from all other measured values ($p < 0.001$).[15]

We have recently observed that the progesterone-binding substance of intact amnion can be extracted into buffers that contain 0.4 M KCI; however, the progesterone-binding substance cannot be extracted from intact chorion laeve under similar conditions. While there are many possible explanations for these observations, the hypothesis that is most appealing to us at the present time is the one illustrated in FIGURE 3. In this Figure, a model is graphically represented in which it is envisioned that the progesterone-binding substance is localized *on* the amnion and *in* the chorion. This localization of the progesterone-binding substance along with the apparent dramatic increase in the amount of progesterone-binding substance before, but near, the time of onset of labor could provide for a system in which progesterone withdrawal could occur at the level of the fetal membranes and not be reflected by maternal plasma progesterone concentrations.

In consideration of these observations, the basic model proposed may be expanded.

CONCLUSION: AN EXPANDED MODEL PROPOSED FOR THE INITIATION OF HUMAN LABOR

FIGURE 4 illustrates the proposed expanded model. Progesterone-binding substance is localized on the amnion. At or near term, a dramatic increase in the amount of progesterone-binding substance causes progesterone withdrawal in the fetal membranes either by preventing further entry of progesterone into the

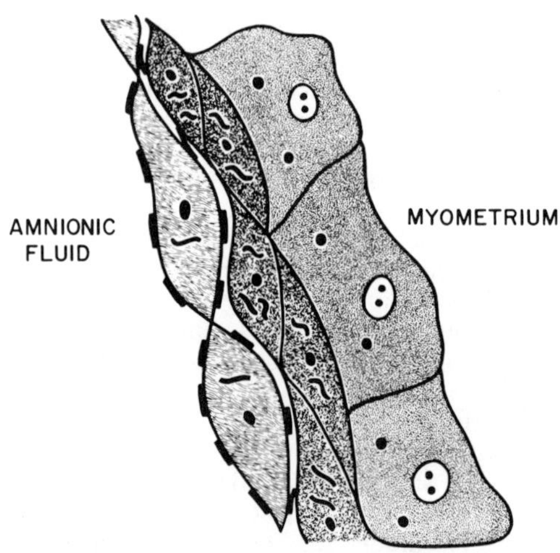

FIGURE 3. A model for the localization of progesterone-binding substance. Progesterone-binding substance illustrated by the short bars is localized on the amnion and in the chorion. The open circles within decidual cell cytoplasm and nuclei represent typical progesterone "receptor" protein, which is presumed to be present in this tissue.

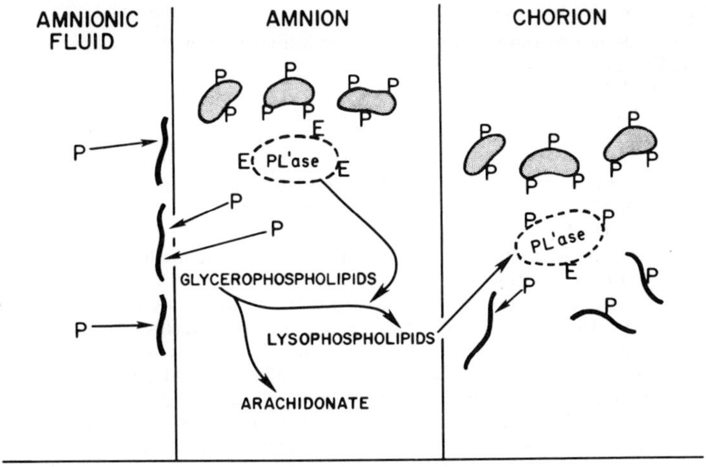

FIGURE 4. An expansion of the proposed basic model for the initiation of human labor. Progesterone-binding substance, as represented by the short bars, is illustrated on the amnion and in the chorion.

amnion cell or by actually removing progesterone from the amnion cell or by a combination of both mechanisms. This progesterone withdrawal is reflected by a decrease in the activity of enzymes that metabolize progesterone. Progesterone withdrawal alone or in concert with continued estrogen stimulation perturbs the fetal membrane lysosomes, allowing accelerated expression of phospholipase A_2 activity and initiating the entire sequence of cascading and self-perpetuating metabolic events that eventuate in human labor. Alternatively, the progesterone-binding substance in the chorion laeve or the protein-progesterone complex may act to provide for the perturbation of the lysosomes. In any event, the demonstration of a unique protein with high affinity for progesterone that appears in the fetal membranes before, but near, the onset of human parturition is of considerable interest in a further definition of the biochemical events that result in human parturition.

REFERENCES

1. KARIM, S. M. M. 1972. Prostaglandins and human reproduction. *In* The Prostaglandins.: 73–164. John Wiley & Sons, Inc. New York, N.Y.
2. SCHWARZ, B. E., F. M. SCHULTZ, P. C. MACDONALD & J. M. JOHNSTON. 1975. Initiation of human parturition: III. Fetal membrane content of prostaglandin E_2 and $F_{2\alpha}$ precursor. Obstet. Gynecol. **46**(5): 564–568.
3. SAMUELSSON, B. 1970. Structure, biosynthesis and metabolism of prostaglandins. *In* Lipid Metabolism. S. J. Wakil, Ed.: 107–153. Academic Press, Inc. New York, N.Y.
4. SCHULTZ, F. M., B. E. SCHWARZ, P. C. MACDONALD & J. M. JOHNSTON. 1975. Initiation of human parturition: II. Identification of phospholipase A_2 in fetal chorioamnion and uterine decidua. Amer. J. Obstet. Gynecol. **123**(6): 650–653.
5. SCHWARZ, B. E., F. M. SCHULTZ, P. C. MACDONALD & J. M. JOHNSTON. 1976. Initiation of human parturition: IV. Demonstration of phospholipase A_2 in the lysosomes of human fetal membranes. Amer. J. Obstet. Gynecol. **125**(8): 1089–1092.

6. Schultz, F. M., P. C. MacDonald & J. M. Johnston. 1975. Initiation of human parturition: demonstration of a unique phospholipase A_2 in chorioamnion. Gynecol. Invest. **6**(1–2): II (Abs.).
7. Carsten, M. E. 1973. Prostaglandins and cellular calcium transport in the pregnant human uterus. Amer. J. Obstet. Gynecol. **117:** 824–832.
8. MacDonald, P. C., F. M. Schultz, J. H. Duenhoelter, N. F. Gant, J. M. Jimenez, J. A. Pritchard, J. C. Porter & J. M. Johnston. 1974. Initiation of human parturition: I. Mechanism of action of arachidonic acid. Obstet. Gynecol. **44**(5): 629–636.
9. Pickles, V. R., W. J. Hall, F. A. Best & G. N. Smith. 1965. Prostaglandins in endometrium and menstrual fluid from normal and dysmenorrhaeic subjects. J. Obstet. Gynecol. Brit. Commonwealth **72:** 185–195.
10. Milewich, L., N. F. Gant, B. Schwarz, R. A. Prough, G. Chen, B. Athey & P. C. MacDonald. 1976. Metabolism of progesterone by the human fetal membranes. Gynecol. Invest. **7**(1–2): 91 (Abs.).
11. Moore, R. J. & J. D. Wilson. 1973. The effect of androgenic hormones on the reduced nicotinamide adenine dinucleotide phosphate:Δ^4-3-ketosteroid 5α-oxidoreductase of rat ventral prostate. Endocrinology **93**(3): 581–592.
12. Tseng, L. & E. Gurpide. 1974. Estradiol and 20α-dihydroprogesterone dehydrogenase activities in human endometrium during the menstrual cycle. Endocrinology **94:** 419–423.
13. Tseng, L. & E. Gurpide. 1975. Induction of human endometrial estradiol dehydrogenase by progestins. Endocrinology **97:** 825–833.
14. Philibert, D. & J. P. Raynaud. 1974. Binding of progesterone and R 5020, a highly potent progestin, to human endometrium and myometrium. Contraception **10**(5): 457–466.
15. Schwarz, B. E., L. Milewich, J. C. Porter, J. M. Johnston & P. C. MacDonald. 1976. Initiation of human parturition: V. Progesterone binding substance in fetal membranes. Obstet. Gynecol. **48**(6): 685–689.
16. Bedford, C. A., J. R. G. Challis, F. A. Harrison & R. B. Heap. 1972. The role of oestrogens and progesterone in the onset of parturition in various species. J. Reprod. Fertil. Suppl. **16:** 1–23.

Discussion

Question: We have performed simpler but similar studies on rhesus monkeys, in which progesterone levels also do not change during gestation and do not decrease prior to parturition. We have also found that progesterone production and clearance rates remain constant throughout gestation. However, we have found that the uterine and umbilical progesterone concentrations decrease drastically during the second half of gestation. Did you measure progesterone levels in these sites, which are more closely related to the uterus?

Dr. Schwarz: We have measured the total progesterone content of amnion and chorion in tissues obtained from cesarian sections, before and after labor, and can find no difference in total progesterone content. We have not yet done the study in which one would differentiate free from bound progesterone to see if their concentrations are different before and after labor.

Dr. P. K. Siiteri: Could you tell us just a little bit more about the protein, Dr. Schwarz?

Dr. Schwarz: The affinity constant is in the neighborhood of 10^8 or 10^9 M^{-1}. The total amount of progesterone-binding substance that we are able to find in association with amnion would account for approximately one-half of the total progesterone content of the amnion. The molecular weight of the progesterone-binding substance on SDS gels appears to be in the neighborhood of 57,000 daltons. Other than that, we have no further characterization to give you.

DR. R. J. B. KING: Studies by Dr. Weissman on the effect of steroids on lysosomal membrane stability have indicated that certain 5α steroids stabilize these membranes, but the Δ^4,3-ketones have no effect. How would you incorporate that information in with your model?

DR. SCHWARZ: More recent studies have actually shown that progesterone will accelerate the release of enzymes from lysosomes rather than stabilize them (Briggs. 1973. J. Steroid Biochem. **4:** 341). Unfortunately, very high concentrations of progesterone were used to see an effect at the lysosomal level. The only additional suggestion that I have is that everybody who has looked at lysosome-progesterone interactions has looked at just that, and, as we said time and time again at this conference, estrogen is there first, and certainly in pregnancy it is there simultaneously. Estrogen is now well known to be capable of labilizing lysosomes (Szego. 1973. Gynecol. Invest. **3:** 63). Progesterone may well modify the labilizing ability of estrogen, even though it may have no action at the level of the lysosome without estrogen stimulation. Nobody has ever looked at it.

DR. SIITERI: Dr. Schwarz, I would just remind you that in a tissue very nearby to that you're speaking of, namely, the placenta, the concentration of free progesterone is 10 μM or higher. This concentration certainly is pharmacologic in most people's minds, but it does happen to be the case in the human placenta.

DR. G. L. FLICKINGER: Dr. Schwarz, with respect to the specificity of your phospholipase A_2, you indicated that this enzyme has a high specificity for cleaving arachidonic acid. I think this finding is somewhat different from what other people have reported. What evidence do you have for this statement, because, obviously you are dealing here with kinetics at an interface and not in a soluble system? I think it would be rather difficult to prove the specificity of such an enzyme.

DR. SCHWARZ: I did not mean to indicate that we had proven a specificity. I said we had some preliminary evidence for specificity. We have the suggestion that if one mixes equimolar concentrations of dipalmitoyl phosphatidylcholine and 1-palmitoyl-2-arachidonoyl phosphatidylcholine with the label in the 2 position of both lecithins, more arachidonic than palmitic acid will be liberated. As you must know, there are people who argue very strongly that the initiation of labor occurs at the decidual site rather than at the fetal membrane site. Indeed, there is a phospholipase in decidua. However, it has not been convincingly demonstrated that this enzyme is a phospholipase A_2. We have shown that the decidual enzyme has no preference for the unsaturated fatty acid when presented with the same substrate mixture.

DR. FLICKINGER: My second question involves whether you have considered the possibility that your binding protein might bind cortisol under physiologic conditions. Removal of cortisol would be, I think, a more attractive possibility for causing a destabilization or a decreased latency of the lysosomal membrane.

DR. SCHWARZ: This situation is somewhat paradoxical. In the sheep, cortisol production by the fetus appears to precede the onset of labor, so that there is an apparent turning on of labor by cortisol production rather than by cortisol withdrawal. That doesn't appear to be the case in the human, because fetuses that are precluded by an enzymatic defect from producing augmented cortisol levels are not delivered post term; they are delivered on time. Whether cortisol has anything to do with the initiation of labor in the human at this point is an open question.

QUESTION: Since an increase in prostaglandins is generally not demonstrated before the onset of labor and not until after labor has begun, why do you hypothesize that they are not simply an energizer rather than an initiator?

DR. SCHWARZ: Although uterine venous blood concentrations of $PGF_{2\alpha}$ do rise prior to the onset of labor in the sheep (Liggins *et al.* 1972. J. Reprod. Fertil. Suppl. **16:** 85), what you suggest is still a possibility. Without uterine contractions, prostaglandins will efface and soften the cervix in the sheep and may have similar effects in the human. Additional evidence that prostaglandins are important in the initiation of labor is the observation that prostaglandins are able to cause rhythmical uterine contractions, which ultimately result in parturition at any stage of human gestation. These contractions are inhibited by drugs that we classically consider to be able to inhibit human labor, whereas oxytocin-stimulated contractions are not.

COMMENT: No, but almost any technique you use to produce uterine contractions will result in prostaglandin synthesis in the uterus.

DR. SCHWARZ: Mostly in the myometrium.

DR. W. H. PEARLMAN (*University of North Carolina School of Medicine, Chapel Hill, N.C.*): I think your binding of a CBG-like material in the fetal membrane is very interesting. I don't know what it's role might be, but it seems rather hard to believe that when as much as 0.25 g of progesterone is being produced daily toward the end of pregnancy that the CBG-like material in the fetal membranes can actually induce a local withdrawal of progesterone. You know the organ is being flooded with progesterone.

DR. SCHWARZ: But the amnion is not. The amnion has no blood supply. The concentration of progesterone in the human amnion is less than that in maternal serum. The concentration of progesterone in amniotic fluid is much less than that in maternal serum. The amnion is not flooded by progesterone by any means. The myometrium is being flooded.

DR. PEARLMAN: Your hypothesis relates to a withdrawal or an unavailability of progesterone to the myometrium.

DR. SCHWARZ: No, to the fetal membranes.

PROGESTERONE AND PROGESTINS IN THE MALE REPRODUCTIVE SYSTEM*

Charles Terner

Department of Biology
Biological Science Center
Boston University
Boston, Massachusetts 02215

Progesterone is a precursor of steroid hormones and is therefore present in the male as an intermediate. But progesterone is not a male sex hormone, and it may seem unnecessary to study its physiologic or pharmacologic effects on the male organism. On the other hand, the discovery of the antiandrogenic effects of synthetic progestins and their suggested uses as male antifertility drugs and in the treatment of cancer of the prostate have stimulated interest in the mechanisms of action of progestational compounds in the male. Because it was expected that the male would lack sensitivity, it has been customary to treat male animals with large doses of progestational compounds. We have found[1] that the male rat is much more sensitive to progestins than had been assumed before and that testicular germ cells contain a progesterone-binding protein for which synthetic progestins compete.[2]

When we attempted to isolate spermatozoa from testis homogenates by means of a filtration technique, we found that it was much easier to recover nonflagellate germ cells than spermatozoa. This paper will describe briefly how these cells are isolated from seminiferous tubules.

We tease the tubules in isotonic Krebs saline and then pass them through two changes of distilled water for 2 min each change. This treatment lyses the interstitial cells outside the tubular walls. We then return the tubules to saline (two changes), grind them in a loosely fitting hand-operated homogenizer, and pass the homogenate through a layer of Sephadex® G-25. The gel retains the spermatozoa and the spermatids with long flagella. The filtrate contains the intact round germ cells. These filtrates are then sedimented and washed by repeated centrifugation at low speed until the wash fluid is free from debris.

The final suspension of nonflagellate germ cells consists mainly of pachytene spermatocytes and spermatids (early and elongating).[3] Sertoli cells, which can be seen in crude homogenates, are absent from the filtered germ cell suspensions, and no spermatogonia are present. It seems that the Sertoli cells and the spermatogonia that are attached to the basement membrane are shredded by the homogenization and that the spermatocytes and spermatids are released intact. The germ cells are metabolically active. They glycolyse and respire. Their Z_{O_2} value (microliters per 10^8 cells per hour) is of the order of -70, whereas that of spermatozoa is about -10. They dismutate pyruvate to lactate and carbon dioxide in the absence of carbohydrate, as do spermatozoa.[4]

The germ cells in the seminiferous tubules are supported by Sertoli cells, and they are connected by intercellular bridges.[5] Those bridges are broken during homogenization, but the cells appear to "heal." The cells are round, and most appear to be undamaged. A recent paper by Romrell *et al.*[6] confirms that isolated

*Supported by National Institute of Child Health and Human Development Contract 69-2102. The Population Council, and the National Science Foundation.

germ cells, despite their broken bridges, are morphologically and functionally intact. Because of the presence of multinucleate cells in the early suspensions, our calculations were based on corrected cell counts obtained by protein determination.

These are the cell suspensions that we used in our earlier work. We have more recently separated the germ cells by density gradient sedimentation and are in the process of isolating cells of single types. However, this paper will describe our earlier work with nonflagellate germ cells. They are prepared easily, and even though our old preparation contained several types of germ cells, it has provided useful leads that we can now pursue in single cell types.

What attracted us most about the germ cells that we had isolated was that they were at the stage of spermatogenesis that is responsive to hormones. Spermatogenesis proceeds to the spermatocyte and early spermatid stages in the immature and in the hypophysectomized rat. Further development to advanced spermatids, however, requires gonadotropic hormones, probably follicle-stimulating hormone and also androgen. In our early attempts to measure metabolic changes, we injected male rats with various progestins and observed that the germ cells isolated from animals that had been treated with progestins showed a reduced capacity to incorporate glucose into lipids. We used the incorporation of [^{14}C]glucose into the lipids of isolated germ cells as a test to determine the minimum dose of progestin that would alter the metabolism of the germ cells. This treatment worked within a few days of injection and showed inhibition of labeling of the glycerides. Our test enabled us to reduce the dose of progestin to 0.5 or 1 mg/day (subcutaneously). Because treatment with progestin resulted in a decrease of testis and accessory gland weights, we tried to prevent this loss in weight by injecting the rats with testosterone at the same time.

We found that quite small amounts of testosterone were sufficient to stimulate growth of the accessory glands without supporting spermiogenesis. In young rats, 10 μg/day was an effective dose; in older animals, we used 50–100 μg/day in combination with 1 mg of Provera® or 0.5 mg of ethynodiol diacetate. After 6 weeks of treatment, the epididymis was free of spermatozoa, but the now infertile males were still capable of mating. By these experiments, we demonstrated in a model system based on the rat that it is possible to arrest spermiogenesis and maintain the accessory glands and libido by carefully adjusting the doses of the administered hormones.[1] A clinical trial in men of a similar treatment was subsequently reported by Frick.[7]

This background was required because it is the basis of our continuing studies. It should be noted that we approached this problem by thinking backward. When progestins are used as antiandrogens, the standard procedure is to treat castrated animals with large amounts of testosterone to build up the accessory glands and then to administer sufficient antiandrogen to suppress the effect of the androgen on the growth of the prostate and seminal vesicles. In our system, we suppressed gonadotropin production in intact animals by progestin treatment and then added only enough testosterone to prevent atrophy of the accessory glands. By stimulating the accessory glands without stimulating spermatogenesis, we separated the action of testosterone on the testes from its effect on the accessory glands. This means that although spermatogenesis is dependent on androgen, the germ cells are much less sensitive to androgen than are the prostate and the seminal vesicles. We wanted to look into the reasons for this phenomenon, and because we had a technique to isolate germ cells, we attempted to study their biochemical properties.

Christensen and Mason[9] had reported that intact seminiferous tubules, stripped free of Leydig cells, can convert progesterone to androgen. Because the cell type within the tubules had not been defined, we thought it would be interesting to see whether our isolated germ cells could produce androgen.

As stated earlier, it was found that we could remove the Leydig cells from the tubules more rapidly and completely by exposure to water than by mechanical stripping. Of course, if intact tubules are to be incubated, they should be stripped mechanically, because exposure of the tubules to water denatures the tubular wall and makes it impermeable. On the other hand, the coagulated walls protect the cells inside the tubules and, when the tubules are homogenized in isotonic saline and the suspension is passed through Sephadex, the filtrate contains germ cells free of Leydig cells.

On incubating the germ cells with ^{3}H-labeled progesterone, we found that they produced testosterone and androstenedione.[3] The experiments were performed by isolation of the products with ^{14}C-labeled carrier and crystallization to constant

TABLE 1

INHIBITION BY PROGESTINS OF PROGESTERONE METABOLISM IN MALE GERM CELLS*

Progestin Concentration (M)	17α-Hydroxyprogesterone		Testosterone	
	Picomoles	Inhibition (%)	Picomoles	Inhibition (%)
0	1.46 ± 0.21	—	4.25 ± 0.28	—
3×10^{-7}	0.96 ± 0.17	34	2.68 ± 0.30	37
3×10^{-6}	0.87 ± 0.25	41	2.46 ± 0.28	42
3×10^{-5}	0.66 ± 0.34	55	2.02 ± 0.42	52

*Nonflagellate germ cells ($2-6 \times 10^8$ cells/ml) were incubated with [1,2-^{3}H]progesterone (2 μCi, 2×10^{-8} M) and a progestin in Krebs-phosphate-saline; total volume, 5 ml; temperature, 37°C; incubation period, 3 hr. ^{14}C-labeled carrier steroid (0.01 mCi, 100 μg) was added at the end of the incubation. Testosterone and 17α-hydroxyprogesterone were purified by thin-layer chromatography and crystallization to a constant ^{3}H/^{14}C ratio. The data represent the means ± SD (picomoles per 10^8 cells per 3 hr) of nine experiments (three experiments with each of the following progestins: ethynodiol diacetate, medroxyprogesterone acetate, and cyproterone acetate).

isotope ratio. Recently, we determined the conversion of progesterone to testosterone by radioimmunoassay of testosterone and confirmed our results.

Production of testosterone is suppressed when rats are injected with progestins, and release of gonadotropins is inhibited. Accessory sex glands undergo atrophy, and spermatogenesis ceases. To support spermatogenesis in rats with suppressed gonadotropin production, high doses of testosterone (0.5–1 mg/day) must be injected. As was mentioned earlier, to maintain the accessory sex glands, it is sufficient to inject much lower doses, which may not support spermiogenesis. Obviously, a high level of intratubular androgen is needed, and we have evidence that at least some of it is produced locally within the tubules by the germ cells. According to Harris and Bartke,[10] testosterone concentration in the testis fluid of the intact, untreated rat is 20 times higher than that in the peripheral blood plasma. We therefore became interested in interactions of natural hormones and progestins at the local level. A local effect of progestins is described in TABLE 1, which illustrates their inhibitory effect *in vitro* on the conversion of [^{3}H]progesterone to androgens by germ cells. This effect is a direct competition of progestins with progesterone locally in the germ cells. We therefore expected the germ cells to have hormone-binding proteins. They should have an androgen receptor if they are target cells for androgens, and a binding protein for progesterone if it is to serve as a precursor of androgen.

It was found that more progesterone than androgen was bound by intact germ cells (FIGURE 1). After incubation with steroids, the cells were reisolated, cell membranes were lysed with Triton® X-100, and the cytosol and nuclei were separated. It was found that progesterone was bound exclusively by the cytosol, whereas considerable amounts of dihydrotestosterone were bound by the nuclei.

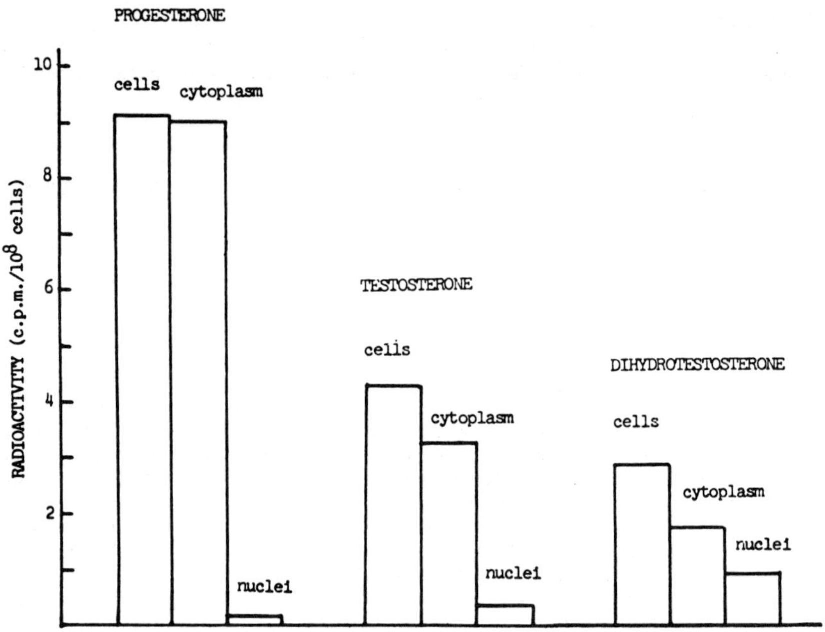

FIGURE 1. Retention of ^3H-labeled steroids by nonflagellate germ cells and their cytoplasmic and nuclear fractions. All flasks contained cells in 5 ml of Earle's medium (2.3×10^8 cells/ml) and ^3H-labeled steroid (1.5×10^{-10} M, 50 Ci/mmol). Additional unlabeled steroid was added to a second set of flasks. The cells were incubated for 30 min at 37°C, washed six times by centrifugation and resuspension, and treated with Triton X-100 to lyse the cell membranes. The nuclei were sedimented, washed twice by resuspension and sedimentation from phosphate saline, and further purified by centrifugation in sucrose. The specifically bound steroid shown in bar graphs was calculated by subtracting the counts per minute per 10^8 cells bound in the presence of unlabeled steroid (total steroid concentration 6.4×10^{-8} M) from that bound by incubation with the undiluted ^3H-labeled steroid (1.5×10^{-10} M).

In extracts of germ cells (TABLE 2) and of prostate and epididymal spermatozoa, bound androgens were displaced by progestins but not by progesterone. Progesterone was not bound by accessory tissues; it was displaced by progestins from the cytoplasmic binding protein of the germ cells (TABLE 3). Progestins are therefore both antiprogesterones and antiandrogens.

TABLE 2

COMPETITIVE DISPLACEMENT OF BOUND ANDROGEN*

Displacing Steroid	^{3}H-Labeled Steroid Displaced			
	Dihydrotestosterone		Testosterone	
	Counts per Minute	Percent	Counts per Minute	Percent
Dihydrotestosterone	318 ± 34	100	255 ± 34	112
Testosterone	213 ± 14	67	228 ± 22	100
Cyproterone acetate	196 ± 25	61	172 ± 40	76
Ethynodiol diacetate	164 ± 21	51	156 ± 21	69
Progesterone	69 ± 26	22	46 ± 18	20
17β-Estradiol	28 ± 18	9	40 ± 10	17
Androstenedione	0	0	0	0
Cortisol	0	0	0	0

*Extracts of nonflagellate germ cells (100,000*g* supernatants) were treated with dextran-coated charcoal to remove endogenous steroid. The extracts were incubated with labeled androgen for 4 hr at 4°C. Portions (5 mg of protein/ml) were equilibrated with 100 ng of displacing steroid for 2 hr at 4°C. Unbound steroid was removed by dextran-coated charcoal. The data are expressed as counts per minute per 5 mg of protein.

When we tested the effect of progestins on the metabolism of testosterone in intact germ cells (TABLE 4), we observed only a slight inhibition of its reduction to dihydrotestosterone (15–30%) but a greater inhibition of production of androstanediol (50–60%). Progestins therefore appear to inhibit the 3α-hydroxysteroid dehydrogenase more strongly than the α-reductase. This finding is in agreement with the observation of Villee *et al.*[11] that the effect of cyproterone acetate on α-reductase in prostate and seminal vesicles is a smaller factor than is its competition with dihydrotestosterone receptors.

It appears that progestins could interfere locally with the conversion of progesterone to testosterone by a mechanism analogous to the inhibition by

TABLE 3

DISPLACEMENT OF [^{3}H]PROGESTERONE BY PROGESTINS AND ANDROGEN*

Displacing Steroid	Reduction of [^{3}H]Progesterone Binding (%)
Progesterone	87
Cyproterone acetate	77
Ethynodiol diacetate	74
Chlormadinone acetate	69
Testosterone	57
5α-Dihydrotestosterone	54
Cortisol	<10
Estradiol benzoate	<10

*The 100,000*g* supernatants of nonflagellate germ cells were equilibrated with 10^{-9} M [^{3}H]progesterone for 2 hr at 4°C. The displacing compounds (10^{-7} M) were added, and equilibration was continued for 2 hr. Bound [^{3}H]progesterone was determined by adsorption on dextran-coated charcoal.

TABLE 4

INHIBITION BY PROGESTIN OF 5α REDUCTION OF TESTOSTERONE*

Progestin Concentration (M)	Dihydrotestosterone		5α-Androstanediol	
	Picomoles	Inhibition (%)	Picomoles	Inhibition (%)
0	13.0 ± 0.1	—	9.6 ± 0.5	—
1.5×10^{-7}	12.0 ± 0.8	7.6	7.6 ± 0.4	21
1.5×10^{-6}	11.4 ± 1.2	12.3	6.0 ± 0.9	37
1.5×10^{-5}	9.5 ± 0.4	27.0	4.0 ± 1.1	58

*Nonflagellate germ cells (2–6 × 10^8 cells) were incubated with [^{14}C]testosterone and a progestin in Krebs-phosphate-saline; total volume, 5 ml; temperature, 37°C; incubation period, 90 min. ^{3}H-labeled carrier androgen (100 μg, 0.01 mCi) was added at the end of the incubation. Dihydrotestosterone and 5α-androstanediol were isolated and purified by thin-layer chromatography and crystallization to a constant $^{14}C/^{3}H$ ratio. The data represent the means of four experiments (picomoles per 10^8 cells/90 min). The progestins were ethynodiol diacetate and cyproterone acetate.

progesterone of 17,20(17-hydroxyprogesterone)-lyase.[12] The relative insensitivity to progestin inhibition of α-reductase explains why we were able to maintain accessory gland function in progestin-treated animals by administration of small doses of testosterone.

The germ cells therefore seem to play a dual role. First, they behave like target cells for androgen. Second, they can use progesterone as a precursor of androgen, and we have seen that progesterone and progestins can interfere with some of these reactions. Normally, the progesterone level in male tissues is so low that it is not inhibitory, whereas the level of administered progestins can be manipulated, and they may therefore have practical clinical applications.

What is the function of the progesterone-binding protein in male germ cells? Obviously, this function is different from that in female target tissues, where it enters the target cell nucleus and controls genomic expression. In the male germ cell, the progesterone-binding protein is localized in the cytoplasm and does not carry progesterone into the nucleus. We determined the association constant of the complex, K_a, to be 2×10^9 liter/mol, the same order of magnitude as that found for progesterone binding in the uterine cytosol, 13–15 which, of course, is a target organ.

We believe that progesterone in the seminiferous tubules serves a specific function, namely, to act as a precursor of intratubular androgen. The progesterone-binding capacity of the germ cells enables them to take up progesterone circulating in low concentration. The germ cells are also target cells for androgen, which is required to support spermiogenesis. Their lower androgen-binding capacity appears to be compensated for by a high concentration of androgen in the testis fluid maintained by an androgen-binding protein.[16,17]

REFERENCES

1. TERNER, C. & J. MACLAUGHLIN. 1973. Effect of sex hormones on germinal cells of the rat testis: a rationale for the use of progestin and androgen combinations in the control of male fertility. J. Reprod. Fertil. **32:** 453–464.
2. GALENA, H. J., A. K. PILLAI & C. TERNER. 1974. Progesterone and androgen receptors in non-flagellate germ cells of the rat testis. J. Endocrinol. **63:** 223–237.

3. Galena, H. J. & C. Terner. 1974. Conversion of progesterone to androgens by nonflagellate germinal cells isolated from seminiferous tubules of rat testis. J. Endocrinol. **60:** 269–276.
4. Melrose, D. R. & C. Terner. 1953. The metabolism of pyruvate in bull spermatozoa. Biochem. J. **53:** 296–305.
5. Dym, M. & D. W. Fawcett. 1971. Further observations on the numbers of spermatogonia, spermatocytes, and spermatids connected by intercellular bridges in the mammalian testis. Biol. Reprod. **4:** 195–215.
6. Romrell, L. J., A. R. Bellvé & D. W. Fawcett. 1976. Separation of mouse spermatogenic cells by sedimentation velocity. A morphological study. Develop. Biol. **49:** 119–131.
7. Frick, J. 1973. Control of spermatogenesis in men by combined administration of progestin and androgen. Contraception **8:** 191–206.
8. Meistrich, M. L., W. R. Bruce & Y. Clermont. 1973. Cellular composition of fractions of mouse testis cells following velocity sedimentation separation. Exp. Cell Res. **79:** 213–227.
9. Christensen, A. K. & N. R. Mason. 1965. Comparative ability of seminiferous tubules and interstitial tissue of rat testes to synthesize androgens from progesterone-4-^{14}C *in vitro*. Endocrinology **76:** 646–656.
10. Harris, M. E. & A. Bartke. 1974. Concentration of testosterone in testis fluid of the rat. Endocrinology **95:** 701–706.
11. Villee, C. A., A. Grigorescu & P. R. K. Reddy. 1975. Androgen regulation of RNA synthesis in target tissues. J. Steroid Biochem. **6:** 561–565.
12. Mahajan, D. K. & L. T. Samuels. 1975. Inhibition of 17,20(17-hydroxyprogesterone)-lyase by progesterone. Steroids **25:** 217–228.
13. Feil, P. D., S. R. Glasser, D. O. Toft & B. W. O'Malley. 1972. Progesterone binding in mouse and rat uterus. Endocrinology **93:** 74–80.
14. Faber, L. E., M. L. Sandmann & H. Stavely. 1973. Progesterone and corticosteroid binding in rabbit uterine cytosols. Endocrinology **93:** 74–80.
15. Rao, B. R., W. G. Wiest & W. M. Allen. 1973. Progesterone 'receptor' in rabbit uterus. I. Characterization and estradiol-17β augmentation. Endocrinology **92:** 1229–1240.
16. Hansson, V., O. Djøseland, E. Reusch, A. Attramadal & O. Torgersen. 1973. An androgen binding protein in the testis cytosol fraction of adult rats. Comparison with the androgen binding protein in the epididymis. Steroids **21:** 457–474.
17. Hansson, V., W. S. McLean, A. A. Smith, D. J. Tindall, S. C. Weddington, S. N. Nayfeh & F. S. French. 1974. Androgen receptors in rat testis. Steroids **23:** 823–832.

Discussion

Dr. P. G. Satyaswaroop (*Mount Sinai School of Medicine, New York, N.Y.*): We have also observed inhibition of spermatogenesis during prolonged treatment of adult rats with Depo-Provera®, with a concomitant reduction in testosterone secretion, but we have some evidence to indicate that this effect cannot be explained solely by a suppressive action of progestin on gonadotropin output. We have observed inhibition of testicular 17β-hydroxysteroid dehydrogenase (17β-DH) and Δ^5-3β-hydroxysteroid dehydrogenase (3β-DH) activities after 1 month of treatment with medroxyprogesterone acetate. Treatment of another group of adult rats with gonadotropins alone, by a similar schedule, produced an increase in 3β-DH and a decrease in 17β-DH activities in the testis.

Therefore, the effect of Provera treatment on 17β-DH activity reveals a local effect of the hormone on the testes.

DR. W. L. MCGUIRE: Dr. Terner, what exactly were your criteria for deciding whether you were measuring a specific progesterone receptor or some other type of progesterone-binding protein, perhaps derived from plasma?

DR. TERNER: As I pointed out, unlike cells of the uterus, testicular cells are not target cells for progesterone, and the progesterone-binding complex does not seem to be transferred to the germ cell nuclei. On the other hand, the binding, although of low specificity, is of high affinity; K_a is of the same order of magnitude as that of the uterine progesterone-receptor complex. There is no reason to assume the presence of a protein derived from plasma. The cells were isolated from seminiferous tubules and carefully washed. As far as we know, it seems that there is a binding protein in testicular germ cells whose principal function is to make progesterone available to the cells.

QUESTION: 5α-Reductase is rather nonspecific as to its substrate, and it would equally use progesterone and testosterone. If you are injecting progesterone, it may simply replace testosterone as the substrate. Could you comment on that?

DR. TERNER: Progesterone has been reported to interfere with the conversion of progesterone to testosterone by inhibiting 17,20(17-hydroxyprogesterone)-lyase.[12] Progestins may be expected to do the same. When we added testosterone to germ cells *in vitro,* however, we found that it was reduced to dihydrotestosterone in the presence of progestins.

QUESTION: You said that your progestin/androgen treatment had maintained the accessory organs. Were you including the epididymis in that statement? If not, how did the epididymis fare during this treatment?

DR. TERNER: The testis and epididymis shrink when the production of spermatozoa is inhibited.

ANDROGENIC, SYNANDROGENIC, AND ANTIANDROGENIC ACTIONS OF PROGESTINS*

Leslie P. Bullock and C. W. Bardin

Departments of Medicine and Comparative Medicine
The Milton S. Hershey Medical Center
The Pennsylvania State University
Hershey, Pennsylvania 17033

INTRODUCTION

Although a sex steroid is usually classified according to its major action, namely, androgenic, estrogenic, or progestagenic, it may also stimulate responses that mimic those induced by other steroid classes. The androgenic action of progestins has been recognized for some time and has been described for embryonic, immature, and adult animals and man. However, the sensitivity and type of response vary with steroid and end point tested. In the adult castrate rat, progesterone and its derivatives are only slightly active in maintaining the male reproductive tract, whereas C_{18} gestagens related to 19-nortestosterone are quite androgenic.[1–4] By contrast, derivatives of both progesterone and 19-nortestosterone will masculinize the external genitalia of the female rat fetus.[5–7] Structure-function differences exist even within classes of progestins, because medroxyprogesterone acetate is equipotent to testosterone propionate in the fetus,[5,6] whereas the structurally similar megestrol acetate is inactive.[8] The variation in species response is well illustrated by the virilization of external genitalia that occurs in the guinea pig but not in the rat after cyproterone acetate treatment.[9,10]

Progestins may also act as antiandrogens.[9,11–13] Of the antiandrogens, cyproterone acetate is the most potent and has been the most extensively studied. In addition to these well-accepted actions, several investigators[14–18] recently described the ability of progestins to enhance androgen action, an effect that has been termed synandrogenic.[17] As is the case for the androgenic effects, manifestation of these other actions of progestins also depends on the steroid and end point studied.

This paper will summarize recent observations on the androgenic, synandrogenic, and antiandrogenic actions of C_{21} progestins in rodents. The report will describe both *in vivo* demonstrations of biologic activity and *in vitro* studies designed to demonstrate the molecular mechanism of these actions. In contrast to much of the previous work on progestin effects on reproductive tissues, these studies will focus primarily on responses in nonreproductive organs.

BIOLOGIC ACTIONS OF PROGESTINS

Androgenic, Synandrogenic, and Antiandrogenic Actions of Progestins in the Mouse

The actions of cyproterone acetate, medroxyprogesterone acetate, megestrol acetate, progesterone caproate, and progesterone were compared in several

*Supported by National Institutes of Health Grant HD 05276 and Contract N01-2-2730.

tissues of male and female mice. The basic protocol for most of the studies to be described in this section consisted of a control group of mice and groups treated for 6 days with 0.1 mg of testosterone, 0.1–10 mg of progestin, or a combination of the two steroids.[17]

Kidney

In the mouse kidney, androgens increased organ weight and stimulated RNA and general protein synthesis.[19–21] Androgens also induced an increase in the specific activity of several proteins, including β-glucuronidase, alcohol dehydrogenase, arginase, and 3-keto-steroid reductase.[15,22,23] The progestin medroxyprogesterone acetate also stimulated kidney weight and a significant dose-dependent increase in all four enzymes.[17,23a] When the other C_{21} progestins were assayed for their effects on β-glucuronidase, megestrol acetate was less active than medroxyprogesterone acetate, while progesterone and progesterone caproate had no effect. Although cyproterone acetate was inactive in six of nine studies, on occasion, it was associated with a slight increase in enzymatic activity that was not dose dependent. These variable results are unexplained but were also noted in studies of other tissues. It is thus evident that some progestins can simulate androgen action at several different end points in the mouse kidney.[17]

Except for progesterone, all progestins studied potentiated testosterone action on kidney β-glucuronidase activity (FIGURE 1). The progestin to androgen ratio at which this synergism was elicited varied with the progestin. This synergism occurred at low ratios for cyproterone acetate and megestrol acetate and at higher ratios for medroxyprogesterone acetate and progesterone caproate. The effect was demonstrated in kidneys of both normal female and castrated male mice. Similar results were obtained when the same ratios but larger amounts of testosterone and cyproterone acetate were administered.[17]

Renal 3-keto-reductase was also studied to determine if the synandrogenic effects of progestins on kidney could be demonstrated at an end point other than β-glucuronidase.[17] Medroxyprogesterone acetate and progesterone caproate potentiated androgen stimulation of this enzyme, whereas megestrol acetate had no effect. Cyproterone acetate was not used. Ohno and Lyon[15] reported potentiation by cyproterone acetate of another testosterone-stimulated renal enzyme, alcohol dehydrogenase. The synandrogenic action of progestins on the kidney is therefore not limited to a single gene product.

Cyproterone acetate and megestrol acetate, synandrogenic at low doses, were antiandrogenic when high doses were combined with testosterone (FIGURE 1). To determine if the synandrogenic activity of these steroids was related to their progestagenic or antiandrogenic actions, similar studies were performed with two steroidal (cyproterone, 6α-bromo-17β-hydroxy-17α-methyl-4-oxa-5α-androstan-3-one) and one nonsteroidal (flutamide) antiandrogen. No synandrogenic activity was observed, in that these compounds manifested only inhibitory effects on androgen-stimulated β-glucuronidase activity. From these studies, we conclude that the synandrogenic action of progestins is associated with a progestational structure-function relationship, whereas the antiandrogenic activity is not.[17]

Submaxillary Gland

To determine if similar responses could be elicited in another organ, the effects of progestins were evaluated on the mouse submaxillary gland. In this tissue,

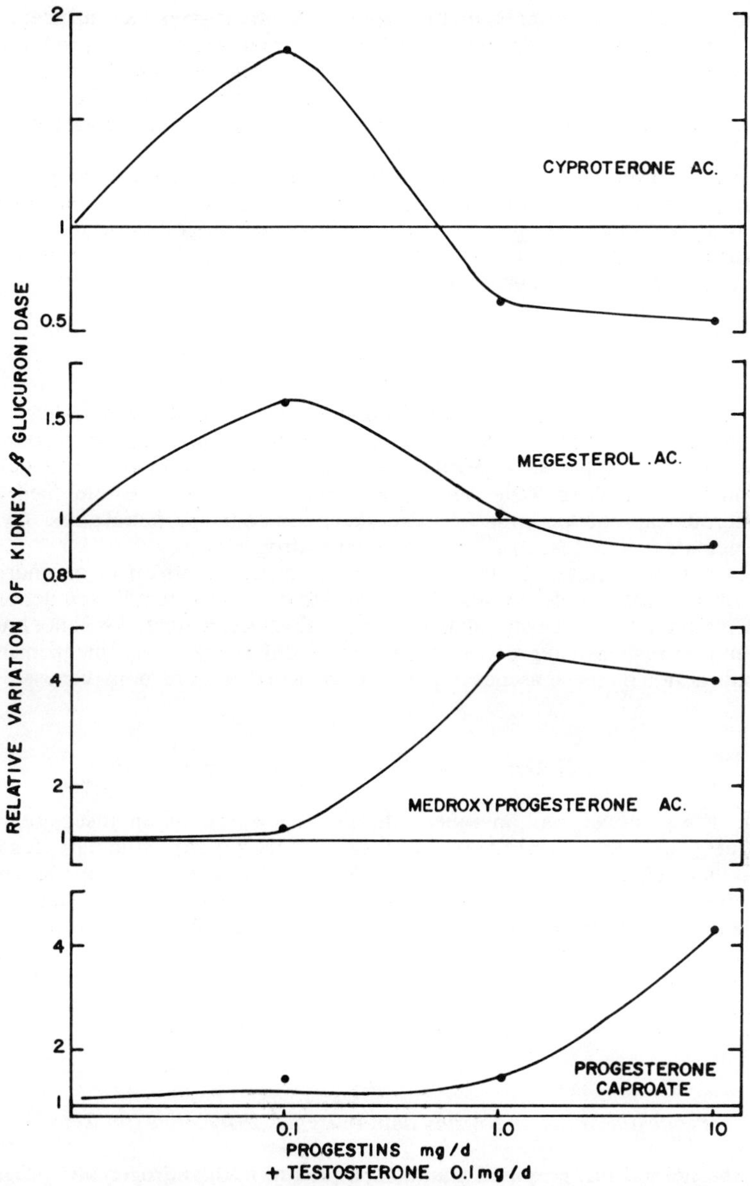

FIGURE 1. Synandrogenic and antiandrogenic effects of progestins on mouse kidney β-glucuronidase. For each steroid, the enzymatic activity induced by 0.1 mg of testosterone alone was taken as unity. The subsequent enzymatic activity that was elicited when testosterone was combined with various doses of each progestin is shown relative to this normalized value. Groups of five female mice were treated daily for 6 days. (From Mowszowicz *et al.*[17] By permission of *Endocrinology*.)

androgens stimulated an increase in organ weight and in the activity of specific proteins, including epidermal growth factor.[24,25] Medroxyprogesterone acetate induced similar responses. Progesterone and megestrol acetate also produced an increase in epidermal growth factor, but the responses were small, and only the megestrol acetate response appeared to be dose dependent. As in the kidney, in some experiments, a small, variable response to cyproterone acetate was detected.[26]

A synandrogenic action was seen only with the highest dose of progesterone caproate. Cyproterone acetate did not enhance testosterone action but, instead, acted as a potent antiandrogen. Megestrol acetate and progesterone were weakly antiandrogenic at the highest dose, whereas medroxyprogesterone acetate did not alter the response to testosterone.[26]

Other Tissues

The effects of progestins on mouse preputial gland and seminal vesicles were less extensively studied.[17,27] Medroxyprogesterone acetate simulated androgen action by increasing preputial gland and seminal vesicle weight and epithelial cell height in the latter gland. When progestins and testosterone were combined, only progesterone caproate potentiated androgen action on the preputial gland. Cyproterone acetate and megestrol acetate were antiandrogenic.

Cyproterone acetate was the only progestin tested for its effect on androgen action on seminal vesicle. Doses of progestin that enhanced androgen action on kidney inhibited androgen stimulation of seminal vesicle weight.[17] It is not known whether this response represents a qualitative difference in the mechanism of hormonal action on these tissues or a difference in end point responsiveness.

Progestin Action in Androgen-Insensitive tfm/y Mice

The tfm/y mouse has an inherited, body-wide end organ insensitivity to androgens such that large doses of testosterone did not stimulate renal or submaxillary gland responses.[15,25,28] It was thus of interest to study the androgenic effects of progestins in these animals. Medroxyprogesterone acetate stimulated renal β-glucuronidase activity and submaxillary gland epidermal growth factor concentration in normal female littermates. By contrast, there was no increase in the activity of either of these proteins in tfm/y mice. Progesterone and cyproterone acetate were also without effects. Thus, tfm/y mice also have an end organ insensitivity to the androgenic action of progestins.[17,26]

Progestin Action in Normal and Androgen-Insensitive tfm Rats

In the normal rat, preputial glands reponded to both androgen and progestin administration with an increase in RNA, DNA, and protein synthesis.[29,30] Specific enzyme synthesis was also stimulated, as evidenced by an increase in β-glucuronidase activity. By contrast, in the androgen-insensitive tfm rat, neither testosterone nor progesterone induced a response in any of these parameters when given in doses sufficient to maximize the response in normal animals.[30]

Progestins can also enhance androgen action in the rat. Carter *et al.*[16] found that cyproterone acetate increased the response of rat prostate DNA polymerase to three daily doses of testosterone if progestin was given 18 hr before animals were killed. If given earlier, cyproterone acetate acted as an antiandrogen. Enhancement by cyproterone of testosterone-stimulated growth of the rat prostate in organ culture was reported by Laznitsky *et al.*[14]

Mechanism of Androgenic Action of Progestins

Although it is possible that the actions of progestins involve separate molecular mechanisms, it would be satisfying to account for all of these actions by a common pathway. The fact that progestins with androgenic, synandrogenic, and antiandrogenic effects bind to androgen receptors[27,31,32] suggests that these actions may be mediated via this protein. The insensitivity of two species of tfm animals, which lack androgen receptors, to both androgens and the androgenic effects of progestins supports this hypothesis.

To elucidate further the interactions of progestins and the androgen receptor, [^{3}H]medroxyprogesterone acetate was synthesized,[33] and a series of *in vivo* and *in vitro* studies were performed with this ^{3}H-labeled steroid.[27] These studies are described below.

Table 1

Nuclear Concentration of [^{3}H]Medroxyprogesterone Acetate (MPA) in Androgen Target Tissues of the Mouse*

Steroid Administered	Route	Number of Experiments	Kidney	Prostate Seminal Vesicle	Submaxillary Gland
[^{3}H]MPA	iv	6	124†	1338	392
[^{3}H]MPA	sc	3	46	710	91
[^{3}H]MPA and MPA	sc	3	17	120	35

*[^{3}H]MPA (60 μCi) $\pm$ a 50-fold excess of unlabeled MPA were administered 30 min before kill to castrate, functionally eviscerated, male BALB/c mice. Nuclear steroid ([^{3}H]MPA) was extracted from purified nuclei by organic solvent and purified by thin-layer chromatography. Tissues from three mice were pooled for each experiment.[27]

†Average counts per minute per 10^7 nuclei.

In Vivo *Nuclear Uptake of [^{3}H]Medroxyprogesterone Acetate*

Mouse

To determine whether medroxyprogesterone acetate, like testosterone, was concentrated by nuclei of androgen-responsive tissues, [^{3}H]medroxyprogesterone acetate was administered intravenously to castrate, functionally hepatectomized mice. Low-capacity retention of unmetabolized [^{3}H]medroxyprogesterone acetate was demonstrated in purified kidney, prostate-seminal vesicle, and submaxillary gland nuclei (Table 1). The role of the androgen receptor as a mediator of this nuclear retention was suggested by inhibition of nuclear concentration of [^{3}H]medroxyprogesterone acetate by excess dihydrotestosterone, suppression of nuclear uptake of ^{3}H-labeled androgen by excess medroxyprogesterone acetate (medroxyprogesterone acetate blocked nuclear androgen accumulation irrespective of whether the predominant steroid was testosterone, as in kidney and submaxillary gland, or dihydrotestosterone, as in prostate-seminal

TABLE 2
NUCLEAR CONCENTRATION OF [^{3}H]MEDROXYPROGESTERONE ACETATE (MPA) IN ANDROGEN TARGET TISSUES OF THE RAT*

Steroid Administered	Number of Experiments	Prostate	Seminal Vesicle
[^{3}H]MPA	6	401†	749
[^{3}H]MPA and MPA	2	102	128

*Conditions were the same as in TABLE 1, except that 150 μCi of [^{3}H]medroxyprogesterone acetate were administered intravenously.[27]
†Average counts per minute per 10^7 nuclei.

vesicle), and by the absence of nuclear concentration of [^{3}H]medroxyprogesterone acetate in nuclei of tfm/y mice.

Rat

Because medroxyprogesterone acetate was androgenic in the rat, studies similar to those described above were repeated in this species. The results suggest that, as in the mouse, medroxyprogesterone acetate was specifically bound *in vivo* by the androgen receptor in prostate and seminal vesicles (TABLE 2).

In Vitro *Binding of Progestins*

[^{3}H]Medroxyprogesterone acetate was bound by macromolecules in mouse kidney cytosol that cosedimented with testosterone in the 8S region of sucrose gradients (FIGURE 2).[34] Androgen, estrogen, and progestins abolished [^{3}H]medroxyprogesterone acetate binding, whereas the glucocorticoid dexamethasone had no effect. This specificity was similar to that reported for [^{3}H]testosterone binding by the androgen receptor.[35] In addition, unlabeled medroxyprogesterone acetate inhibited 8S binding of [^{3}H]testosterone. [^{3}H]Medroxyprogesterone acetate and [^{3}H]testosterone binding were also compared in kidney cytosol from tfm/y mice and their normal littermates. Similar amounts of both steroids were bound by 8S macromolecules in cytosol from males and females. By contrast, there was no evidence of 8S binding in kidney cytosol from tfm/y mice. These findings support the hypothesis, suggested by *in vivo* studies, that medroxyprogesterone acetate is bound by the androgen receptor in mouse kidney. The ability of another progestin, cyproterone acetate, to bind to androgen receptors in mouse kidney[27,35] and other tissues[32] has been well documented.

Progestins are thus bound by androgen receptors in multiple tissues, and this interaction can account for their androgenic and antiandrogenic effects. The mechanism by which progestins either synergize with testosterone or a tissue determines which of these actions will be manifested remains to be elucidated.

Nonreceptor-Mediated Effects of Progestins

While our studies have dealt with the effects of progestins that are mediated through the androgen receptor of target organs, progestins may also affect androgen action in indirect ways. Although these effects have not been discussed specifically in this paper, they should be considered in assessing progestin alteration of androgen response. Progestins may reduce gonadotropin levels in rats[35a] and man,[36,37] which, in intact animals, may affect androgen action by reducing end organ androgen concentration. Progestins may also decrease androgen effects by increasing androgen metabolic clearance rates.[38] Medroxyprogesterone acetate treatment has been associated with an elevation of hepatic Δ^4-keto-steroid reductase activity in rats and man.[38–40] Within different tissues, steroid metabolism and various degrees of sensitivity may also modulate the final response.

Summary

In addition to their action on the uterus and vagina, progestins exert diverse metabolic effects on a variety of tissues. These actions include androgenic, synandrogenic, and antiandrogenic effects on androgen-responsive tissues of rats and mice. The androgenic and antiandrogenic effects of progestins have been demonstrated in multiple tissues. These actions appear to be mediated via the androgen receptor. A synandrogenic effect of progestins has also been detected in some tissues. However, there are few data to indicate how this response is mediated. Progestins may also alter androgen action indirectly through changes in steroid synthesis and metabolism. The overall biologic effect of a steroid may thus be determined by the sum of its actions on a variety of tissues.

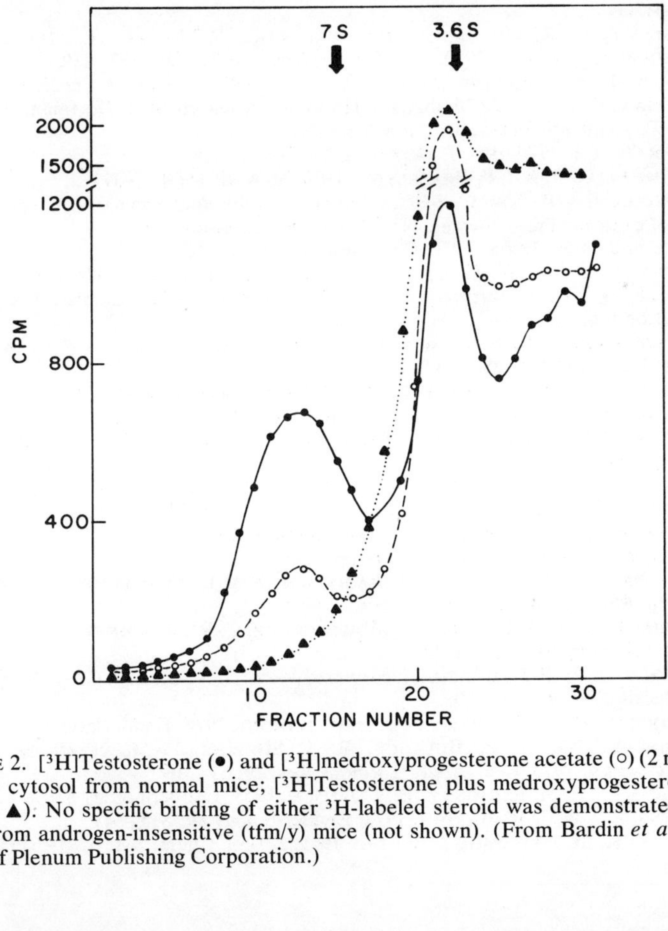

FIGURE 2. [^{3}H]Testosterone (●) and [^{3}H]medroxyprogesterone acetate (○) (2 nM) binding in kidney cytosol from normal mice; [^{3}H]Testosterone plus medroxyprogesterone acetate (200 nM, ▲). No specific binding of either ^{3}H-labeled steroid was demonstrated in kidney cytosol from androgen-insensitive (tfm/y) mice (not shown). (From Bardin *et al.*[34] By permission of Plenum Publishing Corporation.)

ACKNOWLEDGMENTS

We appreciate the secretarial assistance of Marlene Brinser. We also thank The Upjohn, Hoffmann-La Roche, Mead Johnson, Schering AG (Berlin, Germany), and Merrell-National companies for kindly providing the drugs used in this study.

REFERENCES

1. GREENE, R. R., M. W. BURRILL & A. C. IVY. 1939. Endocrinology **24:** 351–357.
2. LYSTER, S. C., G. H. LUND, W. E. DULIN & R. O. STAFFORD. 1959. Proc. Soc. Exp. Biol. Med. **100:** 540–543.
3. EDGREN, R. A., R. C. JONES & D. L. PETERSON. 1967. Fertil. Steril. **18:** 238–256.
4. TISELL, L.-E. & H. SALANDER. 1975. Acta Endocrinol. **78:** 316–324.
5. REVESZ, C., C. I. CHAPPEL & R. GAUDRY. 1960. Endocrinology **66:** 140–144.
6. SUCHOWSKY, G. K. & K. JUNKMANN. 1961. Endocrinology **68:** 341–349.
7. VOMACHKA, A. J., D. C. PAUP, L. P. CONIGLIO, M. J. MCMANUS & L. G. CLEMENS. 1974. J. Reprod. Fertil. **37:** 269–276.
8. DAVID, A., K. EDWARDS, K. P. FELLOWES & J. M. PLUMMER. 1963. J. Reprod. Fertil. **5:** 331–346.
9. NEUMANN, F., R. VON BERSWORDT-WALLRABE, W. ELGER, H. STEINBECK, J. D. HAHN & M. KRAMER. 1970. Rec. Progr. Hormone Res. **26:** 337–410.
10. GRAF, K.-J., R.-L. KLEINECKE & F. NEUMANN. 1974. J. Reprod. Fertil. **39:** 311–317.
11. DORFMAN, R. I. 1965. *In* Methods in Hormone Research. R. I. Dorfman, Ed. Vol. IV: 77–93. Academic Press, Inc. New York, N.Y.
12. DORFMAN, R. I. 1970. Brit. J. Dermatol. **82:** 3–8.
13. MCKINNEY, G. R. & J. P. BRASELTON. 1970. Steroids **15:** 405–411.
14. LAZNITSKI, I. & P. ROBEL. 1969. *In* Advances in the Biosciences. G. Raspé, Ed.: 175–184. Pergamon Press Vieweg. New York and Braunschweig.
15. OHNO, S. & M. F. LYON. 1970. Clin. Genetics **1:** 121–127.
16. CARTER, M. F., L. W. K. CHUNG & D. S. COFFEY. 1972. *In* Urological Research. L. E. King & G. P. Murphy, Eds.: 27–38. Plenum Publishing Corporation. New York and London.
17. MOWSZOWICZ, I., D. E. BIEBER, K. W. CHUNG, L. P. BULLOCK & C. W. BARDIN. 1974. Endocrinology **95:** 1589–1599.
18. PEETS, E. A., M. F. HENSON & R. NERI. 1974. Endocrinology **94:** 532–540.
19. KOCHAKIAN, C. D. 1969. Gen. Comp. Endocrinol. **13:** 146–150.
20. YAMANAKA, H., N. FURUYA, J. SHIMAZAKI & K. SHIDA. 1969. Endocrinol. Japon. **16:** 29–34.
21. FRIEDEN, E. H. & C. KU. 1971. Proc. Soc. Exp. Biol. Med. **137:** 1110–1144.
22. SWANK, R. T., K. PAIGEN & R. E. GANSCHOW. 1973. J. Mol. Biol. **81:** 225–243.
23. MOWSZOWICZ, I. & C. W. BARDIN. 1974. Steroids **23:** 793–807.
23a. BULLOCK, L. P. 1976. Unpublished observations.
24. JUNQUEIRA, L. C., A. FAJER, M. RABINOVITCH & L. FRANKENTHAL. 1949. J. Cell. Comp. Physiol. **34:** 129–158.
25. BARTHE, P. L., L. P. BULLOCK, I. MOWSZOWICZ, C. W. BARDIN & D. N. ORTH. 1974. Endocrinology **95:** 1019–1025.
26. BULLOCK, L. P., P. L. BARTHE, I. MOWSZOWICZ, D. N. ORTH & C. W. BARDIN. 1975. Endocrinology **97:** 189–195.
27. BULLOCK, L. P., M. R. SHERMAN & C. W. BARDIN. 1976. Endocrinology. In press.
28. BARDIN, C. W., L. P. BULLOCK, R. J. SHERINS, I. MOWSZOWICZ & W. R. BLACKBURN. 1973. Rec. Progr. Hormone Res. **29:** 65–109.
29. HUGGINS, C., F. M. PARSONS & E. V. JENSEN. 1955. Endocrinology **57:** 25–32.
30. SHERINS, R. J. & C. W. BARDIN. 1971. Endocrinology **89:** 835–841.
31. FANG, S., K. M. ANDERSON & S. LIAO. 1969. J. Biol. Chem. **244:** 6584–6595.

32. King, R. J. B. & W. I. P. Mainwaring. 1974. *In* Steroid-Cell Interactions.: 41–101. University Park Press. Baltimore, Md.
33. Feil, P. D., M. Miljkovic & C. W. Bardin. 1976. Endocrinology **98:** 1508–1515.
34. Bardin, C. W., O. Janne, L. P. Bullock & S. T. Jacob. 1975. *In* Hormonal Regulation of Spermatogenesis. F. S. French, V. Hansson, E. M. Ritzen & S. N. Nayfeh, Eds.: 237–255. Plenum Publishing Corporation. New York, N.Y.
35. Bullock, L. P. & C. W. Bardin. 1974. Endocrinology **94:** 746–756.
35a. Worgul, T. 1975. Unpublished observations.
36. Warren, M. P., J. H. Mathews, A. Morishima & R. Vande Wiele. 1975. Amer. J. Med. Sci. 269: 375–381.
37. Angeli, A., G. Boccuzzi, D. Bisbocci, D. Fongo, R. Frajria, C. De Sanctis & F. Ceresa. 1976. J. Clin. Endocrinol. Metab. **42:** 551–560.
38. Gordon, G. G., A. L. Southren, S. Tochimoto, J. Olivo, K. Altman, J. Rand & L. Lemberger. 1970. J. Clin. Endocrinol. Metab. **30:** 449–456.
39. Gordon, G. G., K. Altman, A. L. Southren & J. Olivo. 1971. J. Clin. Endocrinol. Metab. **32:** 457–461.
40. Altman, K., G. C. Gordon, A. L. Southren, J. Vittek & S. Wilker. 1972. Endocrinology **90:** 1252–1260.

Discussion

Dr. W. L. McGuire: How do you account for the difference between the β-glucuronidase response elicited by the combination of testosterone and cyproterone acetate or megestrol acetate, in which a biphasic type of response was seen, and the response to androgen plus progesterone caproate or medroxyprogesterone acetate, for which only synergistic effects were observed? What do you think is going on?

Dr. Bullock: At low doses, cyproterone acetate and megestrol acetate synergized with testosterone in increasing β-glucuronidase activity, while at higher doses they inhibited testosterone action. Medroxyprogesterone acetate and progesterone caproate did not affect testosterone action at low doses but were synergistic at the higher doses used. I assume that if we had been able to give even larger amounts of the latter two steroids, some inhibitory effects would have become evident as the β-glucuronidase activity was reduced to that stimulated by the progestin alone. While the inhibitory effects of these progestins are presumably due to binding to the androgen receptor with the subsequent exclusion of testosterone, we have not determined the molecular mechanism by which synergism occurs. Allosteric models have been used to explain the kinetics of an enzyme whose activity is both potentiated and inhibited by the same ligand (Monod, J., J. Wyman & J.-P. Changeux. 1965. J. Mol. Biol. **12:** 88; Rubin, M. M. & J.-P. Changeux. 1966. J. Mol. Biol. **21:** 265). Samuels and Tomkins have suggested a similar model for the glucocorticoid receptor to account for the interaction of various glucocorticoids on the induction of tyrosine aminotransferase in hepatoma tissue culture cells (Samuels, H. H. & J. M. Tomkins. 1970. J. Mol. Biol. **52:** 57).

Dr. M. Lippman: Is there any evidence to suggest that androgens induce a progesterone receptor? Are there any data that indicate that in a normal animal the progesterone effects that you see are really mediated through the androgen receptor? Do you have competition studies or some other kind of evidence that allows one to conclude that there is no progesterone action in these cells that is mediated through a progesterone receptor? Could the tfm/y animals, which lack the androgen receptor, also lack the progesterone receptor because it is not induced?

DR. BULLOCK: We have not looked for progesterone receptors in androgen-treated mice, but there is no evidence of binding of nanomolar amounts of [^{3}H]progesterone to mouse kidney cytosol from normal or acutely castrated males. If a true progesterone receptor were present in these animals, I would expect evidence of binding with these trace amounts of progesterone. The absence of such binding suggests that progesterone receptors are not present in normal males at least. We do see, however, competition for binding of nanomolar amounts of [^{3}H]testosterone by equimolar or larger amounts of a variety of progestins. Progesterone competes only weakly. To me, these data indicate that a true progesterone receptor is not present in the mouse kidney but that progestins are bound by the androgen receptor.

DR. MCGUIRE: The question really is how diligently has a progesterone receptor been searched for in tfm animals. Didn't you do some studies in estrogen-primed tfm animals to determine the effect of progesterone on the breast? Could you comment on that?

DR. BULLOCK: We have examined the response of the breast to progesterone with whole mounts of mammary gland from estrogen-primed normal and tfm rats and mice. The response in tfm animals was similar to that in normals, so, at least in this tissue, progesterone receptors seem to be present and normally effective. Also, although not characterized extensively, carrier female mice with the tfm gene do not seem to have a gross alteration in reproductive physiology. If progesterone receptors were abnormal in these animals, I would expect a significant decrease in fertility.

QUESTION: What is the evidence that the lack of the androgen receptor is the basic defect in the tfm/y mouse? Is it possible that you don't have the receptor because of an abnormality in some other basic mechanism? In other words, might you need an androgen response initially to induce the androgen receptor?

DR. BULLOCK: I cannot comment on the role of androgens in inducing androgen receptors in the fetus. However, in the adult female mouse, in which only low levels of androgen are present, androgen receptor concentration in the kidney is similar to that of males. Thus, androgens do not appear to be important in maintaining androgen receptors in this tissue. There is also no evidence of a significant change in androgen receptor content in acutely castrate versus long-term castrate males.

DR. W. T. SCHRADER: You normalized the β-glucuronidase response to testosterone plus progestins relative to that for testosterone alone, and it is therefore difficult to understand, for example, how much stimulation occurred with cyproterone acetate alone? What do the unnormalized induction curves look like?

DR. BULLOCK: Cyproterone acetate was ineffective by itself in stimulating β-glucuronidase activity. Thus, the increase in β-glucuronidase activity that occurred when cyproterone acetate was combined with testosterone was purely an enhancement of the androgen-stimulated activity. Medroxyprogesterone acetate, on the other hand, had some androgenic activity of its own; it was approximately 10% as potent as testosterone. Nevertheless, the increase in β-glucuronidase activity that occurred when testosterone and medroxyprogesterone acetate were given together was greater than the additive response from the two steroids when given separately.[17]

PROGESTERONE: ITS ROLE IN THE CENTRAL NERVOUS SYSTEM AS A FACILITATOR AND INHIBITOR OF SEXUAL BEHAVIOR AND GONADOTROPIN RELEASE*

H. H. Feder and B. L. Marrone

Institute of Animal Behavior
Rutgers University
Newark, New Jersey 07102

INTRODUCTION

When the action of a hormone on a tissue is studied, the biochemical condition of the tissue or substrate prior to administration of the hormone should always be considered. Diverse factors, such as genetic sex, nutritional state, temperature, time of day, and season of year, may influence the substrate. Only when these and other factors are controlled for can one be sure that experimental samples begin from a relatively homogeneous baseline, and only in this way can one accurately assess the effects of a hormone on this baseline. Extraordinary emphasis on this stricture is required for progesterone and its actions on neural and genital tissues. This is so because the effects of progesterone are very much dependent on the previous, concurrent, and subsequent influences of estrogenic hormones on target tissue substrates. These temporal factors determine whether progesterone will facilitate or inhibit estrogen-dependent processes.

In this paper, we will first describe, at a molar level, the interaction of progesterone with estrogen-sensitive neural tissues that regulate the expression of female sexual behavior and the release of gonadotropic hormones. Later, we will discuss, at a biochemical level, possible mechanisms by which progesterone can exert both facilitatory and inhibitory influences on sexual behavior and gonadotropin release. This section will include data on estrogen and progesterone uptake and on possible mediation of progesterone effects by neurotransmitters. Also included in this discussion will be a comparison between the inhibitory actions of progesterone and those of synthetic antiestrogens on estrogen-dependent neural processes. To conclude, we will suggest that progesterone-sensitive neural systems operate with a precision that is attributable more to interneuronal channeling of information to or from estrogen-sensitive areas than to intranuclear programming of biochemical events.

*Supported by National Institutes of Health Grant HD 04467, National Institute of Mental Health Research Scientist Development Award K2-MH-29006, a grant from the Busch Foundation at Rutgers University (all to H.H.F.), and a National Science Foundation Prodoctoral Research Fellowship (to B.L.M.). This paper is contribution 241 from the Institute of Animal Behavior.

Progesterone and Sexual Behavior

Description of Experimental Designs That Demonstrate Facilitatory and Inhibitory Influences of Progesterone on Female Sexual Behavior in Rodents

Facilitation

When ovariectomized rats,[1] mice,[2] hamsters,[3] and guinea pigs[4] are given estradiol preparations, they display lordosis behavior (a female sexual response characterized by immobilization and concave arching of the back in response to genital stimulation), but when progesterone is given 24–48 hr after the estrogen, this behavioral response is further facilitated. The facilitation by progesterone may take the form of increasing the percentage of behaviorally responsive animals, of increasing the intensity of lordosis in individual animals, or of decreasing the latency of response to a fixed dose of estrogen.[5–7] Progesterone may also facilitate lordosis in terms of permitting a decrease in dosage of estrogen required for elicitation of the behavior.[7] The actions of progesterone are quite rapid. Intravenous injection or intracranial implants of progesterone in estrogen-primed rats and guinea pigs facilitate lordosis within about 1 hr,[8,9] and even subcutaneous injections of progesterone require only about 4 hr before a behavioral effect is manifested.[1,4] This rapidity of progesterone action contrasts with the longer time requirements (about 20 hr) for outward effects of estrogen on lordosis behavior.[10]

The behavior-facilitating effects of progesterone are not artifactual curiosities but are important features of the normal estrous cycles of at least some rodents. This fact has been demonstrated in several ways. Biochemical measurements of plasma progesterone demonstrate a sharp increase in progesterone concentrations at the beginning of lordosis behavior in rats,[11] hamsters,[12] and guinea pigs.[13] This rise of progesterone levels occurs at least 24 hr after the start of increased estrogen secretion.[14] Thus, the schedules of estrogen and progesterone injection into ovariectomized animals that demonstrate facilitatory effects of progesterone run parallel to the pattern of endogenous secretion of the steroids in intact rodents.

Another line of evidence supports the notion that endogenous progesterone plays a role in facilitating female sexual behavior during a normal estrous cycle. Experiments in which cyclic rats[15] or guinea pigs[16] are deprived of ovarian progesterone, just prior to the time at which they are expected to display lordosis behavior, demonstrate a significant diminution of the behavior. Provision of exogenous progesterone to such animals restores their ability to perform the behavior.

Under normal circumstances, the source of the progesterone that facilitates sexual behavior is the preovulatory ovary, more specifically the interstitial tissue and/or unripe graafian follicles. That corpora lutea or ripe preovulatory follicles are not required sources of this progesterone is shown by studies with immature animals. When immature rats[17] or guinea pigs (Table 1) are given gonadotropic stimulation, they secrete increased quantities of progesterone, even though corpora lutea and ripe follicles are absent. Under conditions of stress or adrenocorticotropic hormone (ACTH) treatment, the adrenal cortex of rats and guinea pigs is also capable of secreting progesterone in quantities adequate to facilitate female sexual behavior as long as there has been a sufficient preceding period of estrogen priming.[18]

TABLE 1

PERIPHERAL PLASMA PROGESTERONE CONCENTRATIONS IN PREPUBERTAL (25 days old) FEMALE GUINEA PIGS GIVEN ESTRADIOL BENZOATE (EB, 10 μg per animal) AND/OR LUTEINIZING HORMONE (LH, 4.0 mg per animal)

Group	Number of Animals	Progesterone (ng/ml)*
EB only	5	0.48 ± 0.22
LH only	5	1.19 ± 0.22
EB (0 hr) and LH (36 hr)	5	1.98 ± 0.67

*Measurements were taken on plasma removed 40 hr after EB injection or 4 hr after LH injection. Values are $\bar{X} \pm$ SEM.

All of these data are consistent with the idea that, in rodents, facilitatory effects of progesterone on female sexual behavior are dependent on prior conditioning of neural tissues with estrogen for a period of 24–48 hr (TABLE 2). What happens when progesterone is given *before* a sufficient period of estrogen conditioning has elapsed?

Concurrent Inhibition

One way to study the problem is to ovariectomize animals and given them concurrent (or nearly concurrent) treatment with estrogen and progesterone (TABLE 2). When this procedure is performed, with appropriate doses of hormones, guinea pigs[19] and rats[20] display little or no lordosis behavior. Furthermore, the facilitatory effects of additional progesterone given 24–48 hr later are not manifested or are diminished (TABLE 3). This dose-dependent[21] inhibitory effect of progesterone can be demonstrated in intact and in ovariectomized animals. For example, at certain stages of pregnancy, rats are resistant to induction of lordosis by sequential estrogen and progesterone treatment.[22] This resistance is

TABLE 2

BASIC EXPERIMENTAL DESIGNS THAT DEMONSTRATE FACILITATORY AND INHIBITORY PROPERTIES OF PROGESTERONE ON FEMALE SEXUAL BEHAVIOR OF OVARIECTOMIZED GUINEA PIGS

0 hr	36 hr	40 hr	60 hr	64 hr
Facilitatory properties of progesterone				
Estradiol benzoate	oil	(+)		
Estradiol benzoate	progesterone	+		
Inhibitory properties of progesterone				
	Sequential inhibition			
Estradiol benzoate	oil	(+)	progesterone	+
Estradiol benzoate	progesterone	(+)	progesterone	−
Concurrent inhibition				
Estradiol benzoate	progesterone	+		
Progesterone/estradiol benzoate	progesterone	−		

manifested when hormonal treatment is initiated at times of high levels of progesterone secretion. Additionally, intact guinea pigs given estradiol and then progesterone 36 hr later display lordosis readily, except when this hormonal treatment is initiated at certain stages of pregnancy or at two particular stages of the estrous cycle. One of these stages is the luteal phase of the estrous cycle, when considerable quantities of progesterone are being secreted concurrently with the injection of estrogen.[23] The other refractory stage will be discussed in the next paragraph.

TABLE 3

CONCURRENT INHIBITION IN RATS; EFFECT OF 0.5 mg OR 5.0 mg OF PROGESTERONE GIVEN 1 HR PRIOR TO STANDARD ESTRADIOL BENZOATE (5 μg/kg) AND PROGESTERONE (0.5 mg) FACILITATION TREATMENT

Pretreatment	Number of Animals	$\bar{X}$ Lordosis Quotient (± SEM) Pretest	Time after 0.5 mg of Progesterone 4 hr	5 hr
Oil	10	5.0 ± 3.41	76.0 ± 7.33	89.0 ± 6.57
0.5 mg of Progesterone	10	0.0	62.0 ± 12.45	77.0 ± 12.21
5.0 mg of Progesterone	10	1.0 ± 1.0	9.0 ± 6.90	12.0 ± 7.86

Sequential Inhibition

When lordosis is induced by sequential estrogen and progesterone treatment in ovariectomized guinea pigs, the behavior persists for about 8 hr.[4] If, at the end of this receptive period, one attempts to reinduce lordosis by another injection of progesterone (TABLE 2) or by a second sequence of estrogen and progesterone, one is invariably unsuccessful.[24] This refractoriness lasts for about 36 hr. The same phenomenon of postestrous refractoriness occurs in intact guinea pigs after they have exhibited lordosis under the influence of their own hormonal secretions.[25] This immediately postestrous period is the other stage of the estrous cycle during which it is difficult to elicit lordosis by means of injecting estrogen and progesterone. To what can this postestrous refractoriness be attributed? Evidence indicates that the same progesterone that first facilitated expression of lordosis subsequently causes a transitory period of refractoriness to further hormonal stimulation of sexual behavior.[24] This type of action of progesterone may be termed "sequential inhibition."[26] It differs from concurrent inhibition in that it can occur in the presence of low levels of plasma progesterone[13] and in that it takes effect after an adequate period of estrogen priming has elapsed. Concurrent inhibition by high levels of circulating progesterone[13] occurs before there has been time for adequate estrogen priming of neural tissues that mediate behavior.

We have now described three behavioral actions of progesterone in combination with estrogen: facilitation, concurrent inhibition, and sequential inhibition. In the next sections, we will discuss these actions in terms of anatomic localization, specificity and dosage, and species differences.

Central Neural Sites of Behavioral Actions of Progesterone

Anatomic localization of the facilitatory and inhibitory effects of progesterone on sexual behavior has been studied by implanting the steroid intracranially into ovariectomized estrogen-primed rodents. Facilitatory sites for progesterone that have been found are the midbrain reticular formation,[27] caudate-putamen,[28] and anterior hypothalamus-preoptic area[29,30] in the rat. In guinea pigs, progesterone implants in the basal hypothalamic-premammillary region facilitate lordosis,[9] but more extensive mapping studies are required to determine whether other brain areas might also be involved.

Sequential inhibition in estrogen-primed guinea pigs[31] and mice[32] is seen after bilateral progesterone implants are made in the midbrain. Interestingly, the most effective site for the sequential inhibitory action of progesterone in guinea pigs is the portion of the midbrain that contains cell bodies of the dopamine system.[33]

Attempts in our laboratory to localize the site of concurrent inhibition by progesterone in guinea pigs have been unsuccessful, thus far. We reasoned that the most likely sites would be the areas of the brain most responsive to estrogenic stimulation. Surprisingly, extensive tests with concurrent estrogen treatment and placement of progesterone in the highly estrogen-sensitive area of the medial basal hypothalamus[34] have failed to reveal significant inhibition of lordosis behavior. Future experiments will test the idea that the midbrain may mediate not only the sequential but also the concurrent type of inhibition by progesterone. In rats, concurrent inhibition by progesterone can be demonstrated with implants of this steroid in the medial basal hypothalamus, but these results are still preliminary.[34a]

Specificity and Dosage Factors Involved in Behavioral Effects of Progesterone

Many steroids have been tested for their ability to mimic the lordosis-facilitating properties of progesterone in ovariectomized estrogen-primed guinea pigs. Androgens are relatively ineffective in this respect.[35] Although a second dose of estrogen 24–48 hr after the first dose may have facilitatory effects, these effects have characteristics that distinguish them from the actions of progesterone.[36] Corticoids, such as corticosterone and deoxycorticosterone acetate, can facilitate lordosis in estrogen-primed guinea pigs, but the dosages required are high.[35,37] Other C_{21} compounds are either ineffective (17α-hydroxyprogesterone)[37] or have facilitatory effects that may be attributable to their metabolism to progesterone (pregnenolone, 20α-dihydroprogesterone).[38] The steroid 5α-dihydroprogesterone (5α-DHP) exhibits lordosis-facilitating properties in estrogen-primed guinea pigs.[39] When administered in an oil vehicle, the minimum effective dose of 5α-DHP is about 50 μg per animal, but this minimum can be reduced to about 15 μg per animal by administering the steroid in an alcohol vehicle.[39a] This finding suggests that if administered in a form that does not impede its bioavailability, 5α-DHP is at least as effective as progesterone (threshold dose, 15 μg per animal)[40] in facilitating lordosis in estrogen-primed guinea pigs. The steroids 3α-hydroxy-5α-pregnan-20-one and 5β-pregnane-3,20-dione are only moderately effective in facilitating lordosis.[39]

Not tested for specificity as extensively as the facilitatory action is the sequential inhibitory function of steroids. Estrogens lack this inhibitory function.[41] The progestin 20α-dihydroprogesterone also appears to lack this property in guinea pigs, but a wide dose range has not been tested.[38] Recently, we found that a synthetic compound, norspiroxenone, has facilitatory and sequential inhibitory actions in guinea pigs.[41a]

Concurrent inhibitory properties have been demonstrated in guinea pigs for 5α-DHP, but 3α-hydroxy-5α-pregnan-20-one and 5β-pregnane-3,20-dione are weak in this respect.[39] Unfortunately, no systematic study with a wide range of steroids has been performed to determine whether specificity requirements for sequential and concurrent inhibition are identical.

Generalizations regarding the significance for behavior of particular functional groups on the steroidal molecule are difficult to make. Ring-A unsaturation is not a requirement (as shown by 5α-DHP), nor is the presence of a C-19 methyl group (as shown by norspiroxenone). Presence of an oxygen function at C-3 does not ensure behavioral potency (as shown by 17α-hydroxyprogesterone). A tentative generalization may be made regarding behavioral potency and steroidal polarity; that is, relatively nonpolar compounds (progesterone, 5α-DHP) are more effective than polar steroids in influencing lordosis behavior as long as artifacts that impede bioavailability are avoided. However, no strict correlation between behavioral potency and steroidal polarity obtains for facilitation. For example, corticosterone facilitates lordosis in guinea pigs more effectively than does 17α-hydroxyprogesterone, even though corticosterone is the more polar steroid.[37]

This discussion of dosage and specificity has centered on the guinea pig. In rats, progesterone and 5α-DHP are the most effective facilitators of lordosis in estrogen-primed subjects.[42] Meyerson's laboratory has made the point that degree of lordosis-promoting potency of a steroid is not necessarily correlated with anesthetic potency of a steroid in rats.[43,44] Extensive attempts at correlating anesthetic potency with strength of inhibitory actions of steroids on lordosis have not been made.

Sequential inhibition by progesterone has been demonstrated in rats,[45] hamsters,[46] and mice,[47] and concurrent inhibition by progesterone has been demonstrated in rats[20,48] and hamsters.[49] However, steroidal specificity data are lacking for inhibitory functions in these species. Dosage data strongly indicate that guinea pigs have a much lower threshold than do rats for progesterone-induced facilitation or inhibition of lordosis[40,50] (TABLE 3). Hamsters appear to be intermediate in their sensitivity to the behavioral effects of progesterone.[51] These quantitative differences among rodent species probably do not reflect basic differences in mechanisms of action of progesterone. However, progesterone acts in some nonrodent species in ways that appear to differ qualitatively from the ways in which it acts in rodents. Two examples of these qualitative species differences follow.

Species Differences in Behavioral Actions of Progesterone

For optimal facilitation of lordosis in rodents, estrogen conditioning must precede exposure to progesterone by 24–48 hr. In ovariectomized sheep, female sexual responses are facilitated best when progesterone is administered and then withdrawn 24–48 hr *before* exposure to estrogen.[52] In the normal estrous cycle of the sheep, the corpus luteum provides progesterone until about 48 hr prior to an increase in circulating levels of estrogen.[52] No preovulatory surge of progesterone occurs after estrogen secretion reaches a peak in sheep. Thus, measurements of the endogenous pattern of steroidal secretion and experiments with exogenous hormones support the idea that, in contrast to rodents, sheep require conditioning with progesterone prior to estrogen but do not require progesterone after estrogen to display maximal levels of sexual behavior.

Although rodents and sheep show facilitation of behavior to differing sequences of estrogen and progesterone, they both appear to be affected similarly by concurrent estrogen and progesterone treatment. That is, concurrent treatment of ovariectomized rodents with estrogen and progesterone diminishes female sexual behavior, and failure to withdraw progesterone 24–48 hr prior to estrogen treatment in sheep results in less sexual receptivity than if the progesterone is withdrawn.[52]

Dogs also lack a preovulatory surge of progesterone,[53] yet ovariectomized dogs given estrogen and then progesterone show a facilitation of female sexual behavior.[54] This finding indicates that although a mechanism responsive to facilitatory effects of progesterone in estrogen-primed dogs is not operative during a normal estrous cycle, this mechanism can still be activated by experimental means. On the other hand, dogs can continue to show female sexual behavior in the presence of progesterone of luteal origin in the circulation after ovulation.[53] In this instance, dogs seem to be insensitive to the concurrent inhibitory effects of progesterone. One might say that they possess the hormone but not the mechanism to respond to it behaviorally. This speculation should be tested more rigorously by administering, to ovariectomized dogs, varying doses of progesterone (or other progestins) concurrently with estrogen.

Discussion of these qualitative species differences in progesterone action is intended as a caveat against facile generalization. Progesterone may interact with estrogen in different temporal sequences in different species, it may be present in the circulation but lack behavioral effects, or it may be absent but have a potentially responsive substrate.

Progesterone and Gonadotropin Release

Description of Experimental Designs That Demonstrate Facilitatory and Inhibitory Influences of Progesterone on Gonadotropin Release in Female Rodents

Facilitation

Everett demonstrated that progesterone given to 5-day cyclic rats on the third day of diestrus accelerates ovulation by about 24 hr.[55] Because this effect is dependent on the stage of the estrous cycle, Everett suggested that the critical factor in progesterone acceleration of ovulation is the level of endogenous estrogen. Subsequent studies have shown that for progesterone to induce ovulation, it must be administered after an adequate period of estrogen priming. A synergistic effect of progesterone on ovulation in estrogen-primed subjects has been confirmed in adult and prepubertal rats[56,57] and in rabbits.[58]

As with progesterone facilitation of ovulation, progesterone induction of luteinizing hormone (LH) release cannot be accomplished without adequate estrogen priming. Thus, progesterone given in late diestrus or in proestrus (when estrogen levels are elevated) causes an increase in plasma LH levels within 6 hr of injection.[59] More recently, it has been shown that progesterone injected into ovariectomized rats 2, 3, or 4 days after a priming dose of estrogen induces increased plasma LH within 2 hr.[60] Progesterone may also act to facilitate release of follicle-stimulating hormone (FSH) in estrogen-primed rats[60] and hamsters.[61]

Although it has been demonstrated experimentally that progesterone is able to facilitate ovulation and gonadotropin secretion, some investigators question whether progesterone plays a necessary role in these processes during a normal estrous cycle. For example, *in vivo* administration of antibodies to progesterone on Day 2 of diestrus or on the morning or proestrus fails to interfere significantly with the LH surge or ovulation in rats.[62] Furthermore, in intact rats[63–65] and guinea pigs,[66] release of the preovulatory surge of LH occurs prior to release of large quantities of preovulatory progesterone from the ovary. However, results of studies that utilized *in vivo* binding of hormones by antibodies must be regarded with caution, because binding of the hormone may not prevent the hormone from exerting biologic effects.[67] Additionally, the adrenal cortex of the rat may secrete enough preovulatory progesterone to play a role in the process of ovulation. Thus, estrogen alone does not induce massive LH release in rats ovariectomized and adrenalectomized in late diestrus but does induce LH release in rats that are ovariectomized but not adrenalectomized.[68]

Concurrent Inhibition

In contrast to its facilitatory effects on ovulation and LH secretion in an animal that has had adequate estrogen priming, progesterone treatment initiated before a sufficient period of estrogen conditioning has elapsed exerts inhibitory effects. Experimental evidence for this statement comes from studies in which progesterone was given to intact guinea pigs,[69] rats,[55] and hamsters[70] before significant estrogen secretion had occurred. In each case, cycle length was increased, suggesting a delay in preovulatory LH release.

Another line of evidence suggests the same conclusion. Removal of corpora lutea from cyclic guinea pigs[71,72] shortens the length of the estrous cycle, thereby indicating that removal of this source of concurrent inhibition by progesterone permits acceleration of LH release in quantities sufficient to cause ovulation. Concurrent inhibition of the LH surge and ovulation by progesterone may be attributable to inhibition of estrogen secretion by the ovary.

Sequential Inhibition

Progesterone injection into ovariectomized rats after 3 days of estrogen priming causes an increase in serum LH levels within a few hours.[60] However, 24 and 40 hr after progesterone injection, the levels of LH fall slightly below those of control animals given no progesterone.[60] Furthermore, during this period, progesterone-treated animals are refractory to additional progesterone, in that they do not release a second pulse of LH. The rise in serum LH that can be induced either by progesterone or by estrogen after 4 days of estrogen priming is completely blocked by an injection of progesterone 24 hr before, on Day 3. A similar sequential inhibition of gonadotropin release sufficient for ovulation occurs in hamsters[73] and rabbits.[58]

The experimental designs that demonstrate facilitation and inhibition of gonadotropin release by progesterone bear a fundamental similarity to the experiments on facilitation and inhibition of female sexual behavior by progesterone. In the next sections, we will consider anatomic localization and dosage and specificity parameters of progesterone in the regulation of gonadotropin release.

Central Neural Sites of Action of Progesterone in Regulation of Gonadotropin Release

Lesions of the medial preoptic area (MPOA) -suprachiasmatic nucleus (SCN) render rats insensitive to triggering of ovulation by progesterone.[74,75] However, electrical stimulation of the median eminence (ME)[74] or the ventromedial nucleus (VMN) -arcuate (ARC) area[75] induces ovulation in rats with such lesions. This information indicates that the MPOA-SCN region, while perhaps not progesterone sensitive itself, is necessary for the facilitation of ovulation by progesterone. Consistent with this idea is the finding that implantation of progesterone directly into the MPOA of rats is ineffective in inducing ovulation.[75,76] Progesterone implants into the VMN-ARC area, on the other hand, abolish the ovulation-delaying effect of a systemic injection of progesterone given 2 days earlier to adults and induce ovulation in estrogen-primed prepubertal rats. In addition, the ovulation-inducing effect of electrical stimulation of the VMN-ARC area in MPOA-SCN-lesioned rats is enhanced by appropriately timed systemic injection of progesterone.[75] Progesterone in the ME-ARC region has also been found to advance ovulation whem implanted during the morning of proestrus.[77] Pituitary implants of progesterone were ineffective in inducing ovulation in each of the above experiments.

While suggestive of central neural sites for a facilitatory action of progesterone on gonadotropin release, these experiments are not conclusive, because they fail to rule out the "implantation paradox" objection.[78] It is possible that progesterone, implanted into the "effective sites" mentioned above, is perfusing the pituitary, thereby inducing ovulation through a direct effect on the pituitary rather than on the central nervous system. Intrahypophyseal implants, on the other hand, do not adequately perfuse the pituitary. This "implantation paradox" objection is especially important for progesterone facilitation of ovulation, because the effective implant sites are so close to the hypophyseal-portal system.

Inhibitory effects of progesterone on ovulation have been found when progesterone is implanted into the anterior pituitary or ME region.[79] That the pituitary may be the more direct site of progesterone inhibition of ovulation has been suggested elsewhere.[80] Inhibition by progesterone has also been found when progesterone is implanted in the VMN at appropriate stages of the rat estrous cycle.[76] In the hamster, the MPOA-diagonal band region appears to be most sensitive to progesterone blockade of ovulation.[81]

Extrahypothalamic sites, such as the amygdala and cerebellum, have also been implicated in the facilitation or inhibition of ovulation by progesterone.[82,83] It is possible that these areas, in addition to the hippocampus, may not be progesterone sensitive but rather may be involved in modifying the activity of estrogen- or progesterone-sensitive sites that contribute more directly to the release of gonadotropins.[76]

The effects of progesterone implants on LH and on LH-releasing hormone (LHRH) have been assessed not only intact but also in ovariectomized rats. A decrease in LH levels was found with progesterone implants in the medial basal hypothalamus, but this decrease was not accompanied by a decrease in responsivity of the pituitary to LHRH. This result indicates that the inhibitory effect of progesterone on LH is mediated by hypothalamic tissue and not by the pituitary.[84] Systemically administered progesterone was also found to have an inhibitory effect on the high levels of circulating LH in ovariectomized rats.[85] This inhibition was not overcome by electrical stimulation of the MPOA or ME-ARC area, thereby indicating involvement of other sites. Perhaps the pituitary or VMN responds to progesterone by inhibiting LH release, and this effect may compete with any possible induction of LH release by electrical stimulation.

In general, the anatomic work that has identified sites of progesterone facilitation and inhibition of gonadotropin release lags behind anatomic work on progesterone regulation of sexual behavior. With radioimmunoassay techniques for gonadotropins now readily available, more precise studies of progesterone-sensitive sites for LH release should be forthcoming. Even studies in which facilitation or inhibition of ovulation is used as a criterion of progesterone action have yet to be performed. Loci of progesterone facilitation and inhibition of ovulation in the guinea pig have not been determined, for example.

Specificity and Dosage Factors Involved in Gonadotropin-Regulating Effects of Progesterone

In the rat, 20α-dihydroprogesterone[86] and 17α-hydroxyprogesterone[87] are ineffective in advancing or delaying ovulation. However, in ovariectomized estrogen-primed rats, 20α-dihydroprogesterone, in a dose of 2.5 mg, increases LH and FSH levels in the circulation. An equal dose of 5α-DHP is similarly effective, and actions of this steroid, unlike those of 20α-dihydroprogesterone, cannot be attributed to back-conversion to progesterone. No effect on LH release in ovariectomized estrogen-primed rats has been found with 17α-hydroxyprogesterone or 5α-pregnan-3β-ol-20-one.[87,88] It is not known whether either 20α-dihydroprogesterone or 5α-DHP plays a role in the normal triggering of FSH and LH release, nor is the minimal effective dosage of either of these steroids known.

The smallest effective dose of progesterone for facilitation of ovulation on the morning of proestrus was found by one investigator to be 0.62 mg per rat.[86] Inhibition of ovulation can be achieved with 0.50 mg of progesterone in diestrous rats.[79] In hamsters, Reuter and Lisk have systematically examined the size of progesterone implants in the brain necessary for blockade of ovulation.[81]

In rabbits, 20α-dihydroprogesterone is a principal progestin.[89,90] This metabolite of progesterone may have a positive feedback effect on LH in rabbits.[91]

Species Differences in Actions of Progesterone on Gonadotropin Release

The corpus luteum of the intact sheep provides progesterone until about 48 hr prior to an increase in estrogen; a preovulatory surge of progesterone is absent, and the estrogen rise is followed by a peak in serum LH.[92] In ovariectomized sheep, LH secretion can be stimulated by administering progesterone for several days and estrogen 48 hr after the last progesterone injection.[93] In some cases, a rise in plasma LH is observed after progesterone withdrawal.[93,94] Thus, LH release in ewes appears to be facilitated both by progesterone withdrawal and by estrogen stimulation.

In ewes, studies of concurrent inhibition of ovulation or LH release by progesterone are inconclusive. Estradiol given on Day 10 of the estrous cycle, when high levels of progesterone are being secreted, fails to induce LH release.[95] However, progesterone given to ovariectomized sheep 24, 8, 4, or 0 hr prior to an injection of estradiol has no inhibitory effect on LH release.

Mechanisms by Which Progesterone Might Facilitate Female Behavior and Gonadotropin Release

Is Facilitation by Progesterone a Process That is Identical to Facilitation by Estrogen?

It seems unlikely that the facilitatory actions of progesterone are attributable to processes that are identical to those activated by estrogen. Instances can be cited of progesterone failing to substitute for estrogen and estrogen failing to substitute for progesterone. For example, progesterone cannot be used in rodents as a substitute for estrogen in conditioning neural tissues that regulate behavior.[97] Unlike estrogen, progesterone by itself is ineffective in causing LH release.[59] Conversely, estrogen acts in only some respects as a progesterone mimic in facilitating lordosis behavior in estrogen-primed rodents.[36,97] Although estrogen mimics progesterone by causing release of LH in estrogen-primed rats,[98] there are also examples of failure of estrogen to imitate progesterone action on gonadotropin release. Thus, in rats kept in constant light, progesterone facilitates release of LH and ovulation, but exogenous estrogen, even in relatively large doses, is ineffective.[99] Additionally, anatomic sites of progesterone and estradiol action in the brain are not always identical,[9,34] and the time course of action of the two hormones may differ.[1,10]

At a biochemical level, several differences also seem to exist between estrogen and progesterone action. Scintillation counting studies of whole homogenates readily indicate that the major low-capacity high-affinity uptake system for estradiol is located in the hypothalamic-preoptic area of rats[100] and guinea pigs.[101] By use of precisely the same techniques, very different results have been obtained in studies of progesterone uptake. For progesterone, the major site of uptake in rats, guinea pigs, and hamsters is the midbrain rather than the hypothalamus, and the uptake system appears to be unsaturable.[102,103] The amount of uptake of steroid into the midbrain is correlated, to some extent, with polarity of the steroid. The less polar the steroid, the higher the uptake[104] (an exception is the somewhat lower uptake of 5α-DHP than of progesterone, Table 4). This type of dependence on polarity is not seen in the portion of the estradiol uptake system that is saturable.

When cell fractions rather than whole homogenates are considered, differences between estradiol and progesterone uptake are still evident. With scintillation counting techniques, after an injection of labeled estradiol, a significant portion of the radioactivity in hypothalamic cells of rats[105] and guinea pigs[106] is located in the nuclear fraction, but almost no radioactivity is observed in the nuclear fraction of midbrain or hypothalamic cells after an injection of labeled progesterone (Table 4).[107] Perhaps the inability to demonstrate nuclear concentration of progesterone in these studies is due to the lack of resolution of the techniques employed. Some workers who utilized autoradiographic techniques have shown saturable nuclear uptake of radioactive hormone in the arcuate nucleus, nucleus preopticus periventricularis, and nucleus preopticus suprachiasmaticus of guinea pigs after injection of labeled progesterone.[108] Even if this autoradiographic evidence for saturable nuclear uptake of progesterone in the brain is accepted, it must be acknowledged that such uptake is far less dramatic than that for estrogen. Furthermore, autoradiographic techniques cannot, by themselves, demonstrate the existence of specific nuclear receptors for steroids in the brain, nor have they resolved the question of whether cells that show saturable nuclear uptake of progestin are the same as those that exhibit saturable nuclear uptake of estrogen. Chemical evidence is required for statements about receptors, and this evidence has been forthcoming for estrogen, but not for progesterone, in the brain.[109] Chemical evidence of cytosol receptors for progesterone in the hypothalamus of rats[110] and guinea pigs[111] has been presented, however.

Another difference between the estrogen and progesterone uptake systems in the brain is that 75–80% of the radioactivity recovered from rat or guinea pig hypothalamus 4 hr after injection of labeled estradiol is in the form of estradiol,[101] whereas the radioactivity recovered from the hypothalamus or midbrain 4 hr after injection of labeled progesterone is composed of only 62–73% progesterone in guinea pigs and 26–31% progesterone in rats.[112] Incidentally, the more rapid metabolism of progesterone in rats than in guinea pigs may account for the lesser sensitivity of rats to the facilitatory and inhibitory effects of progesterone.[40,50]

Yet another difference exists between estrogen and progesterone uptake systems. In broad terms, uptake of estrogen in peripheral target tissues, such as the uterus, seems to provide a reasonable parallel for study of estrogen uptake in brain. Both tissues contain saturable, specific receptors that are translocated to the nucleus in association with estradiol.[105,113] However, no such obvious parallel exists between peripheral and brain tissues for progesterone. For example, the guinea pig uterus contains a saturable estrogen-dependent progesterone uptake mechanism, and appreciable quantities of labeled progestin can be found in nuclear fractions of uterine cells (TABLE 4).[114,115] By contrast, saturability, estrogen dependence, and nuclear localization have not been demonstrated for the brain progestin uptake system by methods adequate to demonstrate these characteristics in the uterus (TABLE 4).[102] Only autoradiography, with its advantage of high resolution, has been able to demonstrate these characteristics in the brain,[108] and controversy exists among autoradiographers on this point (cited in Reference 116).

TABLE 4

COMPARISON OF WHOLE HOMOGENATE AND NUCLEAR UPTAKE OF [^{3}H]PROGESTERONE AND [^{3}H]5α-DIHYDROPROGESTERONE IN BRAIN, ANTERIOR PITUITARY, AND UTERUS 2 HR AFTER INJECTION TO OVARIECTOMIZED ESTRADIOL-PRIMED GUINEA PIGS

Tissue	dpm/mg of protein	
	[1,2-^{3}H]5α-Dihydroprogesterone	[1,2-^{3}H]Progesterone
Hypothalamus		
Whole homogenate	119.19 ± 16.09	363.77 ± 125.85
Nuclear pellet	39.74 ± 14.21	32.15 ± 0.79
Uterus		
Whole homogenate	331.79 ± 108.27	3415.06 ± 874.19
Nuclear pellet	46.64 ± 12.53	1837.18 ± 818.31

We conclude that all of these physiologic and biochemical data argue for separable mechanisms of action of estrogen and progesterone in their facilitation of biologic responses. Although these mechanisms may be separable, they are closely intertwined. One may expect considerable anatomic and biochemical overlap in estrogen-sensitive and progesterone-sensitive systems because of the mutual dependence of these systems.

Is Facilitation by Progesterone Referable to Effects on Neurotransmitters?

In guinea pigs, estrogen implants in the medial basal hypothalamus are highly effective in facilitating lordosis.[34] Progesterone implants in the same site facilitate lordosis in estrogen primed guinea pigs.[9] If it is accepted that progesterone and estrogen have different modes of action, what sort of model consistent with this anatomic overlap might be imagined? One possibility is that progesterone activates a noradrenergic system in the hypothalamus by causing release of norepinephrine (NE) from presynaptic vesicles or causing sensitization of NE receptors in postsynaptic membranes. Either of these effects could have facilitatory influences on estrogen-sensitive cells in the vicinity. For example, the activation of a hypothalamic noradrenergic system might enhance neural stimulation of the estrogen-sensitive cells, might amplify output of such cells, or might inhibit nearby cells that normally suppress activity of estrogen-sensitive cells. Some preliminary evidence for the involvement of noradrenergic mechanisms in facilitation of sexual behavior exists in rats[117] and guinea pigs.[118] For example, in estrogen-primed ovarectomized guinea pigs, the NE receptor stimulator clonidine can act additively with[118] or can partially substitute for[118a] progesterone in facilitating lordosis. In terms of gonadotropin release, activation of NE systems has been shown to be facilitatory,[119] and there is evidence for termination of noradrenergic neurons on estradiol-concentrating cells in the diencephalon.[120] Some of these estradiol-concentrating cells may project to cells that synthesize LHRH.[121] Of course, the foregoing speculations require further experimental work for their validation. Neurotransmitters other than NE are also undoubtedly involved in facilitating sexual behavior and gonadotropin release.[122]

Mechanisms by Which Progesterone Might Inhibit Female Sexual Behavior and Gonadotropin Release

Sequential and Concurrent Inhibition: Are They Fundamentally Different?

Until this point, we have treated sequential and concurrent inhibition by progesterone as two independent processes. Recall that the two most obvious differences between these types of inhibition are that one occurs after estrogen conditioning is complete and is accompanied by low levels of endogenous progesterone in the circulation (sequential), whereas the other occurs before estrogen conditioning is complete and is accompanied by high endogenous levels of progesterone in the circulation (concurrent). Subsequent work has indicated that these two types of inhibition might not be as different as they seem. In guinea pigs, injections of radioactive progesterone (given subcutaneously in an oil vehicle) result in retention of radioactivity in brain tissues long after radioactivity is no longer detectable in peripheral blood plasma.[101] Thus, the preovulatory progesterone released into the circulation during a normal estrous cycle may be retained in brain tissue during the immediate postestrous period of sequential inhibition, even though peripheral plasma levels of progesterone are low.[13] Other experiments support this notion. Administration of progesterone in an ethanol vehicle concurrently with estrogen into ovariectomized guinea pigs does not lead to concurrent inhibition. Likewise, sequential administration of progesterone in an ethanol vehicle to ovariectomized estrogen-primed guinea pigs does not result in sequential inhibition. In both cases, the lack of inhibition can be attributed to a rapid clearance of progesterone from brain tissue as a result of dissolving the injected progesterone in ethanol rather than oil (TABLE 5). Similarly, Wallen *et al.* have shown that the degree of sequential inhibition in guinea pigs is related to the quantity of progesterone that remains in the organism at the time that sequential inhibition is manifested.[123] Thus, both concurrent and sequential inhibition are related to increased levels of progesterone in the brain. If this is the case, what is the common biochemical process responsible for inhibitory processes mediated by progesterone?

Does Progesterone Exert Inhibitory Effects by Acting as an Antiestrogen?

Synthetic antiestrogens, such as CI-628 and enclomiphene, can interfere with expression of lordosis in rats when administered prior to or concurrently with estrogen.[124,125] Isomers of antiestrogens can also facilitate lordosis by acting as estrogen mimics in rats.[126] The synthetic antiestrogens also have the capability either to facilitate[127] or to inhibit[128] LH release. Although these facilitatory and inhibitory actions of synthetic antiestrogens appear to parallel actions by progesterone, the parallel does not always exist. Thus, estrogen-primed guinea pigs given progesterone show facilitation of lordosis and sequential inhibition, whereas estrogen-primed guinea pigs given a synthetic anti-estrogen (CI-628, MER-25, or enclomiphene) do not manifest either of these phenomena (TABLE 6). In rats kept in constant light, exogenous progesterone facilitates the occurrence of ovulation, but the antiestrogen CI-628 does not.[128a]

The actions of progesterone and synthetic antiestrogens can also be compared at the biochemical level. In the rat uterus, synthetic antiestrogens and progesterone can both cause failure to completely replenish estradiol receptors.[129,130] However, the antecedents of this effect differ. Synthetic antiestrogens associate with estradiol receptors,[131] but progesterone does not.[132] In the hamster uterus, synthetic antiestrogens deplete estradiol receptors and increase the number of progesterone receptors. In contrast, progesterone acts to deplete progesterone receptors in this tissue.[133] Morin has suggested that inhibitory ac-

TABLE 5

EFFECT OF PROGESTERONE (0.5 mg) VEHICLE AT 36 HR ON FACILITATION AND SEQUENTIAL INHIBITION IN OVARIECTOMIZED GUINEA PIGS PRIMED WITH ESTRADIOL BENZOATE AT 0 HR

Group	Number of Animals	36 hr	In Heat (%)	60 hr	In Heat (%)
I	9	progesterone/oil	89	progesterone/oil	11
II	10	progesterone/ethanol	90	progesterone/oil	80

EFFECT OF PROGESTERONE (0.5 mg) VEHICLE AT −1 hr ON CONCURRENT INHIBITION IN OVARIECTOMIZED GUINEA PIGS PRIMED WITH ESTRADIOL BENZOATE AT 0 hr

Group	Number of Animals	−1 hr	36 hr	In Heat (%)
III	9	progesterone/oil	progesterone/oil	22
IV	9	progesterone/ethanol	progesterone/oil	89

TABLE 6

COMPARISON OF PROGESTERONE AND SYNTHETIC ANTIESTROGENS (MER-25, ZUCLOMIPHENE, ENCLOMIPHENE, AND NORSPIROXENONE): EFFECTS ON FACILITATION AND SEQUENTIAL INHIBITION IN OVARIECTOMIZED ESTRADIOL-PRIMED (1.6 μg) GUINEA PIGS*

Group	Number of Animals	0 hr	39–44 hr	In Heat (%)	60 hr	In Heat (%)
I	7	EB†	oil-oil	0	progesterone	85.7
II	9	EB	progesterone	89.0	progesterone	11.0
III	9	EB	MER-MER	22.2	progesterone	77.7
IV	8	EB	Zuc-Zuc	0	progesterone	75.0
V	8	EB	Enc-Enc	0	progesterone	75.0
VI	8	EB	Nor-Nor	100.0	progesterone	0

*Dosages used: progesterone, 0.5 mg per injection; antiestrogens, 10 mg per injection. All substances were injected subcutaneously in oil.

†Abbreviations: EB, estradiol benzoate; Zuc, zuclomiphene; Enc, enclomiphene; Nor, norspiroxenone.

tions of progesterone on behavior might be similarly attributable to depletion of progesterone receptors in the brain.[49] Whether this suggestion has merit remains to be tested. However, it is clear that synthetic antiestrogens have actions at biochemical levels that are different from those exerted by progesterone.

We therefore propose the existence of two categories of antiestrogenic activity that relate to behavior and gonadotropin release. Some compounds, such as the synthetic antiestrogens, share some crucial aspects of molecular structure with estrogen that permit them to exert their antagonistic influence directly on estrogen-sensitive neurons and to interact specifically with estrogen sensitive elements within these neurons. These compounds might be termed "direct" antagonists. Other compounds, such as progesterone, do not share adequate components of molecular structure with estrogen to permit them to interact with estrogen-sensitive elements of neural cells. These compounds could, then, interact with subcellular elements other than estrogen receptors in neurons that bear estrogen receptors or they could interact with neurons that do not possess estrogen receptors. The inhibitory effects of such compounds as progesterone on estrogen-dependent processes might therefore be described as "indirect." They appear to depend more on transference of information from progesterone-responsive cells to estrogen-responsive cells than on direct impedance of intranuclear programming processes in estrogen-sensitive cells. A possible example of such indirect inhibition is given in the next section.

Is Inhibition by Progesterone Referable to Effects on Neurotransmitters?

In rats and in guinea pigs, stimulation of the dopaminergic or serotonergic system results in diminution of the display of female sexual behavior.[118,134,135] Similar results have been reported for inhibition of gonadotropin release.[119]

The relation of these findings to the inhibitory actions of progesterone is not yet clear. However, progesterone implants in the midbrain, at the point of origin of dopaminergic cells, causes inhibition of lordosis in guinea pigs.[31] We tentatively suggest that progesterone may activate the nigrostriatal dopaminergic system and that such activation plays onto estrogen-sensitive cells in the hypothalamus. Perhaps the resultant inhibition of lordosis (a response in which the animal is immobile) is due to a dopamine-induced increase in locomotor activity.[136] Or perhaps progesterone somehow causes a decrease in overall arousal by acting on monoaminergic systems. It would be of considerable interest to know whether animals that fail to exhibit lordosis because of progesterone are less responsive to external stimuli in general during the period of progesterone-induced inhibition of sexual behavior.

Acknowledgments

We thank W. Crowley, R. W. Goy, M. Johns, J. Rodriguez-Sierra, and W. Walker for their participation in unpublished studies cited in the text. We are grateful to W. Cunningham and C. Banas for preparation of the manuscript. Norspiroxenone was generously provided by Merck, Sharpe and Dohme (Rahway, N.J.), CI-628 by Parke-Davis (Detroit, Mich.), MER-25 and enclomiphene by Merrell National Labs. (Cincinnati, Ohio), and Proluton (progesterone) by Schering Corporation (Bloomfield, N.J.).

References

1. Boling, J. L. & R. J. Blandau. 1939. The estrogen-progesterone induction of mating responses in the spayed female rate. Endocrinology **25:** 359–364.
2. Ring, J. R. 1944. The estrogen-progesterone induction of sexual receptivity in the spayed female mouse. Endocrinology **34:** 269–275.
3. Carter, C. S., S. J. Michael & A. H. Morris. 1973. Hormonal induction of female sexual behavior in male and female hamsters. Hormones Behav. **4:** 129–141.
4. Eaton, G. G., R. W. Goy & J. A. Resko. Brian uptake and metabolism of estradiol benzoate and estrous behavior in ovariectomized guinea pigs. Hormones Behav. **6:** 81–97.
5. Collins, V. J., J. L. Boling, E. W. Dempsey & W. C. Young. 1938. Quantitative studies of experimentally induced sexual receptivity in the spayed guinea pig. Endocrinology **23:** 188–196.
6. Morin, L. P. & H. H. Feder. 1973. Multiple progesterone injections and the duration of estrus in ovariectomized guinea pigs. Physiol. Behav. **11:** 861–865.
7. Whalen, R. E. 1974. Estrogen-progesterone induction of mating in female rats. Hormones Behav. **5:** 157–162.
8. Lisk, R. D. 1960. A comparison of the effectiveness of intravenous, as opposed to subcutaneous, injections of progesterone for the induction of estrous behavior in the rat. Can. J. Biochem. Physiol. **38:** 1381–1383.
9. Morin, L. P. & H. H. Feder. 1974. Hypothalamic progesterone implants and facilitation of lordosis behavior in estrogen-primed ovariectomized guinea pigs. Brain Res. **70:** 81–93.
10. Green, R., W. G. Luttge & R. E. Whalen. 1970. Induction of receptivity in ovariectomized female rats by a single intravenous injection of estradiol-17β. Physiol. Behav. **5:** 137–141.
11. Feder, H. H., J. A. Resko & R. W. Goy. 1968. Progesterone levels in the arterial plasma of pre-ovulatory and ovariectomized rats. J. Endocrinol. **41:** 563–569.
12. Lukaszewska, J. H. & G. S. Greenwald. 1970. Progesterone levels in the cyclic and pregnant hamster. Endocrinology **86:** 1–9.
13. Feder, H. H., J. A. Resko & R. W. Goy. 1968. Progesterone concentrations in the arterial plasma of guinea pigs during the oestrous cycle. J. Endocrinol. **40:** 505–513.

14. NAFTOLIN, F., K. BROWN-GRANT & C. S. CORKER. 1972. Plasma and pituitary luteinizing hormone and peripheral plasma oestradiol concentrations in the normal oestrous cycle of the rat and after experimental manipulation of the cycle. J. Endocrinol. **53:** 17–30.
15. POWERS, J. B. 1970. Hormonal control of sexual receptivity during the estrus cycle of the rat. Physiol. Behav. **5:** 831–835.
16. JOSLYN, W. D., H. H. FEDER & R. W. GOY. 1971. Estrogen conditioning and progesterone facilitation of lordosis in guinea pigs. Physiol. Behav. **7:** 477–482.
17. HASHIMOTO, I. & W. G. WIEST. 1969. Correlation of the secretion of ovarian steroids with function of a single generation of corpora lutea in the immature rat. Endocrinology **84:** 873–885.
18. FEDER, H. H. & K. B. RUF. 1969. Stimulation of progesterone release and estrous behavior by ACTH in ovariectomized rodents. Endocrinology **69:** 171–174.
19. GOY, R. W. & C. H. PHOENIX. 1965. Inhibitory actions of progesterone. Amer. Zool. **5:** 725 (Abs.).
20. EDWARDS, D. A., R. E. WHALEN & R. D. NADLER. 1968. Induction of estrus: estrogen-progesterone interactions. Physiol. Behav. **3:** 29–33.
21. LISK, R. D. 1973. Hormonal regulation of sexual behavior in polyestrous mammals common to the laboratory. *In* Handbook of Physiology. R. O. Greep & E. B. Astwood, Eds. Sec. 7, Vol. II (Part I): 223–344. American Physiological Society. Washington, D.C.
22. POWERS, J. B. & I. Zucker. 1969. Sexual receptivity in pregnant and pseudopregnant rats. Endocrinology **84:** 820–827.
23. BOY, R. W., C. H. PHOENIX & W. C. YOUNG. 1966. Inhibitory action of the corpus luteum on the hormonal induction of estrous behavior in the guinea pig. Gen. Comp. Endocrinol. **6:** 267–275.
24. ZUCKER, I. 1968. Biphasic effects of progesterone on sexual receptivity in the female guinea pig. J. Comp. Physiol. Psychol. **65:** 472–478.
25. YOUNG, W. C. 1969. Psychobiology of sexual behavior in the guinea pig. *In* Advances in the Study of Behavior. D. S. Lehrman, R. A. Hinde & E. Shaw, Eds. Vol. 2: 1–110. Academic Press, Inc. New York, N.Y.
26. POWERS, J. B. & J. MOREINES. 1976. Progesterone: examination of its postulated inhibitory actions on lordosis during the rat estrous cycle. Physiol. Behav. **17:** 493–498.
27. ROSS, J., V. CLAYBAUGH, L. G. CLEMENS & R. A. GORSKI. 1971. Short latency induction of estrous behavior with intracerebral gonadal hormones in ovariectomized rats. Endocrinology **89:** 32–38.
28. YANASE, M. & R. A. GORSKI. 1975. Sites of estrogen and progesterone facilitation of lordosis behavior in the spayed rat. Fed. Proc. **34:** 340 (Abs.).
29. POWERS, J. B. 1972. Facilitation of lordosis in ovariectomized rats by intracerebral progesterone implants. Brain Res. **48:** 311–325.
30. WARD, I. L., W. R. CROWLEY, F. P. ZEMLAN & D. L. MARGULES. 1975. Monoaminergic mediation of female sexual behavior. J. Comp. Physiol. Psychol. **88:** 53–61.
31. MORIN, L. P. & H. H. FEDER. 1974. Inhibition of lordosis behavior in ovariectomized guinea pigs by mesencephalic implants of progesterone. Brain Res. **70:** 71–80.
32. HALL, N. R. & W. G. LUTTGE. 1974. Intracerebral progesterone: effects on sexual behavior in female mice. Society Neuroscience, Fourth Annual Meeting, Abstract 270.
33. DAHLSTRÖM, A. & K. FUXE. 1964. Evidence for the existence of monoamines containing neurons in the central nervous system: I. Demonstration of monoamines in the cell bodies of brain stem neurons. Acta Physiol. Scand. **62** (Suppl. 232): 1–55.
34. MORIN, L. P. & H. H. FEDER. 1974. Intracranial estradiol benzoate implants and lordosis behavior of ovariectomized guinea pigs. Brain Res. **70:** 95–102.
34a. MARRONE, B. L., J. RODRIGUEZ-SIERRA & H. H. FEDER. 1976. Unpublished observations.
35. BYRNES, W. W. & E. G. SHIPLEY. 1955. Guinea pig copulatory reflex in response to adrenal steroids and similar compounds. Endocrinology **57:** 5–9.

36. JOSLYN, W. D. & H. H. FEDER. 1971. Facilitatory and inhibitory effects of supplementary estradiol benzoate given to ovariectomized, estrogen-primed guinea pigs. Hormones Behav. **2:** 307–314.
37. WADE, G. N. & H. H. FEDER. 1972. Effects of several pregnane and pregnene steroids on estrous behavior in ovariectomized estrogen-primed guinea pigs. Physiol. Behav. **9:** 773–775.
38. ZUCKER, I. & R. W. GOY. 1967. Sexual receptivity in the guinea pig: inhibitory and facilitatory actions of progesterone and related compounds. J. Comp. Physiol. Psychol. **64:** 378–383.
39. CZAJA, J. A., D. A. GOLDFOOT & H. J. KARAVOLAS. 1974. Comparative facilitation and inhibition of lordosis in the guinea pig with progesterone, 5α-pregnane-3,20-dione, or 3α-hydroxy-5α-pregnan-20-one. Hormones Behav. **5:** 261–274.
39a. MARRONE, B. L. & H. H. FEDER. 1976. Unpublished observations.
40. MORIN, L. P. & H. H. FEDER. 1974. Independence of progesterone-induced facilitation and inhibition of lordosis behavior in ovariectomized guinea pigs. Hormones Behav. **5:** 7–12.
41. BOLING, J. L., W. C. YOUNG & E. W. DEMPSEY. 1938. Miscellaneous experiments on the estrogen-progesterone induction of heat in the spayed guinea-pig. Endocrinology **23:** 182–187.
41a. WALKER, W. A., B. L. MARRONE & H. H. FEDER. 1976. Unpublished observations.
42. WHALEN, R. E. & B. B. GORZALKA. 1972. The effects of progesterone and its metabolites on the induction of sexual receptivity in rats. Hormones Behav. **3:** 221–226.
43. MEYERSON, B. J. 1967. Relationship between the anesthetic and gestagenic action and estrous behavior-inducing activity of different progestins. Endocrinology **81:** 369–374.
44. MEYERSON, B. 1972. Latency between intravenous injection of progestins and the appearance of estrous behavior in estrogen-treated ovariectomized rats. Hormones Behav. **3:** 1–9.
45. NADLER, R. D. 1970. A biophasic influence of progesterone on sexual receptivity of spayed female rats. Physiol. Behav. **5:** 95–97.
46. CIACCIO, L. A. & R. D. LISK. 1972. The role of progesterone in regulating the period of sexual receptivity in the female hamster. J. Endocrinol. **50:** 201–207.
47. EDWARDS, D. A. 1970. Induction of estrus in female mice: estrogen-progesterone interactions. Hormones Behav. **1:** 299–304.
48. WHALEN, R. E. & K. NAKAYAMA. 1965. Induction of oestrous behaviour: facilitation by repeated hormone treatments. J. Endocrinol. **33:** 525, 526.
49. MORIN, L. P. 1976. Progesterone: inhibition of rodent sexual behavior. Physiol. Behav. In press.
50. POWERS, J. B. & E. S. VALENSTEIN. 1972. Individual differences in sexual responsiveness to estrogen and progesterone in ovariectomized rats. Physiol. Behav. **8:** 673–676.
51. FRANK, A. & R. FRAPS. 1945. Induction of estrus in the ovariectomized golden hamster. Endocrinology **37:** 357–361.
52. ROBERTSON, H. A. 1969. The endogenous control of estrus and ovulation in sheep, cattle, and swine. Vitamins Hormones **27:** 91–130.
53. SMITH, M. S. & L. E. MCDONALD. 1974. Serum levels of luteinizing hormone and progesterone during the estrous cycle, pseudopregnancy and pregnancy in the dog. Endocrinology **94:** 404–412.
54. BEACH, F. A. & A. MERARI. 1968. Coital behavior in dogs, IV. Effects of progesterone in the bitch. Proc. Nat. Acad. Sci. USA **61:** 442–446.
55. EVERETT, J. W. 1948. Progesterone and estrogen in the experimental control of ovulation time and other features of the estrous cycle in the rat. Endocrinology **43:** 389–405.
56. ZEILMAKER, G. H. 1966. The biphasic effect of progesterone on ovulation in the rat. Acta Endocrinol. **51:** 461–468.
57. DÖCKE, F. & G. DÖRNER. 1966. Facilitative action of progesterone in the induction of ovulation by oestrogen. J. Endocrinol. **36:** 209, 210.

58. Sawyer, C. H. & J. W. Everett. 1959. Stimulatory and inhibitory effects of progesterone on the release of pituitary ovulating hormone in the rabbit. Endocrinology **65:** 644–651.
59. Naller, R., J. Antunes-Rodrigues & S. M. McCann. 1956. Effect of progesterone on the level of plasma LH in normal female rats. Endocrinology **79:** 907–911.
60. Caligaris, L., J. J. Astrada & S. Taleisnik. 1971. Biphasic effect of progesterone on the release of gonadotropin in rats. Endocrinology **89:** 331–337.
61. Siegel, H. I., J. D. Bast & G. S. Greenwald. 1976. The effects of phenobarbital and gonadal steroids on periovulatory serum levels of luteinizing hormone and follicle-stimulating hormone in the hamster. Endocrinology **98:** 48–55.
62. Ferin, M., A. Tempone, P. E. Zimmering & R. L. Vande Weile. 1969. Effect of antibodies to 17β-estradiol and progesterone on the estrous cycle of the rat. Endocrinology **85:** 1070–1078.
63. Feder, H. H., K. Brown-Grant & C. S. Corker. 1971. Pre-ovulatory progesterone, the adrenal cortex and the 'critical period' for luteinizing hormone release in rats. J. Endocrinol. **50:** 29–39.
64. Barraclough, C. A., R. Collu, R. Massa & L. Martini. 1971. Temporal interrelationships between plasma LH, ovarian secretion rates and peripheral plasma progestin concentrations in the rat: effects of Nembutal and exogenous gonadotropins. Endocrinology **88:** 1437–1447.
65. Piacsek, B. E., T. C. Schneider & V. L. Gay. 1971. Sequential study of luteinizing hormone (LH) and "progestin" secretion on the afternoon of proestrus in the rat. Endocrinology **89:** 39–45.
66. Croix, D. & P. Franchimont. 1975. Changes in the serum levels of the gonadotrophins, progesterone and estradiol during the estrous cycle of the guinea pig. Neuroendocrinology **19:** 1–11.
67. Niswender, G. D., T. J. Reimers, M. A. Diekman & T. M. Nett. 1976. Blood flow: a mediator of ovarian function. Biol. Reprod. **14:** 64–81.
68. Mann, D. R. & C. A. Barraclough. 1973. Role of estrogen and progesterone in facilitating LH release in 4-day cyclic rats. Endocrinology **93:** 694–699.
69. Dempsey, E. W., R. Hertz & W. C. Young. 1936. The experimental induction of oestrus (sexual receptivity) in the normal and ovariectomized guinea pig. Amer. J. Physiol. **116:** 201–209.
70. Reuter, L. A., L. A. Ciaccio & R. D. Lisk. Progesterone: regulation of estrous cycle, ovulation and estrous behavior in the golden hamster. Endocrinology **86:** 1287–1297.
71. Loeb, L. 1911. Über die Bedeutung des Corpus luteum für die Periodizität des sexuellen Zyklus beim weiblichen Säugetierorganismus. Deut. Med. Wochschr. **37:** 17–21.
72. Dempsey, E. W. 1937. Follicular growth rate and ovulation after various experimental procedures in the guinea pig. Amer. J. Physiol. **120:** 126–132.
73. Goldman, B. D. & M. X. Zarrow. 1973. The physiology of progestins. *In* Handbook of Physiology. R. O. Greep & E. B. Astwood, Eds. Sec. 7, Vol. II (Part 1): 547–571. American Physiological Society. Washington, D.C.
74. Barraclough, C. A., S. Yrarrazaval & R. Hatton. A possible hypothalamic site of action of progesterone in the facilitation of ovulation in the rat. Endocrinology **75:** 838–845.
75. Döcke, F. & G. Dörner. 1969. A possible mechanism by which progesterone facilitates ovulation in the rat. Neuroendocrinology **4:** 139–149.
76. Schuling, G. A., J. A. M. J. van Dieten & G. P. van Rees. 1974. Induction and inhibition of ovulation in the rat by intracerebral progesterone implants. Neuroendocrinology **15:** 38–50.
77. Kobayashi, F., K. Hara & T. Miyake. 1970. Facilitation of luteinizing hormone release by progesterone in proestrous rats. Endocrinol. Japon. **17:** 149–155.
78. Bogdanove, E. M. 1963. Direct gonad-pituitary feedback: an analysis of effects of intracranial estrogenic depots on gonadotropin secretion. Endocrinology **73:** 696–712.

79. Labhsetwar, A. P. & J. G. Bainbridge. 1971. Inhibition of ovulation by intracranial implantation of progesterone in the 4-day cyclic rat. J. Reprod. Fertil. **27:** 445–449.
80. Stevens, K. R., H. G. Spies, J. Hilliard & C. H. Sawyer. 1970. Site(s) of action of progesterone in blocking ovulation in the rat. Endocrinology **86:** 970–975.
81. Reuter, L. A. & R. D. Lisk. 1973. Progesterone-sensitive loci for blockade of ovulation in the hamster. Neuroendocrinology **12:** 17–29.
82. Kaasjager, W. A., D. M. Woodbury, J. A. M. J. van Dieten & G. P. van Rees. 1971. The role played by the preoptic region and the hypothalamus in spontaneous ovulation and ovulation induced by progesterone. Neuroendocrinology **7:** 54–64.
83. Piva, F., P. S. Kalra & L. Martini. 1973. Participation of the amygdala and of the cerebellum in the feedback effects of progesterone. Neuroendocrinology **11:** 229–239.
84. Smith, E. R. & J. M. Davidson. 1974. Location of feedback receptors: effects of intracranial implanted steroids on plasma LH and LRF response. Endocrinology **95:** 1566–1573.
85. Clemens, J. A., C. J. Shaar & E. B. Smalstig. 1972. Effects of electrical stimulation of the hypothalamus on LH release in steroid-treated rats. Neuroendocrinology **10:** 175–182.
86. Brown-Grant, K. 1967. The effects of a single injection of progesterone on the oestrous cycle, thyroid gland activity and uterus-plasma concentration ratio for radio-iodide in the rat. J. Physiol. (London) **190:** 101–121.
87. Brown-Grant, K. 1974. Steroid hormone administration and gonadotrophin secretion in the gonadectomized rat. J. Endocrinol. **62:** 319–332.
88. Swerdloff, R. S., H. S. Jacobs & W. D. Odell. 1972. Synergistic role of progestogens in estrogen induction of LH and FSH surge. Endocrinology **90:** 1529–1536.
89. Hilliard, J., D. Archibald & C. H. Sawyer. 1963. Gonadotropic activation of preovulatory synthesis and release of progestin in the rabbit. Endocrinology **72:** 59–66.
90. Okano, K., K. Matsumoto, K. Kotch, H. Endo & T. Seki. 1966. Progestins in the ovarian vein blood of nonpregnant and pregnant rabbits before and after gonadotropic stimulation. Endocrinol. Japon. **13:** 438–447.
91. Hilliard, J., R. Penardi & C. H. Sawyer. 1967. A functional role for 20α-hydroxypregn-4-en-3-one in the rabbit. Endocrinology **80:** 901–909.
92. Hansel, W. & S. E. Echternkamp. 1972. Control of ovarian function in domestic animals. Amer. Zool. **12:** 225–243.
93. Radford, H. M., I. S. Wheatley & A. L. C. Wallace. 1969. The effects of oestradiol benzoate and progesterone on secretion of luteinizing hormone in the ovariectomized ewe. J. Endocrinol. **44:** 135, 136.
94. McDonald, P. G. & M. T. Clegg. 1967. The effect of progesterone on serum luteinizing hormone concentrations in the ewe. J. Reprod. Fertil. **13:** 75–82.
95. Bolt, D. J., H. E. Kelley & H. W. Hawk. 1971. Release of LH by estradiol in cycling ewes. Biol. Reprod. **4:** 35–40.
96. Yuthasastrakosol, P., B. E. Howland, S. Simaraks & W. M. Palmer. 1974. Estrogen-induced LH release in progesterone-treated ovariectomized ewes. Can. J. Animal Sci. **54:** 565–572.
97. Kow, L.-M. & D. W. Pfaff. 1975. Induction of lordosis in female rats: two modes of estrogen action and the effect of adrenalectomy. Hormones Behav. **6:** 259–276.
98. Kalra, P. S. & S. M. McCann. 1973. Involvement of catecholamines in feedback mechanisms. Progr. Brain Res. **39:** 185–197.
99. Mennin, S. P. & R. A. Gorski. 1975. Effects of ovarian steroids on plasma LH in normal and persistent estrous adult female rats. Endocrinology **96:** 486–491.
100. Eisenfeld, A. J. & J. Axelrod. 1965. Selectivity of estrogen distribution in tissues. J. Pharmacol. Exp. Ther. **150:** 469–475.
101. Feder, H. H., H. Siegel & G. N. Wade. 1974. Uptake of (6,7-^{3}H) estradiol-17β in ovariectomized rats, guinea pigs and hamsters: correlation with species differences in behavioral responsiveness to estradiol. Brain Res. **71:** 93–103.

102. WADE, G. N. & H. H. FEDER. 1972. 1,2-^{3}H Progesterone uptake by guinea pig brain and uterus: differential localization, time-course of uptake and metabolism, and effects of age, sex, estrogen-priming and competing steroids. Brain Res. **45:** 525–543.
103. WHALEN, R. E. & W. G. LUTTGE. 1971. Differential localization of progesterone uptake in the brain. Role of sex, estrogen pretreatment and adrenalectomy. Brain Res. **33:** 139–146.
104. WADE, G. N. & H. H. FEDER. 1972. Uptake of (1,2-^{3}H)20α-hydroxypregn-4-en-one (1,2-^{3}H) corticosterone, and (6,7-^{3}H) estradiol-17β by guinea pig brain and uterus: comparison with uptake of (1,2-^{3}H) progesterone. Brain Res. **45:** 545–554.
105. ZIGMOND, R. E. & B. S. MCEWEN. 1970. Selective retention of estradiol by cell nuclei in specific regions of the ovariectomized rat. J. Neurochem. **17:** 889–899.
106. FEDER, H. H. & G. N. WADE. 1974. Integrative actions of perinatal hormones on neural tissues mediating adult sexual behavior. *In* The Neurosciences. F. O. SCHMITT & F. G. WORDEN, Eds. Vol. 3: 583–586. The M.I.T. Press. Cambridge, Mass.
107. MCEWEN, B. S., R. DE KLOET & G. WALLACH. 1976. Interactions *in vivo* of corticoids and progesterone with cell nuclei and soluble macromolecules from rat brain regions and pituitary. Brain Res. **105:** 129–136.
108. SAR, M. & W. E. STUMPF. 1973. Neurons of the hypothalamus concentrate (^{3}H) progesterone or its metabolites. Science **182:** 1266–1268.
109. ANDERSON, J. N., E. J. PECK, JR. & J. H. CLARK. 1973. Nuclear receptor estrogen complex: accumulation, retention and localization in the hypothalamus and pituitary. Endocrinology **93:** 711–717.
110. SEIKI, K. & M. HATTORI. 1973. *In vivo* uptake of progesterone by the hypothalamus and pituitary of the female ovariectomized rat and its relationship to cytoplasmic progesterone-binding protein. Endocrinol. Japon. **20:** 111–119.
111. IRAMAIN, C. A., B. J. DANZO, C. A. STROTT & D. O. TOFT. 1973. Progesterone binding in the hypothalamus and hypophysis of female guinea pigs and rabbits. Fourth International Congress of the International Society of Psychoneuroendocrinology (Abs.).
112. WADE, G. N., C. F. HARDING & H. H. FEDER. 1973. Neural uptake of (1,2-^{3}H) progesterone in ovariectomized rats, guinea pigs and hamsters: correlation with species differences in behavioral responsiveness. Brain Res. **61:** 357–367.
113. PUCA, G. A. & F. BRESCIANI. 1968. Receptor molecule for oestrogens from rat uterus. Nature (London) **218:** 967–969.
114. FEIL, P. D. & C. W. BARDIN. 1975. Cytoplasmic and nuclear progesterone receptors in the guinea pig uterus. Endocrinology **97:** 1398–1407.
115. WAREMBOURG, M. 1974. Radioautographic study of the guinea pig uterus after injection and incubation with ^{3}H-progesterone. Endocrinology **94:** 665–670.
116. ATGER, M., E.-E. BAULIEU & E. MILGROM. 1974. An investigation of progesterone receptors in the guinea pig vagina, uterine cervix, mammary glands, pituitary and hypothalamus. Endocrinology **94:** 161–167.
117. EVERITT, B. J., K. FUXE, T. HÖKFELT & G. JONSSON. 1975. Studies on the role of monoamines in the hormonal regulation of sexual receptivity in the female rat. *In* Sexual Behavior: Pharmacology and Biochemistry. M. Sandler & G. L. Gessa, Eds.: 147–159. The Raven Press. New York, N.Y.
118. CROWLEY, W. R., H. H. FEDER & L. P. MORIN. 1976. Role of monoamines in sexual behavior of the female guinea pig. Pharmacol. Biochem. Behav. **4:** 67–71.
118a. CROWLEY, W. R. & H. H. FEDER. 1976. Unpublished observations.
119. TERASAWA, E., W. E. BRIDSON, J. W. DAVENPORT & R. W. GOY. 1975. Role of brain monoamines in release of gonadotropin before proestrus in the cyclic rat. Neuroendocrinology **18:** 345–358.
120. GRANT, L. D. & W. E. STUMPF. 1973. Localization of ^{3}H-estradiol and catecholamines in the identical neurons in the hypothalamus. J. Histochem. Cytochem. **21:** 404 (Abs.).
121. PFAFF, D. W. 1973. Luteinizing hormone-releasing factor potentiates lordosis behavior in hypophysectomized ovariectomized female rats. Science **182:** 1148, 1149.

122. McCann, S. M. & R. L. Moss. 1975. Putative neurotransmitters involved in discharging gonadotropin-releasing neurohormones and the action of LH-releasing hormone on the CNS. Life Sci. **16:** 833–852.
123. Wallen, K., R. W. Goy & C. H. Phoenix. 1975. Inhibitory actions of progesterone on hormonal induction of estrus in female guinea pigs. Hormones Behav. **6:** 127–138.
124. Arai, Y. & R. A. Gorski. 1968. Effects of anti-estrogen on steroid-induced sexual receptivity in ovariectomized rats. Physiol. Behav. **3:** 351–353.
125. Ross, J. W., D. C. Paup, M. Brant-Zawadski, J. R. Marshall & R. A. Gorski. 1973. Effects of cis- and trans- clomiphene in the induction of sexual behavior. Endocrinology **93:** 681–685.
126. Ross, J. W., J. Shryne, R. A. Gorski & J. R. Marshall. 1973. Effect of clomiphene citrate and its isomers on sexual behavior in ovariectomized rats. Endocrinology **92:** 1079–1083.
127. Igarashi, M., Y. Ibuki, H. Kubo, J. Kamioka, N. Yokota, Y. Ebara & S. Matsumoto. 1967. Mode and site of action of clomiphene. Amer. J. Obstet. Gynecol. **97:** 120–123.
128. Schally, A. V., W. H. Carter, A. F. Parlow, M. Saito, A. Arimura, C. Y. Bowers & D. E. Holtkamp. 1970. Alteration of LH and FSH release in rats treated with clomiphene or its isomers. Amer. J. Obstet. Gynecol. **107:** 1156–1167.
128a. Johns, M. A. & H. H. Feder. 1976. Unpublished observations.
129. Clark, J. H., E. J. Peck, Jr. & J. N. Anderson. 1974. Oestrogen receptors and antagonism of steroid hormone action. Nature (London) **251:** 446–448.
130. Hsueh, A. J. W., E. J. Peck, Jr. & J. H. Clark. 1975. Progesterone antagonism of the oestrogen receptor and oestrogen-induced uterine growth. Nature (London) **254:** 337–339.
131. Katzenellenbogen, B. S. & E. R. Ferguson. 1975. Antiestrogen action in the uterus: biological ineffectiveness of nuclear bound estradiol after antiestrogen. Endocrinology **97:** 1–12.
132. King, R. J. B. & W. J. P. Mainwaring. 1974. Steroid Cell Interaction. University Park Press. Baltimore, Md.
133. Leavitt, W. W., D. O. Toft, C. A. Strott & B. W. O'Malley. 1974. A specific progesterone receptor in the hamster uterus: physiologic properties and regulation during the estrous cycle. Endocrinology **94:** 1041–1053.
134. Everitt, B. J., K. Fuxe & T. Hökfelt. 1974. Inhibitory role of dopamine and 5-hydroxytryptamine in the sexual behaviour of female rats. Eur. J. Pharmacol. **29:** 187–191.
135. Meyerson, B. J., H. Carrer & M. Eliasson. 1974. 5-Hydroxytryptamine and sexual behavior in the female rat. Advan. Biochem. Psychopharmacol. **11:** 861–865.
136. Bolme, P., K. Fuxe & P. Lidbrink. 1972. On the function of central catecholamine neurons—their role in cardiovascular and arousal mechanisms. Res. Commun. Chem. Pathol. Pharmacol. **4:** 657–697.

Discussion

Dr. U. F. Westphal: You have concentrated on the action of hormones in the brain. We know that behavior of male animals in influenced by pheromones, and we know that distinct compounds are formed under the action of hormones and influence the male. Is it not possible that progesterone given to females acts to produce pheromones that influence the male's sexual interest and that a direct effect of progesterone on the brain of the female is not necessarily involved?

Dr. Feder: I don't think that pheromones are involved in this instance, because the response that we are looking at is the lordosis reflex of the female, and this response can be elicited not only by the male but also by manual stimulation of the female's back and perineal region.

Dr. J. V. Martin *(University of California at Irvine, Irvine, Calif.)*: In Dr. Whalen's laboratory, we found that replenishment of estrogen receptor depletion after cold estrogen administration is unchanged by concurrent progesterone injection in hamster neural tissue.

Dr. Feder: That's interesting in relation to your previous finding [Whalen, Martin & Olsen. 1975. Nature (London) **258:** 742–743] that the synthetic antiestrogens are effective in delaying replenishment in neural tissues. These combined data support our notion of two classes of antiestrogenic activity.

Dr. W. G. Wiest: Concerning the direct action of progesterone by the classic or intranuclear reaction, Harry Karavolas of Wisconsin has shown in rats that progesterone is metabolized by the very tissues you're looking at to the 5α-dihydro derivative. Have you done a similar binding study with the labeled dihydro compound in guinea pigs?

Dr. Feder: We have compared progesterone and 5α-dihydroprogesterone uptake in whole homogenates and in nuclear fractions in guinea pigs. We find that when we administer the same specific activity and the same dose of the two steroid hormones, progesterone is taken up in slightly higher amounts in the whole homogenate, but neither steroid is concentrated in the nucleus of neural tissues. Interestingly, progesterone is taken up very well in the uterine nuclear pellet, but 5α-dihydroprogesterone is not, and the latter result agrees with Dr. Karavolas' findings.

Dr. R. J. B. King: Your suggestion that progesterone may be acting on the membrane is really quite attractive, and I think there is now quite good evidence that steroids can act on things like synaptosomal membranes. But, on the other hand, the kind of data that you are presenting on progesterone binding doesn't rule out that the possibility of cytoplasmic progesterone receptors. I would just like to call your attention to a technique for measuring steroid binding in various brain fractions that has many advantages when looking for steroid binding in the brain as opposed to other kinds of tissues, and this is the technique reported by Ginsburg *et al.* (Ginsburg, Greenstein, MacLusky, Morris & Thomas. 1974. Steroids **23:** 773–792).

Dr. G. S. Richardson *(Massachusetts General Hospital, Boston, Mass.)*: Regarding polarity-dependent binding, have you tried other steroids of comparable polarity? For example, in partition systems, it's very difficult to separate progesterone from 5α-androstanedione and 5β-androstanedione. I presume that 5α-pregnanedione and 5α-dihydroprogesterone are ineffective in inducing lordosis, although they are relatively nonpolar.

Dr. Feder: I agree that the whole story is not polarity dependence. I mentioned that we thought that 5α-dihydroprogesterone, which is slightly less polar than progesterone and approximately as effective as progesterone in facilitating lordosis in guinea pigs, would be expected to have a greater uptake than progesterone in brain tissue. But it doesn't. We also have a situation in which some steroids are behaviorally ineffective (e.g., androstanedione) but, yet, may be as nonpolar as progesterone. So there is some specificity of action of progesterone, and this specificity is not solely due to polarity properties.

Dr. W. L. McGuire: Regarding Dr. King's comment on your progesterone-binding studies, it was fortunate that you used the uterus as a control for some of your *in vivo* work. It's interesting that 2 hr after an injection of progesterone, only

20% of the radioactivity was in the uterine nuclei. I find that result a little surprising, although I don't know the exact dosage and so forth. I would like to suggest the possibility that the binding you're observing in your whole homogenate may represent posthomogenization binding of steroid trapped in the interstitial spaces or some other phenomenon that may be masking some saturable sites because of the large amount of "nonsaturable binding" that you're observing.

DR. FEDER: Yes, I think that we have a lot of nonsaturable binding possibly masking a little bit of saturable binding. That is probably why the only direct evidence for nuclear uptake and saturable uptake in neural tissues has been by high-resolution autoradiographic techniques (Sar, M. & W. E. Stumpf. 1973. Science **182:** 1266–1267).

GLUCOCORTICOID ACTIVITY OF VARIOUS PROGESTERONE ANALOGS: CORRELATION BETWEEN SPECIFIC BINDING IN THYMUS AND LIVER AND BIOLOGIC ACTIVITY*

Dennis DiSorbo, Fred Rosen, Richard P. McPartland,† and Richard J. Milholland

Department of Experimental Therapeutics
Grace Cancer Drug Center
Roswell Park Memorial Institute
New York State Department of Health
Buffalo, New York 14263

INTRODUCTION

Considerable interest in antisteroids has developed because of their present and potential clinical importance and because of the various mechanisms by which they might antagonize the biochemical and physiologic responses to the hormone. It has been shown that certain steroid antagonists compete with their biologically active counterparts for binding to specific receptors and thus inhibit hormonal action. A compound with antiglucocorticoid activity would have widespread application in the treatment of various hormonal imbalances characterized by the oversecretion of cortisol. We have reported that, in a suspension of rat thymocytes, it is possible to block certain aspects of glucocorticoid action by incubating the inactive corticoid cortexolone (11-deoxycortisol) or progesterone together with triamcinolone acetonide.[1,2] However, neither of these steroids is active as an antiglucocorticoid *in vivo*.

The present report describes a structure-activity study aimed at determining the substituent groups in progesterone analogs that are essential for glucocorticoid or antiglucocorticoid activity. To ascertain such activity, the analog was tested for binding to specific glucocorticoid receptors in rat thymus and liver. If binding occurred, the compound was further examined for its ability to either stimulate or block (when injected with cortisol) the induction of hepatic tyrosine aminotransferase or involution of thymus in adrenalectomized rats. The latter condition is essential, because the enzyme that catalyzes 11β hydroxylation of the steroid nucleus, except under special conditions,[3,4] has been found to occur only in the adrenal glands.[5] The results obtained clearly indicate that 6α-methylprogesterone and other analogs of progesterone that contain the 6α-methyl group possess glucocorticoid activity. It appears that the 6α-methyl substituent either in progesterone or in other progestins can replace or enhance the function of the 11β-hydroxyl group in conferring glucocorticoid activity.

*Supported by American Cancer Society Grant CI-130 National Cancer Institute Grants CA-05016 and CA-05671.

†Recipient of a National Cancer Institute Postdoctoral Fellowship.

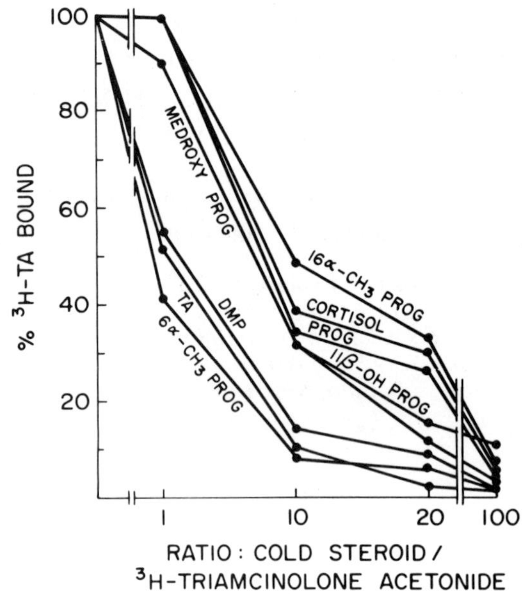

FIGURE 1. Competition among cortisol, progesterone, and several progesterone analogs for the thymic receptor. Steroids were added at various concentrations with [^{3}H]TA (2×10^{-8} M) to a 27,000*g* supernatant and incubated for 4 hr at 4°C. The extent of binding was assayed by the charcoal adsorption method. Percentage of bound [^{3}H]TA represents "specific" binding. Each point is the mean value of triplicate determinations with an individual variation of less than 5%. For details, see MATERIALS AND METHODS.

MATERIALS AND METHODS

Male albino rats of the Sprague-Dawley strain that weighed from 80 to 100g were used in all experiments. Bilateral adrenalectomies were performed under pentobarbital sodium (Nembutal®) anesthesia, and the rats were maintained on 1% NaCl drinking water for 3–5 days before experimental treatment. Steroids to be injected were dissolved in corn oil. The rats were killed by decapitation, and the liver and thymus were removed rapidly and washed free of blood under cold running water. The liver was quickly blotted free of excess water and frozen in a mixture of dry ice and acetone for determination of enzymatic activity at a later date. For the binding analysis, liver and thymus were kept on ice and used within 5 min for the preparation of the 27,000*g* supernatant fraction. The method used to prepare a suspension of thymocytes has been described previously.[6]

[1,2,4-^{3}H]Triamcinolone acetonide ([^{3}H]TA, 34 Ci/mmol) was purchased from Amersham Searle. Cortisol, progesterone, triamcinolone acetonide, testosterone, 5α-dihydrotestosterone, and 17β-estradiol were purchased from Sigma Chemical Co.; 17α-hydroxyprogesterone was obtained from Schwartz-Mann BioResearch; dimethylprogesterone, 11β-hydroxyprogesterone, 6α- and 6β-hydroxyprogesterone, and 16α- and 16β-methylprogesterone were purchased from Steraloids. 6α-Methylprogesterone, 17α-ethynyl-19-nortestosterone diacetate, and 17α-ethynyl-19-nortestosterone were gifts from Searle. Dimethylethynyltestosterone was a gift from Mead Johnson, and 17α-ethynyl-18-ethyl-19-nortestosterone was a gift from Wyeth. For use *in vitro*, all steroids were dissolved in 100% ethanol to yield 10^{-3} M stock solutions.

About 1 g of fresh liver or thymus was weighed and transferred to a Teflon® pestle tissue grinder. Ice-cold Tris buffer was added [0.01 M Tris hydrochloride (pH 7.6), 4 mM disodium EDTA], and the tissue was homogenized with 15 complete strokes of the pestle. To restore the homogenate to isotonicity, a 0.1 vol of cold hypertonic Tris buffer [0.11 M Tris hydrochloride (pH 7.6), 1.43 M NaCl, 0.11 M KCl, and 0.033 M $MgCl_2$] was added. After an additional 10 strokes of the pestle, the homogenate was transferred to 30-ml tubes and centrifuged in a Sorval refrigerated centrifuge for 30 min at 27,000*g*. After centrifugation, 2.0-ml aliquots of cytosol were incubated for 4 hr with either [^{3}H]TA, [^{3}H]TA and cold TA, or [^{3}H]TA plus cold test compound. All procedures, except weighing, were performed at 4°C.

The method used to separate free from bound steroid in the 27,000*g* supernatant was slightly modified from that described by Baxter and Tomkins.[7] Briefly, it was as follows: 0.1 ml of a suspension of charcoal (100 mg/ml of Norit A) pretreated with 5 N HCl, washed with distilled water, followed by treatment with 5 N NaOH, brought to pH 7.6, and resuspended in isotonic Tris buffer, was added to 0.5 ml of incubated cytosol, vortexed for 10 sec, and centrifuged at 4°C at the highest speed in an International clinical centrifuge for 2 min. The supernatant was removed, placed in a 2.0-ml conical tube, recentrifuged for 10 min, and 200-μl aliquots were assayed for radioactivity in 10 ml of Bray's scintillation mixture.[8]

Specific binding is assessed by determining the number of counts that remain after subtracting the count obtained in the presence of [^{3}H]triamcinolone acetonide plus a 100-fold excess of cold steroid from the count obtained with the tritiated steroid alone. When competition between [^{3}H]TA and the test steroid for the receptor was measured, specific binding was calculated by subtracting the nonspecific count obtained in the presence of a 100-fold excess of cold TA from

Table 1

Competition between [^{3}H]TA and Various Progestins for the Glucocorticoid Receptor in Broken and Intact Rat Thymocytes

Compound*	Competition (%) Intact Cells†	Cell Free†
Triamcinolone acetonide	100	100
6α-Methylprogesterone	—	93
6α-Methyl-17α-hydroxyprogesterone	85	93
16α-Methylprogesterone	71	80
Progesterone	65	83
17α-Hydroxyprogesterone	—	55
16α-Methyl-17α-hydroxyprogesterone	46	60
16β-Methylprogesterone	46	45
6α-Hydroxyprogesterone	0	0
6β-Hydroxyprogesterone	0	0

*Intact cells or a 27,000*g* supernatant was incubated with [^{3}H]TA (2×10^{-8} M) plus test compound (10^{-6} M).

†Competition in intact cells was analyzed on a 5–20% sucrose gradient, and the charcoal binding assay was used for the analysis in the cell-free system (see Reference 1 for details of methodology).

TABLE 2

THYMOLYTIC ACTIVITY OF PROGESTERONE ANALOGS

Compound*	Thymus Weight† (g)
Vehicle	0.417 ± 0.026
Cortisol	0.119 ± 0.006‡
6α-Methylprogesterone	0.329 ± 0.025‡
6α-16α-Dimethylprogesterone	0.338 ± 0.017‡
6α-Methyl-17α-hydroxyprogesterone	0.250 ± 0.018‡
17α-Hydroxyprogesterone	0.431 ± 0.034
16α-Methyl-17α-hydroxyprogesterone	0.424 ± 0.016

*Male adrenalectomized rats that weighed between 70 and 80 g were given a single subcutaneous dose (25 mg/kg) of test compound. Forty-eight hours later, the animals were sacrificed, and the thymus was removed and blotted dry.

†Thymus weights are the mean value ± SE for three to five rats in each group.

‡$p < 0.05$.

the count that remained after [^{3}H]TA plus a 10- to 100-fold excess of the test compound were incubated. Competition between [^{3}H]TA and various progestins in intact rat thymocytes was assayed as previously described.[1]

A 48-hr thymus involution test was used to evaluate the thymolytic activity of progesterone analogs and was performed as follows: male adrenalectomized rats that weighed between 70 and 80 g were given a single subcutaneous dose (25.0 mg/kg) of test compound dissolved in corn oil[9]; 48 hr later, the animals were sacrificed, and the thymus was removed and blotted dry. Thymus weights were calculated per 100-g rat.

Tyrosine aminotransferase (E.C. 2.6.1.5) was assayed by a colorimetric

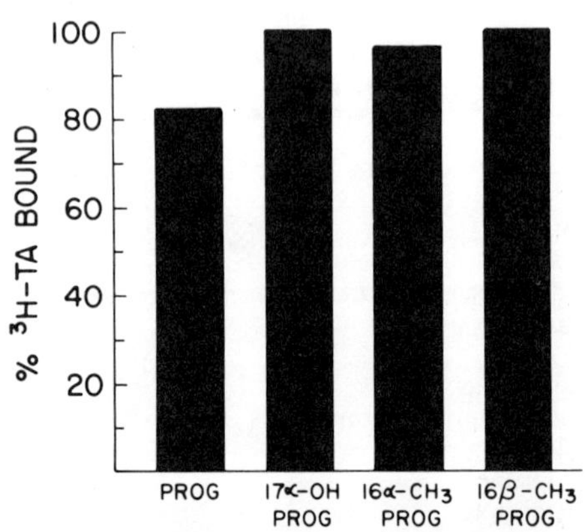

FIGURE 2. Binding of [^{3}H]TA to the liver receptor in the presence of progesterone and three analogs of this steroid. A 27,000*g* supernatant fraction (isotonically buffered protein, 8.6 mg/ml) was incubated with [^{3}H]TA (2×10^{-8} M) alone or in combination with each competing steroid (2×10^{-6} M) for 4 hr at 4°C. Experimental details were the same as in FIGURE 1.

procedure previously described.[10] Protein was determined by the method of Lowry *et al.*[11] with bovine serum albumin used as a standard.

Results

There have been several reports[2,12] that indicate that progesterone is able to block certain biochemical effects of glucocorticoids in rat thymocyte suspensions, and Rousseau *et al.*[13] have observed that progesterone impairs the induction of tyrosine aminotransferase by cortisol in HTC cells. The competition that occurs among different concentrations of progesterone and derivatives of this steroid with [^{3}H]TA for binding to the glucocorticoid receptor in a cell-free preparation of rat thymus is shown in Figure 1. The control value for the specific binding of [^{3}H]TA in the absence of competing steroids was 33,000 dpm per milligram of protein; this value represents 100% binding. The results indicate that 6α-methylprogesterone and 6α,16α-dimethylprogesterone are as effective as similar

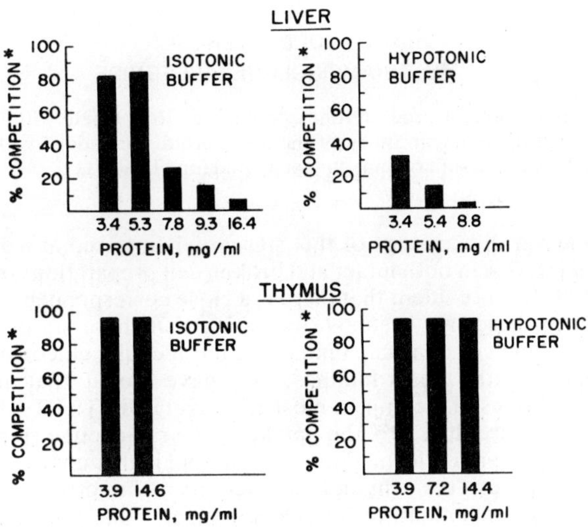

Figure 3. Progesterone binding as a function of protein and salt concentrations. A 27,000*g* supernatant fraction (2.0 ml), which varied in protein and salt concentrations, was incubated with [^{3}H]TA (2×10^{-8} M) alone or in the presence of progesterone (2×10^{-6} M) for 4 hr at 4°C. The hypotonic buffer contained 0.01 M Trishydrochloride and 4 mM disodium EDTA (pH 7.6); isotonicity was achieved by adding 0.1 vol of 0.11 M Trishydrochloride, 1.43 M NaCl, 0.11 M KCl, and 0.033 M $MgCl_2$ (pH 7.6) to the hypotonic cytosol.

concentrations of unlabeled TA in competing with the radioactive glucocorticoid. Somewhat less active in this regard are cortisol and progesterone and some of its analogs, including medroxyprogesterone, which contains a 6α-methyl substituent.

Because our major objective in these studies has been to develop an antiglucocorticoid that would be active *in vivo,* it was important to demonstrate that progesterone derivatives that compete with glucocorticoids for a specific receptor-binding site in a cell-free system are also active in intact cells. A comparison of

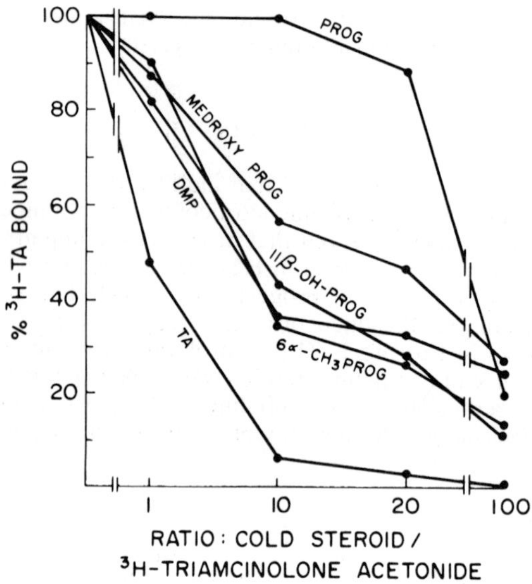

FIGURE 4. Ability of several progesterones derivatives to compete with [^{3}H]TA for the liver receptor. Increasing concentrations of the test steroid were added with [^{3}H]TA (2×10^{-8} M) to a 27,000*g* isotonic supernatant and incubated for 4 hr at 4°C.

progesterone and various analogs of this steroid when tested at a 50-fold higher concentration of [^{3}H]TA in both intact and broken cell preparations of thymocytes is shown in TABLE 1. It is evident that there is a close correspondence between the results obtained in these two systems, indicating that these steroids are readily transported into whole cells and can bind to the intracellular glucocorticoid receptor. In agreement with these findings, we have noted that many of the progesterone derivatives that compete most effectively with [^{3}H]TA for the receptor do not block by more than 10% the uptake of the radioactive steroid ([^{3}H]TA) into the cell, when present in the medium at a 100-fold higher concentration.

TABLE 2 compares the thymolytic activity of cortisol with several progesterone analogs in immature adrenalectomized male rats injected with a single dose of the test compound and killed 48 hr later. It can be seen that while none of these progestins is as active as cortisol, those that contain the 6α-methyl group, in agreement with their greater affinity for the glucocorticoid receptor, are active. The higher activity shown by medroxyprogesterone in contrast to the two other 6α-methyl derivatives that competed more effectively for the glucocorticoid receptor (TABLE 1) might be attributed to the fact that medroxyprogesterone is more polar than are the latter compounds and thus might be released faster from the corn oil diluent that was injected subcutaneously.

Our initial efforts to demonstrate that progesterone and a few of its derivatives that are active in competing with [^{3}H]TA for the thymus receptor are also active in a high-speed liver supernatant fraction were unsuccessful (FIGURE 2). Progesterone showed a minimal inhibitory effect, whereas 17α-hydroxyprogesterone, 16α-methylprogesterone, and 16β-methylprogesterone were inactive. While the results obtained with progesterone in the liver were markedly different from those obtained in the thymus, they agreed with earlier observations by others in the liver.[14] The differences noted between liver and thymus suggested the possibility that progesterone might be metabolized or bound nonspecifically in the liver supernatant fractions. Both the previous work by Beato *et al.*[14] in the liver and our study were performed in supernatant preparations that contained high concentrations of protein and that were hypotonic with respect to their salt concentration. The influence of these factors on competition between progesterone and [^{3}H]TA for the liver and thymus receptors are shown in FIGURE 3.

It is evident that both the buffer salt concentration and the protein concentration in the supernatant fraction determine the competition of progesterone for TA-binding sites. Comparison of homogenates (cytosols) that differed in protein concentration and that were isotonic with regard to salt concentration indicated that progesterone competed much more effectively with TA when the protein concentration was 5.3 mg/ml or lower. Higher concentrations of protein or the use of a hypotonic buffer to prepare the homogenate led to a marked decrease in the affinity of progesterone for the receptor. In contrast to results obtained in the liver, neither the concentration of protein nor the isotonicity of the homogenate altered the ability of progesterone, at a 100-fold higher concentration, to effectively compete for the specific binding of [^{3}H]TA in the thymus supernatant.

FIGURE 4 illustrates the comparative affinity of progesterone and several of its analogs at different concentrations for the liver receptor, as measured by their competition with [^{3}H]TA for a specific binding site. The 27,000*g* isotonic supernatant fraction used in this experiment contained 5.1 mg/ml of protein. Under these conditions, the binding of these compounds in the liver is appreciable but still less than that seen in the thymus (FIGURE 1).

Because various analogs of progesterone bind to the liver receptor with different degrees of affinity, it was of interest to compare their activity with respect to the induction of tyrosine aminotransferase. These data are shown in TABLE 3. It is evident that each of the compounds that contains the 6α-methyl substituent in-

TABLE 3

COMPARISON OF VARIOUS PROGESTINS AS INDUCERS OF LIVER TYROSINE AMINOTRANSFERASE

Compound*	Dose (mg/kg)	Tyrosine Aminotransferase (μmol/mg of protein/hr) Treated/Control†
Vehicle	—	1.0
Cortisol	5	4.5
6α-Methylprogesterone	5	1.7
6α,16α-Dimethylprogesterone	5	4.6
6α-Methyl-17α-hydroxyprogesterone	5	4.5
11β-Hydroxyprogesterone	10	1.7
Progesterone	100	1.0
16α-Methylprogesterone	50	0.5
17α-Hydroxyprogesterone	100	0.7
16α-Methyl-17α-hydroxyprogesterone	25	1.1

*Male adrenalectomized rats were given a single intraperitoneal injection of the test steroid and sacrificed 4 hr later.

†The ratio was calculated from the mean value of five rats in each group.

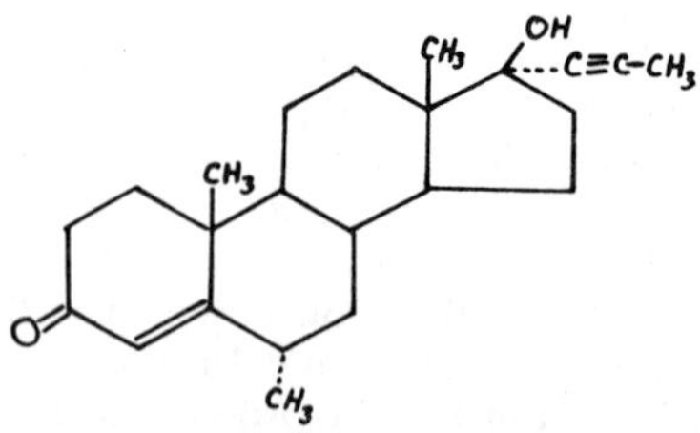

DIMETHYL ETHYNYL TESTOSTERONE

(89%)

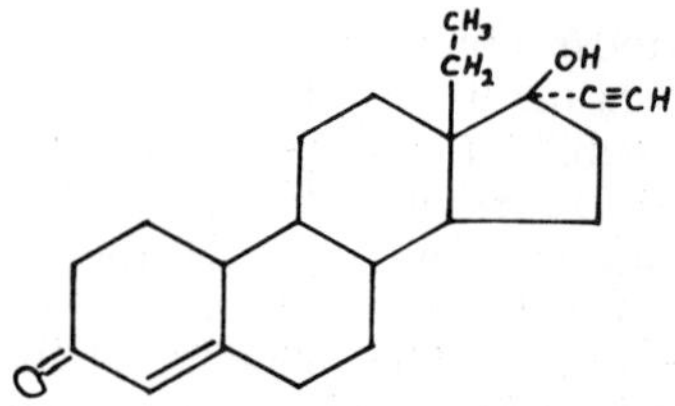

17α-ETHYNYL-18-ETHYL-19 NOR TESTOSTERONE

(70%)

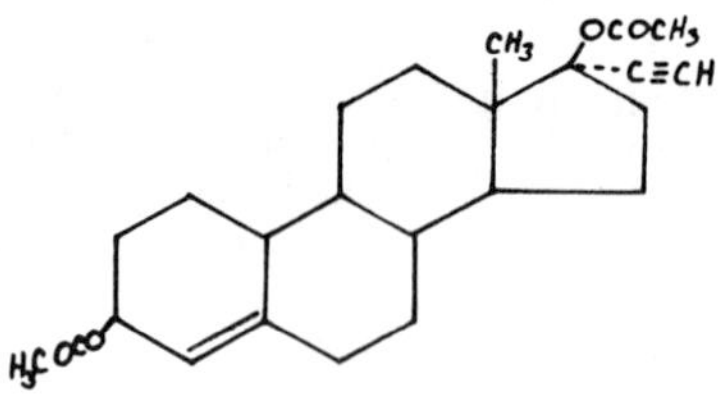

17α-ETHYNYL-19 NOR TESTOSTERONE DIACETATE

(25%)

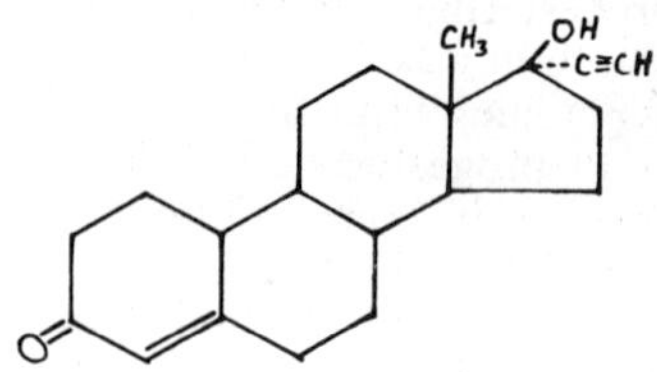

17α-ETHYNYL-19 NOR TESTOSTERONE

(54%)

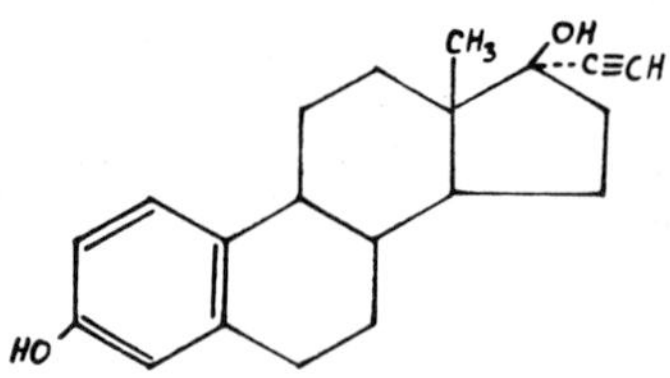

17α-ETHYNYL ESTRADIOL

(22%)

FIGURE 5. Competition among five progestins and [^{3}H]TA for binding to the liver receptor. A 27,000*g* supernatant fraction was incubated with [^{3}H]TA (2×10^{-8} M) and a 100-fold higher concentration of the progestins for 4 hr at 4°C. The values in parentheses are the percentage of inhibition of [^{3}H]TA binding.

duced the enzyme, and some of these analogs were equal in activity to cortisol. 11β-Hydroxyprogesterone also stimulated an increase in tyrosine aminotransferase activity. Progesterone and the other analogs, each of which also binds to the receptor, were inactive, even when tested at relatively high doses. These latter compounds were also inactive in blocking the induction of the enzyme by cortisol (5 mg/kg) when they were injected intraperitoneally into adrenalectomized rats, in amounts 10 times greater than cortisol at −20 min and together with the glucocorticoid at 0 time, and the animals killed 4 hr later.[22]

To further investigate the structural requirements for binding to the glucocorticoid receptor, we evaluated five progestins currently in use as oral

TABLE 4

EFFECT OF SEVERAL SEX STEROIDS ON SPECIFIC BINDING OF [³H]TA IN RAT LIVER

Compound*	Binding† (pmol/mg of protein)	Inhibition (%)
Control	0.324	—
Testosterone	0.244	25
Dimethisterone	0.056	83
5α-Dihydrotestosterone	0.327	0
17β-Estradiol	0.272	16

*A 27,000*g* supernatant was incubated with [³H]TA (2×10^{-8} M) alone or in combination with the test compound (2×10^{-6} M) for 4 hr at 4°C.

†Binding was measured by the charcoal adsorption method.

contraceptive agents. The structures and percentage of competition by these agents for the binding of [³H]TA to the receptor in a 27,000*g* liver supernatant are shown in FIGURE 5. Dimethylethynyltestosterone appears to be as effective as other 6α-methylsubstituted progesterones as a competitor for TA binding. The marked activity of this testosterone analog implicates the 6α-methyl group as an important determinant in the binding of a steroid to the glucocorticoid receptor and for enzymatic induction. The results obtained with this steroid also indicate that neither the 20-ketone nor the 21-methyl or -hydroxymethyl group is essential for binding to the glucocorticoid receptor in the liver. The relatively high binding of the two 19-nortestosterone analogs to the receptor indicates that the 19β-methyl group is not essential for interaction with the receptor, although this substituent has been reported to be required for glucocorticoid activity.[15,16] By analogy with progesterone, these testosterone derivatives might possess antiglucocorticoid activity; to date, we have not tested these compounds for this activity.

The degree of specificity shown by dimethylethynyltestosterone in comparison to other androgens and 17β-hydroxyestradiol for competitive binding with [³H]TA for the rat liver receptor is indicated in TABLE 4. At 100-fold higher concentrations than that of [³H]TA, both testosterone and estradiol competed with TA to a slight extent, whereas 5α-dihydrotestosterone did not compete. Consistent with its high affinity for the glucocorticoid receptor and the presence of the 6α-methyl group in its structure, dimethylethynyltestosterone induced a threefold increase in hepatic tyrosine aminotransferase activity when injected into adrenalectomized rats (TABLE 5).

TABLE 5

INDUCTION OF TYROSINE AMINOTRANSFERASE BY DIMETHYLETHYNYLTESTOSTERONE

Compound*	Tyrosine Aminotransferase† (μmol/mg of protein/hr)
Vehicle	0.488 ± 0.21
Dimethylethynyltestosterone (25 mg/kg)	1.75 ± 0.11

*Adrenalectomized male rats were given a single intraperitoneal injection of the steroid and sacrificed 4 hr later.

†Values are the mean ± SE for four rats in each group.

Discussion

Considerable effort has been devoted in our laboratory to the study of correlations between the molecular structure and biologic activity of steroid analogs to obtain information that may be relevant to the proper design of therapeutically more effective hormones. The present study has focused attention on modifications of the progesterone molecule. Earlier studies had indicated that progesterone exerts antiglucocorticoid activity in a freshly prepared suspension of rat thymocytes[2] but that *in vivo* this steroid was unable to suppress the action of an administered glucocorticoid. In view of these results, and because cortexolone also showed antiglucocorticoid activity *in vitro* but not *in vivo,* we decided to examine various progesterone analogs with the hope of detecting compounds with antiglucocorticoid activity in the whole animal. This goal has not yet been achieved, and the most important conclusion to be drawn from the present work is that progesterone and testosterone modified by a 6α-methyl substituent yield analogs that exhibit high affinity for glucocorticoid receptors in the liver and thymus and, in accordance with their interaction with the receptor, also possess glucocorticoid activity. Thus, the 6α-methyl group appears to fulfill a role similar to that of the 11β-hydroxyl group in the corticosteroid molecule with regard to its essentiality for glucocorticoid activity. The presence of both substituents in a single molecule should lead to a steroid with enhanced activity; several glucocorticoids with this basic structure are known to be potent glucocorticoids.[17] Steroid analogs that lack both the 11β-hydroxyl and 6α-methyl groups can bind to glucocorticoid receptors, and such compounds should act as antiglucocorticoids. However, such compounds as cortexolone and progesterone, which fulfill the above criteria, are active only *in vitro,* presumably because of rapid metabolism[18] or, for cortexolone, possibly because it cannot be concentrated in sufficient amounts in target tissues.[23]

The failure of 6α- or 6β-hydroxyprogesterone to bind to the glucocorticoid receptor, in contrast to the 6α-methyl-substituted derivative, suggests that the nonpolar nature of the methyl group may be an important factor and that hydrophobic interactions occur between the 6α-methyl group and a specific region of the receptor. Whether the sterospecificity or polarity of the substituent in the 6 position is of importance in a steroid that already contains an 11β-hydroxyl group is not entirely clear. For example, fluocinolone acetonide, which contains 6α- and 9α-fluoro substitutents, is one of the most active steroids.[17]

It has been previously reported that progesterone binds weakly to the glucocorticoid receptor in rat liver[14] but that it competes favorably for the receptor in hepatoma cells.[13] Initially, the results we obtained with progesterone in a supernatant prepared from liver were in agreement with these observations. Hepatoma cells in culture appear to contain only one receptor for glucocorticoids,[19] whereas rat liver contains at least five proteins that bind cortisol, only one of which appears to be the receptor that mediates glucocorticoid activity in this tissue.[20] These observations suggested that progesterone might be interacting with one or more of the proteins that bind cortisol nonspecifically. Such a protein might be characterized by low affinity and lack of specificity for progesterone and yet show high capacity for this steroid. Evidence that such a protein(s) may interact with progesterone was found in the present study. Thus, when a 27,000*g* supernatant of a 10:1 liver homogenate was further diluted to contain about 5 mg of protein per milliliter or less, progesterone was found to compete more effectively with [^{3}H]TA for the receptor site. The effect of salt concentration on the binding of dexamethasone to receptors in the liver was first described by

Koblinsky *et al.*[21] In the present work, we were able to confirm the fact that progesterone competes much more favorably with [^{3}H]TA for the liver receptor when the incubation medium is isotonic, rather than of low salt concentration. Thus, aggregation of the monomeric forms of the receptor protein or conformational changes in this macromolecule induced by alterations in the salt content of the medium appear to be involved in the binding of progesterone to the receptor.

Three areas of investigation require further study to better elucidate the relationship between the binding of a steroid to a receptor molecule and biologic activity. These areas include testing additional compounds to determine the effects of diverse modifications of the steroid molecule on its interaction with the receptor, the basis for agonist or antagonist activity after binding of the steroid to the receptor, and more precise information to explain the lack of antisteroid activity *in vivo* for certain compounds with good *in vitro* activity.

Summary

When tested in an *in vitro* assay system, progesterone and various analogs of this steroid were shown to compete with [^{3}H]triamcinolone acetonide (TA) for specific glucocorticoid receptors in both rat liver and thymus. Of these analogs, the following derivatives of progesterone were potent competitors of TA binding and, when injected into adrenalectomized rats, induced regression of the thymus and marked increases in hepatic tyrosine aminotransferase activity: 11β-hydroxyl, 6α-methyl, 6α, 16α-dimethyl, and 6α-methyl-17α-hydroxyl. In contrast, progesterone, 16α-methyl, and 17α-hydroxy progesterone competed with TA *in vitro* but failed to elicit either gluco- or antiglucocorticoid activity *in vivo*. Also, we observed that the oral contraceptive 6α-methyl-17-(1-propynyl)testosterone competes very effectively with TA in a cell-free preparation of rat liver and induces an increase in hepatic tyrosine aminotransferase activity. The 11β-hydroxyl group has previously been thought to be essential for glucocorticoid activity. Our studies indicate that substitution of progesterone or testosterone with a 6α-methyl group negates the need for an 11β-hydroxyl substitutuent as a prerequisite for glucocorticoid activity.

References

1. Kaiser, N., R. J. Milholland, R. W. Turnell & F. Rosen. 1972. Biochem. Biophys. Res. Commun. **49:** 516.
2. Kaiser, N., A. J. Solo, R. J. Milholland & F. Rosen. 1974. J. Steroid Biochem. **5:** 348.
3. Lipsett, M. B., G. A. Sarfaty, H. Wilson, C. W. Bardin & L. M. Fishman. 1966. J. Clin. Invest. **45:** 1700.
4. Finkelstein, M. 1973. Excerpta Med. Int. Congr. Ser. **273:** 845.
5. Heftmann, E. 1970. Steroid Biochemistry. Academic Press, Inc. New York, N.Y.
6. Rosen, J. M., J. J. Fina, R. J. Milholland & F. Rosen. 1970. J. Biol. Chem. **245:** 2074.
7. Baxter, J. D. & G. M. Tomkins. 1971. Proc. Nat. Acad. Sci. USA **68:** 932.
8. Bray, G. A. 1960. Anal. Biochem. **1:** 279.
9. Dorfman, R. I. (Ed.) 1962. Methods in Hormone Research. Vol. 2. Academic Press, Inc. New York, N.Y.
10. Rosen, F., H. R. Harding, R. J. Milholland & C. A. Nichol. 1963. J. Biol. Chem. **238:** 3725.

11. Lowry, O. H., N. J. Rosebrough, A. L. Farr & R. J. Randall. 1951. J. Biol. Chem. **193:** 265.
12. Makman, M. H., B. Dvorkin & A. White. 1966. Fed. Proc. **25:** 768 (Abs.).
13. Rousseau, G. G., J. D. Baxter & G. M. Tomkins. 1972. J. Mol. Biol. **67:** 99.
14. Beato, M., M. Kalimi, W. Beato & P. Feigelson. 1974. Endocrinology **94:** 377.
15. Glenn, E. M., R. O. Stafford, S. C. Lyster & B. J. Bowman. 1957. Endocrinology **61:** 128.
16. Dougherty, T. F. & G. L. Schneebeli. 1955. Ann. N.Y. Acad. Sci. **61:** 328.
17. Sarett, L. H., A. A. Patchett & S. Steelman. 1963. *In* Progress in Drug Research. E. Jucker, Ed. Vol. 5: 13–153. Birkhauser Verlag. Basel and Stuttgart.
18. Fotherby, K. & F. James. 1972. Advan. Steroid Biochem. Pharmacol. **3:** 67.
19. Singer, S., J. E. Becker & G. Litwack. 1973. Biochem. Biophys. Res. Commun. **52:** 943.
20. Litwack, G., R. Filler, S. A. Rosenfield, N. Lichtash, C. Wishman & S. Singer. 1973. J. Biol. Chem. **248:** 7481.
21. Koblinsky, M., M. Beato, M. Kalimi & P. Feigelson. 1972. J. Biol. Chem. **247:** 7897.
22. DiSorbo, D., F. Rosen, R. J. Milholland & R. P. McPartland. 1976. Unpublished observations.
23. Young, D. 1976. Personal communication.

Discussion

Dr. W. L. McGuire: Dr. Rosen, in your summary slide you referred to the receptor. What evidence do you have in the thymus that TA is binding to only one receptor?

Dr. Rosen: Our results provide the usual evidence for the binding of TA (triamcinolone acetonide) to a glucocorticoid receptor in thymus and liver and in mouse lymphosarcoma P1798. In each of these tissues, we have obtained sucrose density profiles for the TA receptor complex in both low- and high-salt buffers, evidence for a temperature-dependent translocation of the steroid-receptor complex and its binding in the nucleus, and data from competition studies with a wide spectrum of steroids that indicate considerable specificity of TA for binding to a glucocorticoid receptor. These results and the fact that each of the above tissues is markedly responsive to glucocorticoid administration strongly implicate a specific glucocorticoid receptor. On the basis of these data, however, we cannot exclude the possibility that TA is binding to more than one receptor in the thymus or other glucocorticoid-responsive tissues.

Dr. McGuire: Let me ask the question in another way. There are data in the literature that would suggest that TA has progestational activity. Have you looked specifically for a progesterone receptor in your tissues that could account for some of the TA binding?

Dr. Rosen: In previous studies by Dr. Nurit Kaiser in our laboratory, the [^{3}H]progesterone-receptor complex in thymus cytosol was found to be relatively unstable; however, it should be noted that its stability was of the same order as that of the [^{3}H]cortisol-receptor complex. Both of these steroids were maximally bound at 4°C in 1 hr, and thereafter there was a gradual decline in binding. Under a variety of conditions used to stabilize the receptor complex. Dr. Kaiser was unable to obtain sucrose gradient profiles with either progesterone or cortisol. When unlabeled cortisol and triamcinolone acetonide (TA) were tested (at 100-fold higher concentrations) as competitors of [^{3}H]progesterone binding in thymus cytosol, cortisol competed for 83% of specific [^{3}H]progesterone binding and TA for 61%. TA did not compete for [^{3}H]progesterone binding in plasma, whereas cortisol competed for 100% of the binding, suggesting that the presence of cortisol-binding globulin could not account for these results. On the basis of our work to date, we cannot exclude the possibility of a progesterone receptor in rat thymus. Tentatively, we have concluded that in addition to binding to a glucocorticoid receptor, progesterone also binds to another site in thymus cytosol. It appears that in the thymus, there are receptors for both glucocorticoids and progesterone and that these steroids show cross-reactivity for these two different binding sites.

Our work in the liver on the specificity of glucocorticoid and progesterone binding is not as comprehensive as that done in the thymus. However, it is not unlikely that there is a progesterone-specific binding site in this tissue and that TA can bind to this site.

Dr. M. R. Sherman: Were the livers perfused *in situ* to minimize the concentration of cortisol-binding globulin (CBG)?

Dr. Rosen: Yes, that was done in all cases.

Dr. Sherman: Can you estimate the relative binding capacities of CBG and the intracellular receptor in the cytosol, and do you have estimates of the relative affinities of the 6α-methyl compounds for CBG and the receptor?

Dr. Rosen: CBG is known to be present in rat liver, so this is an important question. However, we have not compared the relative affinities of any of these 6α-methylprogesterone analogs for CBG and the specific, physiologically important glucocorticoid receptor in the liver.

Dr. Sherman: Was there evidence in the density gradients of a 3S to 4S complex?

Dr. Rosen: Radioactive progesterone analogs would be required to answer this question, and so far we have not attempted to obtain any of these compounds labeled with ^{3}H.

Dr. E. Milgrom: Cortexolone and progesterone are inhibitors of glucocorticoid action in isolated thymus cells. Do these compounds show antiglucocorticoid activity *in vivo*?

Dr. Rosen: Both of these compounds have been extensively tested *in vivo* in the rat as an antiglucocorticoid, but so far such activity has not been demonstrated. In a personal communication, Drs. Munck and Young have told me that when cortexolone is given to the rat, its uptake in the thymus is minimal. Conceivably, this phenomenon may be due to the rapid metabolism and/or excretion of the compound.

Dr. Milgrom: Do any of these progesterone analogs show an antiglucocorticoid effect *in vivo*?

Dr. Rosen: With the assay conditions we have used, none of these compounds has been found to impair cortisol-mediated tyrosine aminotransferase induction in the liver or the thymolytic action of cortisol. In our system, progesterone or its analogs, dissolved in corn oil, are injected in amounts 10–50 times greater than that of cortisol. Both steroids are given intraperitoneally, and the progestins are usually given alone 20 min prior to and simultaneously with cortisol. The induction of the enzyme occurs over a period of 4 hr, whereas a 24-hr test has been used for studying inhibition of thymus involution. It should be noted, however, that many modifications in the test procedure for evaluating these compounds should be tried before we can conclude with certainty that these compounds are without antiglucocorticoid activity *in vivo*.

Dr. N. Orentreich (*Orentreich Medical Group, New York, N.Y.*): There is no question clinically that triamcinolone acetonide has progestational action. Menstrual irregularities are frequently seen when female patients are treated intralesionally with higher doses of this steroid. Conversely, 16,17-dihydroxyprogesterone acetonide (a weak progestin) has antiinflammatory activity. When injected into the wall of a rat granuloma pouch, it is more than two times as potent as hydrocortisone, 13 times as active as cortisone acetate, and 0.3 times as potent as dexamethasone. However, in humans, by topical vasoconstriction assay, it is only 0.5 times as effective as 0.1% triamcinolone acetonide (Bronstein, S., F. Grater, D. Jacobson, N. Orentreich & N. Applezweig. 1966. Arch. Dermatol. **93:** 411–418).

SIGNIFICANCE OF THE PROGESTERONE RECEPTOR IN THE ESTROGEN-INDUCED AND -DEPENDENT RENAL TUMOR OF THE SYRIAN GOLDEN HAMSTER*

Sara Antonia Li, Jonathan J. Li, and Claude A. Villee†

Department of Medicine and Research Service
Veterans Administration Hospital
Minneapolis, Minnesota 55417
Department of Pharmacology
University of Minnesota Medical School
Minneapolis, Minnesota 55455
and† Department of Biological Chemistry
Harvard Medical School
Boston, Massachusetts 02115

INTRODUCTION

The estrogen-induced and -dependent renal adenocarcinoma of the Syrian golden hamster is a rather unique steroid-responsive tissue, in that specific estrogen (8S, 8S + 4S), androgen (8S), and progesterone (7S to 8S) receptors have been identified in our laboratory in the cytosol of this tumor.[1,2] On this basis, the renal tumor provides an excellent model system to investigate the interrelationships among these steroid hormones as they affect tumor growth or regression. Although there is evidence that androgens, like estrogens, play a growth-promoting role in this neoplasm, progesterone is of particular interest, in that this hormone is capable of retarding the growth rate of estrogen-dependent renal tumors.[3,4] Moreover, it has been shown that progesterone is able to prevent estrogen-induced carcinogenesis in the hamster kidney when administered simultaneously with diethylstilbestrol.[3]

Progesterone-binding components have been characterized in the uterine cytosols of a wide variety of mammalian species,[5-10] the chick oviduct,[11] and in human and rat mammary carcinomas.[12,13] An interesting relationship between estrogen and progesterone has emerged from these studies. Estrogen priming has been shown to increase the concentration of progesterone receptor, whereas progesterone treatment can effect the reduction of estrogen receptor levels.[14-18]

The present study was undertaken to more fully describe the progesterone receptor in the renal tumor cytoplasm and to compare this receptor to its counterpart in the hamster uterus. In addition, we have investigated the role of progesterone in tumor induction and regression in the hamster kidney in light of recent studies of more conventional estrogen-sensitive tissues.

*Supported by the Research Service, Veterans Administration Hospital and by Grant CA 16854 from the National Cancer Institute.

Materials and Methods

Chemicals and Reagents

[1,2,6,7-^{3}H]Progesterone (103 Ci/mmol) and 17β-[2,4,6,7-^{3}H]estradiol (105 Ci/mmol) were purchased from New England Nuclear. The purity of the radioactive hormones was determined by thin-layer chromatography in a solvent system described previously.[19] Nonradioactive 17β-estradiol was obtained from Calbiochem, and all other unlabeled steroids were provided by Sigma Chemical Co. All chemicals used in these studies were reagent grade, and buffers were prepared in double-distilled water.

Animals and Treatment

Adult castrated male and ovariectomized female Syrian golden hamsters (LVG:LAK, outbred strain, Charles River Lakeview Hamster Colony, Newfield, N. J.) that weighed 80–100 and 100–110 g, respectively, were used. All male animals were acclimated at least 1 week prior to treatment. Diethylstilbestrol (DES) pellets (20 mg) were prepared by Dr. George M. Krause, Copley Pharmaceutical, Inc., Boston, Mass., and implanted subpannicularly, as reported elsewhere.[20] Additional hormone pellets were implanted every 3 months in each animal to maintain estrogen levels. Although small tumor nodules were occasionally observed after 5 months of treatment, the tumor samples used in these studies were generally taken from animals that had been treated with DES for 8–11 months. All estrogen pellets were removed 48–68 hr prior to sacrifice to clear endogenous hormone. Groups of tumor-bearing male hamsters were subjected to the following regimens prior to study: group A, 8 μg of 17β-estradiol in ethanol-sesame oil (1:10, v/v); group B, 8 μg of 17β-estradiol plus 8 mg of progesterone in aqueous microsuspension (Tilden-Yates Laboratories, Inc.). The hormones were injected subcutaneously in separate sites. All animals were treated for 3–4 days and killed 48 hr after the last injection. Ovariectomized females (48–72 hr) were each treated with 20 μg of DES in sesame oil for 4 days and used 24 hr after the last injection. All animals were decapitated, and the tissues were immediately excised and rinsed twice in cold 0.15 M NaCl in 10 mM Tris hydrochloride, 1.5 mM EDTA, 1 mM dithiothreitol (TED) buffer (pH 7.4). When the tissues were prepared for progesterone receptor studies, the rinse buffer contained 10% glycerol. All subsequent steps were performed at 0–3°C, except as noted.

Cytosol Receptor Preparation

The kidneys and livers obtained from untreated and DES-treated male hamsters and uteri from ovariectomized DES-primed females were weighed, minced, and homogenized in 2.0 or 3.0 vol, respectively, of TED buffer that contained 10% glycerol. Renal tumor tissue was freed of necrotic or hemorrhagic areas, and the tumor fragments were treated similarly. Homogenization was performed in a conical ground-glass apparatus maintained at 0–2°C. Tissue homogenates were then centrifuged in a Spinco L2-65 B ultracentrifuge for 60 min at 3°C and 100,000*g*. After centrifugation, the supernatant fluids (cytosols) were filtered through a Millex® filter (0.45 μm), Millipore Corporation, to remove resi-

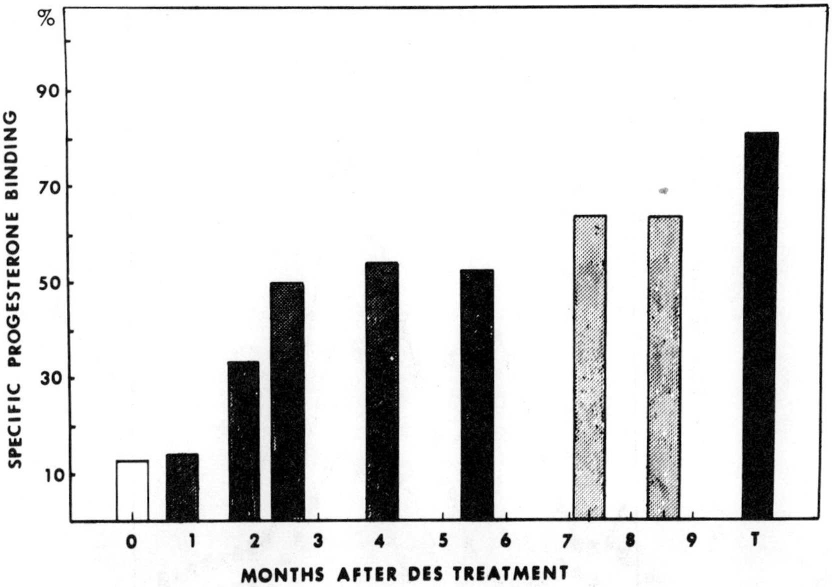

FIGURE 1. Effect of DES treatment on specific progesterone binding activity in the renal cytosols of untreated control (open bar); 0.8-, 1.8-, 2.5-, 4.0-, and 5.7-month DES-treated (dark shaded bars); 7.3- and 8.5-month DES-treated tumor-bearing (light shaded bars) castrate male hamsters; and primary renal tumor (solid bar). Cytosols were incubated *in vitro* with 5 nM tritrated progesterone alone or in combination with nonradioactive progesterone at 5×10^{-7} M at 0–3°C and subsequent dextran-charcoal treatment (15 min). Competition at a 100-fold excess of unlabeled progesterone was taken as specific binding, and the data are expressed as percentage of specific binding relative to the amount bound without added unlabeled hormone for each group. Values are based on the means of two or more determinations with each group containing three animals. The protein concentrations among the various groups were 18–20 mg/ml for control and DES-treated kidneys and 12 mg/ml for pure renal tumor.

dual lipid and particulate matter. Cytosols used in estrogen-binding studies were prepared similarly, except that glycerol was omitted from the buffer medium. The preparation of serum samples has been described elsewhere.[19]

Protein concentration of the cytosols was determined by the method of Lowry *et al.*[21] with bovine serum albumin used as a standard.

Cytosol Treatments

Tumor and uterine cytosols were diluted 1:1 (v/v) in TED buffer that contained 10% glycerol for progesterone receptor studies. Aliquots (0.5 or 1.0 ml) of the cytosol fraction were incubated *in vitro* with 5×10^{-9} M [^{3}H]progesterone or 17β-[^{3}H]estradiol prepared in ethanol-0.15 M NaCl (3:2, v/v). Competition studies were performed with similarly dissolved unlabeled steroids (5×10^{-7} or 2.5×10^{-6} M), which were added immediately prior to the addition of radioactive hor-

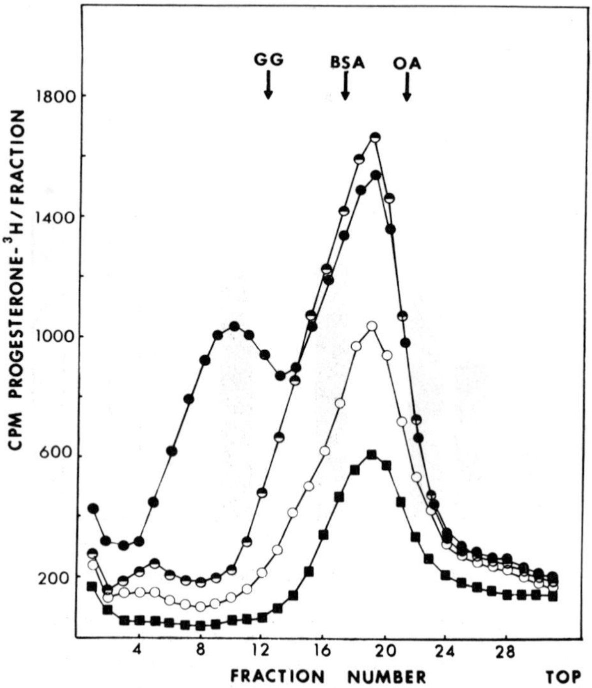

FIGURE 2. Sucrose density gradient centrifugation of renal cytosols from untreated castrate, DES-treated, and renal tumor-bearing male hamsters after *in vitro* incubation with 5 nM [^{3}H]progesterone at 0–3°C. Dextran-charcoal was used to remove free steroid. Aliquots of 0.25 ml were layered on 5–20% sucrose gradients from cytosols of untreated control (■), 2.3-month DES-treated (○), 5.7-month DES-treated (◒), and 8.5-month DES-treated (●) male hamsters. The protein concentrations were 18–20 mg/ml. The kidneys of the 8.5-month DES-treated hamsters contained small tumor nodules. Bovine γ-globulin (GG), bovine serum albumin (BSA), and ovalbumin (OA) served as sedimentation coefficient standards.

mone. The cytosols were incubated at 0–3°C for 90 min with gentle agitation, sampled for radioactivity, and treated with dextran-coated charcoal for 15 min (progesterone binding) for 3–4 hr (estrogen binding), as previously reported.[22] For Scatchard analyses, the cytosol was diluted to 0.6–1.2 mg/ml in the appropriate buffer and incubated with varying concentrations (1–10 nM) of labeled hormone for 22 hr on ice to attain equilibrium, according to Ellis and Ringold.[23]

Sucrose Density Gradient Centrifugation

Tissue extracts (0.25–0.3 ml) were layered on 4.6-ml linear 5–20% sucrose gradients prepared in TED buffer (pH 7.4). Sucrose gradients that contained 0.15 and 0.4 M KCl were prepared similarly. The samples were centrifuged for 17 hr at 39,000 rpm in a Spinco SW50.1 rotor at 4°C. Gradient tubes were pierced with a 20-gauge needle, and nine-drop fractions were collected in scintillation vials. The details of the radioactivity measurements have already been described.[1] Samples were counted at 5°C in a Packard Tri-Carb liquid scintillation spectrometer (model 3375) with a counting efficiency of approximately 38% for tritium.

Sedimentation coefficients were determined by the method of Martin and Ames,[24] with beef liver catalase (11.3S), bovine γ-globulin (7.0S), bovine serum albumin (4.6S), and ovalbumin (3.7S) used as sedimentation markers.

Results

Relative Binding of [^3H]Progesterone in the Untreated and Estrogen-Treated Kidney and Renal Tumor Cytosols

A comparison of progesterone binding activity in renal cytoplasmic fractions from untreated, DES-treated, and tumor-bearing castrate male hamsters was made. If the competition of a 100-fold excess of unlabeled progesterone is taken as

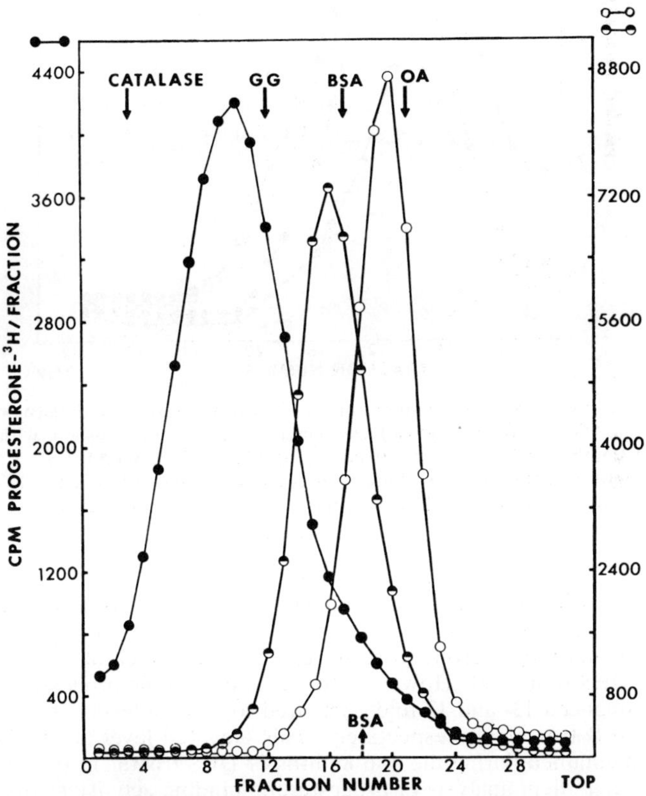

FIGURE 3. Sedimentation patterns of primary renal tumor cytosol from 10-month DES-treated castrate male hamsters incubated *in vitro* with 5 nM tritiated progesterone at 0–3°C and then treated briefly with dextran-charcoal. The protein concentration of the cytosol was 13 mg/ml. Aliquots of 0.3 ml were layered on 5–20% sucrose gradients (●), 5–20% sucrose plus 0.15 M KCl (◒) gradients, and 5–20% sucrose plus 0.4 M KCl (○) gradients. Dotted arrow represents govine serum albumin (BSA) sedimentation in sucrose plus 0.4 M KCl.

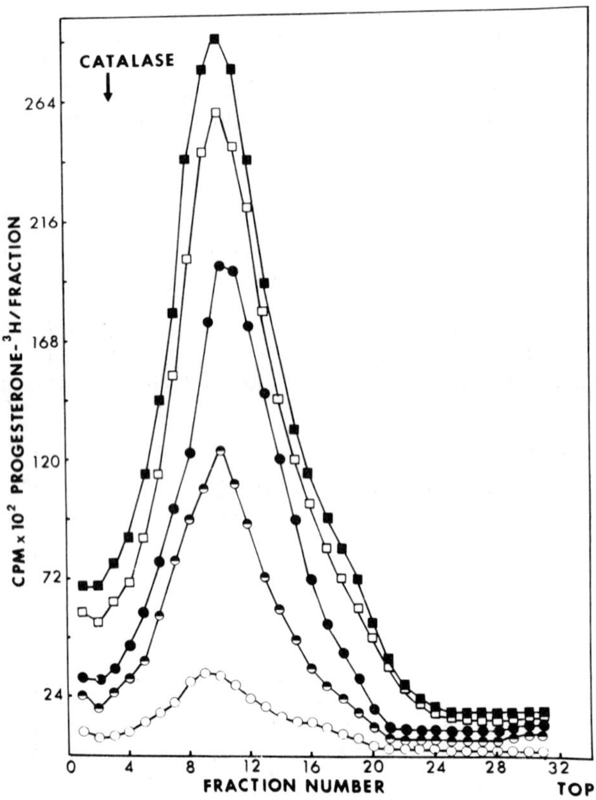

FIGURE 4. Sucrose density gradient patterns of [^{3}H]progesterone binding to primary renal tumor cytosol. Aliquots of the cytosol were incubated *in vitro* at 0–3°C with increasing concentrations of the labeled hormone, from 5×10^{-9} M (○), 10^{-8} M (◓), 5×10^{-8} M (●), 7×10^{-8} M (□), to 10^{-7} M (■). Dextran-charcoal was used to remove free steroid. The protein concentration was 8 mg/ml. Catalase was used as a standard to estimate sedimentation constants.

specific binding, the amount of such binding in the untreated renal cytosol is negligible (< 15%), as illustrated in FIGURE 1. There is only a slight increase in specifically bound progesterone from untreated control levels after approximately 1 month of DES treatment. However, the level of specific progesterone binding activity is enhanced 13- and 17-fold compared to control levels after 1.8 and 2.5 months of DES treatment, respectively. This elevated level of specific binding activity is maintained during the 4–6 months of DES treatment (two pellets) period. Sucrose gradient analysis of progesterone binding activity of the untreated and DES-treated hamster renal cytosols reveals only a 4S binding moiety (FIGURE 2). The appearance of tumor nodules at 7.3 and 8.5 months of DES treatment (three pellets) increases specific progesterone binding activity in renal cytosols 27-fold over control levels, and the presence of both 7S to 8S and 4S binding components is demonstrable in these cytosols after sucrose gradient centrifugation. The amount of specific progesterone binding activity in the pure primary renal tumor cytosol is at least 45- to 50-fold higher than that observed in renal cytosols of castrate animals, and only a single binding peak in the 7S to 8S region of the gradient was detected. Metastases from these animals contained levels of specific progesterone binding activity in their cytosols comparable to those in the primary lesion. The presence of a 500-fold excess of either unlabeled cortisol or corticosterone prior to the addition of [^{3}H]progesterone did not appreciably alter the amount of specific progesterone binding activity in any of the groups studied. The quantity of specific progesterone binding activity in the liver and plasma was comparatively low.

Sedimentation Patterns of Bound Progesterone in Hamster Renal Tumor and Uterine Cytosols

When the progesterone binding activity in the cytosols of hamster renal tumors or their metastases were examined with 5–20% linear sucrose gradients, a discrete 7S to 8S component was observed that sedimented as 6S and 4S components when 0.15 and 0.4 M KCl were present in the gradient, respectively (FIGURE 3). Sucrose density gradient centrifugation of cytosols from the uteri of DES-primed hamsters confirmed the presence of the 7S progesterone receptor in this tissue

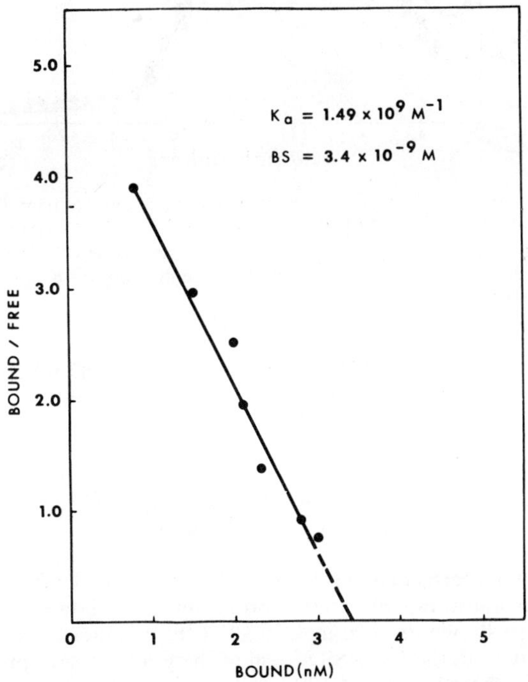

FIGURE 5. Scatchard plot analysis of cytoplasmic receptor binding of tritiated progesterone in the primary renal tumor (1.2 mg of protein/ml) incubated for 22 hr at 0–3°C to attain equilibrium and then treated briefly with dextran charcoal. Each point represents the mean of duplicate determinations.

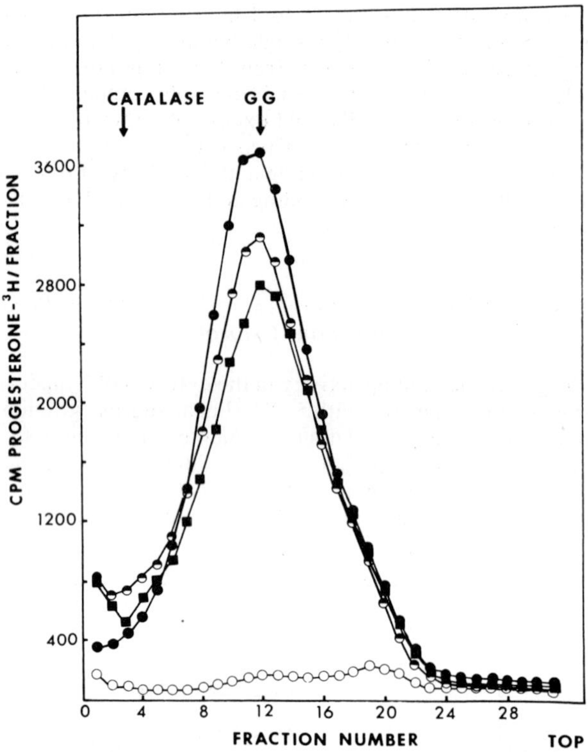

FIGURE 6. Sedimentation profiles of primary renal tumor cytosol from DES-treated male hamsters after incubation with 5 nM tritiated progesterone alone (●), or in combination with unlabeled 17β-estradiol (◓), corticosterone (■), or progesterone (○). The concentration of each competing agent was 2.5×10^{-6} M. Protein concentration was 8 mg/ml, and 0.3 ml was applied to each gradient.

previously reported by others.[9,10] The uterine progesterone receptor, like that of the renal tumor, sedimented as a 6S component in the presence of 0.15 M KCl and as a 4S component in the presence of 0.4 M KCl.

Saturability and Scatchard Analyses of Renal Tumor Progesterone Receptor

Sedimentation patterns of aliquots of renal tumor cytosol after *in vitro* addition of increasing concentrations of tritiated progesterone, followed by dextran-charcoal treatment are shown in FIGURE 4. In all of these patterns, there was a single peak of radioactivity in the 7S to 8S region of the gradient. At approximately 7×10^{-8} M [^{3}H]progesterone, the 7S to 8S binding tended to approach saturation, indicating high-affinity and low-capacity binding. A Scatchard[25] plot of the binding of progesterone (1–10 nM) to renal tumor cytosol fractions substantiates the belief that binding of progesterone to the receptor is of high affinity, with a K_a of 1.49×10^9 M^{-1} and 3.4×10^{-9} M binding sites at a protein concentration of 1.2 mg/ml

(FIGURE 5). Nonspecific binding was subtracted from these data by use of unlabeled progesterone at a 100-fold excess.

Comparison of Progesterone Binding Specificity in Renal Tumor and Uterine Cytosols

The competition by other steroids for progesterone binding in renal tumor and estrogen-primed uterine cytosols *in vitro* is similar, as ascertained by the dextran-charcoal assay and sucrose gradient profiles. The specificity of progesterone binding in these tissues was demonstrated by the inability of androgens (not shown), estrogens, and corticosteroids at 500-fold excess concentrations to compete appreciably with the tritiated progesterone for binding (FIGURE 6 & TABLE 1). In contrast, competition by a 100-fold excess of unlabled progesterone was greater than 80% in both renal tumor and uterine receptors. Although a 100-fold excess of 5α-pregnane-3,20-dione inhibited tritiated progesterone binding in both the renal tumor and uterine cytosol progesterone receptors, the competition was more

TABLE 1

EFFECT OF VARIOUS UNLABELED STEROIDS ON THE BINDING OF [^{3}H]PROGESTERONE TO RENAL TUMOR AND UTERINE CYTOSOLS*

Nonradioactive Steroid	Inhibition (%) Renal Tumor	Uterus
5×10^{-7} M		
Progesterone	83	85
5α-Pregnanedione	62	26
5β-Pregnanedione	16	3
11α-Hydroxyprogesterone	8	10
11β-Hydroxyprogesterone	41	56
17α-Hydroxyprogesterone	7	18
20α-Hydroxy-4-pregnen-3-one	13	12
20β-Hydroxy-4-pregnen-3-one	26	53
5α-Pregnan-3β,20α-diol	0	0
5α-Pregnan-3α,20β-diol	0	0
5β-Pregnan-3β,20α-diol	0	0
5α-Pregnam-3β,20β-diol	6	15
5β-Pregnan-3β-ol-20-one	4	5
5α-pregnan-3β-ol-20-one	10	17
2.5×10^{-6} M		
Cortisol	7	8
17β-Estradiol	29	25
Diethylstilbestrol	0	0
Dihydrotestosterone	26	19
Dexamethasone	0	0
Aldosterone	10	33

*Aliquots of cytosol were incubated at 0–3°C in a total volume of 0.5 ml with 5×10^{-9} M tritiated progesterone alone or in combination with competing nonradioactive steroids for 90 min. Nonlabeled steroids were added at 5×10^{-7} M (100-fold) or 2.5×10^{-6} M (500-fold). Free progesterone was removed by dextran-charcoal adsorption (15 min). [^{3}H]Progesterone concentration in these cytosols, without inhibitor, corresponded to 0% inhibition. Values are based on the means of triplicate determinations in separate experiments.

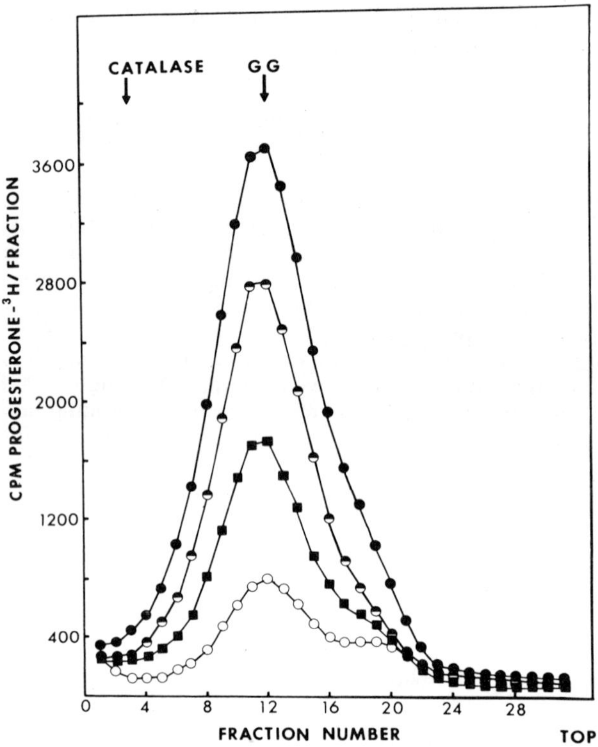

FIGURE 7. Competition by various progestins for [^{3}H]progesterone-binding sites in primary renal tumor cytosol from DES-treated castrate male hamsters. Aliquots of the cytosol were incubated with 5 nM tritiated progesterone alone (●), or in combination with nonradioactive 11β-hydroxyprogesterone (◓), 5α-pregnanedione (■), or progesterone (○). The concentration of each competing agent was 5×10^{-7} M. Protein concentration was 8 mg/ml, and 0.3 ml was applied to each gradient.

marked in the renal tumor (FIGURE 7 & TABLE 1). Both 11β-hydroxyprogesterone and 20β-hydroxy-4-pregnen-3-one had some effect in displacing the labeled hormone from the receptor in these tissues. However, there was no appreciable competition with the other progesterone metabolites tested.

Effect of Progesterone on Estrogen Receptor Levels in Renal Tumor Cytosol

After the DES pellets were removed from tumor-bearing hamsters to clear endogenous estrogen, groups of animals were injected for 4 days with either estradiol or estradiol and progesterone. A modest reduction (22%) in cytoplasmic estrogen receptor was observed in renal tumors of estrogen and progesterone-treated animals, as compared to animals treated with estrogen alone at a protein concentration of 4 mg/ml (FIGURE 8). However, this decrease in estrogen receptor levels is not readily detectable at higher concentrations of cytosol protein. Unlabeled progesterone at a 1000-fold excess did not compete for the tritiated 8S estradiol receptor in the renal tumor.

Discussion

It is now well documented that estrogen pretreatment enhances progesterone receptor concentration in the mammalian uterus and chick oviduct. It is generally conceded that this increase in progesterone binding activity occurs only in estrogen target tissues, because it has been reported that estrogen priming appears to have little effect on the amount of progesterone binding activity in the kidney or diaphragm cytoplasm of castrate rats.[26] In a previous study, we provided evidence that tritiated progesterone does not bind to a significant extent in kidney cytosols of untreated castrate male hamsters.[19] The present results confirm and extend this observation. Our findings demonstrate that estrogen clearly enhances the

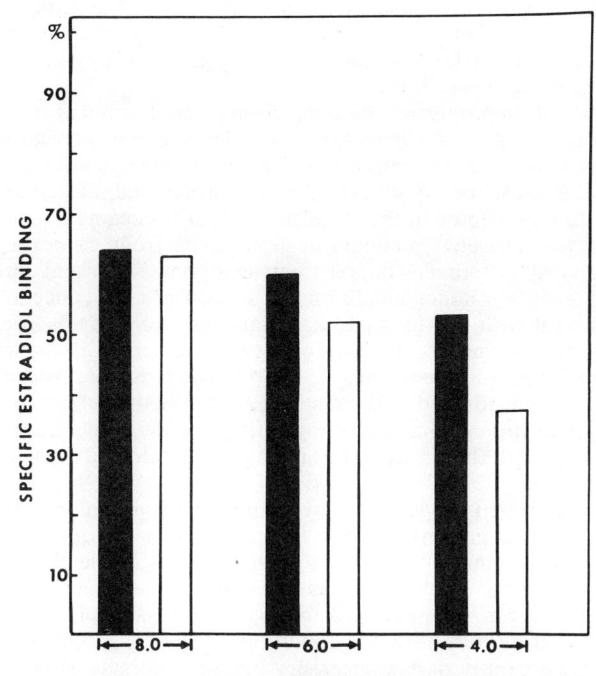

FIGURE 8. Effect of progesterone treatment on the concentration of specific estradiol binding in the renal tumor cytoplasm. Tumor-bearing animals were treated for 4 days with 8 μg of 17β-estradiol (solid bars) or 8 μg of 17β-estradiol plus 8 mg of progesterone (open bars). All animals were killed 48 hr after the last injection. Tumor cytosols were serially diluted, and each dilution was incubated *in vitro* with 5 nM tritiated estradiol alone or in combination with unlabeled estradiol at 5×10^{-7} M at 0–3°C and then treated with dextran-charcoal (3.5 hr). The data are expressed as percentage of specific estradiol binding relative to the amount bound without added unlabeled hormone for each group. Values are based on the mean of two determinations with each group containing at least three animals.

progesterone binding capacity after approximately 2 months of DES treatment. After 2.5 months of estrogen treatment, the amount of specific 4S progesterone-binding component reaches a plateau and remains at a 17-fold higher level than that of untreated controls. The increase in cellular progesterone receptor concentration in response to estrogen treatment in the hamster kidney is not as rapid as in the uterus or chick oviduct.[5–11,27] This marked increase in cytosol progesterone binding activity represents the earliest consistent change thus far reported during the induction period of the Syrian hamster renal tumor and may be related to the prevention of estrogen-induced renal tumorigenesis by progesterone in this species.

With the appearance of renal tumor nodules as a result of renal transformation, the amount of specific progesterone binding activity increases dramatically in the kidney tumor and sediments as a 7S to 8S receptor after sucrose gradient centrifugation. We suggested previously that the carcinogenic process was responsible for the dramatic increase in estrogen, androgen, and progestin receptors and that there may be a common denominator for the expression of these proteins.[2] The observation that the amount of progesterone binding plateaus during the 2.5- and 5.7-month DES treatment periods and remains as a 4S binding component tends to support this contention. In addition, the low amount of specific androgen receptor in the untreated hamster kidney appears to be unaffected by estrogen treatment prior to renal tumorigenesis.[32]

The sedimentation properties, binding affinity, and hormonal specificity of the progesterone receptor in the hamster renal tumor and in uterine cytosols are similar and are comparable to those found in the uterine cytosol fraction of other species.[5–11] The presence of glycerol in the buffer stabilized the binding of progesterone to its receptor in the renal tumor, but it became evident only after prolonged dextran-charcoal incubation. It is clear from competition studies, however, that small differences do exist between renal tumor and uterine cytosol progesterone receptors under conditions of similar protein concentrations. Our data are consistent with previous findings that nonradioactive 5α-pregnane-3,20-dione, 11β-hydroxyprogesterone, 20β-hydroxy-4-pregnen-3-one are capable of inhibiting tritiated progesterone binding.[5,7,9,11,28] Introduction of a hydroxyl group at the 17α, 11α, or 20α position and substitution of a hydroxyl group for the keto group at the 3-position drastically reduce the affinity of progesterone for the receptor. As expected, the greatest steroid hormonal specificity resided with unlabeled progesterone.

It is well known that progestins have an inhibitory action on tumor induction and growth.[3,29–31] Our preliminary data indicate that the progesterone and estradiol-treated kidney tumor cytoplasm has slightly less available 8S estradiol receptor than does that of the renal tumor treated with estradiol alone. The reduction in quantity of the estrogen receptor does not appear to be as rapid or as large as that found for the uterus under similar conditions.[16,17] It is possible that a longer progesterone treatment period is necessary before a more substantial depression of estrogen receptor concentration can be elicited. Nevertheless, this suppression may be important in contributing to progesterone-induced renal tumor regression in the hamster and in other mammalian hormone-dependent tumors.

Acknowledgment

We are grateful for the dedication and excellent technical assistance of Mr. Terry Cuthbertson, Research Service, Veterans Administration Hospital, in these studies.

REFERENCES

1. LI, J. J., D. J. TALLEY, S. A. LI & C. A. VILLEE. 1976. Receptor characteristics of specific estrogen binding in the renal adenocarcinoma of the golden hamster. Cancer Res. **36:** 1127–1132.
2. LI, J. J. & S. A. LI. 1977. Translocation of specific steroid hormone receptors into purified nuclei in Syrian hamster tissues and estrogen-dependent renal tumor. *In* Research on Steroids, 7. A. Vermeulen, P. Jungblut, A. Klopper & F. Sciarra, Eds. North-Holland Publishing Co., Amsterdam, Oxford, The Netherlands and American Elsevier Publishing Co., New York. In press.
3. KIRKMAN, H. 1959. Estrogen-induced tumors of the kidney in the Syrian hamster. Nat. Cancer Inst. Monogr. **1:** 1–59.
4. BLOOM, H. J. G., C. E. DUKES & B. C. V. MITCHLEY. 1963. Hormone-dependent tumours on the kidney: I. The estrogen-induced renal tumor of the Syrian hamster—hormone treatment and possible relationship to carcinoma of the kidney in man. Brit. J. Cancer **17:** 611–645.
5. FEIL, P. D., S. R. GLASSER, D. O. TOFT & B. W. O'MALLEY. 1972. Progesterone binding in the mouse and rat uterus. Endocrinology **91:** 738–746.
6. MILGROM, E., L. THI, M. ATGER & E.-E. BAULIEU. 1973. Mechanisms regulating the concentration and conformation of progesterone receptor (s) in the uterus. J. Biol. Chem. **18:** 6366–6374.
7. RAO, B. R., W. G. WIEST & W. M. ALLEN. 1973. Progesterone "receptor" in rabbit uterus. I. Characterization and estradiol 17β augmentation. Endocrinology **92:** 1229–1240.
8. FREIFELD, M. L., P. D. FEIL & C. W. BARDIN. 1974. The *in-vivo* regulation of the progesterone "receptor" in guinea pig uterus: dependence on estrogen and progesterone. Steroids **23:** 93–103.
9. LEAVITT, W. W., D. O. TOFT, C. A. STROTT & B. W. O'MALLEY. 1974. A specific progesterone receptor in the hamster uterus: physiologic properties and regulation during the estrous cycle. Endocrinology **94:** 1041–1053.
10. REEL, J. R. & Y. SHIH. 1975. Oestrogen-inducible uterine progesterone receptors. Characteristics in the ovariectomized immature and adult hamster. Acta Endocrinol. **80:** 344–354.
11. SHERMAN, M. R., P. L. CORVOL & B. W. O'MALLEY. 1970. Progesterone-binding components of chick oviduct. I. Preliminary characterization of cytoplasmic components. J. Biol. Chem. **245:** 6085–6095.
12. TERENIUS, L. 1973. Estrogen and progesterone binders in human and rat mammary carcinoma. Eur. J. Cancer **9:** 291–294.
13. HORWITZ, K. B. & W. L. MCGUIRE. 1975. Specific progesterone receptors in human breast cancer. Steroids. **25:** 497–505.
14. BRENNER, R. M., J. A. RESKO & N. B. WEST. 1974. Cyclic changes in oviductal morphology and residual cytoplasmic estradiol binding capacity induced by sequential estradiol-progesterone treatment of spayed rhesus monkeys. Endocrinology **95:** 1094–1104.
15. SASAKI, G. H. & B. S. LEUNG. 1975. On the mechanism of hormone action in 7, 12 dimethylbenz(a) anthracene-induced mammary tumor. I. Prolactin and progesterone effects on estrogen receptor *in-vitro*. Cancer **35:** 645–651.
16. HSUEH, A. J. W., E. J. PECK & J. H. CLARK. 1975. Progesterone antagonism of the oestrogen receptor and oestrogen-induced uterine growth. Nature (London) **254:** 337–339.
17. HSUEH, A. J. W., E. J. PECK & J. H. CLARK. 1976. Control of uterine estrogen receptor levels by progesterone. Endocrinology **98:** 438–444.
18. TSENG, L. & E. GURPIDE. 1975. Effect of progestins on estradiol receptor levels in human endometrium. J. Clin. Endocrinol. Metab. **41:** 402–404.
19. LI, J. J., D. J. TALLEY, S. A. LI & C. A. VILLEE. 1974. An estrogen binding protein in the renal cytosol of the intact, castrated, and estrogenized golden hamster. Endocrinology **96:** 1106–1113.
20. LI, J. J., H. KIRKMAN & R. L. HUNTER. 1968. Sex difference and gonadal hormone

influence on Syrian hamster kidney esterase isozymes. J. Histochem. Cytochem. **17:** 386–393.

21. LOWRY, O. H., N. J. ROSENBROUGH, A. L. FARR & R. J. RANDALL. 1951. Protein measurements with Folin phenol reagent. J. Biol. Chem. **193:** 265–275.
22. TALLEY, D. J., J. J. LI, S. A. LI & C. A. VILLEE. 1975. The biochemical comparison of estrogen receptors of the hamster hypothalamus and uterus. Endocrinology **96:** 1135–1144.
23. ELLIS, D. J. & H. J. RINGOLD. 1971. The uterine estrogen receptor: a physiochemical study. *In* The Sex Steroids. K. W. McKerns, Ed.: 73–106. Appleton-Century-Crofts. New York, N.Y.
24. MARTIN, R. G. & B. N. AMES. 1961. A method for determining the sedimentation behavior of enzymes: application to protein mixtures. J. Biol. Chem. **236:** 1372–1379.
25. SCATCHARD, G. 1949. The attraction of proteins for small molecules and ions. Ann. N.Y. Acad. Sci. **15:** 660–672.
26. MILGROM, E. & E.-E. BAULIEU. 1970. Progesterone in uterus and plasma. I. Binding in rat uterus 105,000 g supernatant. Endocrinology **87:**276–287.
27. TOFT, D. O. & B. W. O'MALLEY. 1972. Target tissue receptors for progesterone: the influence of estrogen treatment. Endocrinology **90:** 1041–1045.
28. MCGUIRE, J. L., C. D. BARISO & A. P. SHROFF. 1974. Interaction between steroids and a uterine progestogen specific binding macromolecule. Biochemistry **13:** 319–322.
29. SEGALOFF, A. 1973. Inhibition by progesterone of radiation-estrogen-induced mammary cancer in the rat. Cancer Res. **33:** 1136, 1137.
30. KLEDZIK, G. S., C. J. BRADLEY & J. MEITES. 1974. Reduction of carcinogen-induced mammary cancer incidence in rats by early treatment with hormones or drugs. Cancer Res. **34:** 2953–2956.
31. HOWARD JOHN, A., J. S. CORNES, W. D. JACKSON & P. BYE. 1974. Effect of a systemically administered progestogen on histopathology of endometrial carcinoma. J. Obstet. Gynecol. Brit. Commonwealth **81:** 786–790.
32. LI, J. J., T. L. CUTHBERTSON & S. A. LI. 1977. Specific androgen binding in the kidney and estrogen-dependent renal carcinoma of the Syrian hamster. Endocrinology. In press.

DISCUSSION

DR. W. L. MCGUIRE: Dr. Villee, some human renal tumors are responsive to either progesterone or androgen systemic therapy. Have you had the opportunity to examine human kidney tumors or are you aware of such data?

DR. VILLEE: We have examined more than a dozen specimens of human renal tumors. Dr. Li gave a paper at the Isozyme Conference at Yale about a year ago that summarized our studies with those tumors. There are some remarkable parallels between hamster and human tumors. A progesterone receptor can be demonstrated in the human tumors, and some clinical trials by Bloom have indicated that progesterone can cause some tumor regression. It is interesting that in the human, as in the hamster, the tumor is more common in the male than in the female.

DR. P. C. BEERS (*Columbia University-The Roosevelt Hospital, New York, N.Y.*): The appearance of the 8S receptor in tumor cytosols is very interesting. Dr. Stancel and coworkers (1973. Biochemistry **12:** 2130) have shown that when uterine receptor is incubated with different concentrations of uterine cytosol depleted of receptor, changes occur in sedimentation patterns. These heavier sedimentation patterns are due only to the uterine cytosol itself and do not appear in any other cytosol prepared from other nontarget organs. Have you examined this 8S peak with this point in mind? It is possible that increases in protein synthesis that would accompany tumor development might be responsible for the sedimentation characteristics of this 8S peak appearing in kidney tumor cytosols?

DR. VILLEE: No we haven't examined that kind of problem. It would be interesting.

DR. R. J. B. KING: I was interested in your induction of progesterone receptor in the normal kidney. To my knowledge, this is the first example of something physiologically relevant happening at this stage. Can you find estrogen receptor at any stage through the noninduction period?

DR. VILLEE: Yes.

DR. KING: And does it go up as well?

DR. VILLEE: Yes, it does increase in amount.

DR. G. S. RICHARDSON *(Massachusetts General Hospital, Boston, Mass.):* One always wonders whether the regression response of tumors is receptor mediated. You would think that with this very-high-affinity receptor an amount of steroid sufficient to saturate the receptor could be delivered in quite low dosage. What do you think would be the effective dosage to induce regression of the tumor, and what do you think about the relationships between effective doses and what might be considered sufficient to keep the receptor saturated?

DR. VILLEE: The doses that have been used have always been rather large. They are given *in vivo,* of course, and you have to saturate the whole hamster before you can get an effective level at the tumor receptor. I don't know of any data that would give any dose response *in vivo* for tumor regression.

PROGESTERONE AND MAINTENANCE OF PREGNANCY: IS PROGESTERONE NATURE'S IMMUNOSUPPRESSANT?*

Pentti K. Siiteri, Freddy Febres, L. E. Clemens, R. Jeffrey Chang, Bernard Gondos, and Daniel Stites

Reproductive Endocrinology Center
Departments of Obstetrics and Gynecology,
Pathology, Medicine, and Laboratory Medicine
University of California at San Francisco
San Francisco, California 94143

Introduction

Progesterone derived either from the corpus luteum or the placenta, or both, has been shown to be essential for the maintenance of pregnancy in every species examined. The essential role of the corpus luteum was discovered by Frankel in 1903, and extracts of the corpus luteum were shown to be effective in maintaining pregnancy in rabbits by Allen and Corner about 30 years later. Many more recent studies that utilized elegant immunologic and chemical techniques have further elaborated on the importance of progesterone for pregnancy maintenance. However, the functional role of progesterone remains unclear. The pioneering studies of Csapo led to the concept that progesterone dominance of the uterus suppresses uterine contractility until near the end of gestation. However, other effects of progesterone may be equally as important (for an extensive review of progesterone and pregnancy maintenance, see Reference 1).

More than 20 years ago, it was proposed[2] that a "barrier" exists between fetuses and both normal and sensitized mothers that prevents the mother from developing a state of transplantation immunity to the paternal histocompatibility antigens of the fetus. Much attention has been directed to the possibility that the trophoblast serves this function, simply because it represents the fetal cellular element that, to varying degrees in different species, has direct contact with maternal blood and tissue (decidua). The effectiveness of the placental barrier has been ascribed to nonantigenicity of trophoblastic cells,[3] secretion of fibrinoid or mucopolysaccharide by trophoblasts that masks histocompatibility antigens,[4,5] and suppression of cellular and humoral immunity by trophoblastic hormones.[6] Considering that pregnancy can be terminated by administration of heterologous antiplacental serum, on the one hand, and that interspecies matings have been successful, on the other, it seems obvious that a universal, highly efficient mechanism must prevent the immunologic destruction of the fetus.

The idea that trophoblastic hormones may be important in mediating immunologic tolerance of pregnancy has gained considerable interest recently. Depression of maternal cellular immunity, particularly during the third trimester of human pregnancy, has been observed both *in vivo*[7,8] and *in vitro*. Thymus-dependent lymphocytic proliferation measured after stimulation[9,10] with mitogens (phytohemagglutinin, PHA) or in mixed lymphocyte cultures (MLC)[11,12] is sup-

*Supported in part by a grant from the Rockefeller Foundation and National Institutes of Health Grants HD 3939 and HD 8692.

pressed in pregnancy. Because no depression of response to PHA was observed with gravida lymphocytes in the absence of serum (in fact, they were slightly stimulated),[13] it is apparent that proliferation of T lymphocytes is suppressed by a plasma factor during pregnancy. More recently, several authors have suggested that human chorionic gonadotropin (HCG) may serve this function, because inhibition by HCG of the T-lymphocyte response to PHA[14,15] and in MLC reactions[16-18] has been observed. However, the physiologic significance of these findings is unclear because of the supraphysiologic concentrations required for inhibition. More importantly, the specificity of inhibition of T-lymphocyte activity by HCG has been called into question, because highly purified preparations were found to be without effect.[19] Further doubt about the physiologic importance of HCG in immunosuppression is provided by the observation that massive doses had no demonstrable effect on survival of intrauterine skin allografts in outbred rats.[20]

Placental steriod hormones also have received consideration as possible mediators of immunosuppression during pregnancy because of the immunosuppressive properties of natural and synthetic glucocorticoids. While early studies failed to demonstrate suppressive effects of estradiol or progesterone on allograft rejection, more recently it has been shown that administration of both estradiol and progesterone greatly prolonged survival of intrauterine skin homografts in rats.[21] Indeed, it has been reported that xenogenic cells proliferate indefinitely in hamster uteri during estradiol and progesterone administration.[22] On the other hand, it has been shown that synthetic progestins significantly prolong survival of skin allografts in rabbits[23] and renal allografts in dogs.[24] However, most of these immunosuppressive effects observed in model systems were minimal when compared with those produced by glucocorticoids. For this reason, and also because presensitization of graft recipients usually reduces or obliterates the protective effects of estrogen or progesterone in allograft models, but obviously not in multigravid pregnancy, placental steroids have not been considered to be of primary importance.

However, we propose that progesterone produced by the placenta and/or ovaries may be essential for maintenance of mammalian pregnancy by virtue of its ability to inhibit T-lymphocyte cell-mediated responses involved in tissue rejection. The experiments to be reported below show that progesterone can effectively block cellular immune responses both *in vivo* and *in vitro* under conditions in which the high intrauterine concentrations of human pregnancy are mimicked.

Materials and Methods

The ability of progesterone or other steroids to inhibit cell-mediated immune reactions *in vivo* was tested in rats by use of silastic implants that contained steroid wrapped around with either surgical cotton thread or hamster skin. Host animals were mature female Sprague-Dawley rats, and hamster skin was obtained from female Syrian golden hamsters by full-thickness excision under aseptic conditions. Two-centimeter lengths of Dow Corning silastic tubing (0.078 in. ID × 0.125 in. OD) were filled with steroid, sealed at each end with a wooden plug and silicone cement, and then kept in an oven at 37°C for 24 hr. Surgical blue cotton thread (00) was then wrapped tightly around the silastic tubing, and the assembly was sterilized by dipping in 70% ethanol prior to subcutaneous implantation in one flank of each rat. Similar implants that contained no steroid were placed subcutaneously either in the opposite side of the rat or on the same side at varying

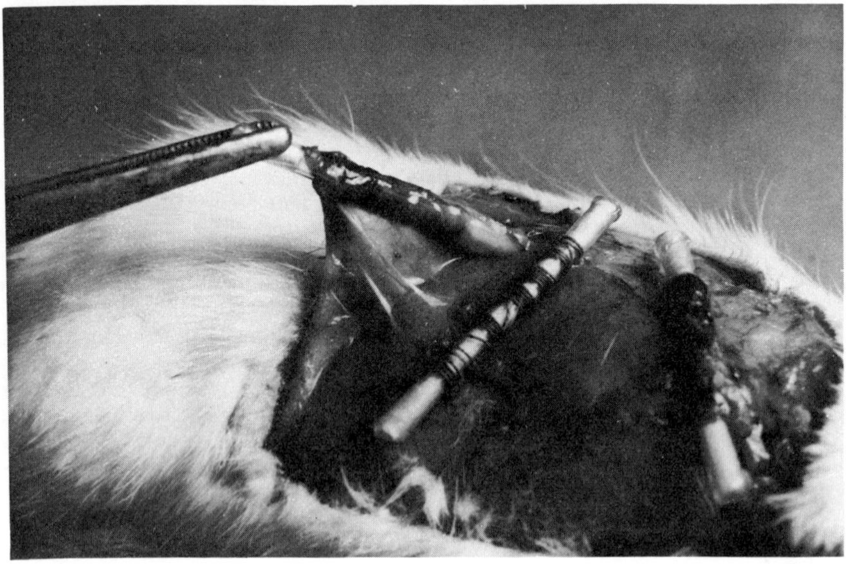

FIGURE 1. Appearance of silastic and cotton thread implants after 1 week in a rat. Only the middle implant contains progesterone.

distance from the steroid-containing implant and served as controls. The incisions were closed with wound clips, and the animals were maintained under normal housing conditions (Purina® rat chow and water ad lib.) until examined 1 week later. Rats were killed by exposure to ether, and the implanted sites were examined for granuloma formation. Animals in which obvious signs of infection were observed around either control or steroid implants were not tested further.

Hamster skin implants were similarly prepared, that is, wrapped around progesterone-containing capsules, or were placed subcutaneously beneath a raft of four to six progesterone capsules that were fastened together at their ends with silastic cement. Skin and capsules were rinsed thoroughly with a saline solution that contained 10,000 units of penicillin (Wyeth) prior to implantation. Skin implants were removed at various times up to 35 days after implantation and were examined grossly and histologically after staining with hematoxylin and eosin.

The effects of estradiol, testosterone, progesterone, and cortisol on antigenically stimulated mitosis were measured in the one-way mixed lymphocyte reaction (MLR). The MLR was performed as described previously,[19] with minor modifications. Briefly, mononuclear cells from normal male donors were purified from heparinized whole blood on a Ficoll/Hypaque density gradient. Cells were cultured in flat-bottomed microtiter plates in RPMI 1640 medium supplemented with 10% heat-inactivated pooled male human serum, antibiotics, and *l*-glutamine. Components were added to five replicate culture wells in the following order: 2×10^5 responding cells, 2×10^5 x-irradiated (2500 R) stimulating cells, and the hormone in the desired concentration. Cultures were incubated at 37°C in 5% CO_2 and air atmosphere for 120 hr. During the last 6 hr of culture, 1 μCi of [^{3}H]thymidine (sp act 6.5 Ci/mmol) was added, and cells were harvested onto glass fiber filters with a multiple automated sample harvester. [^{3}H]Thymidine incorporation into DNA was then determined in a liquid scintillation spectrometer.

The amount of [^{3}H]thymidine incorporated by unstimulated cells was subtracted from that incorporated by the stimulated cultures. The values for steroid-treated cultures were then divided by the proportion of viable cells (compared with controls) in each culture to eliminate any cytotoxic effects of steroids on the cells. These data were then expressed as a percentage of the control cultures.

Stock solutions (1 mg/ml) of each steroid were prepared in ethanol, and appropriate aliquots were evaporated to dryness in sterile test tubes. Normal male serum that had been heated at 60°C for 2 hr was then added, and the tubes were incubated for 60 min at 37°C. The samples were then diluted with RPMI 1640 medium to a 10% serum concentration. Appropriate dilutions of steroid in 10% serum were then prepared for addition to the cultures. All controls were treated in exactly the same manner, except for the addition of steroid.

Steroids were obtained from Steraloids, and purity was checked by thin-layer chromatography. All were found to be greater than 98% pure and were used without further purification. Because the release rates of steroids from silastic polymers are known to vary widely, representative steroids were tested by incubation of 5- to 10-cm lengths that contained steroid in saline at 37°C for 24–48 hr. Spectrophotometric analysis at various times was used to determine relative rates of release.

TABLE 1

LOCAL ANTIINFLAMMATORY ACTIVITY OF STEROIDS

Steroid	Number of Rats	Number of Implants	Granuloma Positive
Control	20	30	30
Control pregnant	4	6	6
Progesterone	20	30	0
Pregnenolone	6	6	6
20α-Hydroxyprogesterone	4	5	5
20β-Hydroxyprogesterone	4	6	6
5α-Dihydroprogesterone	4	6	6
5β-Dihydroprogesterone	4	4	4
17α-Hydroxyprogesterone	5	7	7
d-Norgestrel	4	6	6
Norethisterone acetate	4	6	6
19-Nortestosterone	4	4	4
Desoxycorticosterone	4	5	0
Corticosterone	4	4	0
Cortisol	7	11	11
11-Desoxycortisol	3	5	5
Dexamethasone	4	6	0
Testosterone	7	11	11
Testosterone acetate	4	6	6
Dihydrotesterone	4	6	6
Dihydrotesterone acetate	4	6	6
Androstenedione	4	6	6
5α-Androstanedione	4	6	6
Estrone	4	6	6
Estradiol	7	11	11
Estriol	5	7	7
Diethylstilbestrol	3	4	4

RESULTS

FIGURE 1 shows typical results obtained 1 week after the subcutaneous implantation of one progesterone and two control implants that contained cotton thread. The control implants are surrounded by granulomatous tissue and adhesions that firmly anchor them to the underlying fascia. In marked contrast, the progesterone-containing capsule elicited little if any inflammatory response and lies free at the site of implantation. Neither the control (granuloma) response nor the progesterone response differed if they were placed at more remote sites or in separate animals. The results obtained in this type of assay with a variety of steroids are shown in TABLE 1. Because of the variations in rate of steroid release (and therefore of local concentration), no attempt was made to quantitate activity other than assessing it as either positive or negative. Of the 25 steroids tested, only the following were active: progesterone, desoxycorticosterone, corticosterone, and the synthetic glucocorticoid, dexamethasone. Other closely related derivatives of progesterone, including 17α-hydroxyprogesterone, 11β-hydroxyprogesterone, 5α-, 5β-, 20α-, and 20β-reduced progesterone, and hydrocortisone, were inactive. The fact that hydrocortisone was inactive is probably a result of its slow release rate, because the more potent synthetic steroid dexamethasone and the less polar corticosterone are both active. The progestational steroids 19-nortestosterone, norethisterone acetate (17α-ethynyl-19-nortestosterone acetate), and *d*-norgestrel (13β-ethyl-17α-ethynyl-19-nortestosterone) were inactive. All of the other steroids tested, including androgens and estrogens, were also without effect in the granuloma assay.

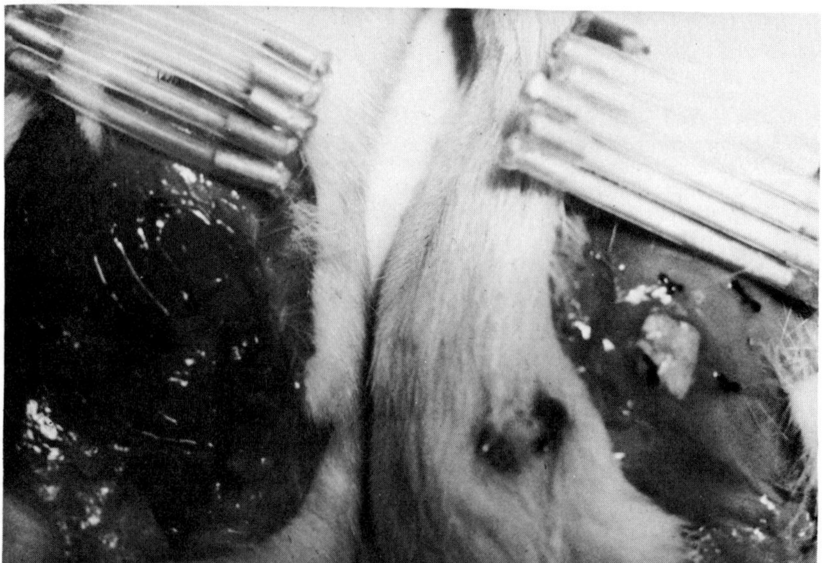

FIGURE 2. Appearance of hamster skin 21 days after implantation in a rat. *Left:* control, no steroid; *right:* progesterone treated.

TABLE 2
SURVIVAL OF SYRIAN GOLDEN HAMSTER SKIN SUBCUTANEOUS IMPLANTS IN FEMALE RATS

Days After Implantation	Number of Viable Implants	
	Control	Progesterone
2	2/2	2/2
3	2/2	2/2
6	2/3	4/4
10	0/2	—
14	0/5	5/5
21	0/5	5/7
35	—	1/1

FIGURE 2 shows hamster skin implants that were removed from subcutaneous sites of a rat 21 days after implantation. Tissue that was adjacent to progesterone-containing capsules remained in a healthy viable state, whereas the control skin was completely destroyed, as expected. FIGURES 3a and 3b show the histologic appearances of progesterone-treated and control skin implants from a similar experiment after 21 and 14 days, respectively. Although some inflammatory cells can be seen in the progesterone section, the epidermal and dermal layers are well preserved. No dermal structures are evident in the control section. TABLE 2 summarizes the results of similar experiments to date. Progesterone promoted the survival of subcutaneous hamster implants in rats up to 35 days. Of the two failures at 21 days, one was clearly associated with bacterial infection. Of 13 progesterone-treated skin implants, all survived for more than 14 days, whereas none of 12 controls survived beyond 10 days. Other steroids have not been tested in this model.

On the basis of the above observations that demonstrated that progesterone in high local concentrations exerts significant antiinflammatory and/or immunosuppressive activity, its ability to inhibit an *in vitro* response of T lymphocytes associated with cell-mediated immunity was examined. FIGURE 4 illustrates a comparison of the suppressive effects of several steroids when added to human MLC. Significant suppression by progesterone was observed in the range of 1–10 μg/ml, and virtually complete (95–98%) inhibition was found at 20 μg/ml in five experiments. On the other hand, testosterone and estradiol caused suppression of only 20–30% at the highest dose tested (10 μg/ml). Of particular interest was a comparison of the activity of progesterone and cortisol in the MLR system. On the basis of the present limited amount of data, it would appear that the two steroids do not differ widely in their immunosuppressive activity in the human MLR system. It should be noted that the data in FIGURE 4 have been corrected for differences in the cell viability at the end of the 5-day culture period and, furthermore, that all of the steroids produced little cytotoxic effects at the concentrations tested.

DISCUSSION

The results obtained with *in vivo* cotton and xenogeneic skin implants clearly demonstrate the potential importance of progesterone as an immunosuppressive

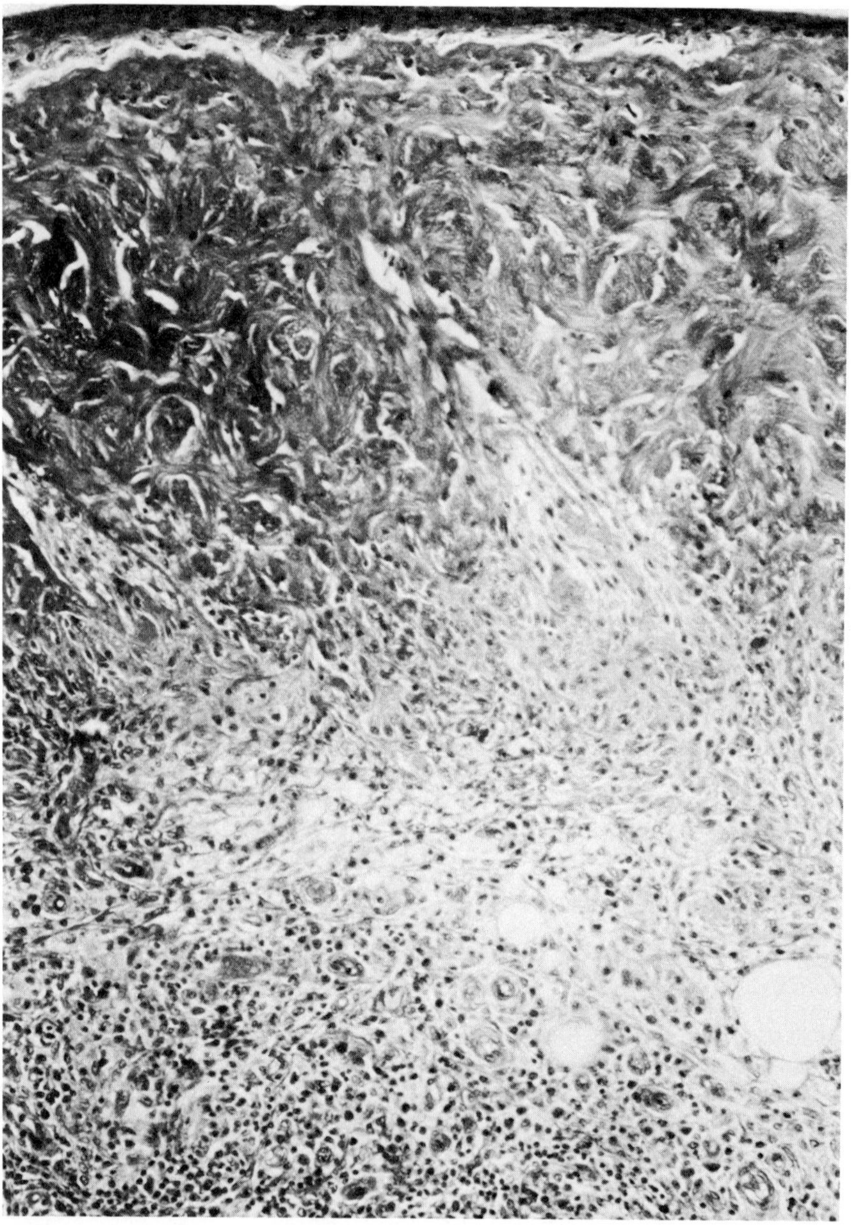

FIGURE 3a. Histologic appearance of hamster skin after implantation in a rat. Section taken after 21 days from the progesterone-treated skin shown in FIGURE 2. Note the well-preserved epidermal and dermal layers with little leukocytic infiltration in this specimen, as compared with virtually complete destruction of the control implant (FIGURE 3b). ×190.

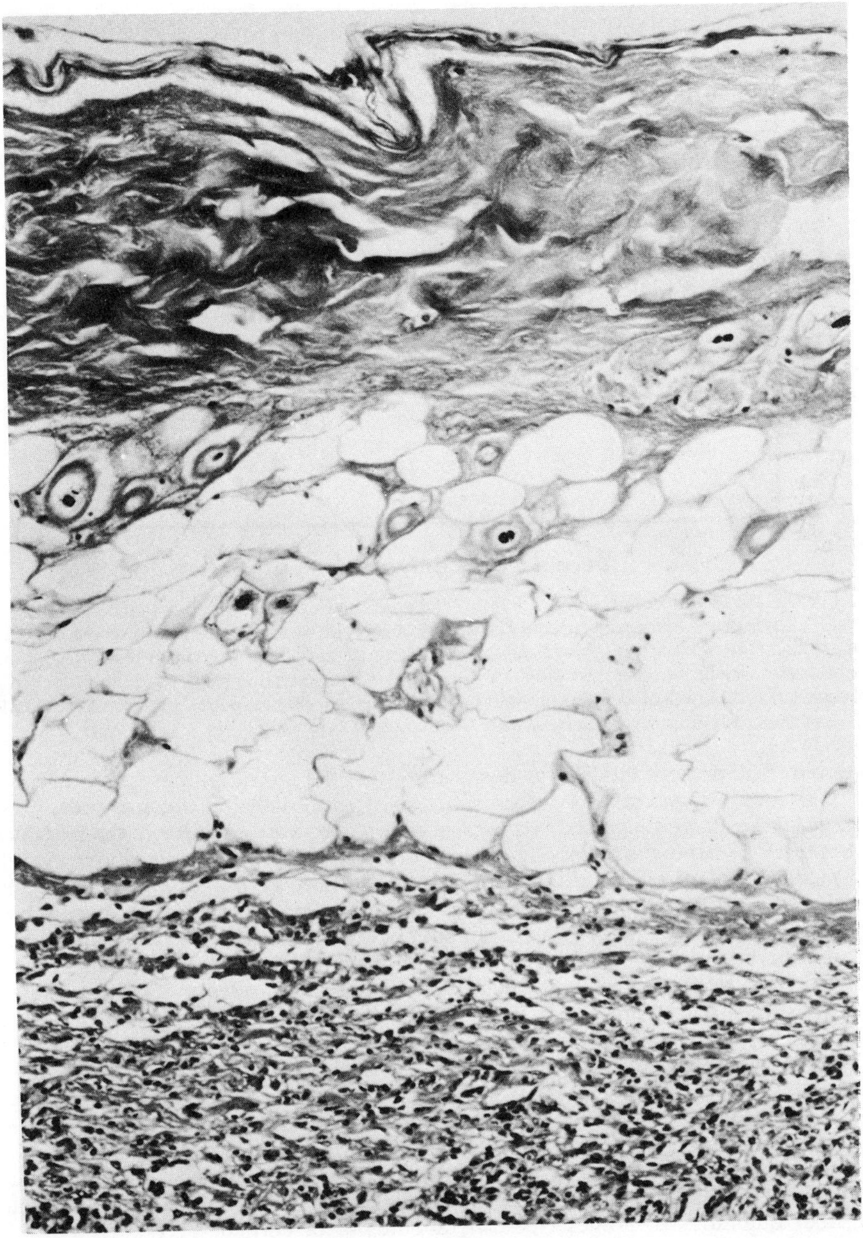

FIGURE 3b. Histologic appearance of control hamster skin implant removed after 14 days. Note the virtually complete destruction of the implant. ×190.

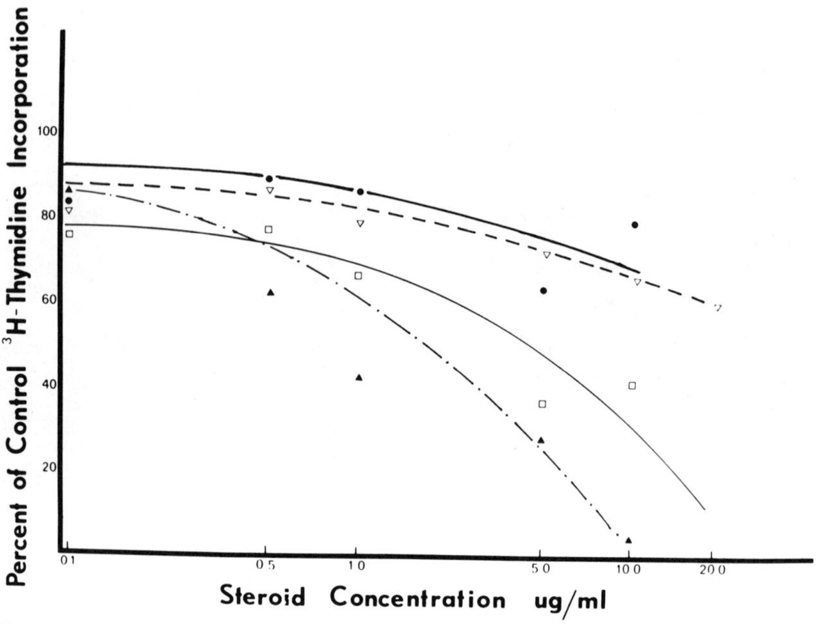

FIGURE 4. Mixed lymphocyte reaction. The response of antigenically stimulated normal male lymphocytes to increasing concentrations of steroid was measured as described under MATERIALS AND METHODS. Viability was measured on Day 5 by the trypan blue dye exclusion assay. At steroid concentrations of 10 μg/ml for progesterone (□), estradiol (●), testosterone (▽), and cortisol (▲), the numbers of living cells were, respectively, 86, 96, 95, and 71% of those of the control cultures, which contained no steroid.

steroid. The present model was designed to test the immunosuppressive activity of high local concentrations of steroids in an *extra*uterine site, because many previous studies have suggested that fetal rejection does not occur due to the fact that the uterus somehow is an immunologically privileged site. While the above model demonstrates rather forcefully the potential activity of progesterone, accurate estimates of relative potencies of steroids are not possible because of variable release rates from silastic. Measurements of local tissue steroid concentrations have not been made. Nevertheless, some meaningful comparisons can be obtained from release rates measured *in vitro*. The rates of release of progesterone, diethylstilbestrol, 19-nortestosterone, desoxycorticosterone (DOC), testosterone, and 20β-reduced progesterone (20β-P) were 7.1, 7.0, 5.7, 2.4, 1.1, and 1.0 μg/hr/cm, respectively. Rates of release of cortisol, dexamethasone, and estradiol were less than 0.1 μg/hr/cm. Thus, it is likely that slow release cannot explain the lack of activity of 19-nortestosterone or diethylstilbestrol when compared with progesterone or of testosterone and 20β-P when compared with DOC.

It is important in this regard to recall that of the steroids measured in human placenta, progesterone is present in the highest concentration, whereas much smaller quantities of progesterone metabolites or of cortisol have been found.[1] Indeed, measurements of the total concentration of progesterone range from 2 to 10 μg/g at term and are similar throughout pregnancy. The effective concentration at the syncytial surface of the trophoblastic villi is likely to be even higher. Moreover, estimates of corticosteroid-binding globulin (CBG) concentrations by

Seal and Doe indicate that the binding capacity in term placenta is about 0.15 μg/g.[26] Therefore, it seems reasonable to assume that maternal lymphocytes in the intervillous blood are exposed to free progesterone concentrations similar to those that we have shown to be suppressive *in vitro* (FIGURE 4). On their return to the peripheral circulation, lymphocytes are exposed to free progesterone concentrations at least two orders of magnitude lower. Thus, an efficient mechanism can be envisaged by which progesterone provides local immune suppression, thereby preventing maternal destruction of the placenta without seriously compromising immune defenses elsewhere. Although the free concentration of progesterone in the fetal circulation is considerably higher than in the maternal circulation because of the much lower CBG levels, it is unlikely that suppression of fetal lymphocytic function occurs. Thus, both maternal and fetal immune systems are functional and undoubtedly destroy the small numbers of cells that cross the placenta in both directions. Thus, the mechanism proposed is consistent with present concepts of immune functions during human pregnancy.

Despite the widespread use of steroids as immunosuppressive agents, their mode of action remains unclear. It has recently been shown, however, that the major effect of glucocorticoid administration in guinea pigs is to cause a profound redistribution of circulating lymphocytes to bone that can be sustained by chronic treatment.[26] Interestingly, the sensitivity of the remaining lymphocytes to stimulation by several mitogens was unaltered. Because the peripheral levels of circulating lymphocytes are not markedly altered during pregnancy, it seems unlikely that a similar mechanism protects the fetus.

Our results with the MLR suggest that progesterone and cortisol have a similar ability to suppresss human T-lymphocyte function. However, with the possible exception of the pregnant guinea pig, free concentrations of cortisol equivalent to those of progesterone found in the human placenta are not encountered in nature. The guinea pig is remarkable in several respects, because an enormous increase in CBG levels and in a specific progesterone-binding globulin occurs during pregnancy. The peripheral concentration of cortisol (about 5 μg/ml), therefore, is extraordinarily high, about 10–20 times higher than that of progesterone. Nevertheless, the free concentrations of both steroids are much lower. Therefore, the role of cortisol in pregnancy maintenance in guinea pigs is unclear, because cortisol bound to CBG is generally regarded as being inactive. It should be noted that the placental progesterone concentration in guinea pigs and most other species is only 1% or less of that found in the human. This information would suggest that progesterone may not be important as an immunosuppressive agent in other species. However, variations in antigenic challenge presented by the fetus, placental structure, and sensitivity of the cellular immune recognition system to suppression by progesterone may be such that much lower concentrations of progesterone are required to protect the fetus. It is likely that the histocompatibility differences between humans are far greater than those between rodents. This possibility may be reflected by the fact that much greater responses are observed in human than in rodent MLC, yet their responses to plant mitogens are similar.[32] Furthermore, in view of the great variation in placental structure, and consequently in the degree of interaction of maternal blood and cells with fetal elements among species, measurements of total placental progesterone concentrations may not accurately reflect local conditions at the sites of trophoblastic progesterone production and immunologic susceptibility. While we have not yet tested the *in vitro* effects of progesterone on lymphocytes of other species, it is well known that glucorticoid effects on lymphoid systems are much greater in rodents than in man.

Other lines of evidence are consistent with the hypothesis that progesterone provides immunosuppression during pregnancy. A fall in progesterone production occurs in many species near the end of normal gestation. For example, in sheep, a dramatic fall in circulating progesterone levels and a concomitant rise in estrogen occur in the last 48 hr of pregnancy, and both phenomena can be induced earlier by glucocorticoid administration.[27] These changes are thought to elicit local prostaglandin formation in the decidua, which leads to tissue destruction and uterine contractions by as yet ill-defined mechanisms. Similar changes in progesterone and estradiol levels in the maternal circulation at the end of normal human pregnancy have not been uniformly observed. However, this situation is not surprising, since a relatively small decline in placental progesterone secretion may be masked in the peripheral circulation by binding to CBG. Indeed, a fall in pregnanediol excretion does occur, normally beginning 2–3 days prior to term.[1] Furthermore, maternal progesterone plasma levels decline, beginning several weeks prior to premature labor,[28] and low placental concentrations of progesterone have also been reported in premature births.[29] Together with the well-described inflammatory changes in the placenta and endometrium associated with normal delivery,[30] these observations are consistent with the concept of parturition and late abortion being due to declining placental progesterone production and the onset of a local immune rejection reaction. Many early attempts to prevent spontaneous abortion in humans by progestin administration have produced equivocal results. More information is clearly needed concerning the mechanisms of progesterone action in pregnancy before the beneficial effects of progestin administration in human pregnancy can be evaluated.

In conclusion, it would seem that local suppression of maternal cellular immune defenses by progesterone may constitute one mechanism that prevents rejection of the products of conception. Other factors, such as the presence of the nonantigenic HCG on the surface of invading trophoblasts and the presence of blocking antibodies,[31] may also contribute to the success of pregnancy.

Acknowledgments

The expert technical assistance of Mr. Laurence Brodkin and Ms. Janice Perlman is greatly appreciated.

References

1. Eichler, O., A. Farah, H. Herken & A. D. Welch. (Eds.) 1968. Handbook of Experimental Pharmacology. Vol. XXII/1. Springer-Verlag New York Inc. New York, N.Y.
2. Medawar, P. B. 1953. Some immunological and endocrinological problems raised by the evolution of viviparity in vertebrates. Symp. Soc. Exp. Biol. **7:** 320–337.
3. Little, C. C. 1924. The genetics of tissue transplantation if mammals. J. Cancer Res. **8:** 75–95.
4. Bardawil, W. A. & B. L. Toy. 1959. The natural history of choriocarcinoma: the problems of immunity and spontaneous regression. Ann. N.Y. Acad. Sci. **80:** 197–261.
5. Bradbury, S., W. D. Billington & D. R. S. Kirby. 1965. A histochemical and electron microscopical study of the fibrinoid of the mouse placenta. J. Royal Microsc. Soc. **84:** 199–211.
6. Billingham, R. E., P. L. Krohn & P. B. Medawar. 1951. Effects of locally applied cortisone acetate on survival of skin homografts in rabbits. Brit. Med. J. **2:** 1049–1053.

7. ANDRESEN, R. H. & C. W. MONROE. 1962. Experimental study of the behavior of adult human skin homografts during pregnancy. Amer. J. Obstet. Gynecol. **84**(8): 1096–1103.
8. NELSON, J. H. & J. E. HALL. 1964. Studies on the thymopathic system in humans. Amer. J. Obstet. Gynecol. **90:** 482–492.
9. FINN, R., C. A. ST, HILL, A. J. GOVAN, I. G. RALFS, F. J. GURNEY & V. DENYE. 1972. Immunological responses in pregnancy and survival of fetal homograft. Brit. Med. J. **8:** 150–152.
10. PURTILO, D. T., H. M. HALLGREN & E. J. YUNIS. 1972. Depressed maternal lymphocyte response to phytohaemagglutinin in human pregnancy. Lancet **I:** 769–771.
11. LEIKIN, S. 1972. The immunosuppressive effects of maternal plasma. *In* Proceedings of the VIth Leukocyte-Culture Conference. M. R. Schwartz, Ed.: 725–740. Academic Press, Inc. New York, N.Y.
12. KASAKURA, S. 1972. The inhibitory effect of pregnant plasmas on the reactivity of mixed leukocyte cultures. *In* Proceedings of the VIth Leukocyte-Culture Conference. M. R. Schwartz, Ed.: 711–721. Academic Press, Inc. New York, N.Y.
13. CARR, M. C., D. P. STITES & H. H. FUDENBERG. 1973. Cellular immune aspects of the human fetal maternal relationship II: in vitro response of gravida lymphocytes to phytohemagglutinin. Cell. Immunol. **8:** 448–454.
14. ADCOCK, E. W., F. TEASDALE, C. S. AUGUST, S. COX, G. MESCHIA, F. C. BATTAGLIA & M. NAUGHTON. 1973. Human chorionic gonadotropin: its possible role in maternal lymphocyte suppression. Science **181:** 845–847.
15. CONTRACTOR, S. F. & H. DAVIES. 1973. Effect of human chorionic somatomammotrophin and human chorionic gonadotropin on phytohaemagglutinin induced lymphocyte transformation. Nature [New Biol.] **243:** 284–286.
16. JENKINS, D. M., M. G. AGRES, J. PETERS & J. RILEY. 1972. Human chorionic gonadotropin and the fetal allograft. Amer. J. Obstet. Gynecol. **14**(1): 13–15.
17. KAYE, M. D. & W. R. JONES. 1971. Effect of human chorionic gonadotropin on *in vitro* lymphocyte transformation. Amer. J. Obstet. Gynecol. **109:** 1029–1031.
18. TEASDALE, F., E. W. ADCOCK, C. S. AUGUST, S. COX, F. C. BATTAGLIA & M. A. NAUGHTON. 1973. Human chorionic gonadotropin: inhibitory effect on mixed lymphocyte cultures. Gynecol. Invest. **4:** 263–269.
19. CALDWELL, J. L., D. P. STITES & H. H. FUDENBERG. 1975. Human chorionic gonadotropin: effects of crude and purified preparations on lymphocyte responses to phytohemagglutinin and allogeneic stimulation. J. Immunol. **115**(5): 1249–1253.
20. KAYE, M. D., W. R. JONES, R. M. Y. ING & R. MARKHAM. 1971. Effect of human chorionic gonadotropin on intrauterine skin allograft survival in rats. Amer. J. Obstet. Gynecol. **110**(5): 640–643.
21. WATNICK, A. S. & R. A. RUSSO. 1968. Survival of skin homografts in uteri of pregnant and progesterone-estrogen treated rats. Proc. Soc. Exp. Biol. Med. **128:** 1–4.
22. MORIYAMA, I. & T. SUGAWA. 1972. Progesterone facilitates implantation of xenogenic cultured cells in hamster uterus. Nature [New Biol.] **236:** 150–152.
23. HULKA, J. F., K. MOHR & M. W. LIEBERMAN. 1965. Effect of synthetic progestational agents on allograft rejection and circulating antibody production. Endocrinology **77:** 897–901.
24. TURCOTTE, J. G., R. F. HAINES, G. L. BORDY, T. J. MEYER & S. A. SCHWARTZ. 1968. Immunosuppression with medroxyprogesterone acetate. Transplantation **6**(2): 248–260.
25. FAUCI, A. S. 1975. Mechanisms of corticosteroid action on lymphocyte subpopulations I. Redistribution of circulating T and B lymphocytes to the bone marrow. J. Immunol. **28:** 669–679.
26. SEAL, U. S. & R. P. DOE. 1967. The role of corticosteroid-binding globulin in mammalian pregnancy. Excerpta Med. Int. Cong. Ser. **132:** 697–706.
27. LIGGINS, G. C., R. J. FAIRCLOUGH, S. A. GRIEVES, J. Z. KENDALL & B. S. KNOX. 1973. The mechanisms of initiation of parturition in the ewe. Recent Progr. Hormone Res. **29:** 111–159.
28. TAMBY RAJA, R. L., A. B. M. ANDERSON & A. C. TURNBULL. 1974. Endocrine changes in premature labour. Brit. Med. J. **4:** 67–71.

29. KUMAR, D., R. S. AZOURY & A. C. BARNES. 1963. Studies on human premature births I. Placental progesterone concentrations. Amer. J. Obstet. Gynecol. **87**(1): 126–129.
30. BURSTEIN, R. H. & H. T. BLUMENTHAL. 1969. Immune reactions of normal pregnancy. Amer. J. Obstet. Gynecol. **104:** 671–678.
31. HELLSTRÖM, K. E., I. HELLSTRÖM & J. BRAWN. 1969. Abrogation of cellular immunity to antigenically foreign mouse embryonic cells by serum factor. Nature (London) **224:** 914, 915.
32. STITES, D. 1976. Personal communication.

DISCUSSION

DR. L. P. BULLOCK: What are your thoughts about reports a few years ago that HCG can suppress the PHA lymphocyte system, and do you think that in the human this suppression might have a greater effect than that of progesterone?

DR. SIITERI: Yes, I'm aware of those reports. Perhaps you're not aware of the recent report by Caldwell *et al.*[19] in which they have shown the pure HCG, as provided by Dr. Canfield, has absolutely no effect on suppressing PHA stimulation of lymphocytes. So it appears that the earlier reports that suggested such activity of HCG may be inaccurate. Commercial HCG (APL) contains many proteins, one of which has the ability to suppress lymphocyte reactivity, but it's not HCG. We, in fact, have confirmed this observation in a totally different system. If you add APL to human fibroblasts in culture, you can shut down protein synthesis virtually completely in a dose-dependent manner. But if you use purified HCG, there is absolutely no effect. More importantly, it seems to me that HCG may be important in another aspect. It has been clearly shown by several workers that the human syncytiotrophoblast has a coating of HCG. It is entirely possible that HCG may be important by virtue of the fact that it is not antigenic and therefore may serve to block access to the paternal histocompatibility antigens of trophoblastic cells that should be rejected in the placenta. Those are the cells that are exposed to the maternal blood circulation and the maternal lymphocytes.

DR. R. B. BILLIAR (*Case Western Reserve University, Cleveland, Ohio*): How are you going to extrapolate this finding to the rat, since you did show in the pregnant rat that it wasn't enough to protect against granuloma formation, especially in early pregnancy, in the rat or in any species where the ovary is a primary source?

DR. SIITERI: Yes, that is a very important question, for which I don't have any firm answers at this time. I can give you some speculations. Clearly, placental structure is important in this regard. Comparative placentation is a fascinating business, because no two species do it exactly the same way. The point is that the degree of interaction of maternal cells with the fetal tissues varies tremendously, so that the challenge of fetal antigens to maternal cells also varies. I'm suggesting that perhaps most species don't need as much progesterone as does the human. The other point is that we have begun to look at the relative susceptibility of lymphocytes from different species to inhibition by progesterone to see whether that may be a variable. It is well known that PHA stimulation of lymphocytes from different species, such as human and rabbit, elicits about the same magnitude of response. But, in mixed lymphocyte reactions, the response with human cells is much greater than it is with mouse cells, suggesting that the intensity of cell-mediated immune reactions may vary according to the antigenic complexity inherent in the species. Finally, it is well known that murine and other species are much more sensitive to glucocorticoids than is the human, and the same may be true for progesterone.

DR. F. ROSEN: I would like to know whether progesterone causes lymphopenia in animals or in man similar to that produced by glucorticoids, because I think the mechanism of this lymphopenia would now appear to be redistribution of lymphocytes into lymph nodes and spleen and not killing of the cells by glucocorticoids. We find a very marked discrepancy between rodent and human lymphocytes in terms of their biochemical response to glucocorticoids. Human lymphocytes require approximately 10^{-4} M cortisol to show a suppression of nucleic acid and protein synthesis, whereas rodent lymphocytes are responsive to 10^{-6} cortisol, so I think this would be an important point.

DR. SIITERI: I absolutely agree with you. Dr. Fauci at the National Institutes of Health has clearly shown in the guinea pig that the reduction in number of cells in the circulation is, in fact, a redistribution to bone.[25] However, this phenomenon obviously does not occur in pregnant animals, including the human and the rat. There is no reduction in circulating lymphocyte concentrations. This is a local system that exists only in the placenta and not elsewhere, which is just exactly what you would want to have if you desired protection of the fetus without endangering the maternal host in terms of susceptibility to infection, for example. I am visualizing this system as one in which lymphocytes are suppressed only while they are in the placenta. Once they escape the placenta, they return to their normal reactivity.

DR. P. BECK: It seems that there is a comparable analogy in humans that might be useful to explore, namely, the model that Dr. Pharriss presented to us yesterday. It is my understanding that the IUDs do tend to generate an inflammatory response. Do you think that there is less of an inflammatory response with these progesterone implants?

DR. SIITERI: If our hypothesis is correct, one would expect that the progesterone-filled IUD would produce very little inflammatory response in the uterus, and, in fact, this may be important as to how it is operating in terms of preventing implantation. An inflammatory response is elicited during the early stages of implantation, which may be essential for success.

DR. BECK: One of the complications that has been reported with the IUDs is an increased incidence of tubular ovarian abscess. I'm not aware of any comparable data from the patients who have these progesterone IUDs.

DR. M. LIPPMAN: I just want to comment on glucocorticoid receptors in various lymphoid cell populations. We've examined peripheral blood lymphocytes, purified T and B subpopulations of lymphocytes, and non-PHA-stimulated human lymphocytes. All of these cells have readily demonstrable glucocorticoid receptors. In all of them, competition studies reveal that progesterone will compete for the glucocorticoid receptor with approximately a 10-fold lower affinity than that of cortisol itself. None of these cells has a specific progesterone receptor, as indicated by the relatively rigid criteria defined in my talk. Whether progesterone action in these cells is effected through the glucocorticoid receptor is not certain, and I think you said that perfectly clearly yourself. We and others have shown, over and over again, that high concentrations of any steroid (10^{-5} M) may very well act on cells through a nonreceptor-mediated mechanism. I think that it simply remains to be seen whether that's the explanation. But I think that doesn't denigrate the very great importance of showing that these progesterone concentrations can exist in the placenta and that they are clearly immunosuppressive.

DR. SIITERI: I agree with everything you said.

STIMULATION OF POLY(ADENOSINE DIPHOSPHATE RIBOSE) SYNTHASE ACTIVITY OF *XENOPUS* GERMINAL VESICLE BY PROGESTERONE*

Luis O. Burzio and S. S. Koide

The Population Council
The Rockefeller University
New York, New York 10021

At the end of oogenesis, the full-grown oocytes are in the diplotene stage of the first meiotic prophase and have completed the major part of their growth and differentiation. After this period, which may take considerable length of time, the oocyte is ready to undergo the first meiotic, or reduction, division. This process is generally referred to as oocyte maturation and involves a perfectly programmed sequence of morphologic and biochemical transformation. An excellent review of this subject was recently published by Schuetz.[1]

In amphibians and fish, this process of oocyte maturation is mediated by progesterone. The most dramatic morphologic change that occurs after the hormone acts is the dissolution of the oocyte nucleus, or germinal vesicle (GV). After germinal vesicle breakdown (GVBD), the partially condensed lambrush chromosomes suffer a more drastic and rapid condensation to finally become the compact metaphase chromosomes, which will undergo the first reductive meiotic division.[1,2] After these changes, a factor appears in the cytoplasm of the maturing oocytes that is capable of inducing chromosomal condensation of a microinjected brain cell nucleus. The appearance of this factor depends on the presence of the GV and has been designated as chromosomal condensation activity, and the phenomenon has been described as "prophasing."[3,4]

In the present study, we have focused our attention on this phenomenon of chromosomal condensation. The *Xenopus* oocyte is an excellent model to study the biochemical transformation that occurs after progesterone-induced condensation of the lampbrush chromosomes. Moreover, we are currently exploring the possibility that poly(adenosine diphosphate-ribose) [poly(ADP-ribose)] synthase activity may participate in this process of chromosomal condensation.[5,6] This enzymatic reaction of ADP-ribosylation results in the modification of chromosomal proteins (histones and nonhistone proteins), which undoubtedly alters the structure and is involved in the condensation of chromosomes. Therefore, the aims of the present study were to determine whether progesterone affected the poly(ADP-ribose) synthase activity located in the GV and to establish the timing of the change in enzymatic activity to GVBD and to the condensation of lampbrush chromosomes.

Materials and Methods

Isolation of Germinal Vesicle

Female frogs (*Xenopus laevis*), 3 years of age or older, were used in this study. These animals belong to a colony maintained for many years in our laboratory at

*Supported in part by National Institute of Child Health and Human Development Grant 5P01 HDO 5671.

The Rockefeller University. The animals are kept at 18–20°C with 12 hr of light and 12 hr of darkness.

The procedure for the preparation of GV from oocytes was described in a previous report.[7] In summary, the female frog is killed by decapitation. The ovary is excised and suspended in amphibian Ringer's solution (AR). The ovary is cut into small pieces and incubated in AR that contains 0.25% collagenase for 90–120 min at 25°C to dissociate the tissue into free oocytes. A mixture of oocytes of different diameters, ranging from previtellogenic oocytes to full-growth or banded oocytes is obtained after this treatment.[7] The suspension of oocytes is then filtered through a 700-μm mesh nylon screen or Nitex® (TET/Kressilk, Elmsford, N.Y.). The oocytes retained by this filter was designated as class-A oocytes, which correspond to stages V and VI of Dumont.[8] The oocytes that passed through this filter were refiltered on 500-μm mesh Nitex. The retained oocytes were designated as class-B oocytes. This class of oocytes is composed of a mixture of stages III and IV. The filtrate of oocytes is then collected on a 53-μm mesh Nitex screen. The retained oocytes correspond to stages I and II of Dumont.[8]

To isolate GV from the oocytes, each class was incubated in 0.25% pronase in AR for 20 min at 25°C. After this treatment, the oocytes were extensively washed with cold AR and once with SMT-1 solution (0.25 M sucrose, 1 mM $MgCl_2$, 0.02% Triton® X-100). The washed oocytes were suspended in SMT-1. The tube of suspended oocytes was set in ice for 10–15 min. The suspension was centrifuged at 250–400g for 3 min. The liberated GV suspended in the supernatant was stabilized by the addition of about 2–4 vol of SMT-2 (0.25 M sucrose, 2 mM $MgCl_2$, 0.1% Triton X-100). The GV were collected by filtering the supernatant through a 26- or 53-μm mesh Nitex screen. The GV retained on the filter were washed with SMT-2 to eliminate yolk granules and pigments. The GV were collected and counted. The usual yield of GV by the procedure described is about 60% of the initial number of oocytes.

Incubation with Progesterone and Determination of Germinal Vesicle Breakdown

About 50–100 class-A or -B oocytes were incubated in 2 ml of AR that contained progesterone at a final concentration of 5 μg/ml. The control sample consisted of oocytes incubated under identical conditions with the same amount of ethanol in the medium, except that the progesterone was omitted. The incubation was performed for varying periods of time at 20°C. Two criteria were used to evaluate the degree of maturation attained by the oocytes induced by progesterone. First, the animal poles were observed for the presence of the white maturation spot, which is indicative of GVBD. The second approach consisted of verifying the presence of the GV by manual dissection of the oocyte. To carry out this procedure, the oocytes were incubated for 15 min in SMT-2 (described under *Isolation of Germinal Vesicle*) and subsequently dissected under the microscope. This method proved to be a very useful and rapid technique to establish the presence or absence of GV.

To study the effect of progesterone on the activity of poly(ADP-ribose) synthase, the following procedure was employed. Batches of 1500–2500 oocytes were incubated with or without progesterone (final concentration 5 μg/ml in AR) for varying periods of time at 20°C. At the end of the incubation period, the medium was removed, and 5 ml of 0.25% pronase in AR was added. After incubating at 20°C for 30 min, the oocytes were washed, and the GV was isolated as described above.

Enzymatic Studies

To measure enzymatic activity, the isolated GV were washed once or twice with SM Buffer [0.25 M sucrose, 2 mM $MgCl_2$, 15 mM Tris hydrochloride (pH 7.5)] by sedimentation. The supernatant was removed by suction, and the final pellet of GV was suspended in TMGED [50 mM Tris hydrochloride (pH 7.9), 25%, glycerol, 5 mM $MgCl_2$, 0.1 mM EDTA, 0.5 mM dithiothreitol]. The suspension of GV was stored at −70°C. Just before assay, the suspension of GV was thawed and sonicated for 10 sec twice at 2°C. This sonicated suspension was used to assay for enzymatic activities.

Poly(ADP-ribose) synthase was assayed as described in a previous report.[9] The assay medium contained, in a final volume of 0.25 ml, 50 mM Tris hydrochloride (pH 7.9), 10 mM $MgCl_2$, 0.1 mM [^{3}H]NAD (110 cpm, equivalent to 1 pmol) or [^{14}C]NAD (45 cpm, equivalent to 1 pmol), and sonicated GV that contained 20–50 μg of protein. The mixture was incubated at 20°C for 15 min, and the reaction was stopped by the addition of 10% (TCA) trichloroacetic acid. The insoluble material that contained the radioactivity was collected on a glass filter and washed with 10% TCA and ethanol. The filter was dried at 110°C for 10 min and placed in a vial to which liquifluor toluene was added. The radioactivity was counted with a Packard scintillation counter.

Other Determinations

Proteins were determined according to Lowry *et al.*[10] with bovine serum albumin used as a standard.

Results

The poly(ADP-ribose) synthase located in the GV exhibits the same characteristics as those of the enzyme described in other eukaryotic cells.[5,6] The product of the reaction (oligomers and polymers of ADP-ribose) showed the same properties as those formed in other tissues.[5,6] A significant finding is the high level of activity in the GV. Although the activity of the enzyme per GV showed considerable variation between different preparations, the values ranged from 0.1 to 1 pmol of NAD incorporated per GV per 15 min at 20°C. This activity is about 1000 times higher than that found in rat liver nuclei[5,6] and about 10,000 times that found in *Xenopus* liver nuclei.[11]

Table 1
Effect of Progesterone on Poly(ADP-ribose) Synthase Activity of Isolated Germinal Vesicles

Expt	Activity (pmol of [^{3}H]NAD/100 GV) Control	Progesterone	Stimulation (%)
1	18.2	91	500
2	15.6	48	310
3	40	92	230
4	11.8	37.5	315

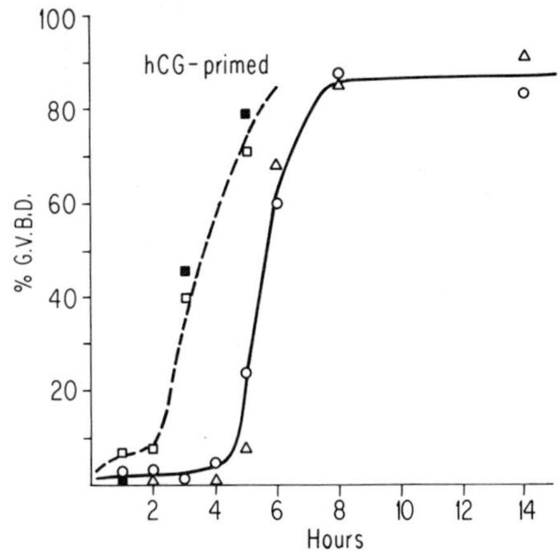

FIGURE 1. Effect of progesterone on GVBD of *Xenopus* oocytes. Human chorionic gonadotropin (hCG) -primed (- - - - -) depicts the response to progesterone of oocytes obtained from female *Xenopus* that were injected 10 days earlier with 250–500 IU of hCG. Progesterone concentration, 5 μg/ml; incubation temperature, 20°C. Two separate experiments were performed, for each group designated as ■ and □ and as ○ and △.

It is of interest to determine whether progesterone can affect this enzymatic activity present in the GV of oocytes. Class-A oocytes were incubated for about 3 hr with or without progesterone (5 μg/ml) in AR at 20°C. After the hormone treatment, the oocytes were incubated in AR that contained 0.25% pronase for about 30 min (described under *Isolation of Germinal Vesicle)*, and the GV were isolated. The isolated GV were washed and resuspended in TMGED. The suspension was sonicated and assayed for poly(ADP-ribose) synthase activity (TABLE 1). For each experiment shown in TABLE 1, the average values of the activity from two controls and two progesterone-treated preparations of GV are presented. Although the enzymatic activities of the control samples varied markedly, duplicate values for each experiment of the control or progesterone preparation of GV did not vary by more than 10–20%. This rather small variation is acceptable, because each preparation of GV came from a pool of 1500–2500 class-A oocytes, which were obtained from three or four ovaries. Nevertheless, aside from the variation in activity between experiments, the most significant finding is that progesterone treatment of GV always resulted in two- to fivefold stimulation of synthase activity.

It is of interest to relate this stimulation of poly(ADP-ribose) synthase activity by progesterone to the time of GVBD induced by the hormone. FIGURE 1 shows the rate of GVBD when class-A oocytes were incubated with progesterone (5 μg/ml in AR) at 20°C. The percentage of GVBD varies markedly among the batches of class-A oocytes prepared from different animals. Nonetheless, with most batches, GVBD commenced after 4 hr of incubation at 20°C and reached nearly 100% within 6–8 hr. On the other hand, in oocytes obtained from frogs that had been primed by administration of human chorionic gonadotropin 10–14 days (250–500 IU per animal) before the date of preparation, GVBD induced by progesterone occurred much earlier; that is, the lag phase was shortened. This phenomenon has also been observed by other investigators.[1]

The stimulation of poly(ADP-ribose) synthase induced by progesterone, as shown in TABLE 1, was measured after a total hormonal treatment time of about 210 min, which consisted of 180 min of actual incubation with progesterone plus 30 min of incubation with pronase. Thus, the stimulatory effect on the enzyme occurs prior to the onset of GVBD. To obtain a clearer picture of the sequence of events, the kinetics of stimulation were studied. The results are depicted in

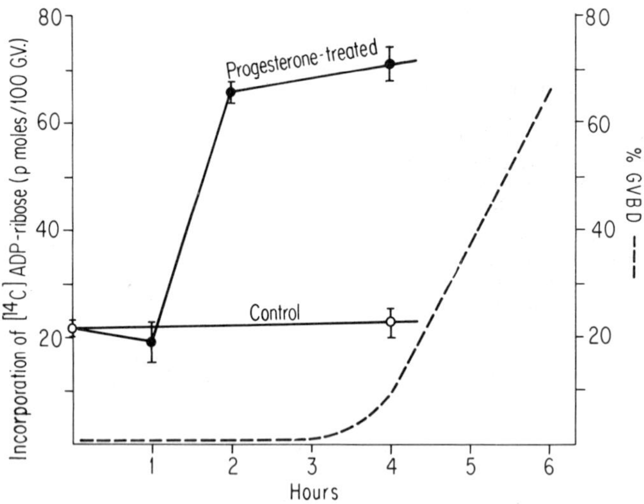

FIGURE 2. Time course of stimulation of poly(ADP-ribose) synthase activity isolated from oocytes incubated with progesterone. Percentage of GVBD, ---.

FIGURE 2. The poly(ADP-ribose) synthase activity of GV isolated from class-A oocytes incubated for 4 hr at 20°C in AR did not vary significantly from the enzymatic activity found in GV isolated from freshly prepared oocytes. After 50 min of incubation with progesterone, the enzymatic activity remained at the control level. After 2 hr of incubation, however, the activity reached a level more than threefold that of the control value. This stimulated activity of poly(ADP-ribose) synthase remained elevated after 4 hr of incubation with progesterone. The most

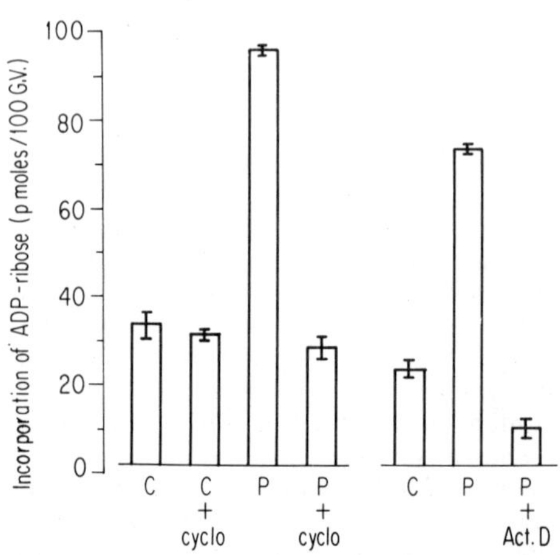

FIGURE 3. Effect of cycloheximide (cyclo) and actinomycin D (Act. D) on poly(ADP-ribose) synthase activity of *Xenopus* oocytes stimulated with progesterone (P). Concentration of cycloheximide, 20 μg/ml; of actinomycin D, 50 μg/ml.

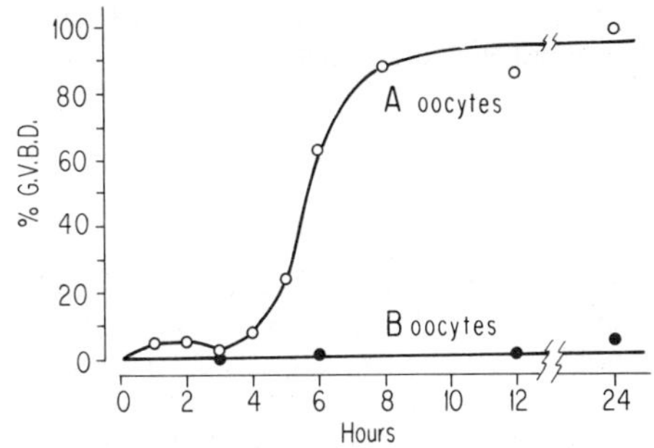

FIGURE 4. Induction of GVBD in class-A (●) and -B (○) oocytes with progesterone.

significant feature of this experiment is that the dramatic increase in enzymatic activity preceded the onset of GVBD.

Obviously, it is very important to establish that the observed stimulation of poly(ADP-ribose) synthase by progesterone is dependent on *de novo* synthesis of the enzyme or is due to an activation step. To answer this question, the effect of cycloheximide and actinomycin D on the stimulation of synthase activity by progesterone was studied (FIGURE 3). Control oocytes incubated for 4 hr with or without cycloheximide (20 μg/ml) showed no difference in activity of poly(ADP-ribose) synthase. When the oocytes were incubated with progesterone for 4 hr, the described stimulation of almost threefold was observed. This induction of poly(ADP-ribose) synthase by progesterone was completely blocked when the oocytes were incubated with cycloheximide (20 μg/ml) added to the suspending medium. Moreover, the stimulatory effect of the hormone was suppressed by actinomycin D (50 μg/ml; FIGURE 3).

An interesting situation exists in the small-sized oocytes with respect to their ability to undergo maturation in response to progesterone. The majority of class-B oocytes did not exhibit GVBD on incubation with progesterone (FIGURE 4). Although the GV of class-A oocytes started to disintegrate after 4 hr of incubation with progesterone, and almost all of the GV were disintegrated between 12 and 25 hr of incubation, most of the GV of class-B oocytes remained intact. A small number of class-B oocyte GV (less than 10%) was disintegrated at 12–24 hr of incubation with progesterone. A similar finding was recently reported by Reynhout and Smith.[12] In view of this observation, it was of interest to test the ability of progesterone to effect poly(ADP-ribose) synthase activity in GV of class-B oocytes. When class-A oocytes were incubated for 225 min with progesterone, the activity of poly(ADP-ribose) synthase in the isolated GV was stimulated by 268% (TABLE 2). However, when class-B oocytes were incubated with progesterone for 270

TABLE 2

EFFECT OF PROGESTERONE ON POLY(ADP-RIBOSE) SYNTHASE ACTIVITY IN CLASS-A AND -B OOCYTES

Oocyte Class	Activity (pmol of [^{3}H]NAD/100 GV) Control	Progesterone	Variation (%)
A	5.9	21.6	+268
B	7.2	4.8	−32

min, the enzymatic activity was not stimulated. On the contrary, a slight inhibition of the activity occurred.

Discussion

Poly(ADP-ribose) synthase is a nuclear enzyme associated with chromatin that catalyzes the transfer of the ADP-ribose moiety of NAD to chromosomal proteins.[5,6] During the second phase of the reaction, new ADP-ribose moieties are linked to the preexisting one, so that oligomers and polymers of ADP-ribose are formed. The chromosomal proteins modified by this novel reaction are histones and nonhistones. Although studies on ADP ribosylation of nonhistone proteins are preliminary, the reported results suggest that several nuclear proteins are modified.[13,14] Among the histones, H_1 is most extensively modified by this reaction, followed by H_3 and probably H_{2B}.[15-17]

In regard to the possible physiologic function of this enzymatic system, so far only two roles have been proposed. One possible role of this enzyme is that it may participate in DNA replication, a hypothesis based on a series of *in vitro* and *in vivo* studies.[15,18-21] However, other studies suggest that the enzyme may modify chromosomal structure and participate in their condensation. As mentioned previously, H_1 is most extensively modified by this reaction, as compared to the other histones or nonhistone proteins.[15-17] We have accumulated preliminary data that show that this modification induces a dramatic change in the structure and probably alters the function of H_1.[7,22] Also, several reports published during the last few years strongly support the thesis that H_1 and its modification play an important role in chromosomal structure and condensation.[23,24]

During meiotic maturation of amphibian oocytes induced by progesterone, a series of biochemical and morphologic changes occur; this topic has been reviewed by Schuetz.[1] During this process of transformation, several dramatic changes occur in the oocytic nuclei or GV, including disintegration of the nuclear membrane, dissolution of thousands of nucleoli, and the dramatic condensation of lampbrush chromosomes to form metaphase chromosomes.[1,2] Although the present results are preliminary and incomplete, one can hypothesize that ADP ribosylation of the lampbrush chromosomal proteins may occur and play a major role during the process of chromosomal condensation. Our preliminary experiments suggest that the enzyme is associated primarily with the lampbrush chromatin.[11] It is of interest, therefore, to determine which types of lampbrush chromosomal proteins undergo modification by this reaction. The *Xenopus* oocyte offers an excellent opportunity to study the distribution of radioactive NAD, which can be microinjected into the oocyte, and to follow the *in vivo* modification of the lampbrush chromosomal proteins during the earliest stages of meiotic maturation induced by progesterone.

In regard to the stimulation of poly(ADP-ribose) synthase by progesterone, the two most significant findings are the marked stimulation of the enzymatic activity and the occurrence of maximal stimulation just before the onset of GVBD. The present findings suggest that ADP ribosylation of nuclear proteins may be required in other nuclear event(s) that occur during or after GVBD. The stimulatory effect of progesterone appears to be dependent on protein and on RNA synthesis. The complete suppression of stimulation by cycloheximide is remarkable, because this antibiotic also completely inhibits GVBD.[1,2,25] The inhibitory effect of actinomycin D on stimulation of the enzyme is difficult to interpret at the present time, because poly(ADP-ribose) synthase is blocked by the drug *in vitro*.[26]

Several reports showed that the maturation of GVBD induced by progesterone is not affected by actinomycin D.[1,27] These reports proved that certain changes induced by progesterone, such as disintegration of the GV and the capacity of the cortical granules to be discharged after activation, are independent of transcription. However, Brachet *et al.*[2] reported recently that even though actinomycin D does not prevent maturation, it induces a marked swelling of the chromosomes. On the other hand, Brown and Littna[27] reported that during maturation of *Xenopus* oocytes, a new burst of RNA synthesis occurs. This RNA is similar to DNA-like RNA, which suggests that a part of this RNA could be messenger RNA that could be transcribed for synthesis of poly(ADP-ribose) synthase and could be induced by progesterone. A recent report of Morrill *et al.*[28] is relevant to this issue. They showed that shortly after progesterone treatment of oocytes, a marked stimulation of RNA synthesis occurred. However, Smith[29] reported that the major type of RNA synthesized during this period of maturation was ribosomal RNA. The present study on the induction of poly(ADP-ribose) synthase by progesterone requires further experimental work to elucidate the mechanisms of action of the hormone.

Finally, we will say a few words in regard to the refractory nature of class-B oocytes to progesterone *in vitro*. Neither GVBD nor stimulation of poly(ADP-ribose) synthase activity was observed when these oocytes were incubated for 4 hr or longer with progesterone (FIGURE 4 & TABLE 2). Similar findings have been reported by Wallace and Ho[30] and Reynhout and Smith.[12] An explanation for these results may be that the "receptor" for progesterone is not synthesized or activated in young oocytes and is induced at a later stage of oogenesis by some unknown mechanism. Thus, the nonresponsiveness of class-B oocytes to progesterone, as reflected by a lack of stimulation of poly(ADP-ribose) synthase and by the failure of GV to undergo disintegration, may be due to the absence of or a deficiency in the progesterone receptor system.

SUMMARY

A practical procedure for the isolation of massive numbers of GV from oocytes of *Xenopus laevis* at various stages of oogenesis was developed. The method is simple, rapid, and easy to perform. The isolated GV possess high activity of poly(ADP-ribose) synthase. Incubation of class-A oocytes (stages V and VI) with progesterone resulted in a stimulation of the poly(ADP-ribose) synthase activity in the GV. The stimulation of enzymatic activity occurred prior to GVBD. This stimulatory effect of progesterone on enzymatic activity was blocked by cycloheximide and actinomycin D, suggesting that induction is dependent on protein and RNA synthesis. Progesterone, however, was unable to cause disintegration of GV or to stimulate poly(ADP-ribose) synthase activity of class-B oocytes (stages III and IV). This finding suggests that the oocytes must progress to a certain stage of differentiation before progesterone can induce GVBD or stimulate poly(ADP-ribose) synthase activity.

REFERENCES

1. SCHUETZ, A. W. 1974. Role of hormones in oocyte maturation. Biol. Reprod. **10:** 150–178.
2. BRACHET, J., E. BALTUS, A. DE SCHUTTER, F. HANOCQ, J. HANOCQ-QUERTIER, E.

HUBERT, S. IACOBELLI & G. STEINERT. 1974. Biochemical changes during progesterone-induced maturation in *Xenopus laevis* oocytes. Mol. Cell. Biochem. **3:** 189–205.

3. ZIEGLER, D. & Y. MASUI. 1973. Control of chromosomal behavior in amphibian oocytes. Devel. Biol. **35:** 283–292.
4. MATSUI, S., H. WEINFELD & A. A. SANDBERG. 1972. Fate of chromatin in interphase nuclei subjected to "prophasing" in virus-fused cells. J. Nat. Cancer Inst. **43:** 1621–1630.
5. HONJO, T. & O. HAYAISHI. 1973. Enzymic ADP-ribosylation of proteins and regulation of cellular activity. Current Topics Cell. Regulation **2:** 87–127.
6. SUGIMURA, T. 1973. Poly(adenosine diphosphate ribose). *In* Progress in Nucleic Acid Research and Molecular Biology. J. Davidson & W. E. Cohn, Eds.: 127–151. Academic Press, Inc. New York, N.Y.
7. BURZIO, L. & S. S. KOIDE. 1976. Isolation and characterization of *Xenopus laevis* oocyte nucleus. Arch. Biol. Med. Exp. In press.
8. DUMONT, J. N. 1972. Oogenesis in *Xenopus laevis* (Daudin). 1. Stages of oocyte development in laboratory maintained animals. J. Morphol. **136:** 153–180.
9. BURZIO, L. O. & S. S. KOIDE. 1970. A functional role of poly ADPR in DNA synthesis. Biochem. Biophys. Res. Commun. **40:** 1013–1020.
10. LOWRY, O. H., N. J. ROSEBROUGH, A. L. FARR & R. J. RANDALL. 1951. Protein measurement with the Folin phenol reagent. J. Biol. Chem. **193:** 265–275.
11. BURZIO, L. O. & S. S. KOIDE. 1976. Biochemical properties of isolated germinal vesicle from *Xenopus* oocyte. In preparation.
12. REYNHOUT, J. K. & L. D. SMITH. 1974. Studies on the appearance of a maturation-inducing factor in the cytoplasm of amphibian oocytes exposed to progesterone. Devel. Biol. **38:** 394–400.
13. BURZIO, L. & S. S. KOIDE. 1973. *In vitro* effect of NAD on DNA synthesis in regenerating liver and Novikoff hepatoma. FEBS Lett. **20:** 29–32.
14. SMULSON, M. & J. ROBERTS. 1973. Biological function of ADP-ribosylation of nuclear projects during the cell cycle of HeLa cell, xeroderma pigmentosum and normal human fibroblasts. *In* Poly(ADP-ribose), An International Symposium. M. Harris, Ed.: 141–160. Fogarty International Center Proceeding 26. Publ. 74–477. Department of Health, Education, and Welfare. Washington, D.C.
15. BURZIO, L. & S. KOIDE. 1973. Activation of the template for DNA synthesis of rat liver nuclei and inhibition by NAD. *In* Poly(ADP-ribose), An International Symposium. M. Harris, Ed.: 117–130. Fogarty International Center Proceeding 26. Publ. 74–477. Department of Health, Education, and Welfare. Washington, D.C.
16. SMITH, J. A. & L. A. STOCKEN. 1975. Chemical and metabolic properties of adenosine diphosphate ribose derivatives of nuclear proteins. Biochem. J. **147:** 523–529.
17. UEDA, K., A. OMACHI, M. KAWAICHI & O. HAYAISHI. 1975. Natural occurrence of poly(ADP-ribose) histone in rat liver. Proc. Nat. Acad. Sci. USA **72:** 205–209.
18. YOSHIHARA, K., Y. TANIGAWA, L. BURZIO & S. S. KOIDE. 1975. Evidence for adenosine diphosphate ribosylation of Ca^{2+}, Mg^{2+}-dependent endonuclease. Proc. Nat. Acad. Sci. USA **72:** 289–293.
19. SMULSON, M. E. & C. RIDEAU. 1972. Nuclear poly adenosine diphosphoribosylation during restricted macromolecular synthesis of HeLa cells. Biochim. Biophys. Acta **111:** 408–416.
20. KIDWELL, W. R. & M. G. MAGE. 1976. Changes in poly(adenosine diphosphate-ribose) and poly(adenosine diphosphate-ribose) polymerase in synchronous HeLa cells. Biochemistry **15:** 1213–1217.
21. CLAYCOMB, W. C. 1976. Inhibition of DNA synthesis in differentiating cardiac muscle by NAD. FEBS Lett. **61:** 231–233.
22. BURZIO, L. & S. S. KOIDE. 1976. Adenosine diphosphate ribosylation of lysine-rich histone (H1) of rat liver. In preparation.
23. DIXON, G. H., E. P. M. CANDIDO, B. M. HONDA, A. J. LOUIE, A. R. MACLEOD & M. T. SUNG. 1975. The biological role of post-synthetic modifications of basic nuclear proteins. *In* The Structure and Function of Chromatin, Ciba Foundation Symposium

28. D. W. Fitzsimons & G. E. W. Wolstenholme, Eds.: 229–250. Elsevier, New York, N.Y.

24. BRADBURY, E. M. & THE BIOPHYSIC'S GROUP. 1975. Histone in chromosome structure and control of cell division. *In* The Structure and Function of Chromatin, Ciba Foundation Symposium 28. D. W. Fitzsimons & G. E. W. Wolstenholme, Eds.: 131–155. Elsevier, New York, N.Y.
25. SMITH, D. L. & R. E. ECKER. 1969. Role of the oocyte nucleus in physiological maturation in *Rana pipiens*. Devel. Biol. **19:** 281–309.
26. KOIDE, S. S. & K. YOSHIHARA. 1973. Purification and characteristics of poly(ADP-Rib) polymerase of rat liver. Biochem. Soc. Trans. **1:** 30–34.
27. BROWN, D. D. & E. LITTNA. 1964. Variations in the synthesis of stable RNA's during oogenesis and development of *Xenopus laevis*. J. Mol. Biol. **8:** 688–695.
28. MORRILL, G. A., F. SCHATZ & V. S. ZABRENETZKY. 1975. RNA and protein synthesis during progesterone-induced germinal vesicle breakdown in *R. pipiens* ovarian tissue. Differentiation **4:** 143–152.
29. SMITH, D. L. 1975. Molecular events during oocyte maturation. *In* The Biochemistry of Animal Development. R. Weber, Ed. Vol. III: 1–46. Academic Press, Inc. New York, N.Y.
30. WALLACE, R. A. & T. HO. 1972. Protein incorporation by isolated amphibian oocytes. II. A survey of inhibitors. J. Exp. Zool. **181:** 303–318.

DISCUSSION

DR. A. W. SCHUETZ: When you inhibition with actinomycin D, do you also get chromosomal condensation?

DR. KOIDE: Actinomycin D inhibits RNA polymerase activity, but germinal vesicle breakdown continues unaffected. Whether there is chromosomal condensation we cannot say. We haven't looked at this problem yet.

QUESTION: Do you think that this change in synthase activity is a direct effect of progesterone, or is it an indirect effect through the induction of the cytoplasmic factor?

DR. KOIDE: We think that probably it's an indirect effect through the induction of cytoplasmic factor. Although we have seen an *in vitro* effect, we would like to confirm this observation before we say yes or no.

DR. E.-E. BAULIEU: Have you tested the activity of the enzyme not in the germinal vesicles but in the cytoplasm?

DR. KOIDE: No, so far we haven't. The activity may be present in the cytoplasm. Robert *et al.* (1975. Arch. Biochem. Biophys. **171:** 305) reported that the activity is in the polyribosomal fraction obtained from HeLa cells, and Kun *et al.* (1975. Proc. Nat. Acad. Sci. USA **72:** 1436) reported that enzymatic activity occurs in the mitochondria. We haven't checked this out at the present time.

INDUCTION OF OOCYTIC MATURATION AND DIFFERENTIATION: MODE OF PROGESTERONE ACTION*

Allen W. Schuetz

Department of Population Dynamics
School of Hygiene and Public Health
The Johns Hopkins University
Baltimore, Maryland 21205

Mechanisms involved in the initiation, mediation, and maintenance of cell differentiation remain central questions of biology. Classically, hormones have been shown to be inducers of cellular differentiation and modulators of cellular synthetic activity in a wide variety of tissues and organs. However, a major difficulty in elucidating the precise role of hormones on differentiation processes is the presence in such tissues of a variety of cell types. It is difficult to assess whether *in vivo* or *in vitro* hormonal effects are due to direct interactions of the hormones with a particular cell type or occur indirectly as a result of cell-cellular interactions. To evaluate and study the hormone-cellular interactions that occur during the process of differentiation, it is advantageous to have a system in which identifiable cells respond to discrete hormones and undergo distinct, readily identifiable morphologic and biochemical transformations. In recent years, the amphibian oocyte and/or ovarian follicle has provided a unique model for the experimental analysis of certain aspects of hormone-cellular interactions, following the demonstration that oocytes were directly responsive to steroidal hormones.[1–4] This system has been particularly helpful in assessing the control and mediation aspects of the fundamental process of meiosis that occurs in the germ cells. Additionally, it has been used to investigate the associated processes of oocytic growth, ovulation, fertilization, activation, and embryogenesis.[6,28–31] Specific characteristics that make the amphibian oocyte and/or follicle a particularly useful model for the analysis of hormone-cellular interactions and for elucidating nucleus-cytoplasmic interactions involved in these processes include their large size and ease of *in vitro* culture, the relative ease of distinguishing different stages of differentiation, the demonstration that differentiation occurs *in vitro,* and the accessibility of oocytes and follicles to microsurgical procedures, including enucleation and microinjection. Studies of oocytic and follicular responsiveness to steroidal and gonadotropic hormones have led to the general hypothesis that gonadotropic hormones initiate meiotic maturation in amphibian oocytes primarily as a result of the local synthesis and/or release of steroidal hormones (progesterone-like) from the follicular cells that surround the individual oocytes within the ovarian follicle.[2–4,12] Although the specific steroids produced by the amphibian ovary have not been identified, recent studies indicate that progesterone synthesis and release occur *in vitro* after addition of human chorionic gonadotropin (HCG) or amphibian pituitary homogenate to ovarian fragments.[5] Induction of ovulation and maturation also occurred in association

*Supported by National Institutes of Health Grants 1-P01 HD05594, 1-R01-HD 07041-01A1, and 5T01 HD00109-09, Population Council Grant 4732.2093.10, and by a grant from the Ford Foundation.

with the secretion of steroidal hormones by the ovarian fragments. Further experimental studies of hormonal effects on amphibian oocytes have established that:

Steroidal induction of nuclear breakdown requires protein synthesis and occurs in the presence of actinomycin D.[2–4]

Estrogenic steroids are ineffective in inducing maturation, even though they are extensively incorporated into oocytes.[1,7,12]

Oocytes sequester large amounts of progesterone and other steroids, and progesterone is extensively metabolized by several pathways.[6–11]

Enucleated oocytes respond to progesterone and undergo subsequent cytoplasmic differentiation, indicating that hormonal effects are not necessarily mediated through the nucleus.[13]

Oocytic cytoplasm acquires new biologic properties after exposure to progesterone and other maturation-inducing steroids. Cytoplasmic factors are transferable to nonhormone-treated oocytes, where they can initiate meiotic maturation and other aspects of physiologic maturation.[14,16,17]

TABLE 1
BIOLOGIC ACTIVITIES ISOLATED FROM AMPHIBIAN OOCYTES DURING INDUCTION OF MEIOTIC MATURATION

Factor	Major Activity	References
Maturation-promoting factor (MPF)	induce germinal vesicle breakdown	14, 15, 17–19, 56, 57
Cytostatic factor	arrest mitosis and cleavage	14
Pseudomaturation-inducing factor (PIF)	abnormal maturation and inhibition of protein synthesis	20, 21
Chromosomal condensation activity (CCA)	induce chromosomal condensation	22–25
DNA synthesis activity	initiate DNA synthesis	22, 26, 27

Significantly, most biologic activities are induced by hormones independent of the presence of the nucleus and appear to require protein synthesis. Recent studies indicate that this maturation-promoting factor(s) is proteinaceous in nature and is heat labile. Its activity is drastically affected by divalent ions.[15] A variety of other biologic activities or factors have also been associated with hormonal treatment and the disintegration of the germinal vesicle. These factors have been designated by the terms cytostatic factor, pseudomaturation factor, chromosomal condensation factor, and substances that initiate DNA synthesis (TABLE 1). These experimental results clearly demonstrate that some of the actions of progesterone and certain other steroids in inducing meiotic maturation in amphibian oocytes are the result of complex interactions between different components of the oocyte and are mediated in many cases by effects on translational rather than transcriptional processes.

In addition to initiating nuclear breakdown and affecting meiotic chromosomal events, progesterone and other maturation-inducing steroids also cause oocytes to change or attain new properties.

Presently being investigated in this laboratory are oocyte cytoplasmic processes that are sensitive to progesterone regulation. These processes include vitellogenin (yolk protein precursor) incorporation into the oocyte and establishment of the conditions for activation and fertilization as a result of changes in the oocyte cortical components. As with nuclear breakdown, mediation of these changes appears to occur in a particular sequence and involves complicated ionic and hormonal, in addition to nuclear and cytoplasmic, interactions, some of which are linked to the nuclear breakdown process. Further studies, to be described, are directed toward elucidating the extent to which steroid-cellular surface interactions are involved in the initiation of maturational changes in the oocyte. In some of the studies discussed here, the steroid desoxycorticosterone acetate (DOCA) was used in place of progesterone to initiate maturation of oocytes. Its effects on maturation appear to be identical to those of progesterone.

Effects of Progestational Steroids on Vitellogenin Incorporation

In amphibians, a major proportion of oocyte growth involves the incorporation of a yolk platelet precursor protein (vitellogenin) across the plasmalemma by a process of micropinocytosis.[31] The precursor protein is produced in the liver under estrogenic stimulation and is transported via the blood to the ovary, where it is subsequently sequestered. Once within the oocyte, vitellogenin undergoes a further molecular rearrangement, with the resultant formation of two distinct yolk proteins, phosvitin and lipovitellin.[32] *In vitro* incorporation and rearrangement of vitellogenin were shown to occur when isolated *Xenopus* oocytes were removed from their outer follicular membranes and incubated with radioactively labeled vitellogenin. Defolliculated *Rana pipiens* oocytes also incorporated *Xenopus*

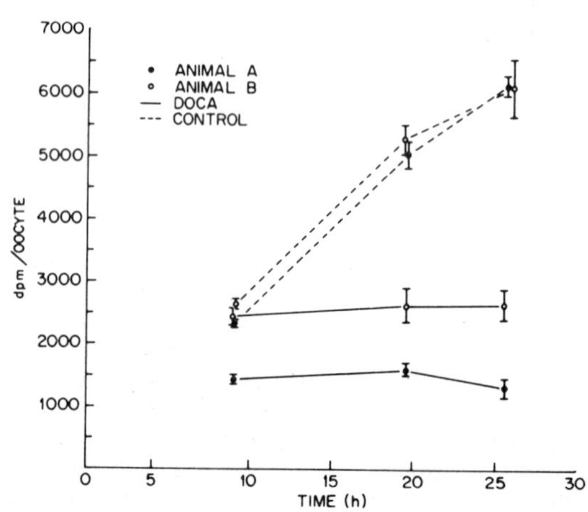

FIGURE 1. Time course effect of desoxycorticosterone acetate on incorporation of [^{3}H]vitellogenin into denuded *R. pipiens* oocytes *in vitro*. Individual oocytes were simultaneously incubated in labeled vitellogenin and either the steroid or the hormone vehicle. Each group consisted of five denuded oocytes obtained from an individual animal. Each point on the graph represents the mean, and the bars represent the standard error of the mean. (From Schuetz *et al.*[33] By permission of *Journal of Cell Biology*.)

TABLE 2

UPTAKE OF [^{3}H]VITELLOGENIN BY ISOLATED OOCYTES OF *R. pipiens* AFTER PREINCUBATION IN THE PRESENCE OR ABSENCE OF STEROID HORMONE*

Animal	Number of Oocytes	dpm/Oocyte	dpm/mm^2
Preincubation with DOCA			
A	5	76 ± 7	8.9
B	5	62 ± 5	7.3
Preincubation controls			
A	5	4427 ± 110	608.9
B	5	3653 ± 568	502.5

*Oocytes were preincubated for 9 hr in amphibian Ringer's solution that contained either DOCA or steroid vehicle (propylene glycol:ethanol, 1:1) before being transferred to medium (50 μl) that contained [^{3}H]vitellogenin. Incubation in [^{3}H]vitellogenin was for 16.5 hr. (From Schuetz *et al.*[33])

vitellogenin *in vitro* over extended periods of time, and this system has been utilized to investigate the effect of steroidal hormones on oocytic capacity to incorporate isotopically labeled vitellogenin.[33] Such studies demonstrate that hormone-induced nuclear breakdown is associated with a marked alteration in the capacity of the oocyte to incorporate vitellogenin. Extensive incorporation of vitellogenin occurred in defolliculated meiotically immature oocytes not exposed to steroidal hormones. Twenty-four hours after the simultaneous addition of [^{3}H]vitellogenin and maturation-inducing steroids (DOCA), suppression of oocytic vitellogenin incorporation was observed. Nuclear breakdown had occurred in these oocytes. If oocytes were simultaneously exposed to steroid and [^{3}H]vitellogenin and subsequently analyzed for vitellogenin incorporation at different times, it was observed that inhibition of incorporation occurred during the later phase of the 24-hr incubation period. During the early period of incubation, vitellogenin incorporation in both control and DOCA-treated oocytes was remarkably similar (FIGURE 1).

Therefore, it appears that oocytic insensitivity to the suppressive effects of DOCA was associated with the presence of the germinal vesicle, whereas sensitivity to suppression was related to the absence of the germinal vesicle. If oocytes were preincubated in steroids prior to exposure to labeled vitellogenin, the lag phase to inhibition was essentially obliterated, which suggests that the alteration in the physiologic activity of the oocyte may be a consequence of the induction of nuclear breakdown (TABLE 2). Ultrastructural studies demonstrated that the oocytic cortex underwent marked structural alterations and that the micropinocytotic process was inhibited in the oocytes that underwent nuclear maturation. Suppressive effects of steroids on vitellogenin uptake were related to the type and dose of steroid with which the oocytes were treated.[34] Both progesterone and DOCA inhibited vitellogenin incorporation, whereas the estrogenic steroid estrone had no suppressive or stimulatory effect. Also, estrone did not induce nuclear breakdown or inhibit micropinocytosis, as determined by ultrastructural analysis.[1,34,35] Doses of active steroids that were insufficient to induce germinal vesicle breakdown appeared to slightly suppress protein incorporation. Ineffectiveness of the estrogenic steroid to inhibit protein incorporation and micropinocytosis or induce maturation was in marked contrast to the capacity of the oocytes to incorporate this steroid.[7] Extended exposure of immature oocytes to ethylenediaminetetraacetate also inhibited vitellogenin incorporation, which suggests that calcium ions may be involved in the sequestration of this protein.[33]

These experimental results indicate that the mechanisms that mediate oocytic maturation and inhibition of vitellogenin incorporation exhibit the same steroidal specificity and are closely linked. Preliminary studies indicate that enucleated immature oocytes also incorporate vitellogenin readily and that maturation-inducing steroids suppress this incorporation.[59] These results provide further evidence for the hypothesis that cytoplasmic factors may also be involved in mediating steroidal inhibition of vitellogenin uptake.

Role of Progesterone in Establishment of Activation Response

In addition to its effects on protein incorporation and induction of germinal vesicle breakdown, progesterone also plays a role in preparing oocytes for activation, fertilization, and embryogenesis. At the time of fertilization, the mature oocyte typically undergoes an activation response that involves elevation of the vitelline membrane and discharge of the cortical granules. These changes are an integral part of the mechanism by which the block to polyspermy is established in amphibians and many other species. Meiotically immature (germinal vesicle) oocytes do not exhibit activation reactions to sperm or to other activating stimuli, such as pricking with a glass needle. Under normal conditions of pituitary-induced ovulation, an activation response can be elicited in the postovulatory period at about the time of second meiotic metaphase arrest.[36,37] After *in vitro* exposure to progesterone and other maturation-inducing steroids, oocytes also attain the capacity to undergo an activation response and fertilization.[4] Strikingly, enucleated meiotically immature oocytes exposed to progesterone undergo cortical granule breakdown (activation) in response to pricking with a glass needle.[13]

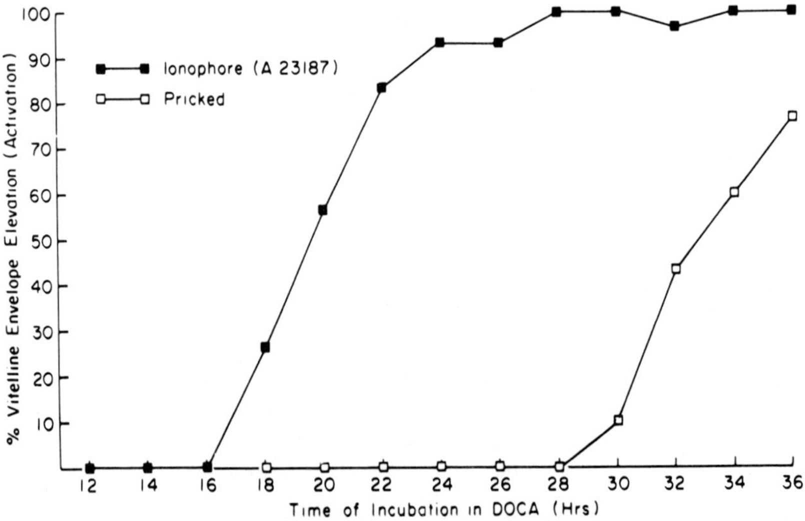

FIGURE 2. Timing of activation in response to ionophore and to pricking after *in vitro* incubation of oocytes with DOCA (1 μg/ml) or pricked with a glass needle at each designated time. After 15 min, the percentage of oocytes that exhibited vitelline envelope elevation was determined. A total of 30 oocytes (10/animal) was examined at each time. (From Belanger & Schuetz.[38] By permission of *Developmental Biology*.)

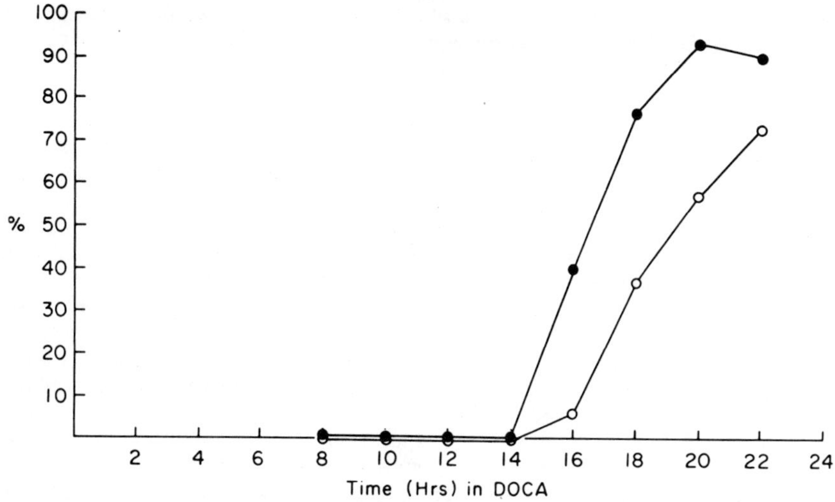

FIGURE 3. Timing of germinal vesicle breakdown and vitelline envelope separation after *in vitro* incubation of oocytes with DOCA (1 μg/ml). Oocytes were fixed in 10% formalin at designated times and were subsequently dissected to determine whether the germinal vesicle was present (•) and/or the vitelline envelope was separated (○) from the oocytic plasma membrane. A total of 30 oocytes (10/animal) was examined at each time. (From Belanger & Schuetz.[38] By permission of *Developmental Biology*.)

However, establishment of the conditions for activation does not appear to occur as an immediate and direct response of the oocyte to progesterone. Time course studies of the onset of the activation response indicate that the hormone-induced differentiation of this response is closely linked to a sequence of nucleus-cytoplasmic interactions and ionic alterations within the oocytes.[38] To study these interrelationships, defolliculated oocytes were exposed to maturation-inducing steroids, and, at regular intervals, groups of oocytes were tested for activation in two ways: by pricking with a glass needle or by treatment with the divalent ionophore A-23187, which is known to initiate an activation response in mature oocytes of a variety of species.[39,40] Activation, as evidenced by vitelline membrane elevation, was scored within 15 min of treatment, and the same oocytes were then fixed and examined to determine if nuclear breakdown and separation of the vitelline membrane from the oocyte plasmalemma had occurred. The results of these studies are depicted in FIGURES 2 and 3. Activation was not observed in any of the hormone-treated oocytes until many hours after initial exposure to the hormones. As anticipated, oocytes attained the capacity to activate in response to pricking many hours after the breakdown of the germinal vesicle. However, in striking contrast, activation was elicited by this ionophore many hours prior to that seen with pricking and was, furthermore, strongly correlated with the time of nuclear breakdown and separation of the vitelline membrane from the oocyte. In none of the hormone-treated oocytes subsequently treated with the ionophore or pricked with a glass needle was there any evidence of activation responses seen before germinal vesicle breakdown. Correlation of the activation process with time of nuclear breakdown and associated vitelline membrane elevation suggests that these events are in some way linked by intermediary processes.

This idea is supported by the fact that both hormone-induced nuclear breakdown and vitelline membrane separation were suppressed by protein synthesis inhibitors[41] and could be induced in immature oocytes by the transfer of cytoplasm from maturing hormone-treated oocytes.[14]

The difference in time of activation onset to ionophore and pricking is particularly striking, and the basis for this difference appears to be of considerable importance in understanding differentiation of the oocyte.[38] Several studies indicate that the ionophore acts by liberating endogenous pools of divalent cations or by transporting such cations across membranes. Thus, these results suggest that hormone-induced changes in oocytes responsive to an ionophore may include increase in the availability of divalent cations or alterations in the sensitivity of the cortical granules and/or oocytic surface. That cortical granules are already present in the immature oocyte at the time of hormone exposure indicates that the effects of the maturation-inducing steroid are not the result of cortical granule formation.

Activation in response to pricking or fertilization is generally considered to be a response that is propagated around the oocyte from the site of sperm entry or pricking. In contrast, some evidence sugggests that an ionophore elicits a cortical reaction only in the portion of the oocytic surface with which it is in direct contact.[58] On the basis of these differences, it was suggested that the interval between activation onset to ionophore or pricking stimulation may include the differentiation of processes related to the ability of the oocytic surface to translate a pricking stimulus into a wave of cortical granule breakdown.[38] Other investigators have shown that contractile elements in the cortex of mature oocytes respond to an ionophore and may also be involved in the activation events in the maturing oocytes.[42–44] Pigment migration and the capping phenomenon were also noted in many of the ionophore-treated oocytes after germinal vesicle breakdown. Although the ionophore data indicate that ionic alterations occur during maturation, analysis of mature and immature oocytes for extractable elements (calcium, sodium, and potassium) by atomic absorption spectrophotometry has to date revealed no significant differences.[60] In contrast, experiments that involved the direct microinjection of calcium into oocytes at various stages of hormone-induced differentiation have been shown to initiate aspects of the activation response, including cortical granule breakdown.[45] The type of response elicited varied with the stage of oocytic differentiation at the time of calcium injection. These results support the idea that ionic alterations occur in response to progesterone.

Steroid-Cell Surface Interactions

The preceding discussion and other data clearly indicate that a multitude of biochemical, morphologic, and functional properties of oocytes are altered after their exposure to maturation-inducing steroids, especially progesterone.[46–53] From early studies, it is clear that the duration of oocytic exposure to steroid required to initiate maturation is very short (minutes) relative to the onset of nuclear breakdown (typically more than 10 hr); however, the site and mechanisms involved in the induction or triggering of these responses remain largely unknown.[2,4] On the basis of the ineffectiveness of progesterone to initiate maturation when injected into oocytes, it has been postulated that steroids effect maturational changes at the cell surface.[13,14] Induction of maturation in *Xenopus* oocytes not previously exposed to progesterone was recently shown to occur in response to organomercurials. Their site of action is also considered to be at the surface.[20]

A question of particular interest is to what extent the initiation of physiologic change in the oocyte is determined by interaction of steroid with the total surface of the oocyte. However, to investigate this question, a method for the localized application or restricted exclusion of steroid from specific areas of the oocytic or follicular surface is required. Additionally, it must not interfere with the capacity of oocytes to undergo maturation. Such a method has recently been devised and involves the placement of follicles and/or oocytes into a vertically held disposable pipette tip of a particular size.[54] After addition of the oocyte or follicle to the pipette tip, a designated volume of incubation medium is added to the upper reservoir. Steroids or other compounds to be locally applied to the oocyte or follicle are dissolved in 200 μl of incubation medium and placed into wells of a spotting plate. The pipette tip that contains the oocyte or follicle is then lowered into this 200-μl reservoir. Treatment of the exposed undersurface of the follicle or oocyte was accomplished by mixing the steroid-containing fluid in the 200-μl reservoir with the small amount of fluid between the lower surface of the follicle and the end of the pipette. To establish what proportion of the oocytic surface was isolated in the lower reservoir and to determine whether leakage between the two media compartments occurred, a concentrated (0.1%) solution of toluidine blue was added to the lower compartment. Under these circumstances, the surface exposed to steroid becomes darkly stained, and even after 24 hr, no evidence of dye leakage into the upper compartment was detected. Furthermore, studies of radioactive progesterone uptake by part of or the total surface of the oocyte demonstrated that incorporation per unit area was essentially identical. These results suggest that accessibility of steroid to the surface in the pipette was not impaired.[55] To determine if oocytes maintained in such pipettes were viable, the whole surface of follicles was exposed to concentrated steroid solution for 10 min prior to being placed in the pipettes. After a 24-hr incubation in pipettes, steroid-treated, but not control, oocytes had undergone nuclear breakdown. In subsequent studies, it was observed that when follicles were exposed over all or part of their surface to equal concentrations of steroid, they underwent maturation to different extents.[55] Exposure of the total follicular surface to steroid was much more effective in inducing nuclear breakdown. A possible explanation for the lesser effectiveness of steroid applied locally was revealed following the assessment of the distribution of progesterone within the oocyte after its local application. Radioactive progesterone was applied to a portion of the surface, and the exposed areas were marked. Oocytes were subsequently fixed by boiling and then divided into approximately equal portions, one of which contained the surface exposed to steroid. Even after 24 hr of incubation, more than 90% of the radioactivity remained localized at the site of application, irrespective of whether it was applied to the animal or vegetable oocytic hemisphere. Clearly, then, diffusion of steroid throughout the oocyte is not a rapid process, and this finding may in part explain why injected steroids are ineffective as inducers of maturation.[55,60]

Summary

Full-grown amphibian oocytes, arrested in prophase I or meiosis, respond *in vitro* to progesterone and certain other steroids. They undergo an apparently normal sequence of nuclear maturation and cytoplasmic differentiation, which are necessary precedents for fertilization and embryogenesis. Individual oocytes or populations of these cells thus provide a model system for investigations concerning the nature and mechanism of hormone-cellular interactions. In this system, previous studies have shown that certain aspects of hormonal (progesterone, DOCA) induction of morphologic and biochemical differentiation in the nucleus can be induced in part, as a result of the formation of secondary cytoplasmic factors, some of which do not require the presence of the nucleus for their formation. In addition to initiating nuclear events, progesterone or DOCA alters the functional activity of the plasma membrane and establishes the conditions necessary for fertilization and activation. Uptake of radioactive vitellogenin, a yolk protein precursor, was inhibited by progesterone and DOCA. Maximum inhibition was dependent on induction of nuclear breakdown, the dose of steroid used, and was correlated with morphologic alterations at the oocytic surface. Estrone neither stimulated nor inhibited vitellogenin incorporation and had no effect on nuclear breakdown. Oocytic capacity to exhibit activation responses (vitelline membrane elevation) was dependent on oocytic exposure to progesterone or DOCA and development subsequent to the initiation of nuclear breakdown. Onset of the activation response after steroid treatment varied with the type of activation stimulus utilized (pricking or divalent ionophore A-23187). The results suggest that hormones cause ionic alterations in oocytes and that ions are directly involved in the activation response. To study steroid interaction with the cell surface, a method was developed for culturing oocytes that permits localized application of steroids to portions of the oocytic or follicular surface. The results obtained suggest that oocytes exposed to steroid over part of their surface do not respond, with regard to nuclear breakdown, in the same manner as do oocytes exposed over their entire surface to similar concentrations of steroid. Studies of isotopic distribution within the oocyte after local application of steroid indicate that hormone does not readily diffuse through the oocyte. Evidence for the role of cytoplasmic factors in the mediation of nuclear and cytoplasmic events is discussed.

Acknowledgments

The contributions of Drs. A. Belanger, J. Cloud, J. Dumont, T. Hollinger, and R. Wallace to the studies reported here are greatly appreciated.

References

1. Schuetz, A. W. 1967. Effect of steroids on the germinal vesicle of oocytes of the frog (*Rana pipiens*) *in vitro*. Proc. Soc. Exp. Biol. Med. **124:** 1307–1310.
2. Schuetz, A. W. 1967. Action of hormones in germinal vesicle breakdown in frog (*Rana pipiens*) oocytes. J. Exp. Zool. **166:** 347–354.
3. Masui, Y. 1967. Relative roles of the pituitary, follicle cells and progesterone in the induction of oocyte maturation in *Rana pipiens*. J. Exp. Zool. **166:** 365–376.
4. Smith, L. D., R. E. Ecker & S. Subtelny. 1968. *In vitro* induction of physiological maturation in *Rana pipiens* oocytes removed from their ovarian follicles. Devel. Biol. **17:** 627–643.
5. Fortune, J. E., P. W. Concannon & W. Hansel. 1975. Ovarian progesterone levels during *in vitro* oocyte maturation and ovulation in *Xenopus laevis*. Biol. Reprod. **13:** 561–567.
6. Schuetz, A. W. 1972. Hormones and follicular functions. *In* Oogenesis. J. D. Biggers & A. W. Schuetz, Eds.: 479–511. University Park Press. Baltimore, Md.
7. Smith, L. D. & R. E. Ecker. 1971. The interaction of steroids with *Rana pipiens* oocytes in the induction of maturation. Devel. Biol. **25:** 232–247.
8. Schatz, F. & G. A. Morrill. 1975. 5β-Reductive pathway of progesterone metabolism in the amphibian ovarian cytosol. Biol. Reprod. **13:** 408–414.

9. OZON, R., R. BELLE', C. SERRES & C. FOUCHET. 1975. Mechanism of action of progesterone on amphibian oocytes. A possible biological role for progesterone metabolism. Mol. Cell. Endocrinol. **3:** 221–231.
10. REYNHOUT, J. K. & L. D. SMITH. 1973. Evidence for steroid metabolism during the *in vitro* induction of maturation in oocytes of *Rana pipiens*. Devel. Biol. **30:** 392–402.
11. THIBIER-FOUCHET, C., D. MULNER & R. OZON. 1976. Progesterone biosynthesis and metabolism by ovarian follicles and isolated oocytes of *Xenopus laevis*. Biol. Reprod. **14:** 317–326.
12. SCHUETZ, A. W. 1971. *In vitro* induction of ovulation and oocyte maturation in *Rana pipiens* ovarian follicles. Effects of steroidal and non-steroidal hormones. J. Exp. Zool. **178:** 377–386.
13. SMITH, L. D. & R. E. ECKER. 1969. Role of the oocyte nucleus in physiological maturation in *Rana pipiens*. Devel. Biol. **19:** 281–309.
14. MASUI, Y. & C. L. MARKERT. 1971. Cytoplasmic control of nuclear behavior during meiotic maturation of frog oocytes. J. Exp. Zool. **177:** 129–146.
15. WASSERMAN, W. J. & Y. MASUI. 1976. A cytoplasmic factor promoting oocyte maturation: its extraction and preliminary characterization. Science **191:** 1266–1268.
16. GURDON, J. B. & H. R. WOODLAND. 1968. The cytoplasmic control of nuclear activity in animal development. Biol. Rev. **43:** 233–267.
17. REYNHOUT, J. K. & L. D. SMITH. 1974. Studies on the appearance and nature of a maturation-inducing factor in the cytoplasm of amphibian oocytes exposed to progesterone. Devel. Biol. **38:** 394–400.
18. MASUI, Y. 1972. Distribution of the cytoplasmic activity inducing germinal vesicle breakdown in frog oocytes. J. Exp. Zool. **179:** 365–368.
19. DETTLAFF, T. A., L. A. NIKITINA & O. G. STROEVA. 1964. The role of the germinal vesicle in oocyte maturation in anurans as revealed by removal and transplantation of nuclei. J. Embryol. Exp. Morphol. **12:** 851–873.
20. BRACHET, J., E. BALTUS, A. PAYS-DESCHUTTER, J. HANOCQ-QUERTIER, E. HUBERT & G. STEINERT. 1975. Induction of maturation (meiosis) in *Xenopus laevis* oocytes by three organomercurials. Proc. Nat. Acad. Sci. USA **72:** 1574–1578.
21. BRACHET, J., E. BALTUS, A. DESCHUTTER, F. HANOCQ-QUERTIER, E. HUBERT, S. JACOBELLI & G. STEINERT. 1974. Biochemical changes during progesterone-induced maturation in *Xenopus laevis* oocytes. Mol. Cell. Biochem. **3:** 189–205.
22. GURDON, J. B. 1967. On the origin and persistence of a cytoplasmic state inducing DNA synthesis in frogs' eggs. Proc. Nat. Acad. Sci. USA **58:** 545–552.
23. GURDON, J. B. 1968. Changes in somatic cell nuclei inserted into growing and maturing amphibian oocytes. J. Embryol. Exp. Morphol. **20:** 401–414.
24. ZIEGLER, D. H. & Y. MASUI. 1973. Control of chromosome behavior in amphibian oocytes. I. The activity of maturing oocytes inducing chromosome condensation in transplanted brain nuclei. Devel. Biol. **35:** 283–292.
25. ZIEGLER, D. & Y. MASUI. 1976. Control of chromosome behavior in amphibian oocytes. II. The effect of inhibitors of RNA and protein synthesis on the induction of chromosome condensation in transplanted brain nuclei by oocyte cytoplasm. J. Cell. Biol. **68:** 620–628.
26. GRAHAM, C. F., K. ARMS & J. B. GURDON. 1966. The induction of DNA synthesis by frog egg cytoplasm. Devel. Biol. **14:** 349–381.
27. BENBOW, R. M. & C. C. FORD. 1975. Cytoplasmic control of nuclear DNA synthesis during early development of *Xenopus laevis:* a cell-free assay. Proc. Nat. Acad. Sci. USA **72**(6): 2437–2441.
28. SCHUETZ, A. W. 1974. Role of hormones in oocyte maturation. Biol. Reprod. **10:** 150–178.
29. SMITH, L. D. & R. E. ECKER. 1970. Regulatory processes in the maturation and early cleavage of amphibian eggs. *In* Current Topics in Developmental Biology. A. A. Moscona & A. Monroy, Eds. Vol. 5: 1–38. Academic Press, Inc. New York, N.Y.
30. SMITH, L. D. 1975. Molecular events during oocyte maturation. *In* Biochemistry of Animal Development. R. Weber, Ed. Vol III: 1–46. Academic Press, Inc. New York, N.Y.
31. WALLACE, R. A. & E. W. BERGINK. 1974. Amphibian vitellogenin: properties,

hormonal regulation of hepatic synthesis and ovarian uptake, and conversion to yolk proteins. Amer. Zool. **14:** 1159–1175.

32. Wallace, R. A., J. M. Nickol, T. Ho & D. W. Jared. 1972. Studies on amphibian yolk. X. The relative roles of autosynthetic and heterosynthetic processes during yolk protein assembly by isolated oocytes. Devel. Biol. **29:** 255–270.
33. Schuetz, A. W., R. A. Wallace & J. N. Dumont. 1974. Steroid inhibition of protein incorporation by isolated amphibian oocytes. J. Cell. Biol. **61:** 26–34.
34. Schuetz, A. W., R. A. Wallace & J. N. Dumont. 1964. Inhibition of protein incorporation by isolated amphibian oocytes: steroid dose and specificity relationships. J. Cell Biol. **63:** 305a (Abs.).
35. Schuetz, A. W. 1972. Effect of estrogens on pituitary and progesterone induced events in ovarian follicles of *Rana pipiens in vitro*. Gen. Comp. Endocrinol. **18:** 32–36.
36. Subtelny, S. & C. Bradt. 1961. Transplantations of blastula nuclei into activated eggs from the body cavity and from the uterus of *Rana pipiens*. II. Development of the recipient body cavity eggs. Develop. Biol. **3:** 96–114.
37. Kemp, N. E. & N. I. Istock. 1967. Cortical changes in growing oocytes and in fertilized or pricked eggs of *Rana pipiens*. J. Cell Biol. **34:** 111–122.
38. Belanger, A. M. & A. W. Schuetz. 1975. Precocious induction of activation responses in amphibian oocytes by divalent ionophore A-23187. Devel. Biol. **45:** 378–381.
39. Steinhardt, R. A., D. Epel, E. J. Carroll, Jr. & R. Yanagimachi. 1974. Activation of sea-urchin eggs by a calcium ionophore. Proc. Nat. Acad. Sci. USA **71:** 1915–1919.
40. Steinhardt, R. A., D. Epel, E. J. Carroll, Jr. & R. Yanagimachi. 1974. Is calcium ionophore a universal activator for unfertilized eggs? Nature (London) **25:** 41–43.
41. Schuetz, A. W. 1972. Hormone induction of structural changes in the preovulatory amphibian ovarian follicle. Biol. Reprod. **6:** 67–77.
42. Schroeder, T. E. & D. L. Strickland. 1974. Ionophore A-23187, calcium and contractility in frog eggs. Exp. Cell Res. **83:** 139–142.
43. Elinson, R. P. 1975. Site of sperm entry and a cortical contraction associated with egg activation in the frog (*Rana pipiens*). Devel. Biol. **47:** 257–268.
44. Schroeder, T. E. 1974. Ionophore-induced contractions in frog eggs: role of action. J. Cell Biol. **63:** 305a (Abs.).
45. Hollinger, T. & A. W. Schuetz. 1976. Cleavage and cortical granule breakdown in *Rana pipiens* oocytes induced by direct microinjection of calcium. J. Cell Biol. **71:** 395–401.
46. Baltus, E., J. Brachet, J. Hanocq-Quertier & E. Hubert. 1973. Cytochemical and biochemical studies on progesterone induced maturation in amphibian oocytes (effects of inhibitors and of a "maturation promoting factor"). Differentiation **1:** 127–143.
47. Wiblet, M. 1974. Protein kinase activities during maturation in *Xenopus laevis* oocytes. Biochem. Biophys. Res. Commun. **60**(3): 991–998.
48. Hanocq, F., A. DeSchutter, E. Hubert & J. Brachet. 1974. Cytochemical and biochemical studies on progesterone-induced maturation in amphibian oocytes. 2. DNA synthesis. Differentiation **2:** 75–90.
49. Brachet, J., E. Baltus, A. DeSchutter, F. Hanocq, J. Hanocq-Quertier, E. Hubert, S. Jacobelli & G. Steinert. 1974. Biochemical changes during progesterone-induced maturation in *Xenopus laevis* oocytes. Mol. Cell. Biochem. **3**(3): 189–205.
50. Jacobelli, S., J. Hanocq, E. Baltus & J. Brachet. 1974. Hormone-induced maturation of *Xenopus laevis* oocytes: effects of different steroids and study of the properties of a progesterone receptor. Differentiation **2:** 129–135.
51. LaMarca, M. J., M. C. Strobel Fidler, L. D. Smith & K. Keem. 1975. Hormonal effects on RNA synthesis by stage 6 oocytes of *Xenopus laevis*. Devel. Biol. **47:** 384–393.
52. Grippo, P., G. Locorotondo & A. Caruso. 1975. Characterization of the two major

DNA polymerase activities in oocytes and eggs of *Xenopus laevis*. FEBS Lett. **51**(1): 137–142.
53. Brachet, J., A. Pays-DeSchutter & E. Hubert. 1975. Studies on maturation in *Xenopus laevis* oocytes. III. Energy production and requirements for protein synthesis. Differentiation **3:** 3–14.
54. Schuetz, A. W. & J. G. Cloud. 1976. Hormone-cell surface interactions *in vitro*: method for simultaneous incubation and application of substances to isolated portions of the surface of individual amphibian ovarian follicles or oocytes. Submitted for publication.
55. Cloud, J. & A. W. Schuetz. 1975. Hormone-cell surface interactions in the induction of amphibian oocyte maturation. J. Cell Biol. **67:** 73a (Abs.).
56. Wasserman, W. J. & Y. Masui. 1975. Effects of cycloheximide on a cytoplasmic factor initiating meiotic maturation in *Xenopus* oocytes. Exp. Cell Res. **91:** 381–388.
57. Schorderet-Slatkine, S. & K. C. Drury. 1973. Progesterone induced maturation in oocytes of *Xenopus laevis:* appearance of a maturation promoting factor in enucleated oocytes. Cell Different. **2:** 247–254.
58. Chambers, E. L., B. C. Pressman & B. Rose. 1974. Parthenogenetic activation of sea urchin eggs by divalent ionophores. J. Cell Biol. **63:** 56a (Abs.).
59. Schuetz, A. W., R. Wallace & J. Dumont. 1976. Unpublished observations.
60. Schuetz, A. W. 1976. Unpublished observations.

Discussion

Dr. S. S. Koide: Recently, it was reported that the progesterone receptor in the frog oocytic cytoplasm may be located in the melanosomes. Do you have any idea as to the function of progesterone interaction with the melanosomes?

Dr. Schuetz: The studies of Ozon and Belle (1973) indicate that progesterone binds to the melanosomal component of oocytes after they are homogenized and fractionated. Although these results have been interpreted in terms of the existence of a progesterone receptor in oocytes, the question of whether this binding is of significance to the meiotic maturation process remains to be demonstrated. It must be remembered that these studies were performed with homogenized oocytes. It has not been shown that progesterone incorporated into intact oocytes is localized in the melanosomal fraction subsequent to homogenization. In our studies (Cloud & Schuetz. 1975–6. J. Cell Biol. Abs.), we find no differential uptake of progesterone by the pigmented portion of the oocyte after local application of steroid to the oocytic surface. The fact that albino frogs reproduce also needs to be considered. Thus, in my view, the question of whether there is a functional interaction of progesterone with the melanosomes has not been resolved.

Dr. E.-E. Baulieu: Would you comment on how you measure what you call "bound" progesterone?

Dr. Schuetz: In our experiments (Cloud & Schuetz. 1975. J. Cell. Biol.), progesterone incorporation or binding to individual oocytes is monitored with the use of isotopically labeled progesterone added to the incubation medium. After incubation, the oocytes are washed, digested in protosol, and the radioactivity is then assayed. Bound progesterone in our experiments thus refers to the radioactivity retained in the oocytes after these procedures rather than to the amount of radioactivity present in progesterone isolated from the oocytes.

Dr. Schatz: Dr. Schuetz, you know progesterone is rapidly metabolized by the oocyte. Do you have any indication that what you are calling progesterone is, in fact, progesterone?

DR. SCHUETZ: No, I assume that progesterone is probably metabolized to a major extent after its entry into the oocyte. Whether progesterone or these metabolites are actually initiating maturation clearly is an important question that needs to be resolved.

DR. G. A. MORRILL (*Albert Einstein College of Medicine, Bronx, N.Y.*): I have one comment that fits in nicely with your story. We found that oocytic plasma membrane depolarizes at the time of germinal vesicle breakdown in response to progesterone. The depolarization occurs in enucleated eggs on the same time course and is blocked by cycloheximide. This finding suggests that progesterone is not acting directly on the membrane but via cytoplasmic factors.

DISCUSSION PAPER: INDUCTION BY PROGESTERONE AND A "MATURATION-PROMOTING FACTOR" OF SOLUBLE PROTEINS IN *XENOPUS LAEVIS* OOCYTES *IN VITRO**

Sabine Schorderet-Slatkine

Experimental Zoology Station
University of Geneva
Geneva, Switzerland

Etienne-Emile Baulieu

Molecular Metabolism and Steroid Physiopathology Research Unit
INSERM, Hospital Bicêtre
University of Paris-Sud
94270 Bicêtre, France

In amphibian eggs, until the blastula stage, protein synthesis is mainly controlled at the translational level.[1] An appropriate hormonal stimulus is needed to trigger the transition of oocytes to eggs. *In vitro*, progesterone and other steroids can induce true maturation (meiosis) of *Xenopus laevis* oocytes.[2] In the present study, germinal vesicle breakdown (GVBD) has been used as a suitable index to follow the process of maturation.

The use of protein synthesis inhibitors has revealed that the physiologic response to progesterone depends on protein synthesis.[3–6] This finding suggests that specific protein(s), essential for the initiation of oocytic maturation and egg development, might be induced by progesterone. We have previously demonstrated the preferential labeling of some proteins in *X. laevis* oocytes after incubation with progesterone ("induced proteins").[7] It has also been established that a "maturation-promoting factor" (MPF) appears during progesterone-induced maturation. MPF is operationally defined by its capability to induce GVBD after transfer into nonhormone-treated recipient oocytes[5,8] and acts even in the presence of cycloheximide.[2,9] Similar transfer experiments have also shown that MPF induces more MPF and that this "autocatalytic"[8,10,11] amplification process is protein synthesis dependent.[2] Finally, it is known that the formation of MPF, induced by progesterone or by MPF itself, can occur in enucleated oocytes.[10]

This paper describes the possible relationship between the progesterone-induced proteins and the synthesis and action of MPF. The induction of specific proteins by progesterone and MPF is an example of the progressive utilization of stored mRNA molecules during development.

Materials and Methods

Oocyte Collection and Induced Maturation

Ovarian tissues were removed from *X. laevis* females through a small incision made on the lateral abdominal wall. To obtain full-grown oocytes free of follicular

*Supported in part by the Ford Foundation, le Fond National Suisse (Grant 3171063), and the World Health Organization.

cells, the ovaries were treated with collagenase,[12] and, if necessary, the last follicle cell layer was removed by hand with watchmaker's forceps. In each experiment, all oocytes were obtained from the same animal. Experiments were conducted at room temperature in Gurdon's solution.[13]

When maturation was induced by steroids, the oocytes were incubated for a 30-min period. Then, they were repeatedly washed and left to mature. Maturation was scored by the appearance of GVBD. Hormones were mostly progesterone (10 μM) and occasionally pregnenolone (5-pregnene-3β-ol-20-one) or cortisol (50 μM). When *p*-chloromercuribenzoate (PCMB, 0.1 mM) replaced the hormone, it was administered throughout the maturation period.

In other experiments, maturation was provoked with MPF-containing cytoplasm. A fraction (approximatively 40 nl) of the cytoplasm of mature (progesterone-treated) oocytes was taken with a micropipette and immediately transferred into each recipient oocyte.

Protein Labeling and Analysis

Injection Experiments

Twenty-five treated oocytes and 25 controls were each injected with 80 nl of radioactive amino acid solution.

Usually, treated oocytes received ^{3}H-labeled amino acids, and controls received ^{14}C-labeled amino acids. The following radiolabeled amino acids were obtained from Amersham: [^{3}H]leucine, 58 or 53 Ci/mmol; [^{14}C]leucine, 324, 330, or 348 mCi/mmol; [^{3}H]lysine, 12 Ci/mmol; [^{14}C]lysine, 348 mCi/mmol; [^{3}H]valine, 2 Ci/mmol; [^{14}C]valine, 280 μCi/mmol.

Appropriate amounts of nonradioactive amino acids were added to obtain identical concentrations of ^{3}H- and ^{14}C-labeled amino acids and a ^{3}H/^{14}C disintegrations per minute (dpm) ratio of about 10. After amino acid injection, oocytes were incubated for 2 hr and then washed. Treated and control oocytes were pooled and homogenized together in 2 ml of the saline solution. The 105,000*g* supernatant was obtained as reported previously.[7]

Incubation Experiments

Oocytes were incubated in a medium that contained radioactive leucine (0.3 mM), with an isotopic dpm ratio of approximately 10 for ^{3}H-treated versus ^{14}C-untreated cells. The oocytes, suspended in 0.1 ml of medium, were usually left for 2 hr at room temperature. The rate of maturation was established by observing additional oocytes from the same animal (see FIGURES 5a & 5b).

Additional Procedures

Enucleation

The germinal vesicles of 50 oocytes were extruded, and 25 enucleated cells were exposed to progesterone for 30 min.

Actinomycin D (AMD)

Twenty-five oocytes were incubated in AMD (50 μg/ml) for 1 hr before the addition of progesterone, and the two drugs were left until 100% GVBD was observed. Then, [^{3}H]leucine was injected. Controls were exposed only to AMD for the same period of time and injected with [^{14}C]leucine.

Ethidium Bromide

Ethidium bromide (20 μg/ml) was used either exactly the same way as AMD or, in other experiments, 80 nl of a 200 μg/ml solution were injected into oocytes 15 min before progesterone; the cells were then further incubated in medium that contained ethidium bromide.

Both AMD and ethidium bromide have already been used under similar conditions. It is known that AMD enters germinal vesicles and that ethidium bromide blocks mitochondrial DNA synthesis.[14] Neither AMD nor ethidium bromide affects the overall protein labeling of nonhormone-treated oocytes.

Cycloheximide

Twenty-five oocytes were incubated in cycloheximide (40 μg/ml) together with progesterone, and the two drugs were left until 100% GVBD was obtained in progesterone-treated oocytes, observed in the absence of inhibitor. Then, [^{3}H]leucine was injected. Control oocytes were exposed only to cycloheximide for the same period of time and injected with [^{14}C]leucine. In other experiments, the maturation inducer was MPF instead of progesterone. Here, 50 oocytes were each injected first with 25 μl of cycloheximide solution (10 mg/ml). After 15 min, MPF was injected into 25 oocytes, and maturation was left to proceed, with the cells remaining in a 40 μg/ml cycloheximide solution. At 100% maturation (2.5 hr), [^{3}H]leucine was injected and left for 2 hr. The other 25 oocytes received inactive cytoplasm instead of MPF and [^{14}C]leucine instead of [^{3}H]leucine.

In all experiments with metabolic inhibitors, we checked that oocytes of the same animal responded normally to progesterone or MPF.

Protein Analysis

Dialysis concentration and electrophoresis were performed as previously described.[7] Sodium dodecyl sulfate (SDS, 0.1%) polyacrylamide gel (6%) electrophoresis was performed at 2 mA per tube for 20 min and then at 5 mA per tube. Gels were reelectrophoresed in 7% acetic acid for 2 hr and immediately sliced. Soluene (0.5 ml) was added, and the suspension was left for 3 hr at 50°C. Ten milliliters of a mixture of PPO (7 g), POPOP (0.6 g), and toluol (1 liter) were added to each vial. In some experiments, mercaptoethanol (2%) was added for 4 min at 100°C to the protein extract before electrophoresis.

RESULTS

Proteins Induced by Progesterone and Other Hormones

During *in vitro* progesterone-induced maturation, several "peaks" are observed along the ^{3}H/^{14}C pattern of soluble proteins. This finding indicates a progesterone-induced increased labeling of discrete entities, in addition to the labeling of many proteins already found in the absence of the hormone (FIGURE 1, *top*). There is no evidence that progesterone increases the labeling of proteins from the particle fractions of the homogenate.[7]

As seen in FIGURE 1, two distinct complex peaks are regularly observed. Both show roughly a 150–200% increase above the mean $^3H/^{14}C$ ratio. Several smaller peaks are observed between the two major fractions. One is often partially superimposed on the largest molecular weight protein peak; four others are found rather regularly, although their $^3H/^{14}C$ ratios are only approximately 20% higher than the baseline. FIGURE 1 (*top*), which presents the protein patterns of progesterone and control oocytes separately, shows that the $^3H/^{14}C$ peaks correspond to an actual increase in ^3H labeling and not to a decrease in ^{14}C-labeled

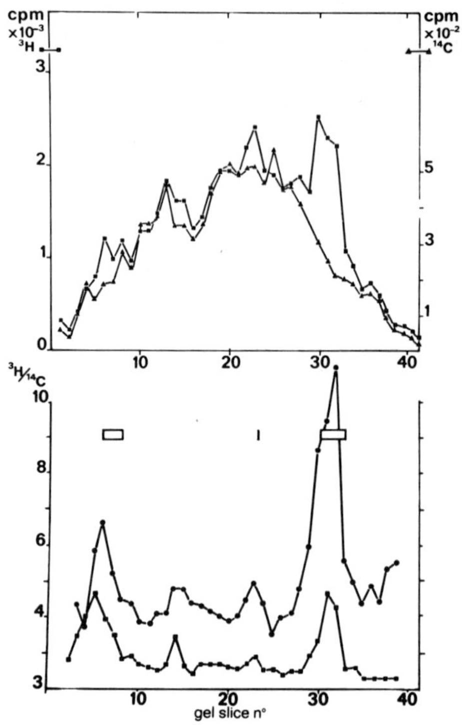

FIGURE 1. Proteins during hormone- and MPF-induced oocytic maturation. Approximately 8 hr after exposure to progesterone, at 100% GVBD, 25 oocytes are injected with [^{3}H]leucine, and 25 untreated oocytes are injected with [^{14}C]leucine. SDS-acrylamide electrophoresis is performed as indicated under MATERIALS AND METHODS (migration toward anode on the left). The upper panel of the Figure represents the labeling pattern of the 105,000*g* supernatant proteins in progesterone-treated oocytic proteins (■) and untreated oocytic proteins (▲). The upper curve (●) of the lower panel shows the corresponding $^3H/^{14}C$ ratio.

Approximately 1.5 hr after transfer of cytoplasm that contains MPF activity into recipient oocytes, 25 oocytes that exhibit GVBD are injected with [^{3}H]leucine for 2 hr. Twenty-five oocytes that have been injected 1.5 hr before with inactive cytoplasm are injected with [^{14}C]leucine for 2 hr. The lower curve (■) of the lower panel shows the $^3H/^{14}C$ ratio of the labeled 105,000*g* supernatant proteins. the two rectangles and the bar indicate the three protein peaks and have been systematically included in other Figures to indicate the reproducibility of the $^3H/^{14}C$ pattern.

proteins. Inversion of the isotopes ([^{14}C]leucine in progesterone-treated cells and [^{3}H]leucine in controls) leads to the same peaks (FIGURE 2, *top*). Replacement of radioactive leucine by radioactive valine or lysine also gives the same pattern (FIGURE 2). Moreover, control/control experiments with injection of the same amino acid in ^3H and ^{14}C forms into nontreated oocytes do not yield any peak (FIGURE 3, *top*). Finally, pretreatment of extracts with mercaptoethanol does not change the electrophoretic pattern, which emphasizes that the two main peaks are not produced by some artificial aggregation.

When cortisol and pregnenolone are used instead of progesterone, 100% GVBD is also obtained, and the oocytes develop the same protein pattern (data not shown).

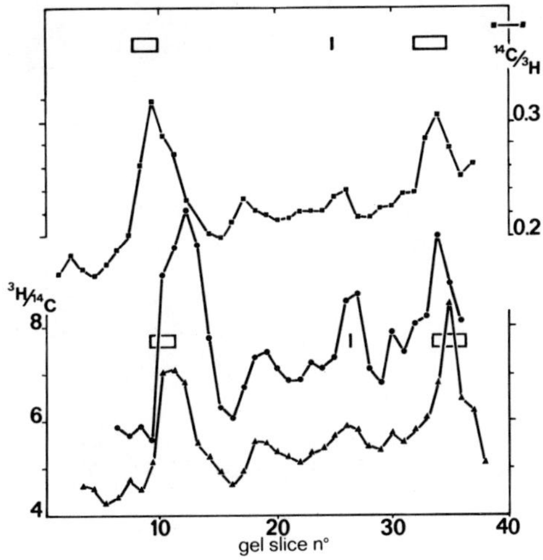

FIGURE 2. Proteins during progesterone-induced oocytic maturation, as revealed by use of differently labeled amino acids. The upper part of the Figure represents the pattern of the $^{14}C/^{3}H$ ratio of 105,000g supernatant leucine-labeled proteins (■) (progesterone treated, ^{14}C; untreated, ^{3}H). The lower part of the Figure represents the $^{3}H/^{14}C$ ratio of the valine-labeled proteins (●) and of the lysine-labeled proteins (▲) (progesterone treated, ^{3}H; untreated, ^{14}C).

Proteins Induced by Organomercurials

Exposure to PCMB induces maturation within the same time as does exposure to progesterone.[17,18] Incubation with PCMB also yields the same induced proteins as does incubation with hormones, although there is a lower $^{3}H/^{14}C$ baseline ratio (FIGURE 3, bottom plot).

Effects of MPF-Containing Cytoplasm

After MPF-containing cytoplasm is transferred into recipient oocytes, amino acids are injected at different times during maturation, left for 2 hr, and proteins are analyzed in comparison with oocytes injected with inactive cytoplasm from

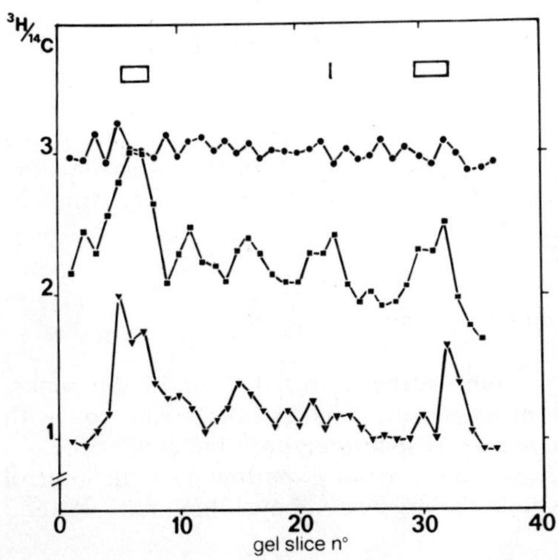

FIGURE 3. Proteins during PCMB-induced maturation. At GVBD, 25 oocytes are injected with [^{3}H]leucine for 2 hr. Twenty-five untreated oocytes are injected with [^{14}C]leucine (▼). Controls are the $^{3}H/^{14}C$ pattern ratio obtained when 25 untreated oocytes are injected with [^{14}C]leucine for 2 hr (●) and proteins when maturation is induced by progesterone (■).

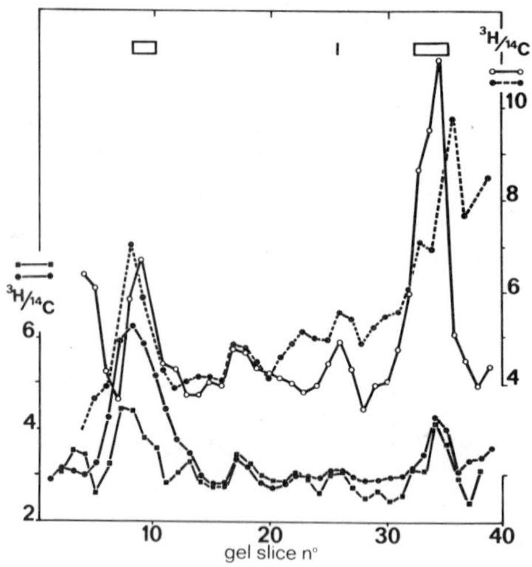

FIGURE 4. Proteins during progesterone-induced maturation in intact, enucleated, AMD- and ethidium bromide-treated oocytes. In the upper part of the Figure, 25 oocytes are injected with [^{3}H]leucine for 2 hr after progesterone treatment around the time showing 100% GVBD. Twenty-five untreated oocytes are injected with [^{14}C]leucine for 2 hr (○). Twenty-five enucleated oocytes, incubated with progesterone for the same time period as above, are injected with [^{3}H]leucine for 2 hr. Twenty-five enucleated untreated oocytes are injected with [^{14}C]leucine for 2 hr (●).

In the lower part of the Figure, 25 oocytes, showing GVBD and having been exposed to AMD 1 hr before progesterone treatment and during the whole maturation time, are injected with [^{3}H]leucine for 2 hr. Twenty-five oocytes exposed to AMD for the same time period as above are injected with [^{14}C]leucine for 2 hr (●). Twenty-five oocytes, showing GVBD and having been treated with ethidium bromide just before exposure to progesterone and incubated during the whole maturation time are injected with [^{3}H]leucine for 2 hr. Twenty-five oocytes not treated with ethidium bromide and incubated for the same time period are injected with [^{14}C]leucine for 2 hr (■).

resting oocytes. The pattern of induced proteins is the same as that obtained with progesterone. This induced pattern is observed as early as after 2–3 hr, whereas progesterone treatment takes 4–5 hr to achieve the same result (FIGURE 1). Similarly, GVBD occurs sooner after MPF injection than after progesterone incubation.[10]

Nontranscriptional Control of Induced Proteins: AMD Treatment and Enucleation

When oocytes are first incubated for 1 hr in AMD (50 μg/ml) and then progesterone is added in the continuous presence of AMD, the same ^{3}H/^{14}C peaks are observed (the controls are exposed to AMD alone) (FIGURE 4). Progesterone also induces the same proteins when the oocytes have been first enucleated. In the view of the possible involvement of mitochondrial DNA in the progesterone-induced proteins, ethidium bromide has also been tested, but no effect was observed.

Cycloheximide Experiments

To evaluate the participation of protein synthesis in induction of the peaks, oocytes have been incubated with progesterone and cycloheximide or with cycloheximide alone. [^{3}H]- and [^{14}C]leucine, respectively, are injected at the expected time of GVBD. This time is estimated from experiments with control oocytes, because GVBD is not observed in the presence of cycloheximide. After 2 hr of incubation, the ^{3}H and ^{14}C counts in each fraction are so low that one cannot measure the ratio of incorporated isotopes (data not shown). In addition, we have first labeled oocytes for 2 hr by injecting radioactive leucine and then injected cycloheximide and exposed oocytes to progesterone for the time required for maturation in control oocytes. No induced proteins were seen (data not shown), suggesting that the peaks do not represent transfer of labeled proteins from one cellular compartment to another.

In other experiments, MPF is introduced into cycloheximide-injected oocytes; 100% maturation is obtained, and at that time, [^{3}H]leucine is injected. These eggs are pooled with cycloheximide-treated oocytes that have received inactive cytoplasm from untreated oocytes and that are then injected with [^{14}C]leucine. Again, only a few counts are obtained, and the $^{3}H/^{14}C$ ratio is meaningless. Therefore, we have confirmed previous findings that MPF can induce GVBD in oocytes that do not synthesize proteins[2] and have also established that MPF-containing cytoplasm does not induce protein peaks in recipients under these conditions. A prelabeling experiment, similar to that described in the preceding paragraph, that involved injection of cycloheximide and MPF-containing cytoplasm was also negative with respect to formation of induced peaks. In all of these experiments, systematic controls have been obtained with progesterone and/or MPF in the absence of cycloheximide; these controls gave the same results shown in FIGURE 1.

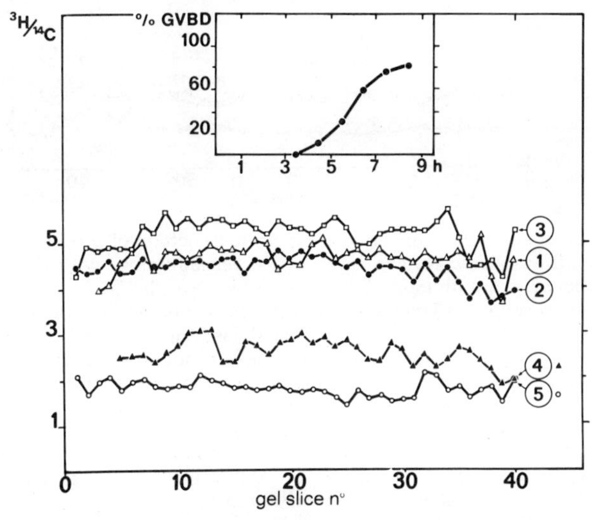

FIGURE 5a. Radioactive leucine uptake experiments: effect of progesterone and MPF on oocytes incubated in radioactive amino acids. Decreased uptake of [^{3}H]leucine by oocytes during progesterone-induced maturation, as shown by evolution of the $^{3}H/^{14}C$ labeling ratio of 105,000*g* supernatant proteins. 1) Untreated oocytes are incubated for 2 hr with [^{3}H]leucine. 2) Progesterone-exposed oocytes are incubated for 2 hr with [^{3}H]leucine. 3) Two hours after exposure to progesterone, oocytes are incubated for 2 hr with [^{3}H]leucine. 4) Four hours after exposure to progesterone, oocytes are incubated for 2 hr with [^{3}H]leucine. 5) Six hours after exposure to progesterone, oocytes are incubated for 2 hr with [^{3}H]leucine. In all cases, untreated oocytes are exposed to ^{14}C for 2 hr. *Inset:* Maturation, as expressed by percentage of GVBD, is plotted as a function of time after progesterone exposure.

Effect of Progesterone and MPF-Containing Cytoplasm on Radioactive Leucine Uptake by Oocytes

For confirmation of previous experiments in which oocytes were incubated in medium that contained either [^{3}H]- or [^{14}C]leucine,[7] it was found that progesterone decreases the uptake of radioactive amino acids after a 4-hr exposure (FIGURE 5a). The incubation conditions are not favorable for the observation of induced protein peaks. To investigate whether MPF-containing cytoplasm also affects leucine uptake, 25 oocytes were so injected and immediately in-

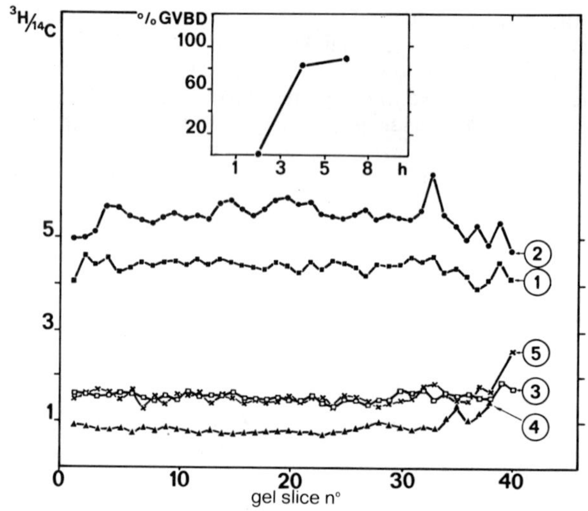

FIGURE 5b. Radioactive leucine uptake experiments: effect of progesterone and MPF on oocytes incubated in radioactive amino acids. Decreased uptake of [^{3}H]leucine by oocytes during MPF-induced maturation, as shown by evolution of the ^{3}H/^{14}C labeling ratio of 105,-000*g* supernatant proteins. 1) Untreated oocytes are incubated for 2 hr with [^{3}H]leucine. 2) MPF-injected oocytes are immediately incubated for 2 hr with [^{3}H]leucine. 3) Two hours after injection of MPF-containing cytoplasm, recipient oocytes are incubated for 2 hr with [^{3}H]leucine. 4) Four hours after injection of MPF-containing cytoplasm, recipient oocytes are incubated for 2 hr with [^{3}H]leucine. 5) Two hours after injection of MPF-containing cytoplasm, recipient oocytes are incubated for 4 hr with [^{3}H]leucine. In all cases, oocytes injected with inactive cytoplasm are exposed after the time indicated to [^{14}C]leucine for 2 hr (except for group 5, exposed for 4 hr). *Insert:* Maturation, as expressed by percentage of GVBD, is plotted as a function of time after MPF transfer.

cubated with [^{3}H]leucine for 2 hr, while control oocytes, injected with inactive cytoplasm, were incubated with [^{14}C]leucine. FIGURE 5b shows that the control ratio is approximately 4.5. When MPF-containing cytoplasm is injected into oocytes that are then immediately incubated for 2 hr with [^{3}H]leucine, the ratio is 5.5, which suggests a global increase in protein synthesis. However, if ^{3}H labeling is performed between 2 and 4 or 4 and 6 hr after MPF injection, the ^{3}H/^{14}C ratios decrease to 2 and 1, respectively. To exclude a possible decrease in the ratio by proteolysis during the 4–6-hr period, we incubated MPF-injected oocytes with [^{3}H]leucine for 4 hr (between 2 and 6 hr after MPF injection), a procedure similar to that previously used in progesterone experiments.[7] The resultant ratio was the same as that found with the 2–4 hr period, a finding that therefore excludes a significant degree of proteolysis. Comparison of FIGURES 5a and 5b also indicates that MPF produces the same effects as does progesterone but 2 hr earlier.

DISCUSSION

We have presented electrophoretic data that suggest synthesis of "induced proteins" during hormone-induced maturation of *X. laevis* oocytes. Well-defined protein peaks were observed after injection of the maturing oocytes with amino acids, by use of a double-labeling technique. These peaks were reproducible with three different radioactive markers (leucine, valine, lysine). They were obtained with cortisol and pregnenolone, with progesterone, and also with PCMB, a maturation-inducing substance.[17,18] The only similar electrophoretic studies have been performed in *Rana*, which showed differences only between proteins obtained at the first meiotic metaphase and those from fertilized eggs.[3]

When oocytic maturation is induced by progesterone, an MPF appears in the oocytic cytoplasm. When cytoplasm that contains MPF is injected into resting oocytes, they mature and produce more MPF, within a time span shorter than that needed to produce the same effects with progesterone. At the same time, induced proteins appear in the cytoplasm of the MPF-treated oocytes, and these proteins are, as far as we are able to determine, identical with those induced by progesterone.

The induction by progesterone of MPF and protein peaks persists in the presence of AMD or ethidium bromide and also after enucleation of the oocytes. Therefore, neither nuclear transcription nor mitochondrial DNA synthesis appears to be responsible for these hormone-induced changes in protein synthesis.

Our results suggest that although progesterone may not cause gross changes in protein synthesis,[20] certain species of proteins appear to be present in larger quantities after progesterone treatment. Caution is needed in interpreting our results in terms of specific protein synthesis, because our methods cannot distinguish between the appearance of new protein species and a change in the turnover of proteins synthesized in the absence of progesterone or MPF. Pulse labeling with radioactive leucine for 30 min revealed the same protein peaks in the same proportions (data not shown); therefore, synthesis of new proteins is a more likely explanation of our findings than is changes in turnover rates. In fact, important physiologically is the biologic significance of eventual new protein(s), and, indeed, the same question applies to a modified rate of synthesis of already existing proteins. Moreover, the peaks appear to depend neither on the transfer of nuclear radioactive proteins to cytoplasm under the influence of progesterone, as shown by experiments with enucleated oocytes, nor on compartmental changes in the cytoplasm, as indicated by studies with prelabeling before cycloheximide administration. The cycloheximide experiments also confirm that the "induced protein" peaks depend on protein synthesis, because labeling does not occur in the presence of the drug, with or without progesterone or MPF-containing cytoplasm. However, even if progesterone does not induce proteins or MPF in oocytes exposed to cycloheximide, MPF can still provoke maturation.[2] Therefore, induction of proteins is not an intermediate step in the events that lead to GVBD after injection of MPF.

The relationship between MPF and induced proteins is unknown. The latter might only be important for postmaturational events. For instance, histone (all but

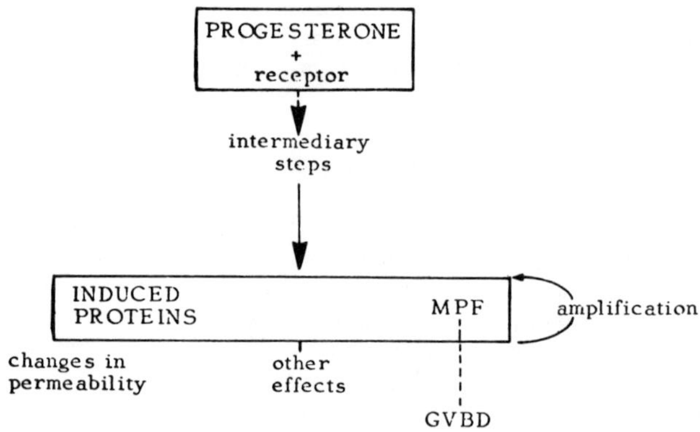

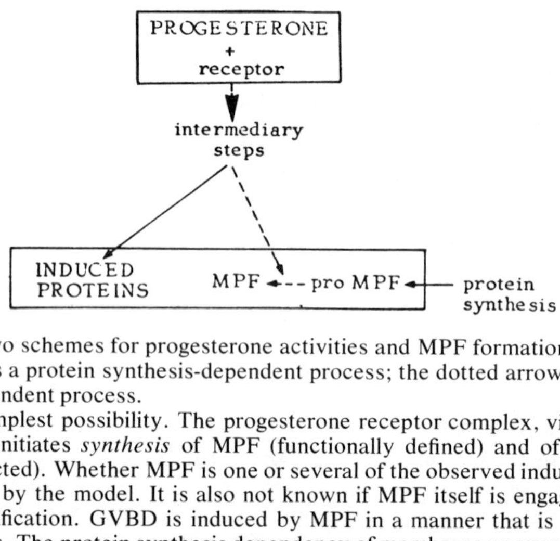

FIGURE 6. Two schemes for progesterone activities and MPF formation in oocytes. Solid arrow represents a protein synthesis-dependent process; the dotted arrow denotes a protein synthesis-independent process.

Top: The simplest possibility. The progesterone receptor complex, via undefined intermediary steps, initiates *synthesis* of MPF (functionally defined) and of induced proteins (physically detected). Whether MPF is one or several of the observed induced protein peaks is not predicted by the model. It is also not known if MPF itself is engaged in its protein-dependent amplification. GVBD is induced by MPF in a manner that is not dependent on protein synthesis. The protein synthesis dependency of membrane permeability changes has not been studied. Other effects, at or after GVBD, may be due to induced proteins.

Bottom: The progesterone-receptor complex does *not* lead *directly* to *synthesis* of MPF. The latter derives from a precursor "pro-MPF" that is activated after progesterone-receptor interaction in a manner that does not depend on protein synthesis. The formation of pro-MPF is not modulated by the hormone but is blocked by cycloheximide. Therefore, the response to progesterone only occurs in the presence of protein synthesis. In the Wasserman and Masui scheme,[9] progesterone provokes the protein synthesis-dependent formation of an "initiator" that activates pro-MPF to MPF. Other features are the same as in the top scheme.

F1) synthesis is stimulated in progesterone-treated oocytes,[21] and these proteins are found in the region of the fast-moving large peak of our electropherograms. Increased DNA polymerase[22] and new cAmp-dependent kinase[23] activities have also been reported.

The present results are actually compatible with the possibility that MPF activity is dependent on one or several of the proteins induced by progesterone or MPF itself. Two hypotheses that relate to the formation of MPF are illustrated in FIGURE 6. First, MPF might be a protein synthesized as a direct consequence of hormone-receptor interaction, with cycloheximide inhibiting a translational step (FIGURE 6, *top*). Alternatively (FIGURE 6, *bottom*), MPF formation observed after progesterone exposure might depend on a permissive action of the hormone; that is, progesterone-receptor interactions might promote the modification of an already synthesized protein ("Pro-MPF") into MPF. Similarly, the positive feedback loop, by which MPF reinforces its own formation, may or may not be directly dependent on protein synthesis.

Another event associated with the action of progesterone on oocytes is the change in membrane permeability, as evidenced by the decrease of leucine uptake from the medium while maturation proceeds (FIGURE 5a). The MPF-containing cytoplasm also reduces leucine uptake; for the other events elicited by progesterone, the difference in timing is revealed by the fact that the change in permeability occurs 2 hr earlier than with progesterone (FIGURE 5b). Whether this permeability change is protein synthesis dependent is not known. Interestingly, these experiments have indicated that, at a time when the decrease in leucine uptake is beginning, the overall mean $^3H/^{14}C$ protein ratio increases (2–4 hr after progesterone administration and 0–2 hr after MPF exposure; see FIGURES 5a and 5b), a finding indicative of a global, even discrete, increase of protein labeling. This result may be compared to the overall increase in protein synthesis originally described in *Rana* oocytes with a different technologic approach[14,20]; however, in *Rana*, this elevation in protein synthesis occurs to a significant extent only later on. Finally, both techniques, incubation and injection of amino acids, indicate a nontranscriptional, hormone-induced early synthesis of many proteins, some of which are preferentially labeled, as indicated by their electrophoretic patterns. Possible changes in amino acid pools do not provide a likely explanation for the present results.

Whether the operationally defined MPF corresponds to physically defined induced protein(s), the mechanism by which progesterone and MPF increase protein synthesis at the translational level, and decrease leucine uptake, remains of interest. In oocytes, the progesterone receptor may be membrane[24] or particulate[16,25] linked, evidence different from that reported for other steroid-sensitive cells.[26,27] Whether steroid actions in somatic cells may include a step at a nontranscriptional level remains a matter of uncertainty.[28,29] The amphibian oocyte may provide a remarkable opportunity to study hormonal actions that have not yet been recognized.

SUMMARY

In vitro incubation of isolated *X. laevis* oocytes with progesterone induces the specific labeling of proteins during maturation. They are detected as several discrete peaks with a double-labeling technique that involves the injection of [^{3}H]leucine into hormone-treated and [^{14}C]leucine into control cells. The peaks are separated by sodium dodecyl sulfate polyacrylamide gel electrophoresis.

Identical proteins are obtained with two other steroids that provoke maturation and with *p*-chloromercuribenzoate. The same progesterone-induced proteins are observed even if oocytes have been treated with actinomycin D or ethidium bromide or have been enucleated.

Cycloheximide suppresses the labeling of proteins that are induced by progesterone, if administered either at the time of radioactive amino acid exposure or after prelabeling the oocytes to determine whether the hormone-induced peaks are due to compartmental changes of the proteins.

A cytoplasmic fraction, obtained from maturing oocytes before GVBD, promotes maturation when injected into resting oocytes and therefore contains an MPF. After this injection, GVBD occurs earlier than during incubation with progesterone and is accompanied by the formation of the same proteins and of MPF, both suppressed by cycloheximide. The possibility that MPF is an induced protein is then discussed.

It has been also found that there is a decrease in membrane permeability, as evidenced by decreased leucine uptake into proteins of oocytes incubated in radioactive amino acids and exposed to progesterone. The same decrease occurs after injection of MPF-containing cytoplasm into oocytes.

Acknowledgments

We thank Prof. A. Bouhuys for his assistance in writing the manuscript, Dr. P. Pennequin for his advice, Dr. Y. Timowska for scientific assistance, and Mrs. M. Romios for technical help.

References

1. Brachet, J., H. Denis & F. de Vitry. 1964. The effects of actinomycin D and puromycin on morphogenesis in amphibian eggs and Acetabularia mediterranea. Devel. Biol. **9:** 398–434.
2. Drury, K. C. & S. Schorderet-Slatkine. 1975. Effects of cycloheximide on the "autocatalytic" nature of the maturation promoting factor (MPF) in oocytes of Xenopus laevis. Cell **4:** 268–274.
3. Ecker, R. E. & L. D. Smith. 1971. The nature and fate of Rana pipiens proteins synthesized during maturation and early cleavage. Devel. Biol. **24:** 559–576.
4. Merriam, R. W. 1972. On the mechanism of action in gonadotropic stimulation of oocyte maturation in Xenopus laevis. J. Exp. Zool. **180:** 421–426.
5. Schorderet-Slatkine, S. 1972. Action of progesterone and related steroids on oocyte maturation of Xenopus laevis. An in vitro study. Cell Different. **1:** 179–189.
6. Baltus, E., J. Brachet, J. Hanocq-Quertier & E. Hubert. 1973. Cytochemical and biochemical studies on progesterone-induced maturation in amphibian oocytes. 1. Ribonucleic acid and protein synthesis effects of inhibitors and of a "maturation promoting factor." Differentiation **1:** 127–143.
7. Pennequin, P., S. Schorderet-Slatkine, K. Drury & E. E. Baulieu. 1975. Decreased uptake of ^{3}H-leucine during progesterone induced maturation of Xenopus laevis oocytes. FEBS Lett. **51:** 156–160.
8. Masui, Y. & C. L. Markert. 1971. Cytoplasmic control of nuclear behavior during meiotic maturation of frog oocytes. J. Exp. Zool. **177:** 129–147.
9. Wasserman, W. J. & Y. Masui. 1975. Effects of cycloheximide on a cytoplasmic factor initiating meiotic maturation in Xenopus oocytes. Exp. Cell Res. **91:** 381–388.
10. Schorderet-Slatkine, S. & K. C. Drury. 1973. Progesterone induced maturation in oocytes of Xenopus laevis. Appearance of a "maturation promoting factor" in enucleated oocytes. Cell Different. **2:** 247–254.

11. Reynhout, J. K. & L. D. Smith. 1974. Studies on the appearance and nature of a maturation-inducing factor in the cytoplasm of amphibian oocytes exposed to progesterone. Devel. Biol. **38:** 394–400.
12. Eppig, J. J., Jr. & J. N. Dumont. 1972. Aminoacid pools in developing oocytes of Xenopus laevis. Devel. Biol. **28:** 531–536.
13. Gurdon, J. B. 1968. Changes in somatic cell nuclei inserted into growing and maturating amphibian oocytes. Embryol. Morphol. **20:** 401–414.
14. Brachet, J. 1974. Le contrôle de la maturation dans l'ovocyte de Xenopus laevis. Ann. Biol. **13:** 403–434.
15. Schuetz, A. W. 1970. Hormones and follicular functions. *In* Oogenesis. J. D. Biggers & A. W. Schuetz, Eds.: 479–512. University Park Press. Baltimore, Md.
16. Jacobelli, S., J. Hanocq, E. Baltus & J. Brachet. 1974. Hormone induced maturation of Xenopus laevis oocytes: effects of different steroids and study of a progesterone receptor. Differentiation **2:** 129–135.
17. Brachet, J. & A. de Schutter-Pays. 1974. Induction de la maturation chez l'oocyte de Xenope par trois inhibiteurs des groupes sulfhydrile de la membrane plasmatique. Compt. Rend. **279:** 2107–2110.
18. Brachet, J., E. Baltus, A. de Schutter-Pays, J. Hanocq-Quertier, E. Hubert & G. Steinert. 1975. Induction of maturation (meiosis) in Xenopus laevis oocytes by three organomercurials. Proc. Nat. Acad. Sci. USA **72:** 1574–1578.
19. Smith, L. D. & R. E. Ecker. 1969. Role of the oocyte nucleus in physiological maturation in Rana pipiens. Devel. Biol. **19:** 281–309.
20. Ecker, R. E. & L. D. Smith. 1968. Protein synthesis in amphibian oocytes and early embryos. Devel. Biol. **18:** 232–249.
21. Adamson, E. D. & H. R. Wooland. 1974. Histone synthesis in early amphibian development. Histone and DNA syntheses are not co-ordinated. J. Mol. Biol. **88:**263–285.
22. Benbow, R. N., R. Q. W. Pestell & C. C. Ford. 1975. Appearance of DNA polymerase activities during early development of Xenopus laevis. Devel. Biol. **43:** 159–174.
23. Wiblet, M. 1974. Protein kinase activities during maturation in Xenopus laevis oocytes. Biochem. Biophys. Res. Commun. **60:** 991–998.
24. Smith, L. D. & R. E. Ecker. 1971. The interaction of steroids with Rana pipiens oocytes in the induction of maturation. Devel. Biol. **25:** 232–247.
25. Ozon, R. & R. Bellé. 1973. Progesterone receptor associated with the "melanosome" fraction in Pleurodeles waltlii oocytes (urodela amphibian). Biochim. Biophys. Acta **320:** 588–593.
26. Jensen, E. V. & E. R. DeSombre. 1972. Mechanism of action of the female sex hormones. Annu. Rev. Biochem. **41:** 203–230.
27. Baulieu, E.-E. 1974. The mode of action of steroid hormones: some recent findings. *In* Physiology and Genetics of Reproduction. Part A. E. M. Coutinho & F. Fuchs, Eds. Vol. 4: 113–141. Plenum Publishing Corporation. New York and London.
28. Tomkins, G. M., T. D. Gelehrter, D. Granner, D. Martin, Jr., H. Samuels & E. B. Thompson. 1969. Control of specific gene expression in higher organisms. Science **166:** 1474–1480.
29. Liang, T. & S. Liao. 1975. A very rapid effect of androgen on initiation of protein synthesis in prostate. Proc. Nat. Acad. Sci. USA **72:** 706–709.

EFFECT OF PROGESTINS ON GLUCOSE AND LIPID METABOLISM*

Paul Beck

Endocrinology Division
Department of Medicine
University of Colorado School of Medicine
Denver, Colorado 80262

Introduction

This paper will present a broad overview of the effect of progesterone and synthetic progestins on carbohydrate and lipid metabolism in mammals. To clarify apparent contradictory results in the literature, the importance of progestin dosage, chemical nature of the progestin, concurrent estrogen administration, and species differences will be assessed. Wherever possible, the alteration of physiologic mechanisms induced by progestins will be described.

Insulin Production

Increased insulin production has been observed after the administration of gestamimetic doses of native progesterone (i.e., doses that simulate pregnancy). In rhesus monkeys, there is a marked rise in the serum insulin response to intravenous glucose after 3 weeks of progesterone treatment (4 mg/kg/day subcutaneously; FIGURE 1), with the total serum insulin response [i.e., the integrated area under the insulin response curve ($\sum$I)] averaging four times greater after progesterone treatment (FIGURE 2).[1] Although the mean serum progesterone concentration that resulted from this dosage of progesterone was four to eight times greater than that reported in nonpregnant rhesus monkeys,[2] a twofold increase in the mean $\sum$I has also been observed in rhesus monkeys treated with 500 μg of progesterone per day.[3] Increased fasting serum insulin concentrations, in addition to serum insulin responses to glucose, have been reported by Kalkhoff *et al.* in men and women after 6 days of progesterone (300–400 mg/day intramuscularly)[4] and in rats after 21 days of progesterone treatment (2.5 mg/day subcutaneously).[5] Similar increases in fasting and glucose-stimulated serum insulin concentrations occur in human and rat pregnancy.[5,6] Finally, Costrini and Kalkhoff[5] have demonstrated increased pancreatic islet size and increased islet insulin production in rats treated with large doses of progesterone.

The extra insulin produced by progesterone treatment appears to be biologically active. As shown in FIGURE 2, concurrent administration of progesterone and hydrocortisone reverses the deterioration of glucose tolerance produced in the rhesus monkey by hydrocortisone alone. Also, Matute and Kalkhoff[7] have demonstrated increased hepatic glycogen and decreased conversion of alanine to glucose in rats treated with gestamimetic doses of progesterone.

The synthetic progestins, the nortestosterone and 17α-acetoxyprogesterone derivatives, produce more variable effects on insulin production. When

*Supported in part by United States Public Health Service Grants HD 02455 and FR 00051 and by a grant from Syntex Corporation.

administered to rhesus monkeys in suprapharmacologic doses, chlormadinone acetate (6-chloro-6-dehydro-17α-acetoxyprogesterone, 750 μg/day) and norethindrone (17α-ethinyl-19-nortestosterone, 2.5 mg/day) enhanced glucose-stimulated $\sum$I, whereas comparable doses of ethynodiol diacetate (17α-ethinyl-3,17-diacetoxy-19-nortestosterone, 1 mg/day) did not (FIGURE 3). Lesser doses of norethindrone and medroxyprogesterone acetate (6α-methyl-17α-acetoxyprogesterone acetate, MPA) produced no consistent changes in glucose-stimulated insulin release in rhesus monkeys.[3] In women, Spellacy *et al.* have reported increased plasma insulin responses to glucose in women treated with two different nortestosterone derivatives, namely, norethindrone only (350 μg/day for 1 year)[8]

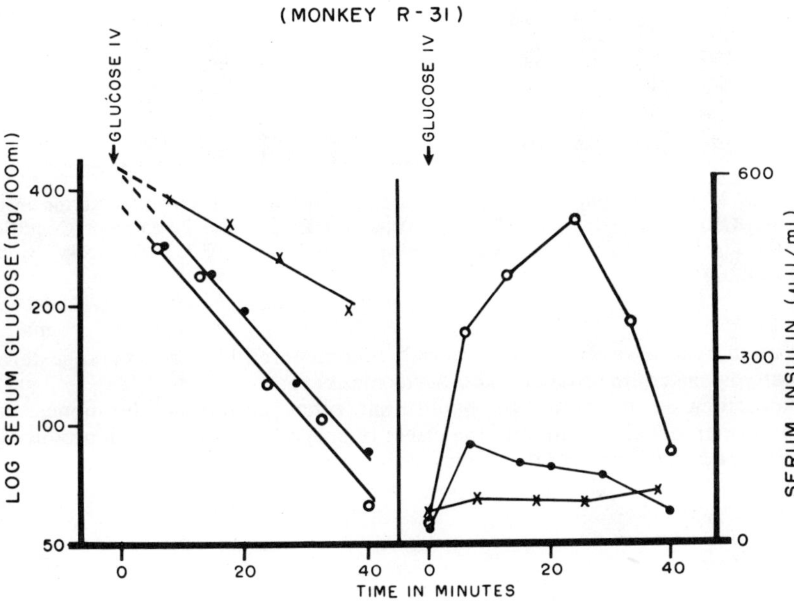

FIGURE 1. Serum glucose and insulin responses to intravenous glucose in female rhesus monkeys after progesterone or hydrocortisone treatment. Progesterone in olive oil (○, 4 mg/kg/day) was administered subcutaneously for 3 weeks, or hydrocortisone phosphate (×) was administered intramuscularly 2 and 12 hr before the administration of glucose intravenously (1 g/kg). The monkeys were anesthetized with phencyclidine hydrochloride (8 mg) and atropine (0.1 mg) immediately before glucose administration. Solid circles represent controls. (From Beck.[1] By permission of *Diabetes*.)

and norgestrel only (17α-ethinyl-13-ethyl-19-nortestosterone, 75 μg/day for 6 months).[9] By contrast, Goldman[10] found no change in insulin production in women treated with another nortestosterone derivative, ethynodiol diacetate. Whereas oral administration of 17α-acetoxyprogesterone derivatives produces no changes in insulin production,[11–16] several investigators have observed a modest increase in circulating insulin after parenteral administration of depot preparations of MPA to human subjects.[17–19] We have observed a similar discrepancy in the ef-

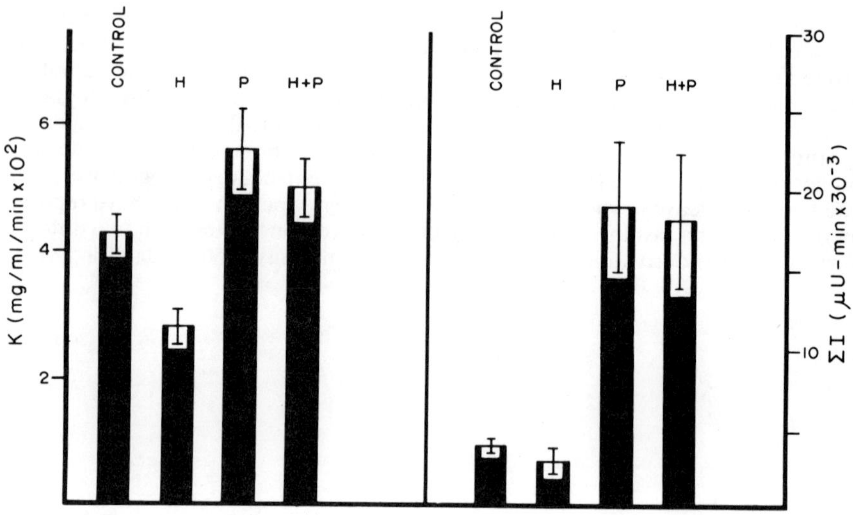

FIGURE 2. Mean serum glucose disappearance rates (K) and integrated serum insulin responses (ΣI) after progesterone (P), hydrocortisone (H), or H plus P treatment. Conditions were the same as in FIGURE 1. Horizontal bars represent ± SEM.[1] (From Beck.[1] By permission of *Diabetes*.)

fects of short-term orally and parenterally administered 17α-acetoxyprogesterone derivatives on insulin production in rhesus monkeys.[3]

Nevertheless, it should be noted that other gestational hormones, and synthetic estrogens, may modify the effect of progesterone on insulin production. Kalkhoff *et al.* have shown that concurrent estradiol plus progesterone treatment

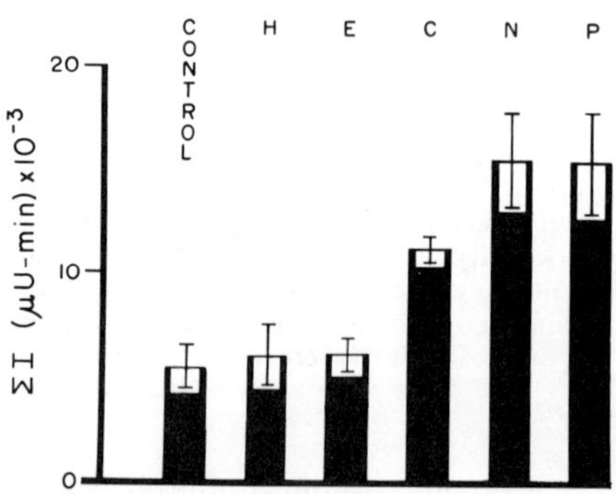

FIGURE 3. Effect of synthetic progestins on the mean serum integrated insulin responses (ΣI) to glucose. Progesterone (P), hydrocortisone (H), and anesthesia were administered as in FIGURE 1. Ethynodiol diacetate (E, 1.0 mg), chlormadinone acetate (C, 0.75 mg), or norethindrone (N, 2.5 mg) was administered in olive oil daily for 3 weeks to four, nine, and four monkeys, respectively. Horizontal bars represent ± SEM. (From Beck.[1] By permission of *Diabetes*.)

increases pancreatic islet diameter and isolated islet insulin secretion[5] and increases fasting plasma insulin concentrations in the rat[7] to a greater extent than does progesterone treatment alone. In rhesus monkeys, concurrent treatment with norethindrone plus mestranol or ethinylestradiol produced a greater fasting serum insulin concentration and a greater $\sum$I after intravenous glucose administration than did treatment with any of these three synthetic steroids alone (FIGURE 4). On the other hand, addition of human chorionic somatomammotropin to the treatment regimen neutralized the insulinotropic effect of progesterone alone in intact rhesus monkeys[20] and of progesterone plus estriol in isolated rat pancreatic islets.[21] By contrast, we have observed no augmentation of insulin production when gestamimetic doses of estriol were added to progesterone treatment

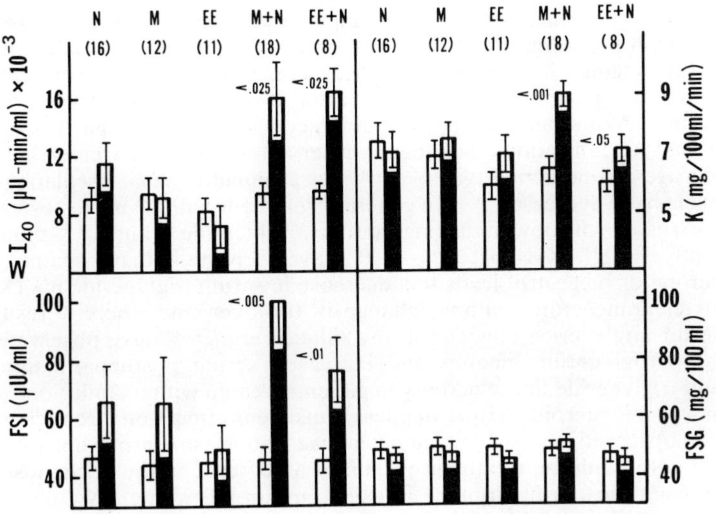

FIGURE 4. Mean integrated serum insulin responses to glucose (ΣI), serum glucose disappearance rates (K), and fasting serum insulin (FSI) and glucose (FSG) concentrations during intravenous glucose tolerance tests in female rhesus monkeys after treatment with norethindrone (N, 500 μg/day), mestranol (M, 10 μg/day), ethinylestradiol (EE, 10 μg/day), or M plus N and EE plus N for 3 weeks. (From Beck *et al.*[3] By permission of *Journal of Clinical Endocrinology and Metabolism.*)

regimens in monkeys[22] or in women[23] or when mestranol was added to an MPA treatment regimen in rhesus monkeys[3] or to chlormadinone acetate treatment in women.[23]

In summary, progesterone and synthetic progestins generally enhance insulin production, when administered in gestamimetic or suprapharmacologic doses. In lesser or contraceptive doses, only nortestosterone derivatives and parenterally administered medroxyprogesterone acetate promote insulin production. Concurrent estrogen administration may potentiate the effects of progesterone and norethindrone on insulin secretion. The magnitude of these insulinotropic effects appears to be modified by the route of progestin administration and the species in which the progestin is tested.

Triglyceride Metabolism

Many *in vivo* and *in vitro* studies demonstrate that insulin stimulates triglyceride synthesis,[24,25] when free fatty acids (FFA) are used as a substrate that has been mobilized from adipose tissue.[26] Growth hormone enhances adipose tissue lipolysis[27] and increases circulating FFA concentrations.[28] Conversely, glucagon inhibits hepatic triglyceride synthesis.[25,29] In women who use combinations of ethinylestradiol plus nortestosterone derivatives, fasting serum growth hormone levels[30–32] and insulin levels are elevated,[33] their insulin response to glucose stimulation is increased,[11,33] and their plasma glucagon response to an aminogenic stimulus is blunted.[34] Similarly, their fasting serum triglyceride concentrations are also increased.[11,34,35] Thus, one might anticipate an increase in hepatic triglyceride production and serum triglyceride concentrations in progestin-treated subjects with increased insulin production and/or glucagon deficiency.

Surprisingly, no increase in circulating triglycerides has been observed after treatment with progesterone or synthetic progestins. In the rat, Kalkhoff *et al.*[36] observed no change in plasma triglyceride concentration or in net triglyceride entry into the plasma compartment after treatment with large doses of progesterone. With one exception,[37] no increase in fasting plasma or serum triglyceride concentrations has been observed in women treated with 17α-acetoxyprogesterone derivatives[11,14,15,19,38]; occasionally, basal circulating triglyceride levels have decreased.[18,39] In general, treatment with 19-nortestosterone derivatives results in lower fasting serum triglyceride values,[8,9] though not consistently.[38,40–43] Kissebah *et al.*[44] have reported that treatment with progesterone or megestrol leads to a decrease in serum triglyceride pool size and apparent clearance rate, without change in turnover rate, thereby resulting in lower serum triglyceride concentrations. Glueck *et al.*[45,46] have observed similar changes in triglyceride kinetics and increased serum postheparin lipoprotein lipase and triglyceride lipase activity in patients treated with oxandrolone (an anabolic-androgenic steroid). However, less consistent effects on circulating lipases have been observed in normal women who use 19-nortestosterone derivatives.[42,43] Although norethindrone treatment produced a decrease in the serum insulin:glucagon molar ratio during arginine infusions in normal women, we observed no consistent correlation with their changes in basal plasma triglyceride concentrations.[34] Thus, these data suggest that pathologic hypertriglyceridemia is likely to develop only in progestin-treated women in whom there is a preexisting defect in plasma-clearing lipases or in whom there is excessive basal insulin production with limited glucagon secretory reserve.

Glucose Metabolism

Because of progesterone-enhanced insulin production, one would expect increased tissue utilization of glucose, in addition to acceleration of plasma glucose clearance rates, in subjects treated with progesterone. As noted previously, there are increased hepatic glycogen formation and decreased hepatic gluconeogenesis in rats treated with gestamimetic doses of progesterone.[7] On the other hand, we have observed decreased sensitivity to the hypoglycemic action of exogenous insulin in rhesus monkeys treated with gestamimetic doses of progesterone[1] and with mestranol plus norethindrone.[3] In actuality, no consistent changes in plasma glucose disappearance rates (during glucose tolerance tests) occur in rats, monkeys, or human subjects treated with pregnancy levels of progesterone.[1,4,5]

Nevertheless, in some species, the concurrent administration of an estrogen with gestamimetic doses of progesterone produces changes in glucose metabolism that are beyond those seen with progesterone treatment alone. Matute and Kalkhoff[7] observed more glycogen formation and more apparent inhibition of gluconeogenesis in rats treated with estradiol plus progesterone than with either steroid alone. In rhesus monkeys, addition of estriol to a progesterone treatment regimen resulted in acceleration of the mean serum glucose disappearance rates after intravenous glucose administration.[22] By contrast, no change in glucose disappearance rates was seen during treatment with estriol alone[47] or with estradiol plus progesterone.[22] In women, we have observed no change in plasma glucose concentrations after oral ingestion of glucose during treatment with gestamimetic doses of estriol or estriol plus progesterone.[23]

The use of 17α-acetoxyprogesterone derivatives as the sole contraceptive agent has generally resulted in no discernible change in glucose tolerance in women. We found no change in glucose tolerance in nondiabetic or subclinical diabetic women treated with chlormadinone acetate for 6 months.[11] Larsson-Cohn *et al.*[12] and Vermeulen *et al.*[13] observed no changes in the intravenous glucose tolerance of women treated for up to 1-year with chlormadinone acetate. No consistent changes in plasma glucose have been found in women treated with megestrol acetate for 3–6 months.[14,15] Similarly, Goldman *et al.*[48] and Tuttle and Turkington[19] observed no significant changes in carbohydrate tolerance in normal women treated with MPA. Although Spellacy *et al.*[17] found a slight deterioration in glucose tolerance in normal women 6 months after receiving a single large injection of a depot preparation of MPA, Vermeulen and Thiery[18] observed greater than normal intravenous glucose assimilation constants in women receiving the same preparation every 3 months for more than 3 years.

The use of 19-nortestosterone derivatives may actually lead to deterioration of glucose tolerance and higher blood glucose levels, and these effects may be potentiated by concurrent ingestion of a synthetic estrogen. Spellacy *et al.*[49] reported deterioration of *oral* glucose tolerance in 13% of normal women after 6 months of treatment with ethynodiol diacetate; the same workers observed significant elevations of blood glucose concentrations after 6 months of norgestrel contaception.[9] In women who used mestranol plus ethynodiol diacetate concurrently, Spellacy *et al.*[33] observed glucose tolerance deterioration in 41%. On the other hand, no change in *intravenous* glucose tolerance was observed during treatment with ethynodiol diacetate[10] or norethindrone[12] or in *oral* glucose tolerance during norethindrone treatment.[8]

Contrary effects on carbohydrate metabolism have been observed in nonhuman species treated with testosterone derivatives. In rhesus monkeys, we have observed an acceleration of serum glucose disappearance rates during mestranol plus norethindrone treatment, which was not observed after treatment with either steroid alone (FIGURE 4). Undoubtedly, the improved glucose tolerance in these monkeys resulted from their increased basal and glucose-stimulated insulin production, because other animal studies suggest that large amounts of insulin may neutralize the hyperglycemic effect of testosterone. In castrated rats 95% pancreatectomized, Lewis *et al.*[50] demonstrated that estrogen administration could reverse the excessive incidence of glycosuria produced by long-term testosterone treatment, presumably because of estrogen-mediated hyperplasia of the remaining islets of Langerhans.[51] Also, Kochakian and Costa[52] have demonstrated that fasting blood glucose levels decrease in totally pancreatectomized-castrated dogs when insulin is administered concurrently with testosterone.

The effect of 17α-acetoxyprogesterone derivatives on glucose metabolism in nonhuman species is contradictory. Sloan and Oliver[53] reported the development

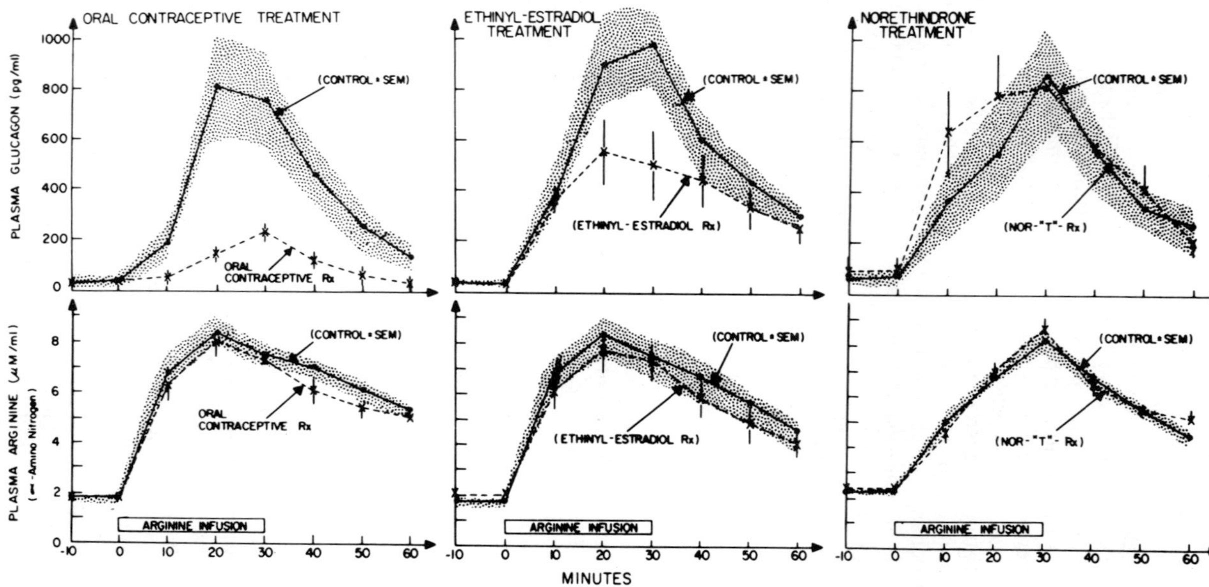

FIGURE 5. Effect of gonadal steroid administration on the plasma glucagon response to intravenous *l*-arginine in 18 normal women studied in groups of six [*left*, mestranol (80 μg/day) plus norethindrone (1 mg/day); *middle*, ethinylestradiol (100 μg/day); *right*, norethindrone (10 mg/day)]. The rise in plasma α-amino nitrogen in response to arginine infusion is plotted below. All values represent the mean ± SEM, with the control study values shown by the dotted area. (From Beck *et al.*[34] By permission of *Metabolism*.)

of overt diabetes in two of 16 beagles treated with suprapharmacologic doses of chlormadinone acetate for 1 year. By contrast, we observed improvement in intravenous glucose tolerance in rhesus monkeys treated with the same compound (200 μg/kg/day) for 3 weeks.[54] With lesser doses (125 μg/kg/day), we observed accelerated serum glucose disappearance rates in rhesus monkeys treated for 1 week with parenteral MPA or oral MPA, chlormadinone acetate, or megestrol acetate; however, glucose tolerance was unchanged after 3 weeks of oral MPA, either alone or in combination with mestranol.[3] The reasons for these discrepancies are obscure.

It is tempting to speculate about the reasons for the occasional deterioration of glucose tolerance in human subjects treated with 19-nortestosterone derivatives, despite generally increased insulin production. One possible explanation may be the failure of some individuals to reduce endogenous glucagon secretion and hepatic glucose production during contraceptive steroid treatment. We have recently observed marked blunting of arginine-stimulated glucagon secretion in normal women after 2 weeks of treatment with mestranol plus norethindrone or mestranol only but not with norethindrone alone (FIGURE 5). It is of interest that Gerich *et al.*[55] have reported lower blood glucose concentrations (despite ingestion of breakfast) in insulin-dependent diabetic subjects whose circulating glucagon concentrations were reduced by somatostatin. An enhanced insulin response to glucose, together with blunting of glucagon secretion, would reduce hepatic glucose output and could effectively neutralize other contraceptive steroid-induced contrainsulin factors.

Accelerated insulin degradation may be a second explanation for the apparently decreased sensitivity to insulin in 19-nortestosterone-treated human subjects. Srivastava *et al.*[56] observed a fixed metabolic clearance rate for plasma insulin in birth control pill users that was greater than normal at elevated plasma insulin concentrations. The plasma half-life ($t_{1/2}$) was longer than normal in the oral contraceptive users, and these users showed less than normal hypoglycemia after administration of exogenous insulin. These data suggest increased capillary permeability to insulin and increased peripheral degradation in birth control pill users. Consistent with these findings is the decreased *in vivo* conversion of blood glucose to adipose tissue fatty acids in rats treated with mestranol plus norethynodrel.[57]

SUMMARY

Gestamimetic amounts of progesterone enhance basal and glucose-stimulated insulin production.

Contraceptive doses of synthetic progestins cause a moderate increase or no change in glucose-stimulated insulin production, depending on route of administration and species tested.

Estrogens potentiate the insulinotropic effects of progesterone and the synthetic progestins.

Basal serum triglyceride concentrations are generally unaffected by progesterone or 17α-acetoxyprogesterone treatment but may decrease during 19-nortestosterone administration.

Glucose tolerance does not change during treatment with gestamimetic doses of progesterone alone but may improve in rats and monkeys during concurrent estrogen administration.

By contrast, deterioration of glucose tolerance is observed in women treated concurrently with synthetic estrogen plus 19-nortestosterone derivatives and, occasionally, with 19-nortestosterone derivatives alone.

No consistent changes in glucose metabolism have been observed after treatment with 17α-acetoxyprogesterone derivatives alone.

The cause of the species-related differences in glucose metabolism during 19-nortestosterone treatment is obscure.

References

1. Beck, P. 1969. Progestin enhancement of the plasma insulin response to glucose in rhesus monkeys. Diabetes **18:** 146–152.
2. Neill, J. D., E. O. B. Johansson, J. K. Datta & E. Knobil. 1967. Relationship between the plasma levels of luteinizing hormone and progesterone during the normal menstrual cycle. J. Clin. Endocrinol. Metab. **27:** 1167–1173.
3. Beck, P., R. L. Venable & D. L. Hoff. 1975. Mutual modification of glucose-stimulated serum insulin responses in female rhesus monkeys by ethinyl estradiol and nortestosterone derivatives. J. Clin. Endocrinol. Metab. **41:** 44–53.
4. Kalkhoff, R. K., M. Jacobsen & D. Lemper. 1970. Progesterone, pregnancy and the augmented plasma insulin response. J. Clin. Endocrinol. Metab. **31:** 24–28.
5. Costrini, N. V. & R. K. Kalkhoff. 1971. Relative effects of pregnancy, estradiol and progesterone on plasma insulin and pancreatic islet insulin secretion. J. Clin. Invest. **50:** 992–999.
6. Kalkhoff, R. K., D. S. Schalch, J. L. Walker, P. Beck, D. M. Kipnis & W. H. Daughaday. 1964. Diabetogenic factors associated with pregnancy. Trans. Ass. Amer. Physicians **77:** 270–278.
7. Matute, M. L. & R. K. Kalkhoff. 1973. Sex steroid influence on hepatic gluconeogenesis and glycogen metabolism. Endocrinology **92:** 762–768.
8. Spellacy, W. N., W. C. Buhi & S. A. Birk. 1975. Effects of norethindrone on carbohydrate and lipid metabolism. Obstet. Gynecol. **46:** 560–563.
9. Spellacy, W. N., W. C. Buhi & S. A. Birk. 1974. Norgestrel and carbohydrate-lipid metabolism: glucose, insulin and triglyceride changes during six months time of use. Contraception **9:** 615–625.
10. Goldman, J. A. 1975. Effect of ethynodiol diacetate and combination-type oral contraceptive compounds on carbohydrate metabolism. I. Six month intravenous glucose tolerance study. Diabetologia **11:** 45–48.
11. Beck, P. 1970. Comparison of the metabolic effects of chlormadinone acetate and conventional contraceptive steroids in man. J. Clin. Endocrinol. Metab. **30:** 785–791.
12. Larsson-Cohn, U., B. Tengstrom & L. Wide. 1969. Glucose tolerance and insulin response during daily continuous low-dose oral contraceptive treatment. Acta Endocrinol. **62:** 242–250.
13. Vermeulen, A., R. Daneels & M. Thiery. 1970. Effects of oral contraceptives on carbohydrate metabolism. Diabetologia **6:** 519–523.
14. Adams, P. W. & V. Wynn. 1972. The effects of progestogen, megestrol acetate, on carbohydrate and lipid metabolism. J. Obstet. Gynaecol. Brit. Commonwealth **79:** 744–752.
15. Spellacy, W. N., R. E. Newton, W. C. Buhi & S. A. Birk. 1973. Carbohydrate and lipid studies during six months' treatment with megestrol acetate. Amer. J. Obstet. Gynecol. **116:** 1074–1078.
16. Beck, P., D. Zimmerman & R. P. Eaton. 1976. Effect of contraceptive steroids on arginine-stimulated glucagon and insulin secretion in women. III. Oral medroxyprogesterone acetate. Current Topics in Diabetes Research. Abstracts of the IXth Congress of the International Diabetes Foundation: 34. Excerpta Medica. Amsterdam, The Netherlands.
17. Spellacy, W. N., A. G. W. McLeod, W. C. Buhi, S. A. Birk & S. A. McCreary. 1970. Medroxyprogesterone acetate and carbohydrate metabolism: measurement of glucose, insulin, and growth hormone during six months time. Fertil. Steril. **21:** 457–463.

18. VERMEULEN, A. & M. THIERY. 1974. Hormonal contraceptives and carbohydrate tolerance. II. Influence of medroxyprogesterone acetate and chronic oral contraceptives. Diabetologia **10:** 253–259.
19. TUTTLE, S. & V. E. TURKINGTON. 1974. Effects of medroxyprogesterone acetate on carbohydrate metabolism. Obstet. Gynecol. **43:** 685–692.
20. BECK, P. 1970. Reversal of progesterone-enhanced insulin production by human chorionic somatomammotropin. Endocrinology **87:** 311–315.
21. HAGER, D., R. H. GEORG, J. W. LEITNER & P. BECK. 1972. Insulin secretion and content in isolated rat pancreatic islets following treatment with gestational hormones. Endocrinology **91:** 977–981.
22. BECK, P. & D. L. HOFF. 1971. Estriol modification of the effects of progesterone and human chorionic somatomamotropin on glucose tolerance and plasma insulin in rhesus monkeys. Diabetes **20:** 271–275.
23. BECK, P. 1972. Unpublished observations.
24. REAVEN, G. M., R. L. LERNER, M. P. STEIN & J. W. FARQUHAR. 1967. Role of insulin in endogenous hypertriglyceridemia. J. Clin. Invest. **11:** 1756–1767.
25. POLEDNE, R. & P. A. MAYES. 1970. Lipolysis and the regulation of fatty acid metabolism in the liver. Biochem. J. **119:** 47P–48P.
26. HAVEL, R. J. 1961. Conversion of plasma free fatty acids into triglycerides of plasma lipoprotein fractions in man. Metabolism **12:** 1031–1034.
27. FAIN, J. N., V. P. KOVACEV & R. O. SCOW. 1965. Effect of growth hormone and dexamethasone on lipolysis and metabolism in isolated fat cells of the rat. J. Biol. Chem. **240:** 3522–3529.
28. RABEN, M. S. & C. H. HOLLENBERG. 1959. Effect of growth hormone on plasma free fatty acids. J. Clin. Invest. **38:** 484–488.
29. HEIMBERG, M., I. WEINSTEIN & M. KOHOUT. 1969. The effects of glucagon, dibutyryl cyclic adenosine 3,5 monophosphate, and concentration of free fatty acid on hepatic lipid metabolism. J. Biol. Chem. **244:** 5131–5139.
30. SPELLACY, W. N., K. L. CARLSON & S. L. SCHADE. 1967. Human growth hormone levels in normal subjects receiving an oral contraceptive. J. Amer. Med. Ass. **202:** 451–454.
31. DAVIDSON, M. B. & G. B. HOLZMAN. 1973. Role of growth hormone in the alteration of carbohydrate metabolism induced by oral contraceptive agents. J. Clin. Endocrinol. Metab. **36:** 246–255.
32. SPELLACY, W. N., W. C. BUHI & S. A. BIRK. 1972. The effect of estrogens on carbohydrate metabolism: glucose, insulin, and growth hormone studies on one hundred seventy-one women ingesting Premarin, mestranol, and ethinyl estradiol for six months. Amer. J. Obstet. Gynecol. **114:** 378–390.
33. SPELLACY, W. N., W. C. BUHI & S. A. BIRK. 1971. Studies of ethynodiol diacetate and mestranol on blood glucose and plasma insulin. II. Twelve month oral glucose tolerance test. Contraception **3:** 185–194.
34. BECK, P., R. P. EATON, D. M. ARNETT & R. N. ALSEVER. 1975. Effect of contraceptive steroids on arginine-stimulated glucagon and insulin secretion in women: I. Lipid physiology. Metabolism **24:** 1055–1065.
35. STOKES, T. & V. WYNN. 1971. Serum-lipids in women on oral contraceptives. Lancet **2:** 677–680.
36. KALKHOFF, R. K., N. V. COSTRINI, M. L. MATUTE & H. J. KIM. 1975. Metabolic modifications by the hormones of pregnancy. *In* Early Diabetes in Early Life. R. A. Camerini-Davalos & H. S. Cole, Eds.: 323–331. Academic Press, Inc. New York, N.Y.
37. SHAHANI, S. M. & K. L. PATEL. 1974. Effects of different oral contraceptives (combined and mini pill) on lipid metabolism. Contraception **10:** 263–272.
38. LARSSON-COHN, U., R. BERLIN & O. VIKROT. 1970. Effects of combined and low-dose gestagen oral contraceptives on plasma lipids; including individual phospholipids. Acta Endocrinol. **63:** 717–735.
39. GOWLAND, E. & R. A. JONES. 1973. The effect of oral norethisterone on serum lipid levels in premenopausal women. J. Obstet. Gynaecol. Brit. Commonwealth **80:** 357–359.
40. SPELLACY, W. N., W. C. BUHI, S. A. BIRK & R. CABAL. 1973. The effects of

estrogens, progestogen, oral contraceptives, and intrauterine devices on fasting triglyceride and insulin levels. Fertil. Steril. **24:** 178–184.

41. Danowski, T. S., H. R. Wilson, R. C. Khurana, Y. Jung, A. R. Gonzalez & J. H. Sunder. 1973. Effects of a progestin, quingestanol, in older diabetic women. Hormone Res. **4:** 84–96.
42. Glueck, C. J., S. Ford, Jr., P. Steiner, S. Buxton & R. Fallat. 1973. Amer. J. Obstet. Gynecol. **116:** 689–693.
43. Glueck, C. J., R. I. Levy & D. S. Frederickson. 1971. Norethindrone acetate, post-heparin lipolytic activity, and plasma triglycerides in familial types I, III, IV, and V hyperlipoproteinemia. Ann. Intern. Med. **75:** 345–352.
44. Kissebah, A. H., P. Harrigan & V. Wynn. 1973. Mechanism of hypertriglyceridemia associated with contraceptive steroids. Hormone Metab. Res. **5:** 184–190.
45. Glueck, C. J. 1971. Effects of oxandrolone on plasma triglycerides and post-heparin lipolytic activity in patients with types III, IV, and V familial hyperlipoproteinemia. Metabolism **20:** 691–702.
46. Glueck, C. J., S. Ford, Jr., P. Steiner & R. Fallat. 1973. Triglyceride removal efficiency and lipoprotein lipases: effects of oxandrolone. Metabolism **22:** 807–814.
47. Beck, P. & S. A. Wells. 1969. Comparison of the mechanisms underlying carbohydrate intolerance in subclinical diabetic women during pregnancy and during postpartum oral contraceptive treatment. J. Clin. Endocrinol. Metab. **29:** 807–818.
48. Goldman, J. A., J. L. Ovadia & B. Eckerling. 1968. Effect of progesterone on glucose tolerance in women. Israel J. Med. Sci. **4:** 878–882.
49. Spellacy, W. N., W. C. Buhi & S. A. Birk. 1972. The effect of the progestogen ethynodiol diacetate on glucose, insulin, and growth hormone after six months treatment. Acta Endocrinol. **70:** 373–384.
50. Lewis, J. T., V. G. Foglia & R. R. Rodriguez. 1950. The effects of steroids on the incidence of diabetes in rats after subtotal pancreatectomy. Endocrinology **46:** 111–121.
51. Houssay, B. A. 1951. Action of sex hormones on experimental diabetes. Brit. Med. J. **2:** 505–510.
52. Kochakian, C. D. & G. Costa. 1959. The effect of testosterone propionate on the protein and carbohydrate metabolism in the depancreatized-castrated dog. Endocrinology **65:** 298–309.
53. Sloan, J. M. & I. M. Oliver. 1975. Progestogen-induced diabetes in the dog. Diabetes **24:** 337–344.
54. Beck, P. 1969. Effects of gonadal hormones and contraceptive steroids on glucose and insulin metabolism. *In* Metabolic Effects of Gonadal Hormones and Contraceptive Steroids. H. A. Salhanick, D. M. Kipnis & R. L. Vande Wiele, Eds.: 97–125. Plenum Publishing Corporation. New York, N.Y.
55. Gerich, J. E., M. Lorenzini, V. Schneider, J. H. Karam, J. Rivier, R. Guillemin & P. H. Forsham. 1974. Effects of somatostatin on plasma glucose and glucagon levels in human diabetes mellitus. N. Engl. J. Med. **291:** 544–547.
56. Srivastava, M. C., N. W. Oakley, C. V. Tompkins, P. H. Sönksen & V. Wynn. 1975. Insulin metabolism, insulin sensitivity and hormonal responses to insulin infusion in patients taking oral contraceptive steroids. Eur. J. Clin. Invest. **5:** 425–433.
57. Lei, K. Y., M. G. Yang, D. Oberleas & A. S. Prasad. 1975. Oral contraceptives: effect on plasma insulin response to glucose and on the response to insulin and 2-deoxyglucose uptake by peripheral tissue. Proc. Soc. Exp. Biol. Med. **149:** 417–421.

Discussion

Dr. W. G. Wiest: Has anyone attempted to study these interactions *in vitro* utilizing isolated β-cell preparations?

DR. BECK: There have been several studies. Costrini and Kalkhoff have shown that both estradiol and progesterone in large doses will enhance glucose-stimulated insulin secretion.[5] In our laboratory, we have confirmed the stimulatory effect of progesterone on glucose-stimulated insulin secretion in isolated islets. However, the addition of human placental lactogen to an estriol plus progesterone treatment regimen resulted in neutralization of that stimulatory effect on insulin production.

REMINISCENCES AND COMMENTS ON PROGESTERONE RESEARCH

Walter G. Wiest

Department of Obstetrics and Gynecology
Washington University School of Medicine
St. Louis, Missouri 63110

Dr. Gurpide and the organizing committee have asked me to conclude this Conference with appropriate and provocative remarks. I appreciate their invitation. For about the past 24 years, I've "worked with" progesterone. During this time, it's been my privilege on certain occasions to be closely associated with people and events when pivotal changes took place in the direction and thrust of progesterone research. From the vantage point provided by this Conference, it is possible to look back along the trail of effort and achievement and clearly identify some of these landmarks. I'd like to now retrace that trail for a closer look at some of those significant events. Such a trip will be an enjoyable one for me, and I hope it may be generally entertaining.

The introduction of radiolabeling methodology into steroid endocrine research provided a significant turning point in the trail and facilitated the transition in research emphasis from physiologic considerations of progesterone response to a consideration of biochemical events involved in the mode of hormonal action. Synthesis of the progesterone molecule that contained ^{14}C in position 21 of the side chain was accomplished in 1948 by Byron Riegel and F. S. Prout.[1] Riegel *et al.*'s studies[2] of progesterone metabolism and distribution in rats and mice were performed within the following two years. These studies provided the first biochemical evidence of side-chain cleavage and the role of progesterone as a precursor for androgen and estrogen biosynthesis. Riegel *et al.*'s studies also established more precisely the rapidity of progesterone metabolism and the tendency for radioactivity to accumulate in brain, adrenal, and ovarian tissues. It seemed surprising at the time that progesterone did not appear to accumulate in uterine tissue.

In 1950, George Fujimoto, then at the University of Utah, along with J. Prager, successfully synthesized progesterone with ^{14}C localized in the ring structure.[3] Their achievement was to benefit me significantly. I joined the Biochemistry Department at the University of Utah in 1952, having just received my Ph.D. from the University of Wisconsin. I had worked under Charles Heidelberger on the mechanism of polycyclic hydrocarbon carcinogenesis, and we had observed the binding of ^{14}C-labeled dibenzanthracene derivatives to tumor-bearing tissues. On my arrival at Utah, Leo Samuels, head of the department, presented me with 200 mg of [4-^{14}C]progesterone and the challenge to do something with it.

Past experience with the polycyclic hydrocarbons made the impulse very strong to look into the biochemistry of progesterone interaction with the uterus. Administration of the labeled hormone to eviscerated rats whose uteri were potentiated toward the formation of deciduomata was one of our first experiments. The objective was twofold: to determine the extent of metabolic degradation of progesterone in extrahepatic tissues and to determine to what extent progesterone would accumulate in the uterus. It was hoped that by correlating these two observations with the progress of the progesterone-mediated decidual cell reaction, some key insight could be gained into the biochemical mechanism responsible for the hormonal effects. These and subsequent experiments provided a knowledge of the metabolic pathways open to progesterone in extrahepatic tissues and gave strong indication that when the steroid was hormonally effective in the uterus, it tended to be sequestered there.

I had gone to Utah after being much impressed by the experiments then being conducted by Gerald Mueller at Wisconsin. Gerry occupied the laboratory just next to mine at the McArdle Memorial Laboratory, and I often had the benefit of his keen perception and reports of his progress on the early effects of estrogen on the immature and castrate rat uterus. However, a way to apply his approach to the progesterone problem did not seem apparent, because the progesterone response was always preceded by a necessary exposure to estrogen.

I believe the first instance in which the question of the mechanism of action of steroid hormones was explored in conference was at the Endicott House in May 1960.[4] Claude Villee played a primary role in its organization and conduct. To begin the conference, Lewis Engel presented the state of understanding of the problem and introduced two hypotheses that were considered to be most likely explanations for the mechanism of action of steroid hormones. The first stated that steroid hormones exerted their effects at either the cell surface or some intracellular phase boundary, altering the rates of passage of key metabolic intermediates, thus regulating cell function and synthetic capacity. The second stated that "steroid hormones exert their effects by interaction with enzyme systems," possibly as coenzymes or by an alteration, in some imprecisely defined manner, of the rates of key metabolic reactions.

During the meeting, appropriate attention was given to the significant work performed by Ulrich Westphal on steroid-protein interactions. It took some years before the value of these contributions was fully appreciated. Very significant contributions were also made during discussion periods as the meeting progressed. William Pearlman reported his use of tritiated progesterone synthesized with much higher specific activities than had previously been available with ^{14}C-labeled progesterone. Prolonged infusions of this labeled steroid into rats fixed the effective concentration of the hormone in target tissues at less than 10^{-7} M. His report effectively negated suggested mechanisms that were based on effects that required considerably higher concentrations of progesterone. I reported the finding that progesterone did not participate as a cosubstrate or coenzyme in transhydrogenase reactions that involved NAD and NADP. This conclusion followed from observations that the purified 20α-hydroxysteroid dehydrogenase did not possess dual pyridine nucleotide specificity during its interconversion of progesterone and 20α-dihydroprogesterone.

The role of estrogen as a possible enzyme modifier of transhydrogenation was presented at the Endicott Conference as a plausible hypothesis for the mechanism of estrogen action. However, remarks made in discussion by Gerry Mueller focused everyone's attention on a much more attractive possibility. He reported the effect of the antibiotic puromycin on the early action of estrogen in the rat uterus. By blocking protein synthesis at the level of the transfer of activated amino acids from transfer RNA, puromycin suppressed the acceleration of early hormonal events without suppressing the metabolic process per se. Mueller summarized his findings in these words[5]:

> . . . the primary action of the hormone is concerned with the modification of the environment around the protein-synthesizing machinery of the uterine cell in such a manner so as to facilitate protein synthesis in this tissue. It is quite possible that the hormone acts as an inducer in the synthesis of specific protein catalyzing such a change of state.

Mueller's remarks provided a point of transition for the conference and an introduction to a line of research that has been embellished by several reports at this Conference. Another point of interest to me personally was Mueller's acknowledgment of the contribution of John Gorski in the puromycin work. Gorski's involvement set the stage for his many valuable contributions made since then. It pleases me to realize that Gorski went to work with Mueller at my suggestion after he concluded some postdoctoral training at Utah.

During a sabbatical leave in 1960–61, I had an opportunity to see at close range another development that was later to mark the progesterone research trail. I visited the Max Planck Institute for Biochemistry in Munich where I met Professor Adolph Butenandt whose participation in the early days of progesterone have been outlined by Professors Greep and Allen at this Conference. Butenandt called my attention to work being done in the Institute by Peter Karlson. Karlson showed me the procedure he was using to induce maturation of insect pupa by injections of the steroid hormone ecdysone. He also described the "puffing" phenomenon, which occurred on insect salivary gland chromosomes after ecdysone treatment. Generalizing from the concept of Jacob and Monod (1961), he later suggested[6] that ecdysone combined with gene repressors, resulting in derepression of the genetic message, and that this interaction was the basis of steroid hormonal regulation. Many presentations made during this Conference illustrate the magnitude of the developments in this area since that time.

The progress made in the 1960s by Mueller, Elwood Jensen, Gorski, and others toward clarifying the mechanism of estrogen action in the uterus was not rapidly duplicated by workers with progesterone. During much of this time, my efforts were spent trying to devise analytic methods capable of measuring endogenous progesterone in tissues. The evidence still was not convincing that progesterone actually concentrated in the uterus. In time, a double-isotope assay was developed[7] that allowed us to show that progesterone did, indeed, concentrate in target tissues and that endogenous tissue levels did correlate appropriately with the physiologic state of the animal during pregnancy.[8] Simultaneous measurements of a progestationally inactive steroid indicated that the capacity to sequester progesterone was both hormone and tissue specific. Fortunately, the tedious double-isotope procedure was soon superseded by assay methods based on the high-affinity binding of progesterone to plasma proteins and antibodies.

It was inevitable that the focus of attention on steroid-protein interactions, along with the accompanying methodology, would ultimately result in the characterization of uterine proteins capable of selectively binding progesterone with high affinity. In 1970, I had the opportunity to approach another research landmark by attending the Schering Workshop on Steroid Hormone "Receptors"[9] held in Berlin in December of that year. At this meeting, it was evident that progesterone could now be included together with other steroid hormones for which cytosol receptors had been characterized. I presented the work of my associate Dr. Ramanath Rao[10] regarding the characterization of progesterone-binding proteins found in rabbit uterus and human endometrium and the capacity of estrogen to increase progesterone receptor concentration. For me, the most significant part of the Schering meeting was Bert O'Malley's report on progesterone regulation of avidin synthesis in the chick oviduct. Not only did his report[11] provide identification and characterization of the oviduct receptor but its partial purification and role in the intercompartmental transfer of progesterone from cytosol to nucleus as well. O'Malley also gave details on the nature of the specific interaction of the progesterone-receptor complex with the genome. As evidenced by the reports from his laboratory given at this conference, the progress continues.

The choice of a good model system with which to study progesterone's mechanism of action obviously has been of crucial importance in the past. Although much has been learned of the physiologic and cytologic consequences of progesterone action in uteri from the decidual cell reaction model, and I have benefited materially from its use, the decidual cell model has proved too complex to give the type of definitive information derived from the oviduct model. Of course, success with the oviduct system has been due not only to its simplicity but also certainly to the intellectual acumen and the technical prowess of O'Malley, Schimke, and their coworkers. However, the need for a better mammalian model still remains of paramount importance for future progress. Perhaps the systems described by Feil, Bullock, and Feigelson can be developed and exploited sufficiently to fill the need.

I will conclude my remarks by extending my sincere compliments to the authors and participants whose presentations and comments have added this Conference to the list of landmarks in progesterone research. I also thank the organizing committee for making it possible.

References

1. Riegel, B. & F. S. Prout. 1948. The synthesis of progesterone-21-C^{14}. J. Organic Chem. **13:** 933–936.
2. Riegel, B., W. L. Hartop, Jr. & G. W. Kittinger. 1950. Studies on the metabolism of radio-progesterone in mice and rats. Endocrinology **47**(5): 311–319.
3. Fujimoto, G. & J. Prager. 1953. A synthesis of progesterone labeled in position 4. J. Amer. Chem. Soc. **75:** 3259–3261.
4. Villee, C. A. & L. L. Engel. (Eds.) 1961. Mechanism of Action of Steroid Hormones. Pergamon Press. New York, Oxford, London, Paris.
5. Villee, C. A. & L. L. Engel. (Eds.) 1961. Mechanism of Action of Steroid Hormones: 184. Pergamon Press. New York, Oxford, London, Paris.
6. Karlson, P. 1961. Biochemische Wirkungsweise der Hormone. Deut. Med. Wochschr. **86:** 668–674.
7. Wiest, W. G. 1967. A double isotope derivative assay for progesterone and 20α-hydroxypregn-4-en-3-one. Steroids **10:** 257–278.
8. Wiest, W. G. 1970. Progesterone and 20α-hydroxypregn-4-en-3-one in plasma, ovaries, and uteri during pregnancy in the rat. Endocrinology **87:** 43–48.
9. Raspé, G. (Ed.) 1971. Advances in the Biosciences 7. Pergamon Press Vieweg. Oxford, Edinburgh, New York, Sydney, Braunschweig.
10. Raspé, G. (Ed.) 1971. Advances in the Biosciences 7.: 251. Pergamon Press Vieweg. Oxford, Edinburgh, New York, Sydney, Braunschweig.
11. Raspé, G. (Ed.) 1971. Advances in the Biosciences 7.: 213. Pergamon Press Vieweg. Oxford, Edinburgh, New York, Sydney, Braunschweig.